# Register Now for Online Access to Your Book!

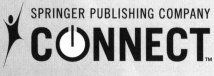

**SPRINGER PUBLISHING COMPANY**

# CONNECT™

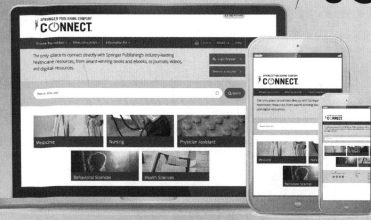

Your print purchase of *Middle Range Theory for Nursing, Fourth Edition* **includes online access to the contents of your book**—increasing accessibility, portability, and searchability!

## Access today at:

**http://connect.springerpub.com/content/book/978-0-8261-5992-2
or scan the QR code at the right with your smartphone
and enter the access code below.**

**8781G719**

*Scan here for quick access.*

**SPRINGER / PUBLISHING COMPANY**

View all our products at springerpub.com

**Mary Jane Smith, PhD, RN, FAAN,** earned her bachelor's and master's degrees from University of Pittsburgh and her doctorate from New York University. She has held faculty positions at the following nursing schools: University of Pittsburgh, Duquesne University, Cornell University-New York Hospital, and The Ohio State University. Currently, Dr. Smith is a professor of nursing at West Virginia University School of Nursing; she has been teaching theory to master's and doctoral nursing students for over four decades.

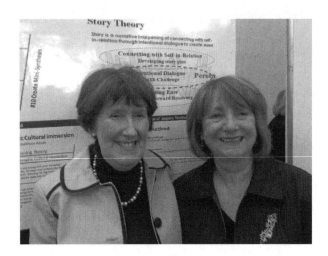

**Patricia R. Liehr, PhD, RN,** graduated from Ohio Valley Hospital, School of Nursing in Pittsburgh, Pennsylvania. She completed her bachelor's degree in nursing at Villa Maria College, her master's in family health nursing at Duquesne University, and her doctorate at the School of Nursing, University of Maryland, Baltimore. She did postdoctoral education at the University of Pennsylvania as a Robert Wood Johnson scholar. Currently, Dr. Liehr is a professor of nursing at the Christine E. Lynn College of Nursing at Florida Atlantic University; she has taught nursing theory to master's and doctoral students for over three decades.

# Middle Range Theory for Nursing

## Fourth Edition

*Mary Jane Smith, PhD, RN, FAAN*

*Patricia R. Liehr, PhD, RN*

Editors

**SPRINGER** **PUBLISHING COMPANY**

Springer Publishing Company, LLC
11 West 42nd Street
New York, NY 10036
www.springerpub.com

*Acquisitions Editor:* Joseph Morita
*Compositor:* Exeter Premedia Services Private Ltd.

*ISBN:* 978-0-8261-5991-5
*e-book ISBN:* 978-0-8261-5992-2

*Instructors Materials: Qualified instructors may request supplements by emailing textbook@springerpub.com*
*Instructors Manual:* 978-0-8261-2584-2

19 20 21 22 23 / 8 7 6 5 4

The author and the publisher of this Work have made every effort to use sources believed to be reliable to provide information that is accurate and compatible with the standards generally accepted at the time of publication. Because medical science is continually advancing, our knowledge base continues to expand. Therefore, as new information becomes available, changes in procedures become necessary. We recommend that the reader always consult current research and specific institutional policies before performing any clinical procedure. The author and publisher shall not be liable for any special, consequential, or exemplary damages resulting, in whole or in part, from the readers' use of, or reliance on, the information contained in this book. The publisher has no responsibility for the persistence or accuracy of URLs for external or third-party Internet websites referred to in this publication and does not guarantee that any content on such websites is, or will remain, accurate or appropriate.

**Library of Congress Cataloging-in-Publication Data**

Names: Smith, Mary Jane, 1938- editor. | Liehr, Patricia R., editor.
Title: Middle range theory for nursing / Mary Jane Smith, Patricia R. Liehr,
  editors.
Description: Fourth edition. | New York, NY : Springer Publishing Company,
  LLC, [2018] | Includes bibliographical references and index.
Identifiers: LCCN 2017053506 | ISBN 9780826159915
Subjects: | MESH: Nursing Theory | Nursing Research
Classification: LCC RT84.5 | NLM WY 86 | DDC 610.7301—dc23
LC record available at https://lccn.loc.gov/2017053506

Contact us to receive discount rates on bulk purchases.
We can also customize our books to meet your needs.
For more information please contact: sales@springerpub.com

Printed in the United States of America by McNaughton & Gunn.

# Contents

### III: CONCEPT BUILDING FOR RESEARCH—THROUGH THE LENS OF MIDDLE RANGE THEORY

### IV: CURRENT STATE OF MIDDLE RANGE THEORY

# Contributors

**Melinda S. Bender, PhD, RN, PNP-BC,** Assistant Professor, School of Nursing, University of California, San Francisco, California

**Heeseung Choi, PhD, MPH, RN,** Professor, College of Nursing and The Research Institute of Nursing Science, Seoul National University, Seoul, Korea

**Margaret F. Clayton, PhD, APRN,** Associate Professor, College of Nursing, University of Utah, Salt Lake City, Utah

**Marleah Dean, PhD,** Assistant Professor in Health Communication, University of South Florida, Tampa, Florida

**Linda S. Franck, PhD, RN, FRCPCH, FAAN,** Jack and Elaine Koehn Endowed Chair in Pediatric Nursing, Professor, Department of Family Health Care Nursing, University of California, San Francisco, California

**Shelley J. Greif, PhD, MPH, RN, CBIS,** Senior Registered Nurse Supervisor, Florida Department of Health, Children's Medical Services, Ft. Lauderdale, Florida

**Eun-Ok Im, PhD, MPH, RN, CNS, FAAN,** Mary T. Champagne Professor of Nursing, Duke University School of Nursing, Durham, North Carolina

**Susan L. Janson, PhD, RN, ANP-BC, CNS, FAAN,** Professor Emerita, University of California, San Francisco, California

**Tiny Jaarsma, PhD, RN, FAAN, FAHA, NFESC,** Professor in Caring Sciences, Faculty of Health Sciences, University of Linköping, Sweden; Professorial Fellow, Mary MacKillop Institute for Health Research, Australian Catholic University, Melbourne, Australia

**Kathryn Aldrich Lee, PhD, RN,** University of Southern California-San Francisco, School of Nursing, San Francisco, California

**Elizabeth R. Lenz, PhD, RN, FAAN,** Professor and Dean Emerita, The Ohio State University, College of Nursing, Columbus, Ohio

**Patricia R. Liehr, PhD, RN,** Professor of Nursing, Christine E. Lynn College of Nursing at Florida Atlantic University, Boca Raton, Florida

**John Lowe, PhD, RN, FAAN,** Endowed McKenzie Professor for Health Disparities Research, Florida State University College of Nursing, Tallahassee, Florida

**Merle Mishel, PhD, RN, FAAN,** Professor Emerita, School of Nursing, The University of North Carolina at Chapel Hill, Chapel Hill, North Carolina

**Misako Nagata, RN, HNP, MA, APHN-BC, CCRN,** Christine E. Lynn College of Nursing, Florida Atlantic University Graduate College, Boca Raton, Florida

**Alvita K. Nathaniel, PhD, APRN-BC, FNP, FAANP,** Professor, Charleston Division, West Virginia University, Health Sciences Center, Charleston, West Virginia

**Linda C. Pugh, PhD, RNC, FAAN,** Professor, University of North Carolina Wilmington, Wilmington, North Carolina

**Marilyn A. Ray, PhD, RN, MS, MA, CTN-A, FSfAA, FAAN,** Colonel (Retired) United States Air Force, Nurse Corps; Professor Emerita, Florida Atlantic University, The Christine E. Lynn College of Nursing, Boca Raton, Florida

**Pamela G. Reed, PhD,RN,FAAN,** Professor, The University of Arizona, College of Nursing, Tucson, Arizona

**Barbara Resnick, PhD, RN, CRNP, FAAN, FAANP,** Professor, OSAH Sonya Ziporkin Gershowitz Chair in Gerontology, University of Maryland School of Nursing, Baltimore, Maryland

**Barbara Riegel, PhD, RN, FAAN, FAHA,** Edith Clemmer Steinbright Professor of Gerontology, University of Pennsylvania School of Nursing, Philadelphia, Pennsylvania

**Teresa Daniel Ritchie, DNP, APRN, FNP-BC,** Assistant Clinical Professor, West Virginia University School of Nursing, Morgantown, West Virginia

**April L. Shapiro, PhD, RN,** Chair, Bachelor of Science in Nursing Program, West Virginia University School of Nursing, Potomac State College, Keyser, West Virginia

**Marlaine C. Smith,** PhD, RN, FAAN, Dean and Professor, Christine E. Lynn College of Nursing, Florida Atlantic University, Boca Raton, Florida

**Mary Jane Smith, PhD, RN, FAAN,** Professor, West Virginia University School of Nursing, Morgantown, West Virginia

**Patricia Starck, DSN, RN, FAAN,** Professor Emerita, University of Texas Health Science Center at Houston, Houston, Texas

**Anna Stromberg, PhD, RN, FAAN, NFESC,** Professor of Nursing Science, Linköping University and Linköping University Hospital, Sweden

**Kimberly Ann Wallace, MSN, FNP-C,** Lecturer, West Virginia University School of Nursing, Morgantown, West Virginia

**Suzy Mascaro Walter, PhD, FNP-BC,** Assistant Professor, School of Nursing, West Virginia University, Morgantown, West Virginia

# Foreword

This fourth edition of *Middle Range Theory for Nursing* by Mary Jane Smith and Patricia R. Liehr deepens our understandings of the importance of theory in developing the science of nursing. Particularly noteworthy is the extent to which the editors and chapter contributors articulate the relevance of the theoretical content for both research and professional nursing practice.

Smith and Liehr were pioneers in nursing knowledge development with the publication of the first edition of this middle range theory book. The demand for information about middle range theories has substantially increased since the publication of the first edition, and Smith and Liehr have remained in the forefront in expanding the boundaries of knowledge development, sustaining their focus on middle range theories. In the first edition of their book, eight middle range theories for nursing were presented. In this latest edition of the book, 13 theories are included, several of which were included in prior editions. For each of the theories there is an update provided; the new theories include the most recent supportive background literature. Each chapter includes the relevance of the theory to professional practice and research. Thus, for each of the theories, faculty and graduate students will have access to the most recent developments in disciplinary knowledge. Further, this book ensures ease of understanding through the consistent structure within each chapter. Each theory is connected to a paradigmatic perspective within nursing, thus offering the reader a view of how knowledge development in nursing moves from the broad philosophical and conceptual perspective to the pragmatic use in professional practice and research. This comprehensive view of theoretical development in nursing will be especially useful for graduate students new to theoretical thinking as well as to expert clinicians who are challenged to embed their practice in the disciplinary perspective of nursing. Throughout the chapters there is evidence that the discipline has moved forward in the development of theoretical knowledge, a heartening and welcomed development and a testament to the maturing of the nursing discipline.

As with the prior edition, the focus on concept building is particularly instructive, especially to nurses newly introduced to the theory development process. This process of concept building enhances our understandings of the concepts relevant to nursing and represents a complementary process to concept analysis. Yet an important distinguishing factor between concept building and concept analysis is the origin of the concept. The concept building process unfolds through a practice story, thus directly linking to clinical knowledge that is familiar to nurses. Through the rigorous 10 step process of concept building clinicians are led from the identification of an important clinical phenomenon to the development and expansion of their conceptual understandings. In this fourth edition, two chapters are included in which authors demonstrate use of the concept building process and in two other chapters, authors describe the movement of concept building to research proposal development. This concept building process continues to hold great potential for future theoretical and scientific development of the discipline, and should be introduced in all introductory courses in nursing theory development.

Smith and Liehr continue to focus attention on the theory lens of nursing knowledge development, an undertaking that is particularly relevant at a time when the focus has drifted to empirical and practical knowledge development. As with prior editions there are key dimensions of the work that make it especially useful to new students of nursing theory, at the graduate and undergraduate levels. Smith and Liehr present their ideas succinctly and raise important discussions about the nature of theoretical thinking within the discipline. The structured format that is used across all of the chapters focused on specific theories provides the reader with a consistent level of explanation and analysis, and is especially useful for those trying to understand the similarities and differences in the theories. This structure facilitates assessment of knowledge development content components, and provides a detailed model for evaluation of the internal and external validity of the theories. And, importantly, each of the chapters includes delineation of the relevance of the theory in research and professional practice.

Particularly noteworthy in this fourth edition is an added section that documents the historical development of middle range theory in nursing. Two articles from *Advances in Nursing Science* have been reprinted as they provide the historical insight into middle range theory development. The editors thus demonstrate the continuing value of middle range theory development as embedded within nursing science.

Overall, this fourth edition is an important contribution to our nursing science literature. Smith and Liehr provide depth to our understandings of middle range theory and set the stage for further theory development within the discipline. Nurses in practice as well as students of nursing at all educational levels will benefit greatly from this scholarly work. This contribution extends our understandings and presents new opportunities for expanding the science of nursing through theory development, research and professional practice.

*Joyce J. Fitzpatrick, PhD, MBA, RN, FAAN, FNAP*
Elizabeth Brooks Ford Professor of Nursing
Frances Payne Bolton School of Nursing
Case Western Reserve University
Cleveland, Ohio

# Preface

The interest in middle range theory continues to grow as demonstrated by the increased number of published theories as well as the desire among nursing faculty and researchers to use theories at the midrange level to guide practice and research. The book is based on the premise that students come to know and understand a theory as the meaning of concepts is made clear and as they experience the way a theory informs practice and research in the everyday world of nursing. Over the years, we continue to hear from students and faculty telling us that the book is user friendly and truly reflects what they need as a reference to move middle range theory to the forefront of research and practice.

Middle range theory can be defined as a set of related ideas that are focused on a limited dimension of the reality of nursing. These theories are composed of concepts and suggested relationships among the concepts that can be depicted in a model. Middle range theories are developed and grow at the intersection of practice and research to provide guidance for everyday practice and scholarly research rooted in the discipline of nursing. We use the ladder of abstraction to articulate the logic of middle range theory as related to a philosophical perspective and practice/research approaches congruent with theory conceptualization.

The middle range theories chosen for presentation in this book cover a broad spectrum—from theories that were proposed decades ago and have been used extensively to theories that are newly developed and just coming into use. Some of the theories were originated by the primary nurse–author who wrote the chapter, and some were originally created by persons outside of nursing. After much thought and discussion with colleagues and students, we have come to the conclusion that theories for nursing are those that apply to the unique perspective of the discipline, regardless of origin, as long as they are used by nurse scholars to guide practice or research and are consistent with one of the paradigms presented by Newman and colleagues (Newman, Sime, & Corcoran-Perry, 1991). These paradigms, which are recognized philosophical perspectives unique to the discipline, present an ontological grounding for the middle range theories in this book. By connecting each theory with a paradigmatic perspective, we offer a view of the middle range theory's place within the larger scope of nursing science. We have structured the book in four sections.

The first section includes three chapters that present a meta-perspective on middle range theory, thereby setting the stage for the subsequent sections. The first chapter in this section, "Disciplinary Perspectives Linked to Middle Range Theory," elaborates on the structure of the discipline of nursing as a present and historical context for the development and use of middle range theories. The second chapter, "Understanding Middle Range Theory by Moving Up and Down the Ladder of Abstraction," offers a clear and formal way of presenting the theories. The ladders were created by the editors and represent the editors' view of the philosophical grounding of the theory rather than the chapter authors' view. We have found that a ladder of abstraction can provide a starting place to guide students' thinking when they are trying to make sense of a theory. In addition, moving ideas up and down the ladder of abstraction generates scholarly dialogue that spurs reflective critique of ideas in a structured and manageable way. The third chapter in this section is titled "Evaluation of Middle Range Theories for the Discipline of Nursing." Students have told us that understanding the way in which theory is evaluated helps further understanding of the theory. So, we have included this chapter in the first section of the book. Certainly, evaluation of theory is a critical skill required for those who strive to move a theory onward in their own work. A unique feature of the evaluation process described in this chapter is that it is based on postmodern assumptions in which context is appreciated as an essential dimension thus, creating an always tentative theory critique.

In the second section of the book, thirteen middle range theories are included. Eleven of these were presented in the third edition: Uncertainty, Meaning, Self-Transcendence, Symptom Management, Unpleasant Symptoms, Self-Efficacy, Story, Transitions, Self-Reliance, Cultural Marginality, and Moral Reckoning. Two new theories are included in this fourth edition: Bureaucratic Caring and Self-Care of Chronic Illness. Although both focus on caring, one addresses system issues affecting a culture of care and the other addresses individual issues of self-care across chronic conditions.

Each chapter describing a middle range theory follows a standard format. This includes purpose of the theory and how it was developed, concepts of the theory, relationships among the concepts expressed as a model, use of the theory in nursing research, use of the theory in nursing practice, and conclusion. We believe this standard format facilitates a complete understanding of the theory and enables a comparison of the theories presented in the book.

The third section contains five chapters that frame a systematic approach for concept building and provide exemplars that highlight the approach. The first chapter in this section, "Concept Building for Research—Through the Lens of Middle Range Theory," is one that was first introduced in the second edition. It has been further developed to refine a 10-phase process, guiding conceptualization of ideas for research. The process presented in the chapter can be used by faculty who teach courses on concept development, students who are working to establish their ideas for research, and scholars who are seeking to systematically shape ideas. Included in this section are two chapters written by students demonstrating use of the concept building process and two chapters that describe the movement of concept building to research proposal development. While this concept-building effort shares some of the processes of concept development, it is distinguished by its foundation in nursing practice stories, use of a theoretical lens that shapes concept structure, and the systematic inclusion of inductive and deductive processes that culminate in a newly created model to be used in research.

A fourth section of the book has been added in this fourth edition. It contains two articles from *Advances in Nursing Science* that document a historical meta-perspective about middle range theory development over decades. We believe that the guidance derived from this meta-perspective provides direction for scholars wishing to ensure that disciplinary knowledge remains a lively dimension of research and practice.

The reader will notice when reading this book and comparing the theory descriptions from one edition of the book to the next that some theories have had ongoing development and use while others have received less attention and use during the past 5 years. The vibrancy of theory is dependent on its use by scholars who critique and apply it, testing its relevancy to real-world practice and research. Proliferation of middle range theory without ongoing critique, application, and development is a concern that requires ongoing attention.

As noted in the third edition of the book, there are beginning clusters of middle range theories around important ideas for the discipline, such as symptoms (Theories of Unpleasant Symptoms and Symptom Management) and moving through difficult times (Theories of Meaning, Self-Transcendence, and Transitions), and this edition adds the cluster of caring (Bureaucratic Caring and Self-Care of Chronic Illness). It would be useful to evaluate theory clusters, noting the common ground of guidance emerging from the body of scholarly work documented in the theory cluster. An advantage of this effort would be that the thinking of unique nurse scholars would come together around a central idea. One might expect that essential dimensions of the discipline could be made explicit by distilling and synthesizing ideas from a theory cluster. Although the analysis of theory clusters is not undertaken in this book, the information about middle range theory provided here creates a foundation for considering theory-cluster analysis.

In the appendix to the book, readers will find a table of middle range theories published from 1988 to 2017 in which the year, full citation, and name of the theory is noted. This table is useful as a starting place for scholars who want to find additional middle range theories in the literature.

In conclusion, this fourth edition presents an organization of chapters by meta-theory, middle range theories for nursing, concept building through a theoretical lens, and historical meta-perspective. The added theory chapters focused on dimensions of caring introduce a core element expressive of the disciplinary perspective (Newman, Sime, & Corcoran-Perry, 1991).The addition of the section describing the historical meta-perspective provides a dimension of context for scholars wishing to advance the body of nursing knowledge articulated through middle range theory. As with previous editions, we have edited and written with the intention of clarifying the contribution of middle range theory. We believe this clarification serves established as well as beginning nurse scholars seeking a theoretical foundation for practice and research.

*Mary Jane Smith, PhD, RN, FAAN*
*Patricia R. Liehr, PhD, RN*

## ■ REFERENCE

Newman, M. A., Sime, A. M., & Corcoran-Perry, S. A. (1991). The focus of the discipline of nursing. *Advances in Nursing Science, 14*, 1–6. Retrieved from http://journals.lww.com/advancesinnursingscience/Citation/1991/09000/The_focus_of_the_discipline_of_nursing_.2.aspx

# Acknowledgments

An endeavor like this book is always the work of many. We are grateful to our students, who have prodded us with thought-provoking questions; our colleagues, who have challenged our thinking and writing; our contributors, who gave willingly of their time and effort; our publishers, who believed that we had something to offer; and our families, who have provided a base of love and support that makes anything possible.

# SECTION ONE

## Setting the Stage for Middle Range Theories

*This section describes metaperspectives that create a context for the middle range theories in this book. In the first chapter, a connection is made between middle range theory and the unique focus of the discipline of nursing, the structure of the discipline, and grand theories in nursing. In the second chapter, middle range theory is described according to philosophical, theoretical, and empirical levels of abstraction along with ladders depicting the assumptions, concepts, and practice/research applications. The editors have created the ladders of abstraction, thereby interpreting each theorist's perspectives to provide the reader an opportunity for visualizing, comparing, and contrasting each middle range theory as related to the others. The third chapter describes the purpose, structure, and process for evaluating middle range theory. In this chapter, a framework for evaluating the substantive foundations, structural integrity, and functional adequacy of middle range theory is provided emphasizing thoughtful consideration of the theory with empathy, curiosity, honesty, and responsibility.*

# CHAPTER 1

## Disciplinary Perspectives Linked to Middle Range Theory

Marlaine C. Smith

Each discipline has a unique focus for knowledge development that directs inquiry and distinguishes it from other fields of study. The knowledge that constitutes the discipline has organization. Understanding this organization or the structure of the discipline is important for those engaged in learning the theories of the discipline and for those developing knowledge expanding the discipline. Perhaps this need is more acute in nursing because the evolution of the professional practice based on tradition and knowledge from other fields preceded the emergence of substantive knowledge of the discipline. Nursing knowledge is the inclusive total of the philosophies, theories, research, and practice wisdom of the discipline. As a professional discipline this knowledge is important for guiding practice. Theory-guided, evidence-informed practice is the hallmark of any professional discipline. The purpose of this chapter is to elaborate the structure of the discipline of nursing as a context for understanding and developing middle range theories.

While the disciplinary focus of nursing has been debated for decades, there now seems to be a growing consensus. In 1978, Donaldson and Crowley stated that a discipline offers "a unique perspective, a distinct way of viewing . . . phenomena, which ultimately defines the limits and nature of its inquiry" (p. 113). They specified three recurrent themes as the nexus of the discipline of nursing:

1. Concern with principles and laws that govern the life processes, well-being, and optimum functioning of human beings, sick or well;
2. Concern with the patterning of human behavior in interaction with the environment in critical life situations; and
3. Concern with the processes by which positive changes in health status are affected. (p. 113)

Nursing is a professional discipline (Donaldson & Crowley, 1978). Professional disciplines such as nursing, psychology, and education are different from academic disciplines such as biology, anthropology, and economics in that they have a professional practice associated with them. According to the authors, professional disciplines include the same knowledge, namely descriptive theories and basic and applied research, common to academic disciplines. In addition to the knowledge inherent in academic disciplines, professional disciplines include prescriptive theories and clinical research. So the differences between academic and professional disciplines are the additional knowledge required for professional disciplines. This is important, because many refer to nursing as a practice discipline. This seems to imply that the knowledge is about the practice alone and not about the substantive phenomena of concern to the discipline.

Failure to recognize the existence of the discipline as a body of knowledge that is separate from the activities of practitioners has contributed to the fact that nursing has been viewed as a vocation rather than a profession. In turn, this has led to confusion about whether a discipline of nursing exists (Conway, 1985, p. 73).

Although we have made significant progress in building the knowledge base of nursing, this confusion about the substantive knowledge base of nursing lingers with nurses, other professions, and in the public sphere.

Fawcett's (1984) explication of the nursing metaparadigm was another model for delineating the focus of nursing. According to Fawcett, the discipline of nursing is the study of the interrelationships among human beings, environment, health, and nursing. Although the metaparadigm is widely accepted, the inclusion of nursing as a major concept of the nursing discipline is tautological (Conway, 1985). Others have defined nursing as the study of the life process of unitary human beings (Rogers, 1970, 1992), human care or caring (Boykin & Schoenhofer, 2001, 2015; Leininger, 1978, 1984; Watson, 1985, 2008), human–universe–health interrelationships (Parse, 1998, 2014), and "the health or wholeness of human beings as they interact with their environment" (Donaldson & Crowley, 1978, p. 113). Newman, Sime, and Corcoran-Perry (1991) created a parsimonious definition of the focus of nursing that synthesizes the unitary nature of human beings with caring: "Nursing is the study of caring in the human health experience" (p. 3).

My definition uses similar concepts but shifts the direct object in the sentence: "Nursing is the study of human health and healing through caring" (M. C. Smith, 1994, p. 50). This definition can be stated even more parsimoniously: Nursing is the study of healing through caring. Healing comes from the same etymological origin as "health," *haelen*, meaning whole (Quinn, 1990, p. 553). Healing captures the dynamic meaning that health often lacks; healing reflects the wholeness of person–environment; healing implies a process of changing and evolving. Caring is the path to healing. In its deepest meaning, it encompasses one's connectedness to all, that is, a person–environment relatedness. Nursing knowledge focuses on the wholeness of human life and experience and the processes that support relationship, integration, and transformation. This is the focus of knowledge development in the discipline of nursing.

Defining nursing as a professional discipline does not negate or demean the practice of nursing. Knowledge generated from and applied in practice is contained within this description. The focus of practice comes from the definition of the discipline. Nursing has been defined as both science and art, with science encompassing the theories and research related to the phenomena of concern (disciplinary focus) and art as the creative application of that knowledge (Rogers, 1992). Newman (1990, 1994, 2008) and others, perhaps influenced by critical/postmodern scholars, have used the term praxis to connote the unity of theory–research–practice lived in the patient–nurse encounter. Praxis breaks down the boundaries between theory and practice, researcher and practitioner, art and science. Praxis recognizes that the practitioner's values, philosophy, and theoretical perspective are embodied in the practice. Chinn (2013) defines praxis as "thoughtful reflection and action that occur in synchrony, in the direction of transforming the world" (p. 10). Praxis reflects the embodied knowing that comes from the integration of values and actions and blurs the distinctions among the roles of practitioner, researcher, and theoretician.

Middle range theories are part of the structure of the discipline. They address the substantive knowledge of the discipline by explicating and expanding on specific phenomena that are related to the caring–healing process. For example, the Theory of Self-Transcendence (Reed, 2015) explains how aging or vulnerability propels humans beyond self-boundaries to focus intrapersonally on life's meaning; interpersonally on connections with others and the environment; temporally to integrate past, present, and future; and transpersonally to connect with dimensions beyond the physical reality. Self-transcendence is related to well-being or healing, one of the identified foci of the discipline of nursing. This theory has been examined in research and used to guide nursing practice. With the expansion of middle range theories, nursing is enriched.

Several nursing scholars have organized knowledge of the discipline into paradigms (Fawcett, 1995; Newman et al., 1991; Parse, 1987). The concept of *paradigm* originated in Kuhn's (1970) treatise on the development of knowledge within scientific fields. He asserted that the sciences evolve rather predictably from a preparadigm state to one in which there are competing paradigms around which the activity of science is conducted. The activity of science to which he is referring is the inquiry that examines the emerging questions and hypotheses surfacing from scientific theories and new findings. Paradigms are schools of shared assumptions, values, and views about the phenomena addressed in particular sciences. It is common for mature disciplines to house multiple paradigms. If one paradigm becomes dominant and if discoveries within it challenge the logic of other paradigms, a scientific revolution may occur.

Parse (1987) described nursing with two paradigms: totality and simultaneity. For her, the theories in the totality paradigm assert the view that humans are bio psycho social–spiritual beings responding or adapting to the environment, and health is a fluctuating point on a continuum. The simultaneity paradigm portends a unitary perspective. Unitary refers to the distinctive conceptualization of Rogers (1970, 1992) that human beings are whole and integral with their environment. Health is subjectively defined by the person (group or community) and reflects well-being, the process of evolving or human becoming. Parse locates only two nursing conceptual systems/theories: the Science of Unitary Human Beings (Rogers, 1970, 1992) and the Theory of Human Becoming (Parse, 1998, 2014) in the simultaneity paradigm. For Parse, all nursing knowledge is related to the extant grand theories or conceptual models of the discipline. While she agrees that theories expand through research and conceptual development, she disagrees with the inclusion of middle range theories within the disciplinary structure if they are not grounded in the more abstract theoretical structure of an existing nursing grand theory or conceptual model.

Newman et al. (1991) and Newman (2008) identified three paradigms. These paradigms are conceptualized as evolving because the more complex paradigms encompass and extend the knowledge in a previous paradigm. The three paradigms are particulate–deterministic, integrative–interactive, and unitary–transformative. From the perspective of the theories within the particulate–deterministic paradigm, human health and caring are understood through their component parts or activities; there is an underlying order with predictable antecedents and consequences; and knowledge development progresses to uncover these causal relationships. Reduction and causal inferences are characteristics of this paradigm. The integrative–interactive paradigm acknowledges contextual, subjective, and multidimensional relationships among the phenomena central to the discipline. The interrelationships among parts and the probabilistic nature of change are assumptions that guide the way phenomena are conceptualized and studied. The third paradigm is the unitary–transformative. Here, the person–environment unity is a patterned field within larger patterned fields. Change is characterized by fluctuating rhythms of organization disorganization, toward more complex organization. Subjective experience is primary and reflects a pattern of the whole (Newman et al., 1991, p. 4).

Fawcett (1995, 2000) joined the paradigm dialogue with her version of three paradigms. She named them: reaction, reciprocal interaction, and simultaneous action. This model was synthesized from the analysis of views of mechanistic versus organismic, persistence versus change, and Parse and Newman and colleagues' nursing paradigmatic structures. In the reaction worldview, humans are the sum of the biological, psychological, sociological, and spiritual parts of their nature. Reactions are causal and stability is valued; change is a mechanism for survival. In the reciprocal interaction worldview, the parts are seen within the context of the whole, and human–environment relationships are reciprocal; change is probabilistic based on a number of factors. In the simultaneous action worldview, human beings are characterized by pattern and are in a mutual rhythmic open process with the environment. Change is continuous, unpredictable, and moves toward greater complexity and organization (Fawcett, 2000, pp. 11–12).

Each middle range theory has its foundations in one paradigmatic perspective. The philosophies guiding the abstract views of human beings, human–environment relationships, and health and caring are reflected in each of the paradigms. This influences the meaning of the middle range theory, and for this reason, it is important that the theory has a philosophical link to the paradigm clearly identified.

Figure 1.1 illustrates the structure of the discipline of nursing. This is adapted from an earlier version (M. C. Smith, 1994). The figure depicts the structure as clusters of inquiry and praxis surrounding a philosophic paradigmatic nexus. The levels of theory within the discipline, based on the breadth and depth of focus and level of abstraction, are represented. Theory comes from the Greek word, *theoria*, meaning "to see."

A theory provides a particular way of seeing phenomena of concern to the discipline. Theories are patterns of ideas that provide a way of viewing

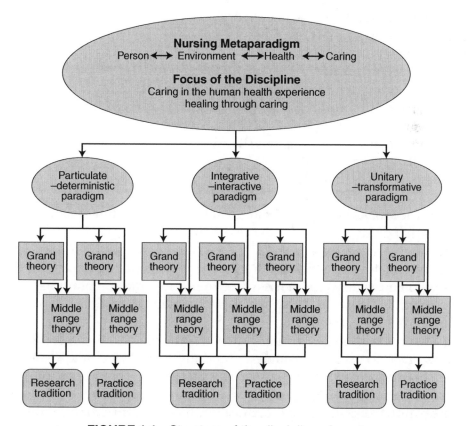

**FIGURE 1.1**   Structure of the discipline of nursing.

a phenomenon in an organized way. Walker and Avant (2010) describe these levels of theory as metatheory, grand theory, middle range theory, and practice theory.

The figure depicts five levels of abstraction. The top oval includes the nursing metaparadigm and focus of the discipline of nursing. These are the agreed-upon phenomena of concern that delineates nursing from other disciplines. Grand theories are at the next level of the figure and include the abstract conceptual systems and theories that provide perspectives on the central phenomena of the discipline, such as persons as adaptive systems, self-care deficits, unitary human beings, or human becoming. These grand theories are frameworks consisting of concepts and relational statements that explicate abstract phenomena. In the figure, the grand theories cluster under the paradigms. Middle range theories are more circumscribed, elaborating more concrete concepts and relationships such as uncertainty, self-efficacy, meaning, and the other middle range theories addressed throughout this text. The number of middle range theories is growing. Middle range theory can be specifically derived from a grand theory or can be related directly to a paradigm. At the bottom level of the figure are the research and practice traditions related to grand and middle range theories. Walker and Avant (2010) refer to this most specific level of theory as practice theory. Practice theories specify guidelines for nursing practice; in fact, the authors state that the word "theory" may be dropped to better conceptualize this level as "nursing practices" (p. 12) or what can be considered practice traditions. Both grand theories and middle range theories have practice traditions associated with them.

A practice tradition contains the activities, protocols, guidance, and practice wisdom that emerge from these theories. Models such as the LIGHT Model (Andersen & Smereck, 1989) or the Attendant Nurse Caring Model (Watson & Foster, 2003) are examples. M. J. Smith and Liehr (2013) refer to these as micro-range theories, those that closely reflect practice events or are more readily operational and accessible to application in the nursing practice environment. Research traditions are the associated methods, procedures, and empirical indicators that guide inquiry related to the theory.

Some differentiate between grand theories and conceptual models. Fawcett (2000) differentiates them by how they address the metaparadigm concepts as she has defined them. Those that address the metaparadigm of human beings, environment, health, and nursing are labeled conceptual models, whereas those that do not are considered grand theories. Using Fawcett's criteria, Human Caring Theory (Watson, 1985, 2008) and Health as Expanding Consciousness (Newman, 1986, 1994) are considered grand theories. Walker and Avant (2010) include conceptual models under the classification of grand theories, and it seems more logical to define conceptual models by scope and level of abstraction instead of their explicit metaparadigm focus. In this chapter, the grand theories are referred to as theories rather than conceptual frameworks.

The grand theories developed as nursing's distinctive focus became more clearly specified in the 1970s and 1980s. Earlier nurse scholars contributed to theoretical thinking without formalizing their ideas into theories. Nightingale's (1860/1969) assertions in *Notes on Nursing* about caring for those who are ill through attention to the environment are often labeled theoretical. Several grand theories share the same paradigmatic perspective. For example, the theories of Person as Adaptive System (Roy, 1989, 2008), Behavioral Systems (Johnson, 1980), and the Neuman (1989; Fawcett & DeSanto-Madeya, 2013; Newman & Fawcett, 2010) Systems Model share common views of the phenomena central to nursing that might locate them within the integrative–interactive paradigm. Others, such as the Science of Unitary Human Beings (Rogers, 1970, 1992), Health as Expanding Consciousness (Newman, 1986, 1994), and Human Becoming (Parse, 1998, 2014), cluster in the unitary–transformative paradigm.

There may be an explicit relationship between some grand theories and middle range theories. For example, Reed's (1991, 2015) middle range theory of Self-Transcendence and Barrett's (1989, 2015) Theory of Power are directly linked to Rogers's Science of Unitary Human Beings. Other middle range theories may not have such direct links to grand theories. In these instances, the philosophical assumptions underpinning the middle range theory may be located at the level of the paradigm rather than of the grand theory. Nevertheless, this linkage is important to establish the theory's validity as a nursing theory. Theoretical work is located in the discipline of nursing when it addresses the focus of the discipline and shares the philosophical assumptions of the nursing paradigms or the grand theories.

Some grand theories in nursing have developed research and/or practice traditions. Laudan (1977) asserts that sciences develop research traditions or schools of thought such as "Darwinism" or "quantum theory." In addition, Laudan's view includes the "legitimate methods of inquiry" open to the researcher from a given theoretical system (p. 79). Research traditions include appropriate designs, methods, instruments, research questions, and issues that are at the frontiers of knowledge development. The traditions reflect logical and consistent linkages among ontology, epistemology, and methodology. Ontology refers to the philosophical foundations of a given theory and is the essence or foundational meaning of the theory. Epistemology is about how one comes to know, and incorporates ways of understanding and studying the theory. Methodology is a systematic approach for knowledge generation and includes the processes of gathering, analyzing, synthesizing, and interpreting information. The correspondence among ontology (meaning), epistemology (knowing), and methodology (investigating) gives breadth and depth to the theory.

Examples of the connection among ontology, epistemology, and methodology are evident in several grand theories. For instance, the research-as-praxis method was developed by Newman (1990, 2008) for the study of phenomena from the Health as Expanding Consciousness perspective, and a research method was developed from the theory of Human Becoming (Parse, 1998, 2014). Tools have been developed to measure theoretical constructs such as self-care agency (Denyes, 1982) or functional status within an adaptive systems perspective (Tulman et al., 1991), and debates on the appropriate epistemology and methodology in a unitary ontology (Cowling, 2007; M. C. Smith & Reeder, 1998) characterize the research traditions of some extant theories. These examples reflect the necessary relationship among theory, knowledge development, and research methods.

Practice traditions are the principles and processes that guide the use of a theory in practice. The practice tradition might include a classification or labeling system for nursing diagnoses, or it might explicitly eschew this type of labeling. It might include the processes of living the theory in practice such as Barrett's (2015) health patterning, or the developing practice traditions around Watson's theory such as ritualizing handwashing and creating quiet time on nursing units (Watson & Foster, 2003). Practice traditions are the ways that nurses live the theory and make it explicit and visible in their practice.

Middle range theories have direct linkages to research and practice. They may be developed inductively through qualitative research and practice observations, or deductively through logical analysis and synthesis. They may evolve through retroductive processes of rhythmic induction–deduction. As scholarly work extends middle range theories, research and practice traditions continue to develop. For example, scholars advancing Uncertainty Theory will continue to test hypotheses derived from the theory with different populations. Nurses in practice can take middle range theories and develop practice guidelines based on them. Oncology nurses whose worldviews are situated in the integrative–interactive paradigm may develop protocols to care for patients receiving chemotherapy using the Theory of Unpleasant Symptoms. The use of this protocol in practice will feed back to the middle range theory, extending the evidence for practice and contributing to ongoing theory development. The use of middle range theories to structure research and practice builds the substance, organization, and integration of the discipline.

The growth of the discipline of nursing is dependent on the systematic and continuing application of nursing knowledge in practice and research. Few grand theories have been added to the discipline since the 1980s. Some suggest that there is no longer a need to differentiate knowledge and establish disciplinary boundaries because interdisciplinary teams will conduct research around common problems, eliminating the urge to establish disciplinary boundaries. Even the National Institutes of Health rewards interdisciplinary research enterprises. This emphasis can enrich perspectives through interdisciplinary collaboration, but it is critical to approach interdisciplinary collaboration with a clear view of nursing knowledge to enable meaningful weaving of disciplinary perspectives that can create new understandings.

Nursing remains on the margin of the professional disciplines and is in danger of being consumed or ignored if sufficient attention is not given to the uniqueness of nursing's field of inquiry and practice. There are hopeful indicators that nursing knowledge is growing. The blossoming of middle range theories signifies a growth of knowledge development in nursing. Middle range theories offer valuable organizing frameworks for phenomena being researched by interdisciplinary teams. These theories are useful to nurses and persons from other disciplines in framing phenomena of shared concern. Hospitals seeking Magnet® status are now required to articulate some nursing theoretic perspective that guides nursing practice in the facility. The quality of the practice environment is important for the quality of care and the retention of nurses. Theory-guided practice elevates the work of nurses leading to fulfillment, satisfaction, and a professional model of practice.

The role of the doctor of nursing practice has the potential to enrich the current level of advanced practice by moving it toward true nursing practice guided by nursing theory. The movement toward translational research and enhanced integration of research findings into the front lines of care will demand practice models that bring coherence and sense to research findings. Isolated, rapid cycling research can result in confusion and chaos if not sensibly synthesized into a model of care that is informed not only by evidence but also guided by a compass of values and a framework that synthesizes research into a meaningful whole. This is the role of theory. With this continuing shift to theory-guided practice and research, productive scientist–practitioner partnerships will emerge committed to the application of knowledge to transform care and to improve quality of life for patients, families, and communities.

## ■ REFERENCES

Andersen, M. D., & Smereck, G. A. D. (1989). Personalized nursing LIGHT model. *Nursing Science Quarterly*, 2, 120–130.

Barrett, E. A. M. (1989). A nursing theory of power for nursing practice: Derivation from Rogers' paradigm. In J. Riehl-Sisca (Ed.), *Conceptual models for nursing practice* (3rd ed., pp. 207–217). Norwalk, CT: Appleton & Lange.

Barrett, E. A. M. (2015). Barrett's theory of power as knowing participation in change. In M. Smith and M. Parker (Eds), *Nursing theories and nursing practice* (4th ed., pp. 495–531). Philadelphia, PA: F. A. Davis.

Boykin, A., & Schoenhofer, S. O. (2001). *Nursing as caring*. Sudbury, MA: Jones & Bartlett.

Boykin, A., & Schoenhofer, S. O. (2015). Theory of nursing as caring. In M. Smith and M. Parker (Eds.), *Nursing theories and nursing practice* (4th ed., pp. 341–356). Philadelphia, PA: F. A. Davis.

Chinn, P. L. (2013). *Peace and power: New directions for community building* (8th ed.). Burlington, MA: Jones & Bartlett.

Conway, M. E. (1985). Toward greater specificity of nursing's metaparadigm. *Advances in Nursing Science, 7*(4), 73–81.

Cowling, W. R. (2007). A unitary participatory vision of nursing knowledge. *Advances in Nursing Science, 30*(1), 71–80.

Denyes, M. J. (1982). Measurement of self-care agency in adolescents (Abstract). *Nursing Research, 31*, 63.

Donaldson, S. K., & Crowley, D. M. (1978). The discipline of nursing. *Nursing Outlook, 26*, 113–120.

Fawcett, J. (1984). The metaparadigm of nursing: Current status and future refinements. *Image: Journal of Nursing Scholarship, 16*, 84–87.

Fawcett, J. (1995). *Analysis and evaluation of contemporary nursing knowledge: Nursing models and theories* (3rd ed.). Philadelphia, PA: F. A. Davis.

Fawcett, J. (2000). *Analysis and evaluation of contemporary nursing knowledge: Nursing models and theories.* Philadelphia, PA: F. A. Davis.

Fawcett, J., & DeSanto-Madeya, S. (2013). *Contemporary nursing knowledge: Analysis and evaluation of nursing models and theories* (3rd ed.). Philadelphia, PA: F. A. Davis.

Johnson, D. E. (1980). The behavioral system model for nursing. In J. P. Riehl & C. Roy (Eds.), *Conceptual models for nursing practice* (2nd ed., pp. 207–216). New York, NY: Appleton-Century-Crofts.

Kuhn, T. S. (1970). *The structure of scientific revolutions* (2nd ed.). Chicago, IL: University of Chicago Press.

Laudan, L. (1977). *Progress and its problems: Toward a theory of scientific growth.* Berkeley, CA: University of California Press.

Leininger, M. (1978). *Transcultural nursing: Concepts, theories and practices.* New York, NY: Wiley.

Leininger, M. (1984). *Care: The essence of nursing and health.* Thorofare, NJ: Slack.

Neuman, B. (1989). *The Neuman systems model* (2nd ed.). Norwalk, CT: Appleton & Lange.

Neuman, B. & Fawcett, J. (2010). *The Neuman systems model* (5th ed.). Norwalk, CT: Appleton & Lange.

Newman, M. A. (1986). *Health as expanding consciousness.* St. Louis, MO: Mosby.

Newman, M. A. (1990). Newman's theory of health as praxis. *Nursing Science Quarterly, 3*(1), 37–41.

Newman, M. A. (1994). *Health as expanding consciousness* (2nd ed.). St. Louis, MO: Mosby.

Newman, M. A. (2008). *Transforming presence: The difference that nursing makes.* Philadelphia, PA: F. A. Davis.

Newman, M. A., Sime, A. M., & Corcoran-Perry, S. A. (1991). Focus of the discipline of nursing. *Advances in Nursing Science, 14*(1), 1–6.

Nightingale, F. (1969). *Notes on nursing: What it is and what it is not.* London, UK: Lippincott, Philadelphia, 1946.

Parse, R. R. (Ed.). (1987). *Nursing science: Major paradigms, theories and critiques.* Philadelphia, PA: Saunders.

Parse, R. R. (1998). *The human becoming school of thought: A perspective for nurses and other health professionals* (2nd ed.). Thousand Oaks, CA: Sage.

Parse, R. R. (2014). *The humanbecoming paradigm: A transformational worldview.* Pittsburgh, PA: Discovery International Publications.

Quinn, J. A. (1990). On healing, wholeness and the haelen effect. *Nursing and Health Care, 10*(10), 553–556.

Reed, P. G. (1991). Toward a nursing theory of self-transcendence: Deductive reformulation using developmental theories. *Advances in Nursing Science, 13*(4), 64–77.

Reed, P. G. (2015). Pamela reed's theory of self-transcendence. In M. Smith and M. Parker (Eds.), *Nursing theories and nursing practice* (4th ed., pp. 411–433). Philadelphia, PA: F. A. Davis.

Rogers, M. E. (1970). *An introduction to the theoretical basis of nursing.* New York, NY: F. A. Davis.

Rogers, M. E. (1992). Nursing science and the space age. *Nursing Science Quarterly, 5,* 27–34.

Roy, C. (1989). The Roy adaptation model. In J. P. Riehl & C. Roy (Eds.), *Conceptual models for nursing practice* (2nd ed., pp. 179–188). New York, NY: Appleton & Lange.

Roy, C. (2008). *The Roy adaptation model* (3rd ed.). Upper Saddle River, NJ: Prentice-Hall Health.

Smith, M. C. (1994). Arriving at a philosophy of nursing. In J. F. Kikuchi & H. Simmons (Eds.), *Developing a philosophy of nursing* (pp. 43–60). Thousand Oaks, CA: Sage.

Smith, M. C., & Reeder, F. (1998). Clinical outcomes research and Rogerian science: Strange or emergent bedfellows. *Visions: Journal of Rogerian Nursing Science, 6,* 27–38.

Smith, M. J., & Liehr, P. R. (2013). *Middle range theory for nursing* (3rd ed.). New York, NY: Springer Publishing.

Tulman, L., Higgins, K., Fawcett, J., Nunno, C., Vansickel, C., Haas, M. B., & Speca, M. M. (1991). The inventory of functional status-antepartum period: Development and testing. *Journal of Nurse-Midwifery, 36*(2), 117–123.

Walker, L., & Avant, K. (2010). *Strategies for theory construction in nursing* (5th ed.). Upper Saddle River, NJ: Prentice Hall.

Watson, J. (1985). *Nursing: The philosophy and science of caring.* Boulder, CO: Associated University Press.

Watson, J. (2008). *Nursing: The philosophy and science of caring* (2nd ed.). Boulder: University Press of Colorado.

Watson, J., & Foster, R. (2003). The attending nurse caring model: Integrating theory, evidence and advanced caring-healing therapeutics for transforming professional practice. *Journal of Clinical Nursing, 12,* 360–365.

# CHAPTER 2

## Understanding Middle Range Theory by Moving Up and Down the Ladder of Abstraction

Mary Jane Smith and Patricia R. Liehr

Every discipline has a process of reasoning that is rooted in the philosophy, theories, and empirical generalizations that define it. The reasoning process is logical when all levels come together and make sense in an orderly and coherent manner. The ladder of abstraction is a logical system for locating and relating three different and distinct levels of discourse: the philosophical, theoretical, and empirical. The purpose of this chapter is to describe the ladder of abstraction as central to understanding and using middle range theory in research and practice. The ladder of abstraction is a structure that maps the connection between levels of discourse (see Figure 2.1). If one pictures a ladder with three rungs, the highest is the philosophical, the middle the theoretical, and lowest is the empirical. These rungs represent levels of discourse, or differing ways of describing ideas.

### ■ PHILOSOPHICAL LEVEL

The philosophical is the highest level, representing beliefs and assumptions that are accepted as true and fundamental to any theory. It represents belief systems essential to understanding the reasoning found in the theoretical and empirical expression of middle range theories. The philosophical level includes assumptions, beliefs, paradigmatic perspectives, and points of view. Reasoning through a nursing situation for practice and for research is based on assumptions and beliefs accepted as true about what constitutes reality.

A paradigm is a worldview including disciplinary values and perspectives that are at the philosophical level. Multiple paradigmatic schemas have been developed in nursing, and several of these are discussed in Chapter 1. The schema used to guide discussion of the theories in this book is the one developed by Newman, Sime, and Corcoran-Perry (1991), who identified caring in the human health experience as the focus of the discipline of nursing. They also identified three paradigms that structure the disciplinary perspective: the particulate–deterministic, interactive–integrative, and unitary–transformative.

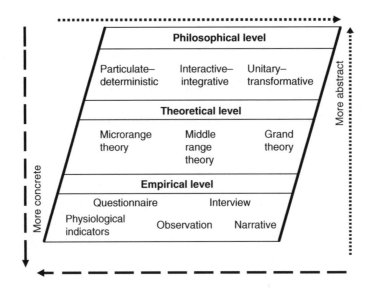

**FIGURE 2.1** Ladder of abstraction.

Each paradigm incorporates unique values about the person, change, and the knowledge base of the paradigm. In the particulate–deterministic paradigm, the person is viewed as an isolated entity, change is primarily linear and causal, and the knowledge base is grounded in biophysical sciences. The interactive–integrative paradigm describes persons as reciprocal interacting entities, change is probabilistic and related to multiple factors, and the knowledge base is that of the social sciences. In the unitary–transformative paradigm, the person is viewed as unitary evolving in a mutual and simultaneous process, change is creative and unpredictable, and the knowledge base is grounded in the human sciences.

One can clearly see that the three paradigms are at differing levels of philosophical abstraction. All three hold assumptions, values, and a point of view at differing levels of abstraction. The most abstract is the unitary–transformative, next is the interactive–integrative, and lowest in level of abstraction is the particulate–deterministic. This is an example of levels of abstraction within the philosophical rung of the ladder. Although theorists may not explicate their assumptions or paradigmatic perspective, a careful reading of the theory will lead to understanding where each stands in relation to what are the philosophical underpinnings of the proposed theory. The ladder of abstraction (Figure 2.1) depicts the highest level of abstraction as the philosophical level, including the particulate–deterministic, interactive–integrative, and unitary–transformative paradigms.

The middle range theories presented in this book have been placed by the editors in one of these paradigms on the philosophical rung of the ladder. This was a judgment reflecting the view of two people that was made through scholarly discourse. It is important for the reader to understand that different judgments may be made by different people who have a different understanding of the theory and the paradigms. There isn't a "right" way to link a theory with a paradigm, but there are always reasons for the linking decisions that are based on logical coherence. The editors made the decision about the theory–paradigm link based on an understanding of the knowledge roots of the middle range theories.

The middle range theories of Uncertainty, Bureaucratic Caring, Unpleasant Symptoms, Self-Efficacy, Symptom Management, Cultural Marginality, Transitions, Moral Reckoning, and Self-Care of Chronic Illness, are rooted primarily in the social sciences and relate to a multidimensional and contextual reality. These nine theories have links to the interactive–integrative paradigm. The middle range theories of Story, Meaning, Self-Transcendence, and Self-Reliance are primarily rooted in the human sciences encompassing a process of mutual and creative unfolding. These four theories describe values consistent with the unitary–transformative paradigm. There is usefulness in understanding the paradigmatic perspective of a theory because it helps to lay out a starting point by establishing the philosophical foundation.

## ■ THEORETICAL LEVEL

Ideas are languaged to explain and describe their essence. Ideas at the theoretical level are concepts specific to a theory. Concepts are the essential ideas that build a theory; concepts characterize properties that describe and explain the theory at a middle range level of discourse. Levels of discourse are differing ways of expressing, defining, and specifying an idea. If one idea is more abstract than another, then it is more encompassing, enveloping a broader scope. On the other hand, if an idea is less abstract it is more concrete. This notion of the relationship between levels of abstraction is key to understanding and making sense of the theoretical. Levels of abstraction apply to each rung of the ladder in relation to the other rungs. That is to say, the philosophical is at a higher level than the theoretical rung of the ladder. When one is grappling with understanding the theoretical or middle level on the ladder, the process is to move the idea up to evaluate the philosophical premise and move down to empirical indicators, where the theory connects to the world of practice and research. To have a complete understanding one moves the theoretical idea back and forth, along the rungs of the ladder and within the rungs of the ladder. For example, if trying to understand a theory, a start at the middle rung of the ladder would lead to the question: How is the theory defined conceptually? What are the concepts, and what do the concepts mean? Then given the answers to the first set of questions, move to a lower ladder rung and ask: What does this mean to me and how does it connect with what I already know, namely my experience? Then one might look at how personal experience fits with the description of the theory. One might also question what values and beliefs are included in the assumptions of the theory, thus moving the theory up the ladder of abstraction. The point is that in coming to know the realm of the theoretical, one thinks through the theory by moving up and down the rungs of the ladder. The theory becomes understandable through personal reflection and discourse with others; processes that include reading, thinking, and dialogue. Coming to understand a theory requires both tacit and explicit knowing. This means that a person can begin to describe in words the meaning of an abstract idea and at the same time hold tacitly more knowledge about the idea than can be made explicit. Each time the idea is described through talking, writing, and discussion, a greater grasp of the theoretical is achieved.

The theoretical is in the realm of the abstract, consisting of symbols, ideas, and concepts. Many of the theories in this book are known by a central abstraction. For instance, uncertainty, meaning, and self-transcendence are some of the theoretically abstract ideas that will be discussed in this book. Implicit in abstraction is an outer shadow of vagueness that enables the ongoing development of the idea. This bit of vagueness can throw a person off guard and engender confusion about the meaning of an idea. However, the abstract nature of theory is not intended to be confusing or abstruse. In deciphering the abstract and differentiating ideas according to the philosophical, theoretical, and empirical, one figures out meaning and comes to know what is explicit about an abstract idea.

The theoretical rung on the ladder of abstraction includes concepts, frameworks, and theories. A theoretical concept is different from an everyday concept because it is a mental image of an aspect of reality that is put into words to describe and explain the meaning of a phenomenon significant to the discipline of nursing. A theoretical framework is a structure of interrelating concepts that describe and explain the meaning of a phenomenon. What then is a theory? Theory is described in the literature at all levels of abstraction. The accepted definition of a theory rests in the eye of the beholder. Chinn and Kramer (1999, p. 258) define theory as "a creative and rigorous structuring of ideas that project a tentative, purposeful and systematic view of phenomena." Im and Meleis (1999, p. 11) define theory as "an organized, coherent and systematic articulation of a set of statements related to significant questions in a discipline that are communicated in a meaningful whole to describe or explain a phenomenon or set of phenomena." McKay (1969), on the other hand, describes theory as a logically interrelated set of confirmed hypotheses. Chinn and Kramer's definition of theory is at the highest level of abstraction, next is Im and Meleis, and at the lowest level is McKay. Given this array of theory definitions it is easy to understand why one could argue several ways about whether a particular theory is indeed a theory: it all depends on the way theory is defined.

Furthermore, there are levels of theory within the theoretical rung of the ladder. At the most abstract level, there are the grand theories. These are theories that have a very broad scope. The conceptual focus of some of these grand theories includes goal attainment (King, 1996), self-care (Orem, 1971), adaptation (Roy & Andrews, 1991), becoming (Parse, 1992), and unitary human field process (Rogers, 1994). Each of these grand theories shares the common ground of offering a structure that enables description and explanation of essential conceptualizations of nursing. However, even on the common ground of grand theory, some are more abstract than others. For instance, becoming is more abstract than goal attainment.

Middle range theories, the subject of this book, are described by Merton (1968, p. 9) as those "that lie between the minor but necessary working hypotheses that evolve in abundance during day-to-day research and the all-inclusive systematic efforts to develop unified theory." He goes on to say that the principal ideas of middle range theories are relatively simple. Simple, here, means rudimentary straightforward ideas that stem from the focus of the discipline. Thus, middle range theory is a basic, usable structure of ideas, less abstract than grand theory and more abstract than empirical generalizations or microrange theory.

Microrange theories, described as situation-specific by Im and Meleis (1999, p. 13), are theories that focus on "specific nursing phenomena that reflect clinical practice and that are limited to specific populations or to particular fields of practice." These theories "offer a blue print that is more readily operational and/or has more accessible utility in clinical situations" (p. 19). Microrange theory is lower on the ladder of abstraction than middle range theory. While Im's Theory of Transitions (see Chapter 11) is at the middle range level of abstraction, the population-specific theories that emerge from it are at a lower level of abstraction and identified as situation-specific theories. Examples of situation-specific theories are menopausal transition of Korean immigrant women, learned response to chronic illness of patients with rheumatoid arthritis, and women's responses when dealing with their multiple roles (Im & Meleis, 1999). In this case, a middle range theory has spawned situation-specific theories that have direct application to particular nursing practice situations.

The ladder of abstraction depicts microrange theory, middle range theory, and grand theory on ascending levels of discourse (Figure 2.1). The ladders for each theory presented in this book show a description of the philosophical, conceptual, and empirical connections. Each chapter's author has specifically identified theory concepts, so the inclusion of concepts on the ladder was a straightforward process. This may not always be true; sometimes the authors of published articles on middle range theory do not clearly identify concepts. In that instance, the reader is left to decipher what the concepts of the theory are and how they are defined. For some middle range theories it may be necessary to differentiate concepts by a very careful reading of the manuscript and examination of the model. When this interpretative process is needed, there is always a risk that the concepts identified by the reader are not exactly what the author of the theory intended.

## ▪ EMPIRICAL LEVEL

The empirical level represents discourse that brings a theory to research and practice. Empirics include physiologic indicators, questionnaires, observation, interview, and narrative (Figure 2.1). Like other rungs on the ladder, the empirical level of discourse moves from the most concrete (physiologic indicators) to the most abstract (narrative). Even at this lowest level of discourse there is a range of abstraction. The empirical is the lowest rung on the ladder, at a concrete level of discourse. The empirical represents what can be observed through the senses and moves beyond to include perceptions, symbolic meanings, self-reports, observable behavior, biological indicators, and personal stories (Ford-Gilboe, Campbell, & Berman, 1995; Reed, 1995).

Whether practicing or doing research, the nurse connects with the empirical level. The advanced practice nurse may use physiologic indicators, interview, and observation while applying theory to caring in the human health experience. The nurse researcher may use observation and narrative in a single study while applying theory to examine caring in the human health experience. Decisions about empirics are guided by philosophy and theory. It is important that the nurse choose empirics that fit with philosophical and theoretical perspectives, thus providing a match between all levels of abstraction.

## ▪ CARING IN THE HUMAN HEALTH EXPERIENCE

All theories in the book comply with the focus of nursing as presented by Newman et al. (1991), who say that nursing "is the study of caring in the human health experience" (p. 3). They go on to say "A body of knowledge that does not include caring and human health experience is not nursing knowledge" (p. 3). Caring is described as a moral imperative having a service identity. All 13 middle range theories described in this work have a focus of caring in the human health experience. Application of any one of these theories in practice or in research aims at facilitating change in the human health experience.

The human health experience is explicit in each of the theories as experiencing: uncertainty, suffering, spiritual–ethical caring, vulnerability, symptoms, decisions to make behavioral change, a health challenge that complicates everyday living, life transitions, being responsible, disciplined and confident, living at the margin of cultures, caring for self, and situational binds that demand moral reckoning. It is noteworthy that two of the middle range theories, Unpleasant Symptoms and Symptom Management, share the common human experience of symptoms. There is also common ground for the theories of meaning and self-transcendence through their respective focus on suffering and vulnerability, which are intricately connected human health experiences. Furthermore, the theories of Cultural Marginality and Self-Reliance are rooted in unique cultural perspectives. It should also be noted that Self-Care of Chronic Illness and Bureaucratic Caring hold caring as a central focus.

Caring in the human health experience requires consideration of how the nurse lives relationships with people regarding health. Based on these theories, some of the ways that caring transpires in the context of nursing are through: promoting structure and order in uncertain circumstances; intentionally engaging in dialogue to address what matters most; supporting inner resources to move beyond vulnerability; exploring symptom experience; and discussing situational binds with practicing nurses.

The middle range theories in this book add to the body of knowledge about nursing regardless of their discipline of origin. All of the theories have been applied in nursing practice and research to enhance caring in the human health experience. Theories belong to many disciplines. What is important to nursing science is that the research and practice based on a theory can be grounded in the focus and paradigmatic perspective of the discipline of nursing.

## ■ MIDDLE RANGE THEORIES ON THE LADDER OF ABSTRACTION

There are 13 middle range theories in the book, presented in chronological order according to when the chapter author introduced the idea in a refereed publication. This approach to ordering the chapters places explicit emphasis on the continued work necessary to grow ideas over time. Nursing scholars must be willing to persist with the sometimes tedious work of theory building that often occurs with spurts and stalls over decades.

The first middle range theory is Uncertainty in Illness and conceptualized for both acute and chronic illness. Mishel and Clayton coauthored the chapter on uncertainty in the first and second editions of this book. The chapter in this fourth edition was coauthored by Clayton and Dean. Clayton was a student of Mishel and Dean has published on uncertainty. The original uncertainty theory pertains to acute illness while the reconceptualized theory pertains to the continual uncertainty experienced in chronic illness. On the ladder, the reconceptualization is represented in bold print at the philosophical and theoretical level. The theories are consistent with beliefs associated with the interactive–integrative paradigm.

Persons experience uncertainty during diagnosis and treatment and when illness has a downward trajectory, and persons experience continual uncertainty in ongoing chronic illness and also with the possibility of recurrence of an illness. Concepts at the theoretical level in both theories are antecedents of uncertainty, appraisal of uncertainty, and coping with uncertainty. Concepts added in the reconceptualized theory include self-organization and probabilistic thinking. Moving to the empirical level with practice is offering information and explanation, providing structure and order, and focusing on choices and alternatives. An instrument has been developed that is directly related to the theory, the uncertainty in illness scale (see Figure 2.2).

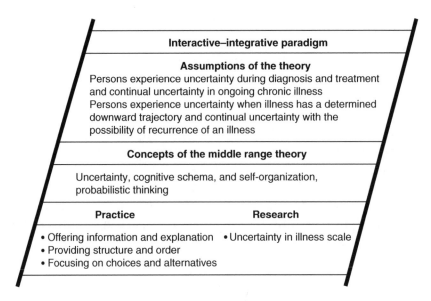

**FIGURE 2.2** Ladder of abstraction: Uncertainty in Illness.

The second middle range theory is the Theory of Meaning, based on the work of Viktor Frankl. The theory was authored by Patricia Starck in all three of the previous editions of this book. When Dr. Starck was invited to revise the chapter for this edition, she graciously requested that authors be found who were interested in the theory. Teresa Ritchie and Suzy Walter, the coauthors of the theory in this fourth edition, have been teaching and applying the theory to their advanced practice. This theory is grounded in the unitary–transformative paradigm. It is assumed that through a transformative process, persons find meaning. When confronted with a hopeless situation, meaning can be freely and responsibly realized in every moment. Concepts at the theoretical level are life purpose, freedom to choose, and suffering. Practice approaches at the empirical level include dereflection, paradoxical intention, and Socratic dialogue. Empirical indicators for research are questionnaires, interviews, and other narrative approaches (see Figure 2.3).

The third middle range theory of Bureaucratic Caring developed by Ray is a new theory in the fourth edition and is supported by assumptions of the inter-active–integrative paradigm. Caring is humanistic, spiritual, and ethical; and bureaucratic systems are political, economic, technological, legal, and sociocultural. The merger of caring and bureaucratic values distinguishes this theory. Concepts include the social–cultural, legal, technological, economic, political, educational, and physical dimensions of spiritual–ethical caring. It allows for both quantitative and qualitative approaches to research. The theory has been used in Magnet® hospital designation processes. Most recently, it has been adopted by the U.S. Air Force to serve as a foundation for an interdisciplinary practice model (see Figure 2.4).

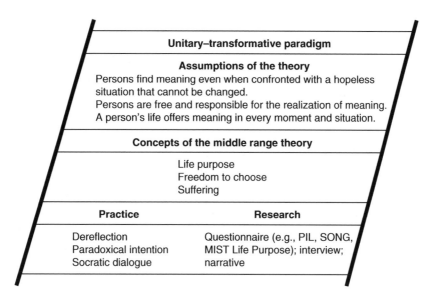

**FIGURE 2.3** Ladder of abstraction: Meaning.

The fourth middle range theory, Self-Transcendence developed by Reed, is grounded in assumptions of the unitary–transformative paradigm. Self-transcendence is a unitary process. The theory assumes that persons are integral and coextensive with their environment and capable of an awareness that extends beyond physical and temporal dimensions. Concepts at the theoretical

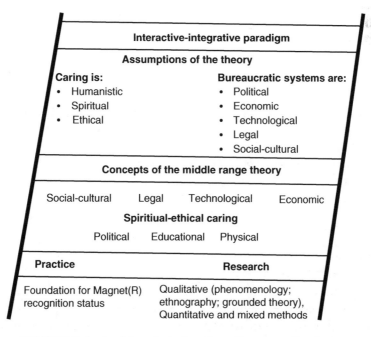

**FIGURE 2.4** Ladder of abstraction: Bureaucratic Caring.

level of discourse include vulnerability, self-transcendence, and well-being. Taking the theory to the empirical level with practice includes integrative spiritual care, support of inner resources, and expansion of intrapersonal, interpersonal, temporal, and transpersonal boundaries. Like the Theory of Uncertainty, a research instrument has been developed that is directly related to the theory, the self-transcendence scale (see Figure 2.5).

The fifth theory presented in the book is Symptom Management Theory by Bender, Janson, Franck, and Lee. These four authors, like the author group in the third edition, are members of the University of California, San Francisco Symptom Management Faculty Group. The theory is grounded in assumptions of the interactive–integrative paradigm, in which persons manage their symptoms in interaction with the environment. The specific assumptions of the theory are that: health and illness affect symptom management, improvement in symptoms extends beyond personal health, and symptoms are subjective and experienced in clusters. There are three concepts at the middle range level of discourse. The concepts are symptom experience, symptom management strategies, and symptom status outcomes. At the empirical level, practice application occurs with patient–provider communication marked by an understanding of the symptom experience and implementation of effective strategies. Research application includes measurement of symptom-specific outcomes and contextual factors related to the symptom under study (see Figure 2.6).

The sixth middle range theory is Unpleasant Symptoms by Lenz and Pugh. The theory is grounded in the beliefs and assumptions associated with the interactive–integrative paradigm. Specific beliefs of the theory are that there

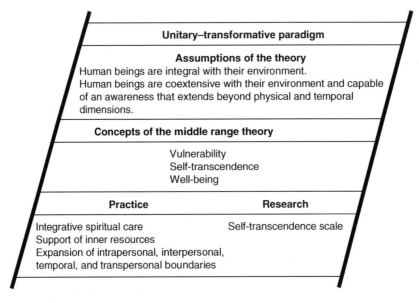

**FIGURE 2.5** Ladder of abstraction: Self-Transcendence.

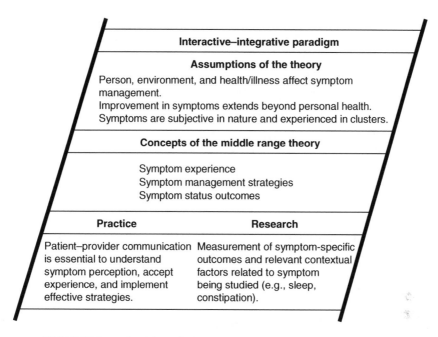

**FIGURE 2.6**   Ladder of abstraction: Symptom Management.

are commonalities across different symptoms experienced by persons in varied situations, and that symptoms are subjective phenomena occurring in family and community contexts. Concepts at the theoretical level include symptoms, influencing factors, and performance. Practice application at the empirical level includes assessment of the symptom, symptom management, and relief intervention. Empirical measurements are gathered through scales and observations that capture the symptom experience (see Figure 2.7).

The seventh middle range theory is Self-Efficacy by Resnick, grounded in the assumptions of the interactive–integrative paradigm. Persons change in a reciprocal interactive process when they exercise influence over what they do and decide how to behave. Concepts at the theoretical level include self-efficacy expectations and self-efficacy outcomes. Examples of practice applications at the empirical level include learning about exercise, addressing unpleasant sensations, and cueing to exercise. Research based on this middle range theory uses self-efficacy scales (see Figure 2.8).

The eighth middle range theory presented is Liehr and Smith's Story Theory, which is grounded in the assumptions of the unitary– transformative paradigm where change is viewed as creative and unpredictable. Story is a narrative happening in the unitary nurse–person process. The specific assumptions of the theory are that persons change in interrelationship with their world as they live in an expanded present and experience meaning. There are three concepts at the theoretical level: intentional dialogue, connecting with self-in-relation, and creating ease. At the empirical level the health story is the basis for both

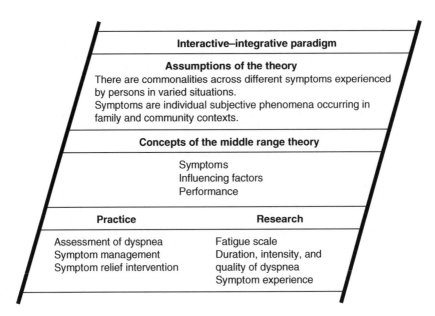

**FIGURE 2.7**  Ladder of abstraction: Unpleasant Symptoms.

practice and research. Examples of empirical approaches in practice include creation of a story path and family tree. Health story data may be analyzed using phenomenological, linguistic, case study, or story inquiry methods (see Figure 2.9).

The ninth theory found in the book is the Theory of Transitions presented by Im. This theory is in keeping with the assumptions of the interactive–integrative paradigm and describes circumstances related to change in health/illness,

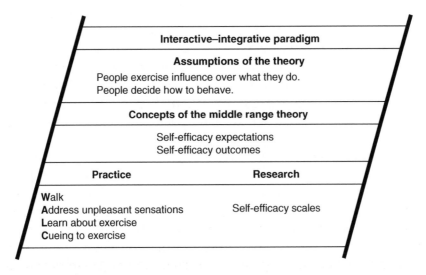

**FIGURE 2.8**  Ladder of abstraction: Self-Efficacy.

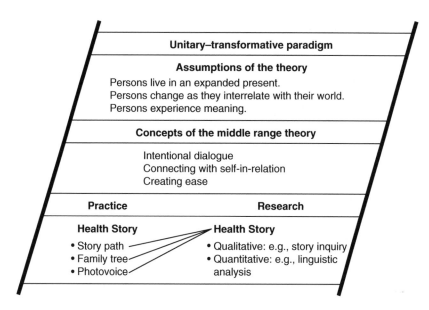

**FIGURE 2.9**  Ladder of abstraction: Story.

life situations, and developmental stages. Assumptions include the centrality of transitions to nursing practice, reciprocity of the nurse/client relationship, and the complexity of patterns and processes of transitions. Nursing therapeutics incorporate the phases of assessment of readiness, preparation for transition, and role supplementation. Research studies have produced situation-specific theories on the pain experience of Caucasian and Asian American cancer patients and the menopausal experience of Asian women (see Figure 2.10).

The tenth theory is the Theory of Self-Reliance developed by Lowe. This theory is in keeping with the unitary–transformative paradigm and is rooted in the author's Native American Cherokee values. Assumptions specific to the theory are the value of being true to oneself and being connected with others. Concepts of the theory are being responsible, disciplined, and confident. This theory articulates a process for promoting well-being with attention to appreciation of one's culture. The Talking Circle offers an approach to nursing practice through honoring the process of life and growth. A 24-item self-reliance instrument has been developed and used in research, including intervention studies (see Figure 2.11).

The eleventh theory presented in this book is the Theory of Cultural Marginality developed by Choi. This theory is embedded in the interactive–integrative paradigm and describes the experience of people who are caught between two cultures. Concepts specific to the theory include marginal living, across-cultural conflict recognition, and easing cultural tension. Examples of practice applications include promoting parent–child engagement through across-cultural understanding and being sensitive to the struggle of

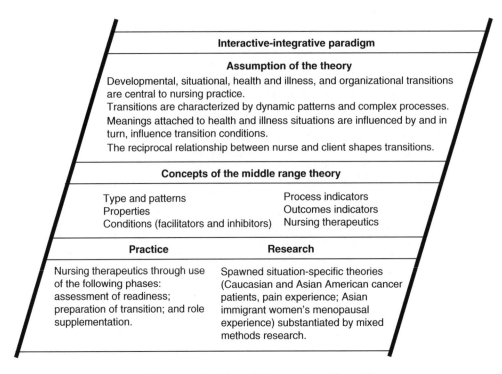

**FIGURE 2.10** Ladder of abstraction: Transitions.

immigration. Research activities are aimed at developing an instrument to measure cultural marginality and studying mental health outcomes of persons living through across-culture conflict (see Figure 2.12).

The twelfth theory is Nathaniel's Theory of Moral Reckoning, grounded in the interactive–integrative paradigm. According to this theory persons engage in a social process of deliberating when faced with a moral dilemma.

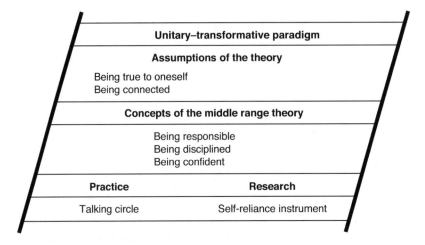

**FIGURE 2.11** Ladder of abstraction: Self-Reliance.

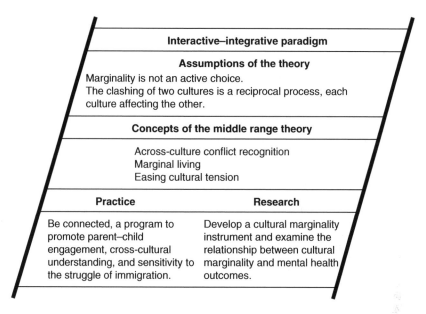

**FIGURE 2.12** Ladder of abstraction: Cultural Marginality.

Assumptions supporting the theory include facing a moral dilemma where no one choice is right or wrong and experiencing situational binds that are inherent to being human. Concepts in the theory are ease, situational bind, resolution, and reflection. Practice based on the theory includes providing structured discussion with nurses about situational binds and introduction of moral reckoning in nursing education courses. Research guided by the theory includes study of moral reckoning with other professionals. Because moral reckoning is a human experience that is increasingly common in this day and age, it warrants consideration for guiding nursing practice and structuring study for people who are in a moral bind (see Figure 2.13).

The thirteenth theory is Self-Care of Chronic Illness by Riegel, Jaarsma, and Stromberg. The theory is aligned with the interactive–integrative paradigm. Assumptions are in keeping with a holistic view, and the unique perspective required for multiple chronic conditions with an understanding that similar self-care behaviors occur across varying chronic illnesses. Concepts are self-care monitoring, maintenance, and management. Practice includes applying self-care approaches with persons experiencing multiple chronic conditions. Research studies center on self-care (see Figure 2.14).

There is one final ladder of abstraction in this book in the evaluation chapter (see Chapter 3) by Smith. In this chapter, Smith offers a process for understanding and evaluating middle range theories based on postmodern beliefs (see Figure 2.15). Overall, the ladders of abstraction provide a structure to guide the student in deciphering theory so that it can be used productively in advanced nursing practice and research. So, we urge you to

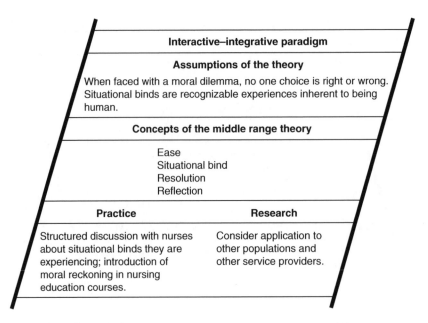

**FIGURE 2.13** Ladder of abstraction: Moral Reckoning.

begin climbing the ladders . . . stay long enough on each rung to get comfortable, and spend enough time on all three rungs to get the whole picture of any theory. Also, expect to be uncomfortable when a rung is new to you. Discomfort is a space for growing and connecting what you know with what you are learning.

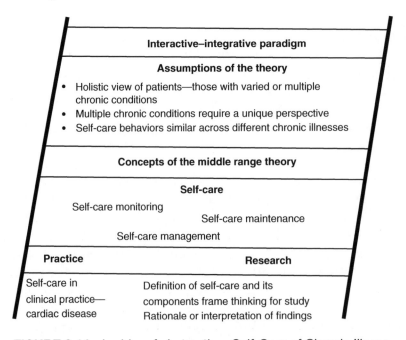

**FIGURE 2.14** Ladder of abstraction: Self-Care of Chronic Illness.

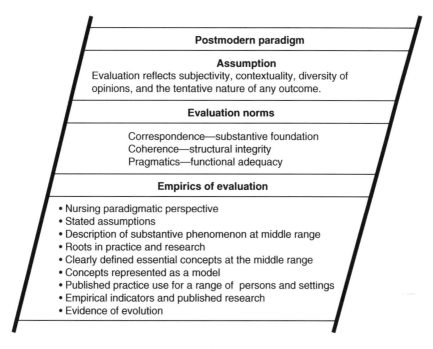

**FIGURE 2.15**  Ladder of abstraction: Evaluation.

It should be pointed out that failure to move around all the rungs of the ladder deters understanding and limits ability to use the theory in practice or research. Sometimes scholars may choose to stay on the rung that is most comfortable. For example, theorists may stay on the theoretical rung, and researchers may stay on the empirical rung, while meta-theorists may be more comfortable on the philosophical rung. It is a premise of this work on middle range theory that in order to move nursing science to the front lines of practice and research, nurses must be skilled in moving up and down and back and forth on the ladder of abstraction when studying, practicing, and researching the science of nursing.

When all levels of an idea can be mapped on the ladder of abstraction and the levels cohere with each other, theory is guided by a logical process that provides clarity and facilitates understanding and use of the theory in research and practice. To understand a theory at all levels of abstraction requires a process of reasoning. By moving from the lower rung of the ladder to the middle and then the upper rung, one is making sense of phenomena through inductive reasoning. And conversely, movement from the upper philosophical rung to the theoretical and then to the empirical requires deductive reasoning. The substantive knowledge of the discipline structured by logic guides thinking through nursing research and advanced nursing practice. This point flies in the face of the notion that theory is bewildering logic, abstruse, and rather incomprehensible. There is logic to the abstract that can be reasoned through with the ladder of abstraction.

# ■ REFERENCES

Chinn, P., & Kramer, M. K. (1999). *Theory and nursing: Integrated knowledge development*. St. Louis, MO: Mosby.

Ford-Gilboe, M., Campbell, J., & Berman, H. (1995). Stories and numbers: Coexistence without compromise. *Advances in Nursing Science, 18*(1), 14–26.

Im, E., & Meleis, A. I. (1999). Situation-specific theories: Philosophical roots, properties, and approach. *Advances in Nursing Science, 22*(2), 11–24.

King, I. (1996). The theory of goal attainment in research and practice. *Nursing Science Quarterly, 9,* 61–66.

McKay, R. P. (1969). Theories, models, and systems for nursing. *Nursing Research, 18,* 393–399.

Merton, R. K. (1968). *Social theory and social structure.* New York, NY: Free Press.

Newman, M., Sime, A. M., & Corcoran-Perry, S. A. (1991). The focus of the discipline of nursing. *Advances in Nursing Science, 14*(1), 1–6.

Orem, D. (1971). *Nursing: Concepts of practice.* New York, NY: McGraw-Hill.

Parse, R. R. (1992). Human becoming: Parse's theory of nursing. *Nursing Science Quarterly, 5*(1), 35–42.

Reed, P. (1995). A treatise on nursing knowledge development for the 21st century: Beyond postmodernism. *Advances in Nursing Science, 17,* 70–84.

Rogers, M. E. (1994). The science of unitary human beings: Current perspectives. *Nursing Science Quarterly, 7,* 33–35.

Roy, C., & Andrews, H. A. (1991). *The Roy adaptation model: The definitive statement.* Norwalk, CT: Appleton & Lange.

# CHAPTER 3

## Evaluation of Middle Range Theories for the Discipline of Nursing

**Marlaine C. Smith**

Theories are patterned ideas that provide a coherent way of viewing complex phenomena. Middle range theories have a more limited view of circumscribed phenomena than do grand theories. However, because nursing is a professional discipline, all the theories within it should be evaluated from a perspective that considers the salient elements of the discipline in the evaluation. Although there are many sets of criteria for evaluating nursing conceptual models and grand theories (Chinn & Kramer, 2014; Fawcett & DeSanto-Madeya, 2013; Fitzpatrick & Whall, 2004; Parse, 1987; Stevens, 1998), few focus particularly on theories at the middle range. In addition, there has been little guidance for beginning nursing scholars on the purpose and the process of critical analysis and evaluation of theories. A common course assignment on the evaluation of nursing theory becomes a pedantic exercise, ending in a rather cynical view of theory development. One is reminded of the aphorism: When our only tool is a hammer, all we see are nails. In other words, the tool of critical evaluation taught to students is often weighted toward finding the faults, errors, and inconsistencies within the theoretic structures. It is no wonder that there is evidence of some devaluation of nursing theory and a reticence to engage in its development.

The theoretical measurement of outcomes of practice, while a worthy endeavor, has eclipsed the compelling need to create systems of thought with potential to describe and explain the nature of phenomena of concern to nursing science. The nursing scholars who contribute to the development of theory for the discipline—including those who are featured in this text—are innovative pioneers who courageously offer their ideas for the advancement of the discipline and the betterment of healthcare. It is important, then, to balance the identification of theoretic weaknesses with the aspects of appreciation, recognition, and affirmation of strengths. The purpose of this chapter is to provide tools for a balanced and reasoned evaluation of middle range theory for the discipline of nursing. Describing the purposes of theory evaluation, articulating a set of criteria to guide evaluation of middle range theory, and elaborating a process for conducting this evaluation organize this chapter.

## ■ THE PURPOSE OF THEORY EVALUATION: TOWARD A POSTMODERN VIEW

Evaluation is one of the most popular indoor sports of the organizations in which we live. Because these organizations are accountable to various stake-holders, evaluation is used as a measure of assurance and accountability. The meaning of evaluation carries an onerous tone because of the baggage that is often attached to it. Students receive grades that reflect evaluation of achievement in a course. A score or category is received when one is evaluated for job performance. Often this evaluation is attached to some reward. The memory of the evaluation of papers, projects, and practice may be more often marked by the red ink of what was done wrong than by what was achieved or done well.

The common, modern definition of evaluation is a process of determining or fixing the value, worth, or significance of something. This definition reflects the anxieties that are experienced surrounding evaluation, connoting the determination of a static and absolute outcome of worth or value. A postmodern meaning of evaluation is quite different. It reflects the presence of subjectivity and contextuality, the diversity of opinions from a community, and, ultimately, the tentative nature of any outcome. It becomes an informed and flawed opinion rendered at a particular moment in time by a person with inherent biases and values. This opinion, which one hopes is not arbitrary or capricious, is based on some sound, reasonable measures or criteria that can be applied consistently. However, it is important to note that the criteria and the evaluator's application of them are value laden. In this way, they should be viewed not as absolute judgments of worth, but as one honest examination by a member of a community.

The evaluation of theory, then, is a process of coming to an opinion about its worth or value. Kaplan (1964)—in his discussion of the validation of theory—states that its purpose is to examine a theory's value or worth for advancement by the scientific community. When evaluating nursing theory, we ask questions about its worthiness to be used as a guide for inquiry and practice and to be taught to students.

Theory, by its definition in any paradigm of science, is a creative constellation of ideas, offered as a possible explanation or description of an observed or experienced phenomenon. In the process of evaluation, one is not determining the truth of the theory, but rather its value for further exploration within the scientific community. History affirms the tentative nature of theory evaluation. Theories that were judged by the scientific community as valid were often later abandoned. Ptolemaic theory on the geocentric nature of the planetary system was abandoned later for the Copernican theory that the Earth and the planets revolve around the Sun.

Many revolutionary ideas of our time were evaluated initially as worthless. Rogers's (1970) conceptual system—describing the integral nature of human–environment energy fields—was an object of ridicule in the early 1970s. Nearly 50 years later, its correspondence to burgeoning contemporary thought is stunning.

Members of a disciplinary community bear the responsibility to participate in authentic dialogue around ideas within the field of study. The purpose of evaluation of theory in this context is to share in the evolution of the discipline through reflection and comment on the ideas offered within the community. The greater value of evaluating theory is to participate as individuals in the community's structuring of ideas. Although the theory is given to the community, the community reforms it through critique, testing, and application. The life of any theory is determined by the scientific community's engagement with it. Evaluation of theory is essential to the life of the theory, leading to its extension, revision, and refinement. Based on the preceding discussion, it is important that the evaluator stay true to the purpose of evaluation of theory. The stance of one who is evaluating theory from a postmodern perspective is characterized by intellectual empathy, curiosity, honesty, and responsibility. The empathic stance is the attempt to understand the perspective of the theorist and is defined by Paul (1993) as "to imaginatively put oneself in the place of others in order to understand them" (p. 261). Here, the evaluator listens carefully to the point of view. Listening is being aware of one's own biases but trying to put them aside to thoughtfully consider others' ideas, even if the evaluator does not share them. The stance of empathy requires an appreciation of others' points of view and a seeking out of the origin and context of those points of view. Curiosity is the second characteristic of the critical stance. Here, the evaluator raises questions in the process of studying the theory that are born from a quest to understand. The evaluator plays with the theory in different circumstances and imagines ways of testing or understanding it more deeply. The evaluator engages fully in trying to understand and acquire a range of sources on the theory and its application. The third stance is one of honesty. The evaluator trusts individual inner wisdom and recognizes the need to honor that wisdom in sharing the evaluation. Knowing personal biases and limitations, the evaluator is still willing to share reflections on the theory. One of the major hurdles in learning to evaluate theory is to rely on one's own opinions rather than jumping on the bandwagon of others who are considered wiser or more learned. From the postmodern perspective, each evaluation should stand on its own, one voice among many diverse ones in the community. It may be difficult to publish negative comments, but it is important to remember that these may be the needed stimuli to make important clarifications or changes in the theory. Finally, the evaluator must be a responsible steward of the discipline. As a member of the scientific community, the evaluator has an obligation to care about the nature of evolution of nursing knowledge. That responsibility entails a thoughtful and scholarly response to the critique, applying the criteria fairly and drawing conclusions that can be useful in the revision or extension of the theory as others use it. Once a theory is published, it no longer belongs to the theorist. The voice of the theorist becomes one of many in the community using the theory to guide processes of knowledge development and practice.

In summary, the purpose of a postmodern approach to the evaluation of middle range theory in nursing is to come to a decision about the merits and limitations of the theory for nursing science. The evaluator approaches the evaluation from a stance of empathy, curiosity, honesty, and responsibility. Evaluation of theory is acknowledged as necessary to the evolution of the theory in the context of the scientific community.

## ■ THE ORIGIN OF EVALUATIVE FRAMEWORKS

Theories are the language of science. "Science is the process of systematically seeking an understanding of phenomena through creating some unifying or organizing frameworks about the nature of those phenomena. In addition, science involves the evaluation of these frameworks for their credibility and empirical honesty" (M. C. Smith, 1994, p. 50). The organizing or unifying frameworks of science are theories. Rigorous and systematic standards of inquiry govern the development and testing of theories. Theories are evaluated for their credibility and empirical honesty by judging them against established standards.

The nature of science and, therefore, the theories of science have undergone change. Philosophies of science have evolved from a sole reliance on the assumptions of logical–positivist views toward expanding philosophies of the postpositivist or postmodern era (M. C. Smith, 1998). For example, the traditional or empirical–analytic view of science defines theories as sets of interrelated propositions that describe, explain, or predict the nature of phenomena (Kerlinger, 1986). In the human science view, which encompasses phenomenology, hermeneutics, and critical and poststructural perspectives, the purpose of theory is to create an understanding of phenomena through description and interpretation. Therefore, the structural rules, which apply to traditional science, do not apply to human science. For this reason, the frameworks used to evaluate theories must be inclusive enough to encompass these differences.

Kaplan's (1964) perspective on the "validation" of theories is open enough to encompass a diversity of theoretic forms. He emphasizes that the evaluation of any theory is not a matter of pronouncement of its truth: "At any given moment a particular theory will be accepted by some scientists, for some of their purposes, and not by other scientists, or not for other contexts of possible application" (p. 311).

The evaluation of theory involves the exercise of good judgment in determining a relative and tentative truth, and is by its nature normative in that the community ultimately determines the outcome. "The validation of a theory is not the act of granting an imprimatur but the act of deciding that the theory is worth being published, taught, and above all, applied—worth being acted on in contexts of inquiry or of other action" (Kaplan, 1964, p. 312). Kaplan identifies three major philosophical conceptions or norms of truth that can be exercised in the process of evaluating theory: correspondence or semantic norms, coherence or syntactic norms, and pragmatics or functional norms.

The norm of correspondence refers to the substantive meaning of the theory. Through application of this norm, one judges the degree to which the theory fits the facts. Although facts are in themselves understood through a theoretic lens, Kaplan argues that this does not necessarily present a tautology. Any theory must in some way pass the test of common sense. Although he acknowledges that significant discoveries have flown in the face of common sense, these discoveries in some way could be explained through their relationship to accepted knowledge or some convergence of evidence that supported the plausibility of the theory. Through the norm of correspondence, one evaluates the extent to which the theory fits comfortably within the nexus of existing knowledge.

The norm of coherence relates to the integrity of the theory's structure. Kaplan describes the experience of the "click of relation, when widely different and separate phenomena suddenly fall into a pattern of relatedness, when they click into position" (p. 314).

This experience of truth or wholeness occurs when all the fragments of the theory come together to form an integrated whole. Simplicity is the most widely applied norm of coherence. Descriptive simplicity is the quality of expressing the complex ideas of the theory parsimoniously. Inductive simplicity refers to the phenomenon being described by the theory. The theory must encompass a manageable number of ideas; too many will overwhelm the capacity of the theory to serve its purpose to provide a framework for understanding. Kaplan warns that a theory can be too simple in that it goes too far in reducing the complexities. Theories should introduce the degree of complexity necessary for clear understanding, nothing more. He quotes Whitehead's axiom: "Seek simplicity and distrust it" (p. 318). Another norm of coherence is aesthetics, that is, the beauty perceived upon the contemplation of the theory. The beauty of the theory involves some sense of symmetry and balance, but Kaplan warns, "Beauty is not truth" (p. 319). The process of developing theory is creative and that creativity is expressed in a product that possesses an aesthetic quality.

The final norm is pragmatics and refers to the effectiveness or functional capability of the theory. In a professional discipline, the norm of pragmatics instructs us to consider the degree to which the theory can guide practice and research to advance the goals of the discipline. On the other hand, Kaplan states that the theory is not judged by the extent to which it makes some external difference alone; he acknowledges that other factors might interfere with or enhance the success of application. The theory is also judged by what it can do for science, "how it guides and stimulates the ongoing process of scientific inquiry" (pp. 319–320). So the degree to which the theory has spawned research questions is relevant: "The value of the theory lies not only in the answers it gives but also in the new questions it raises" (p. 320).

A theory is validated when it is put to good use in the application of concerns to the discipline. The evaluative framework for middle range theories is based on these norms. Criteria will be clustered into the following three categories: substantive foundation, structural integrity, and functional adequacy.

A plethora of evaluative frameworks for nursing theories, some mentioned earlier in this chapter, have evolved over the past several decades. Some of these frameworks are applicable to middle range theories, whereas others are not. Liehr and Smith (1999; M. J. Smith & Liehr, 2013) summarized the literature about the nature of middle range theories and concluded that middle range theories are identified by their scope, level of abstraction, and proximity to empirical findings. Scope refers to the breadth of phenomena addressed by the theory. Compared to conceptual models and grand theories, middle range theories offer constellations of ideas or concepts about more circumscribed phenomena of concern to the discipline. In this way, they are intermediate in scope, focusing on a limited number of concepts focused on a limited aspect of reality (Liehr & Smith, 1999; M. J. Smith & Liehr, 2013). Level of abstraction locates middle range theories between the abstract level of conceptual models and grand theories and situation-specific theories. The language of middle range theories describes concepts and relationships between them more concretely. Finally, middle range theories are more proximal to empirical findings than conceptual models and grand theories. They are developed through an analysis of empirical findings or at a level of immediate testability. These three qualities of middle range theories should be represented in the evaluative frameworks for them.

The criteria in Table 3.1 have been developed from Kaplan's norms for validating theories and are informed by the essential qualities of middle range theories to create an evaluative framework specific to theories of the middle range.

## Substantive Foundation

Substantive foundation is the first category of criteria for the evaluation of middle range theory in nursing. This category includes criteria based on Kaplan's norm of correspondence and leads to questions about the meaning or semantic elements of the theory. A middle range theory in nursing contributes to the knowledge of the discipline of nursing and is developed from assumptions that are clearly specified. The theory provides knowledge that is at the middle range level of abstraction. There are four major criteria related to substantive meaning: (1) the theory is within the focus of the discipline of nursing; (2) the assumptions are specified and are congruent with the focus of the discipline of nursing; (3) the theory provides a substantive description, explanation, or interpretation of a named phenomenon at the middle range level of

**TABLE 3.1** Framework for the Evaluation of Middle Range Theories

**Substantive Foundation**
1. The theory is within the focus of the discipline of nursing.
2. The assumptions are specified and congruent with focus.
3. The theory provides a substantive description, explanation, or interpretation of a named phenomenon at the middle range level of discourse.
4. The origins are rooted in practice and research experience.

**Structural Integrity**
1. The concepts are clearly defined.
2. The concepts within the theory are at the middle range level of abstraction.
3. There are no more concepts than needed to explain the phenomenon.
4. The concepts and relationships among them are logically represented with a model.

**Functional Adequacy**
1. The theory can be applied to a variety of practice environments and client groups.
2. Empirical indicators have been identified for concepts of the theory.
3. There are published examples of use of the theory in practice.
4. There are published examples of research related to the theory.
5. The theory has evolved through scholarly inquiry.

discourse; and (4) the origins are rooted in practice and research experience. Each of these criteria and the questions that guide the application of the criteria in evaluating the theory are discussed. The first criterion emphasizes that a middle range theory in nursing is judged by its location in and contribution to the discipline of nursing. The question "What makes a middle range theory in nursing a *nursing* theory?" is interesting to consider. Some (Fawcett, 2004; Parse, 1987) assert that nursing theories are only those identified as the conceptual models and grand theories developed by nurses in the 1960s through the 1980s. From this perspective, legitimate middle range theories in nursing are those deduced from or inductively developed within existing conceptual models and grand theories of nursing. This is problematic in that it fixates theory development in what has been considered legitimate in the past. It is important to leave space for the possibility of emergent conceptual models or grand constructions that may be articulated as sets of foundational assumptions on which middle range theories are constructed. The evaluator should expect that a middle range theory in nursing contributes to knowledge about human–environment–health relationships, caring in the human health experience, and/or health and healing processes (Fawcett, 2004; Newman, Sime, & Corcoran-Perry, 1991; M. C. Smith, 1994). It should be possible to locate the theory within a paradigmatic perspective endorsed by nursing, such as the particulate–deterministic, integrative–interactive, or unitary–transformative schemas (Newman et al., 1991), the totality or simultaneity paradigm (Parse, 1987), or the reaction, reciprocal interaction, or simultaneous action worldview (Fawcett, 2004).

The second criterion regarding the specification of assumptions in the category of substantive foundation is that the origins and ontological foundations of the theory are specified. The developer of the middle range theory holds philosophical assumptions that are either explicitly stated or implied by the meaning of the theory. Fawcett (2004) argues that the belief that middle range theory is developed outside the context of a conceptual frame of reference is absurd. She emphasizes the contextual nature of theory building. The assumptions of a middle range theory identify the context for theory building and should be identifiable. A stronger middle range theory would explicate the assumptions.

The ideas of parent theories or models should be clearly identified in the explication of the meaning of the theory. The developers should cite primary sources from any parent theories that may be accessed for greater depth in understanding. Although some middle range theories will not be explicitly derived from nursing conceptual models or grand theories, parent ideas that shaped theory development would be clearly described.

Finally, the meaning of the theory should be consistent with its foundational assumptions. This consistency is essential. If Rogers's Science of Unitary Human Beings (SUHB) forms the assumptions of a middle range theory, the meaning of the concepts within the theory should not violate these assumptions. One would not use the language of adaptive responses in a theory purportedly derived from the SUHB. If the assumptions are not derived from an existing conceptual model/grand theory, one is left to analyze inferred foundations about how the assumption corresponds with the meaning of the middle range theory.

The third criterion related to substantive foundation states that the middle range theory provides substantive knowledge about a named circumscribed phenomenon of concern to nursing. Liehr and Smith (1999) contend that a middle range theory is known by the way it is named and that it should be "named in the context of the disciplinary perspective and at the appropriate level of discourse" (p. 86). Middle range theory is defined by its focus on providing knowledge about a specific phenomenon of concern to nursing. The theory should offer a substantive description, explanation, or interpretation of this particular phenomenon that leads to a new understanding or different way of considering the phenomenon. It is incumbent on the developer of the theory to provide adequate explanation substantiated by logical reasoning and reference to existing knowledge sources that lead to a full understanding of the meaning of the concepts and their relationships to each other.

Finally, the theory should capture the complexities of the phenomenon that it addresses. A theory is a map of some aspect of reality; like a map, it cannot capture the landscape. However, to the extent possible, the theory should approximate the fullest range of conceptual relationships that it addresses.

The fourth criterion deals with the rooting of the origins of the theory in practice and research experience. Middle range theory grows out of the research and practice experiences of nurses, who articulate a set of concepts to describe and explain a phenomenon that they have observed in their work. The evaluator will seek out the practice and research roots of the theory. It may be that one set of roots (practice or research) is sturdier than the other. This assessment may indicate the next direction for further application of the theory. Well-developed middle range theory will have documented development related to both practice and research that evolves over time.

## Structural Integrity

A middle range theory is a framework that organizes ideas. Like any framework, it has a structure. The structure provides strength, balance, and the aesthetic qualities that ensure its integrity. Structural integrity is the category that was derived from Kaplan's (1964) norm of coherence. There are four criteria for evaluation of the structural integrity of middle range theories: (a) the concepts are clearly defined; (b) the concepts of the theory are at the middle range level of abstraction; (c) there are no more concepts than are needed to explain the phenomenon; and (d) the concepts and relationships among them are logically represented with a model. The four criteria for structural integrity and their application are discussed in the following.

The first criterion is that the ideas and the relationships among them are clearly presented within the theory. Concepts are the names given to the abstract ideas that constitute the theory. The relationships among the ideas are developed into statements or propositions. In any middle range theory, the concepts within it should be clearly defined. Any neologisms (newly coined terms) should be adequately defined. The relationship statements, whether called propositions or not, should articulate the relationships among the central ideas or concepts within the theory. Concepts, even within the context of middle range theory, are abstractions, and, as such, it takes some willingness to understand them. However, the definitions should lead to this understanding and provide precise meaning.

The second criterion related to structural integrity is that the ideas of the theory are at the middle range level of abstraction. All concepts should be on the ladder of abstraction at a similar level. For example, health may be considered a concept at the metaparadigm level; adaptation, at the level of grand theory; and anxiety, at the level of the middle range. Mixing these as concepts within one theory would be an example of concepts at differing levels of abstraction. Similarly, the concepts in the theory should consistently be presented at the middle range level, more concrete and circumscribed than concepts at a higher level of abstraction. The deductive or inductive processes of theory development should be transparent in the presentation of the theory. Movement up the ladder of abstraction to paradigms or down the ladder to empirical indicators should be logical, reasoned, and clear.

The third criterion is that there should be no more concepts than necessary to describe the theory as named. The theory should be organized and presented parsimoniously. That means that the ideas should be synthesized and communicated in the simplest, most elegant way possible. Extraneous concepts or unclear differentiation of concepts creates complexity that confuses rather than clarifies.

The fourth or final criterion is that the ideas of the theory are integrated to create an understanding of the whole phenomenon, which is presented in a model. This criterion leads to consideration of the internal consistency, balance, and aesthetics of the theory. The concepts and statements of the theory should be logically ordered so that they lead to an appreciation and apprehension of the theory's meaning. The relationships among the ideas can be represented in a schema, a model, or a list of logically ordered statements. In any case, it is the responsibility of the developer to make these relationships accessible. All ideas (concepts and related statements) in the theory should have semantic congruence, that is, the meanings should not be contradictory. Middle range theories are creative products of science. As such, there should be balance and harmony in the way they are presented.

## Functional Adequacy

For a professional discipline, functional adequacy is arguably the acid test of a middle range theory. Middle range theories are closely tied to research and practice. They may be generated from research findings or deduced from larger models to form a set of testable hypotheses. They may have been developed in relation to a practice dilemma and can be used to create practice guidelines. Middle range theories build nursing knowledge and are valuable in and of themselves for this contribution. There are five criteria for functional adequacy of middle range theories: (a) the theory can be applied to a variety of practice environments and client groups; (b) empirical indicators have been identified for concepts of the theory; (c) there are published examples of use of the theory in practice; (d) there are published examples of research related to the theory; and (e) the theory has evolved through scholarly inquiry. Each of these criteria is described in the following.

The first criterion of functional adequacy is that the theory provides guidance for a variety of practice populations and environments. One would expect literature that documents use of the theory with more than one population and in more than one setting. Because the theory is middle range rather than situation-specific, this generality criterion is important and limited to the central phenomenon of the theory.

The second criterion is that there are empirical indicators identified for the concepts of the theory. Empirical adequacy is an essential aspect of middle range theory. Empirics are meant to go beyond empiricism and include perceptions, symbolic meanings, self-reports, observable behavior, biological indicators, and personal stories (Ford-Gilboe, Campbell, & Berman, 1995; Reed, 1995). Researchers working with the middle range theory may have selected empirical indicators for measurement of theoretical constructs, or they may have developed the middle range theory from descriptions and stories. Both of these examples support the theory's empirical adequacy. Empirical adequacy is an indication of the maturity of the theory.

The third criterion is that there are published examples of how the theory has been used in practice. This criterion offers evidence to support that the theory makes a difference in the lives of people. Published reports of the theory should demonstrate that use of the theory enhances well-being and quality of life. When the middle range theory is taken to practice there are expectations about emergent outcomes. These outcomes may be identified and tested by those conducting evaluation studies on theory-guided practice.

The fourth criterion is that there are published examples of research related to the theory. This criterion is a strong indicator of functional adequacy. The research findings can be examined for the level of support of the theory. In addition, middle range theories may generate hypotheses or research questions. Any refinements to the theory based on research findings should be examined; this indicates that the theory is open enough to change through the incorporation of further testing or development of ideas. In the process of evaluating this criterion, it is important to examine the evolution of the theory over time through inquiry and reflection.

The fifth criterion is that the theory has evolved through scholarly inquiry. Theories should evoke thinking, raise questions, invite dialogue, and urge us toward further exploration. This engaging quality of the theory is a hallmark of its potential for advancing the discipline. In order for the theory to grow, a community of scholars must engage with it in practice and research. Middle range theories build the discipline of nursing through expanding knowledge related to specific phenomena. The speculations offered by the theory push the boundaries of what is currently known and invite continuing systematic inquiry. In this way, the theory evolves and contributes to the development of nursing science and art.

## ■ APPLYING THE FRAMEWORK TO THE EVALUATION OF MIDDLE RANGE THEORIES

The evaluation of middle range theory involves preparation, judgment, and justification. In the preparation phase, those evaluating the theory should spend time understanding the theory as fully as possible through dwelling with it. Dwelling with it is investing time in reading and reflecting on the theory. The elements of the critical stance—empathy, curiosity, honesty, and responsibility, as articulated earlier in this chapter—are applied during preparation. It is important to gather a variety of sources on and about the theory, including primary sources written by the author of the theory, research reports, critiques, and practice papers. Reading the theory repeatedly to understand the ideas is the first step. In this process of beginning analysis, it is important to identify the central ideas and the structure of the theory. Middle range theories are developed from parent theories, empirical findings, or practice insights. Depth in understanding a theory may require going to the source documents that were critical to its development. Critical evaluation requires attending to questions and reactions to the theory that surface during the reading. It is important to record these questions and reactions. The next step in preparation is studying the practice and research reports related to the theory. Note how the theory was tested or extended through research. Examine how the theory has been applied in practice and any outcome studies that relate to the application of practice approaches or models based on the theory. Written critiques by others will provide another source of information. Because they may interfere with or unduly influence one's own evaluation, it is preferable to read those critiques or evaluations after one's own is completed.

The judgment phase is the heart of the evaluative process. In this phase, the evaluator reads and reflects on the criteria in the evaluative framework. The evaluator trusts himself or herself as the instrument of judgment, one who has seriously and rigorously engaged in studying the theory. The evaluator reflects on and refers to the notes and responses created during the analysis process. The criteria in the evaluative framework are a guide toward making decisions about the meaning, structure, practice, and research applications. The strengths and weaknesses of the theory should receive equal weight in the judgment phase. Both of these elements of the evaluation can contribute to the development of the theory. In the justification phase, the evaluator supports judgments with explicit reasons for the decisions and with examples that illustrate points. In this phase, the evaluator can refer to other written critiques that may support or refute judgments about the theory. The evaluation is written in a narration structured by the criteria in the framework. Each criterion is addressed through weaving judgments and support of those judgments. A balanced evaluation identifies both the strengths and limitations of the theory and suggests specific recommendations for clarification, extension, or revision.

The goal of this chapter was to explicate the purpose, structure, and process of evaluating middle range theories. Middle range theories are at the frontier of nursing science. The development of substantive knowledge through middle range theories promises movement toward disciplinary maturity. These theories will direct and spawn new inquiry and will stimulate the development of nursing practice approaches to enhance health and well-being. The evaluation of nursing theory is an essential activity within the scientific community. It leads to the advancement, refinement, and extension of substantive knowledge in the discipline. It is a critical skill of any scholar and is honed through practice and mentoring.

## ■ REFERENCES

Chinn, P. L., & Kramer, M. K. (2014). *Knowledge development in nursing: Theory and process* (9th ed.) St. Louis, MO: Elsevier-Mosby.

Fawcett, J. (2004). *Analysis and evaluation of contemporary nursing knowledge* (2nd ed.). Philadelphia, PA: F. A. Davis.

Fawcett, J., & DeSanto-Madeya, S. (2013). *Contemporary nursing knowledge: Analysis and evaluation of nursing models and theories* (3rd ed.). Philadelphia, PA: F. A. Davis.

Fitzpatrick, J. J., & Whall, A. L. (2004). *Conceptual models of nursing.* Stamford, CT: Appleton & Lange.

Ford-Gilboe, M., Campbell, J., & Berman, H. (1995). Stories and numbers: Coexistence without compromise. *Advances in Nursing Science, 18*, 14–26.

Kaplan, A. (1964). *The conduct of inquiry.* San Francisco, CA: Chandler.

Kerlinger, F. N. (1986). *Foundations of behavioral research* (3rd ed.). New York, NY: Holt, Rinehart & Winston.

Liehr, P., & Smith, M. J. (1999). Middle range theory: Spinning research and practice to create knowledge for the new millennium. *Advances in Nursing Science, 21*(4), 81–91.

Newman, M. A., Sime, A. M., & Corcoran-Perry, S. A. (1991). Focus of the discipline of nursing. *Advances in Nursing Science, 14*(1), 1–6.

Parse, R. R. (1987). *Nursing science: Major paradigms, theories, and critiques.* Philadelphia, PA: W. B. Saunders.

Paul, R. (1993). *Critical thinking: How to prepare students for a rapidly changing world.* Santa Rosa, CA: Foundation for Critical Thinking.

Reed, P. (1995). Treatise on nursing knowledge development for the 21st century: Beyond postmodernism. *Advances in Nursing Science, 17*, 70–84.

Rogers, M. E. (1970). *An introduction to the theoretical basis of nursing.* Philadelphia, PA: F. A. Davis.

Smith, M. C. (1994). Arriving at a philosophy of nursing: Discovering? constructing? evolving? In J. Kikuchi & H. Simmons (Eds.), *Developing a philosophy of nursing* (pp. 43–60). Thousand Oaks, CA: Sage.

Smith, M. C. (1998). Knowledge building for the health sciences in the twenty-first century. *Journal of Sport and Exercise Psychology, 20*, S128–S144.

Smith, M. J., & Liehr, P. (2013). *Middle range theory for nursing* (3rd ed.) New York, NY: Springer Publishing.

Stevens, B. (1998). *Nursing theory: Analysis, application, evaluation.* Boston, MA: Little, Brown.

# SECTION TWO

## Middle Range Theories Ready for Application

*Thirteen middle range theories are presented in this section. Each theory is organized by the topics of purpose of the theory and how it was developed, concepts of the theory, a model showing relationships among the concepts, and use of the theory in research and practice. Therefore, the organizational structure of each theory chapter provides consistent information relevant to developing a deepened understanding of the theory. We have found that a consistent organization structure provides a strong foundation for scholars wishing to compare, contrast, and understand the theories. The reader will notice connections between some of the middle range theories in the book. For instance, the theories of Self-Transcendence and Meaning share the same unitary–transformative paradigmatic perspective and they also share a common spirit of finding ways to move on in the midst of difficult circumstances. Several of the middle range theories in the book have cultural roots or links; these include Cultural Marginality, Transitions, and Self-Reliance. The theories of Unpleasant Symptoms and Symptom Management provide two approaches to the important topic of symptoms. Two theories on caring have been added; these are Self-Care of Chronic Illness and Bureaucratic Caring. Scholars wishing to choose a theory to guide research and practice will appreciate the organizational structure of the chapters, where one theory can be readily considered in relation to another. The middle range theories in this book are human constructions rooted in extant literature, personal knowing, and research/practice experience of the authors. The theories have been explicated through defined concepts, modeled to show logical relationships, and applied directly to practice and research.*

# CHAPTER 4

## Theories of Uncertainty in Illness

Margaret F. Clayton, Marleah Dean, and Merle Mishel

In this chapter, theories of uncertainty in illness are described. The original uncertainty in illness theory (UIT) was developed by Mishel to address uncertainty during the diagnostic and treatment phases of an illness or an illness with a determined downward trajectory (Mishel, 1988). Subsequently a reconceptualized uncertainty in illness theory (RUIT) was developed by Mishel to address the experience of living with continuous uncertainty in either a chronic illness requiring ongoing management or an illness with a possibility of recurrence (Mishel, 1990). Since development of the original theory, the concept of uncertainty has been used in many disciplines including nursing, medicine, and health communication with slightly differing definitions, extensions, and applications. Companion instruments to measure uncertainty in illness have been translated into many languages and used extensively (Mishel 1983a, 1997c).

The UIT proposes that uncertainty exists in illness situations, which are ambiguous, complex, and unpredictable. Uncertainty is defined as the inability to determine the meaning of illness-related events. It is a cognitive state created when the individual cannot adequately structure or categorize an illness event because of insufficient cues (Mishel, 1988). The theory explains how patients cognitively structure a schema for the subjective interpretation of uncertainty with treatments and outcomes. It is composed of three major themes: (a) antecedents of uncertainty, (b) appraisal of uncertainty, and (c) coping with uncertainty. Uncertainty and cognitive schema are the major concepts of the theory.

The RUIT retains the definition of uncertainty and major themes, as in the UIT, but adds the concepts of self-organization and probabilistic thinking. The RUIT addresses the process that occurs when a person lives with unremitting uncertainty found in chronic illness or in illness with a potential for recurrence. The desired outcome from the RUIT is a growth to a new value system, whereas the outcome of the UIT is a return to the previous level of adaptation or functioning (Mishel, 1990).

## ■ PURPOSE OF THE THEORIES AND HOW THEY WERE DEVELOPED

The purpose of each theory is to describe and explain uncertainty as a basis for practice and research. The UIT applies to the prediagnostic, diagnostic, and treatment phases of acute and chronic illnesses. The RUIT applies to enduring uncertainty in chronic illness or illness with the possibility of recurrence that requires self-management. The theories focus on the ill individual and on the family or parent of an ill individual. The use of theory within groups or communities is not consistent.

The finding that uncertainty was reported to be common among people experiencing illness or receiving medical treatment led to the creation of the UIT (Mishel, 1988). Although the concept was cited in the literature, there was no substantive exploration of how uncertainty developed and was resolved. It was a personal experience with Mishel's ill father that catalyzed the concept for her as she relays in earlier editions of this chapter and to me (Clayton). During my dissertation studies with Dr. Mishel as dissertation chair (Mishel & Clayton, 2003, 2008), Mishel's father was dying from colon cancer. His body was swollen and emaciated. He did not understand what was happening, so he focused on whatever he could control to provide some degree of predictability. The effort he spent on achieving understanding crystallized the significance of his uncertainty.

Developing the UIT included a synthesis of the research on uncertainty, cognitive processing, and managing threatening events. The UIT was revised from the original measurement model published in 1981, to the RUIT published in 1988. During Mishel's doctoral study, she focused on the development and testing of a measure of uncertainty. At that time she was influenced by the literature on stress and coping that discussed uncertainty as one type of stressful event (Lazarus, 1974) and by the work of Norton (1975), who identified eight dimensions of uncertainty. His work—along with that of Moos and Tsu (1977)—formed a framework leading to the development of the Mishel Uncertainty in Illness Scale (Mishel, 1997c).

Mishel's early ideas were further influenced by Bower (1978) and Shalit (1977), who described uncertainty as a complex cognitive stressor, and by Budner (1962), who described ambiguous, novel, or complex stimuli as sources of uncertainty. The ideas of these cognitive psychologists influenced Mishel's view of uncertainty as a cognitive state rather than as an emotional response. This distinction directed ongoing theory development. Uncertainty as a stressor or threat was based on the work of both Shalit (1977) and Lazarus (1974). The descriptions of coping as a primary appraisal of uncertainty and response to uncertainty as a secondary appraisal were adapted from the work of Lazarus (1974). The original 33-item Uncertainty in Illness Scale (Mishel, 1981) incorporated the work of these primary sources to conceptualize uncertainty in illness. Other population-specific forms have been developed, for example a 23-item version for community dwelling adults (Mishel, 1997c, 1997b), a 22-item version for cancer survivors (Mishel, 1997c), a 22-item version for children and adolescents (the USK, Uncertainty Scale for Kids; Stewart, Lynn, & Mishel, 2010), and a version for use with parents of hospitalized children (Mishel, 1983b). More recently, a 5-item short form for use with adults has been developed and validated (Hagen et al., 2015).

When the Uncertainty in Illness Scale was published, a body of findings on uncertainty quickly emerged in the nursing literature (Mishel, 1983a, 1984; Mishel & Braden, 1987, 1988; Mishel & Murdaugh, 1987; Mishel, Hostetter, King, & Graham, 1984). Research findings on uncertainty substantiated the antecedents of the theory. The stimuli frame variable, composed of familiarity of events and congruence of events, was formed from research on uncertainty in illness and research in cognitive psychology. Symptom pattern was developed from qualitative studies (Mishel & Murdaugh, 1987) describing the importance of consistency of symptoms to form a pattern. The antecedent of cognitive capacities was based on cognitive psychology (Mandler, 1979), and practice knowledge about instructing patients when cognitive processing abilities were compromised. The final antecedent of structure providers was developed from research on uncertainty in illness.

The appraisal section of the theory was developed using sources from the original 1981 model and based on clinical data and discussions with colleagues. Personality variables were thought to be important in the evaluation of uncertainty, and clinical data indicated that uncertainty could be a preferred state under specific circumstances. This led to inclusion of inference and illusion as two phases of appraisal (Mishel & Braden, 1987; Mishel & Murdaugh, 1987).

The RUIT was developed through discussion with colleagues, qualitative data from chronically ill individuals, and an awareness of the limitations of the UIT. The UIT was linear and explained uncertainty in the acute and treatment phases of illness, but did not address life changes over time expressed by persons with chronic illness. Qualitative interviews with chronically ill individuals revealed continuous uncertainty and a new view of life that incorporated uncertainty. From the perspective of Critical Social Theory (Allen, 1985), the patient's desire for certainty may reflect the goals of control and predictability that form the sociohistorical values of Western society (Mishel, 1990). Clinical data revealed that those who chose to incorporate uncertainty into their lives were living a value system on the edge of mainstream ideas. To explain the clinical data, a framework that conceptualized uncertainty as a preferred state was initiated using the process of theory derivation described by Walker and Avant (1989). Chaos was chosen as the parent theory to reconceptualize uncertainty. Chaos theory emphasizes disorder, instability, diversity, disequilibrium, and restructuring as the healthy variability of a system (Prigogine & Stengers, 1984). The reconceptualized theory included ideas of disorganization and reformulation of a new stability to explain how a person with enduring uncertainty emerges with a new view of life.

Drawing from chaos theory (Prigogine & Stengers, 1984), uncertainty is viewed as a force that spreads from illness to other areas of a person's life and competes with the person's previous mode of functioning. As uncertain areas of life increase, pattern disruption occurs, and uncertainty feeds back on itself and generates more uncertainty. When uncertainty persists, its intensity exceeds a person's level of tolerance. There is a sense of disorganization that promotes personal instability. With a high level of disorganization comes a loss of a sense of coherence (Antonovsky, 1987). A system in disorganization begins to reorganize at an imperceptible level that represents a gradual transition from a perspective of life oriented to predictability and control to a new view of life in which multiple contingencies are preferable.

## ■ CONCEPTS OF THE THEORIES

Uncertainty is the central theoretical concept, defined as the inability to determine the meaning of illness-related events inclusive of inability to assign definite value and/or to accurately predict outcomes (Mishel, 1988). Another concept central to the uncertainty theory is cognitive schema, which is defined as the person's subjective interpretation of illness-related events (see Figure 4.1). The UIT is organized around three major themes related to the concepts: (a) antecedents of uncertainty, (b) appraisal of uncertainty, and (c) coping with uncertainty.

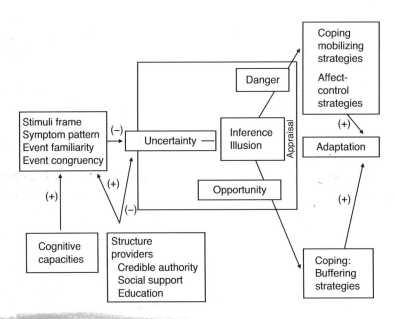

**FIGURE 4.1** Perceived uncertainty in illness.

*Source:* Reprinted with permission from Mishel, M. H. (1988). Uncertainty in illness. *The Journal of Nursing Scholarship, 20*(4), 225–232.

The ideas included in the antecedent theme of the theory include stimuli frame, cognitive capacity, and structure providers. Stimuli frame is defined as the form, composition, and structure of the stimuli that the person perceives. The stimuli frame has three components: symptom pattern, event familiarity, and event congruence. Symptom pattern refers to the degree to which symptoms are present with sufficient consistency to be perceived as having a pattern or configuration. Event familiarity is the degree to which the situation is habitual, repetitive, or contains recognized cues. Event congruence refers to the consistency between the expected and the experienced illness-related events. Cognitive capacity and structure providers influence the three components of the stimuli frame. Cognitive capacity is the information-processing ability of the individual.

Structure providers are the resources available to assist the person in the interpretation of the stimuli frame. Structure providers include education, social support, and credible authority.

The second major theme in the UIT is appraisal of uncertainty, which is defined as the process of placing a value on the uncertain event or situation. There are two components of appraisal: inference or illusion. Inference refers to the evaluation of uncertainty using related examples and is built on personality dispositions, general experience, knowledge, and contextual cues. Illusion refers to the construction of beliefs formed from uncertainty that have a positive outlook. The result of appraisal is the valuing of uncertainty as a danger or an opportunity.

The third theme in the UIT is coping with uncertainty and includes danger, opportunity, coping, and adaptation. Danger is the possibility of a harmful outcome. Opportunity is the possibility of a positive outcome. Coping with a danger appraisal is defined as activities directed toward reducing uncertainty and managing the emotion generated by a danger appraisal. Coping with an opportunity appraisal is defined as activities directed toward maintaining uncertainty. Adaptation is defined as biopsychosocial behavior occurring within the person's individually defined range of usual behavior.

The RUIT includes the antecedent theme in the UIT and adds the two concepts of self-organization and probabilistic thinking. Self-organization is the reformulation of a new sense of order, resulting from the integration of continuous uncertainty into one's self-structure in which uncertainty is accepted as the natural rhythm of life. Probabilistic thinking is a belief in a conditional world in which the expectation of certainty and predictability is abandoned. The RUIT proposes four factors that influence the formation of a new life perspective: prior life experience, physiological status, social resources, and healthcare providers. In the process of reorganization, the person reevaluates uncertainty by gradual approximations, from an aversive experience to one of opportunity. Thus, uncertainty becomes the foundation for a new sense of order and is accepted as the natural rhythm of life. There is an ability to focus on multiple alternatives, choices, and possibilities; reevaluate what is important in life; consider variation in personal investment; and appreciate the impermanence and fragility of life. The theory also identifies conditions under which the new ability is maintained or blocked.

The concepts of both theories tie clearly to nursing, and other healthcare-related disciplines by describing and explaining human responses to illness situations. Uncertainty crosses all phases of illness from prediagnosis symptomatology to diagnosis, treatment, treatment residuals, recovery, potential recurrence, and exacerbation. Thus, the theories are pertinent to the health experience for all age groups. Uncertainty is experienced by ill persons but also caregivers and parents of ill children. Moreover, the theories incorporate a consideration of the healthcare environment as a component of the stimuli frame and the broader support network. Nursing care is represented under the concept of structure providers. Because an important part of nursing involves explaining and providing information, it follows that nursing actions are interventions to help patients manage uncertainty. The outcomes of both theories are directly related to health. The health outcome is to regain personal control, as in adaptation (UIT) or consciousness expansion (RUIT).

## ■ RELATIONSHIPS AMONG THE CONCEPTS: THE MODELS

As seen in Figure 4.1, the UIT is displayed as a linear model with no feedback loops. According to this model, uncertainty is the result of antecedents. The major path to uncertainty is through the stimuli frame variables. Cognitive capacities influence stimuli frame variables. If the person has a compromised cognitive capacity due to fever, infection, pain, or mind-altering medication, the clarity and definition of the stimuli frame variables are likely to be reduced, resulting in uncertainty. In such a situation, it is assumed that stimuli frame variables are clear, patterned, and distinct, and only become less so because of limitations in cognitive capacity. However, when cognitive capacity is adequate, stimuli frame variables may still lack a symptom pattern or be unfamiliar and incongruent due to lack of information, complex information, information overload, or conflicting information. The structure provider variables then come into play to alter the stimuli frame variables by interpreting, providing meaning, and explaining. These actions serve to structure the stimuli frame, thereby reducing or preventing uncertainty. Structure providers may also directly impact uncertainty. The healthcare provider can offer explanations or use other approaches that directly reduce uncertainty. Similarly, uncertainty can be reduced by one's level of education and resultant knowledge. Social support networks also influence the stimuli frame by providing information from similar others, providing examples, and offering supportive information.

Uncertainty is viewed as a neutral state and is not associated with emotions until evaluated. During the evaluation of uncertainty, inference and illusion come into play. Inference and illusion are based on beliefs and personality dispositions that influence whether uncertainty is appraised as a danger or as an opportunity. Because uncertainty renders a situation amorphous and ill-defined, positively oriented illusions can be generated from uncertainty, leading to an appraisal of uncertainty as an opportunity. Uncertainty appraised as an opportunity implies a positive outcome, and buffering coping strategies are used to maintain it. In contrast, beliefs and personality dispositions can result in uncertainty appraised as danger. Uncertainty evaluated as danger implies harm. Problem-focused coping strategies are employed to reduce it. If problem-focused coping cannot be used, then emotional coping strategies are used to respond to the uncertainty. If the coping strategies are effective, adaptation occurs. Difficulty in adapting indicates inability to manipulate uncertainty in the desired direction.

In contrast to the more linear nature of the UIT, the RUIT (Figure 4.2) represents the process of moving from uncertainty appraised as danger to uncertainty appraised as an opportunity and resource for a new view of life. As noted earlier in this chapter, the reconceptualized theory builds on the original theory at the appraisal portion. The RUIT describes enduring uncertainty that is initially viewed as danger due to its invasion into broader areas of life resulting in instability. The jagged line within the arrow represents both the invasion of uncertainty and the growing instability. The patterned circular portion of the line represents the repatterning and reorganization resulting in a revised view of uncertainty. The bottom arrow indicates that this is a process that evolves over time.

## ■ USE OF THE UNCERTAINTY THEORIES

Beginning with the publication of the Uncertainty in Illness Scale (Mishel, 1981), there has been extensive research into uncertainty in both acute and chronic illnesses. The research on uncertainty includes studies in nursing and other disciplines. Several comprehensive reviews of research have

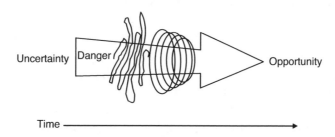

**FIGURE 4.2** Uncertainty in chronic illness.

*Source:* Reprinted with permission from Bailey, D. E., & Stewart, J. L. (2001). Mishel's theory of uncertainty in illness. In A. M. Mariner-Tomey & M. R. Alligood (Eds.), *Nursing theorists and their work* (5th ed., pp. 560–583). St. Louis, MO: Mosby.

summarized and critiqued the current state of the knowledge on uncertainty in illness (Bailey & Stewart, 2001; Barron, 2000; Dean & Street, 2015; Mast, 1995; McCormick, 2002; Mishel, 1997b, 1999; Neville, 2003; Shaha, Cox, Talman, & Kelly, 2008; Stewart & Mishel, 2000). Other authors have attempted to develop an expanded definition of uncertainty (Penrod, 2001) or have critiqued the current work based on a misunderstanding of the reconceptualized uncertainty theory (Parry, 2003).

Although some studies focus on components of the UIT or RUIT, more recent studies have used uncertainty as the conceptual framework for the study and directly tested major sections of the UIT, elaborated on the UIT, or elaborated on selected antecedents and outcomes adding richness to the theory (Clayton, Mishel, M. H., & Belyea 2006; Dimillo et al., 2013; Farren, 2010; Hebdon, Foli, & McComb, 2015; Jurgens, 2006; Kang, 2005, 2006, 2011; Kang, Daly, & Kim, 2004; Kim, Lee, & Lee, 2012; Lin, Yeh, & Mishel, 2010; McCormick, Naimark, & Tate, 2006; Sammarco, 2001; Sammarco & Konency, 2010; Santacroce, 2003; Stewart, Mishel, Lynn, & Terhorst, 2010; Wonghongkul, Dechaprom, Phumivichuvate, & Losawatkul, 2006). Mishel's Uncertainty in Illness Scale—Community Form has demonstrated validity and reliability for measuring uncertainty in men undergoing active surveillance for early-stage prostate cancer (Bailey et al., 2011) and ethnically diverse female breast cancer survivors (Hagen et al., 2015; Liao, Chen, Chen, & Chen, 2008; Sammarco & Konecny, 2010). The theory has also been used as the basis for revising the Parent's Perception of Uncertainty Scale (Santacroce, 2001). In a study by Kang et al. (2004), researchers operationalized and tested the antecedents of social support and education as structure providers along with the stimuli frame variable of symptom pattern on uncertainty in patients with atrial fibrillation. Symptom severity was the strongest predictor of uncertainty, whereas the structure provider variables of education and social support reduced uncertainty. An unusual grounded theory study explored children's perception of uncertainty during treatment for cancer, citing the uncertainty theory as the sensitizing theory (Stewart, 2003). A study in children and adolescents with cancer used the uncertainty theory to guide a conceptual model that served as the study framework; a strong relationship was found between children's uncertainty and psychological distress (Stewart, Mishel, Lynn, & Terhorst, 2010).

The uncertainty theory has grown through research studies in the areas of credible authority and social support as the theory has been used by investigators in nursing and health communication (Brashers et al., 2003; Brashers, Neidig, & Goldsmith, 2004; Clayton et al., 2006; Miller, 2014; Middleton, LaVoie, & Brown, 2012). For example, Brashers, a health communication scholar (colleague of Mishel and a member of Clayton's dissertation committee), expanded Mishel's work into the field of health communication, developing the Uncertainty Management Theory, which was heavily influenced by Mishel's theoretical conceptualization of uncertainty. This expanded uncertainty theory has been used in HIV populations, noting that management of uncertainty may preserve hope (Brashers et al., 2000). Brashers's work is important as it illustrates *how* theoretical development can bridge disciplines, in this case nursing and health communication, contributing to team and interdisciplinary science. Clayton's work in nursing science also addresses the role of structure providers evaluating the contribution of patient–provider communication (contribution of structure providers as a credible authority) as a way to influence the appraisal of uncertainty among breast cancer survivors (Clayton & Dudley, 2009; Clayton, Mishel, & Belyea, 2006). Many studies have focused on the antecedents of stimuli frame and structure providers. For instance, three aspects of illness have been found to cause uncertainty: (a) severity of illness, (b) erratic nature of symptoms, and (c) ambiguity of symptoms. Severity of illness and ambiguity of symptoms correspond to the stimuli frame component of symptom pattern, whereas the erratic nature of symptoms corresponds to the stimuli component of event congruence.

Studies that focus on severity of illness and uncertainty are classified as those that address the theoretical link between symptom pattern and uncertainty. Severity of illness refers to symptoms with such intensity that they do not clearly reflect a discernable, understandable pattern. Several studies have shown that severity of illness is a predictor of uncertainty, although the indicators of severity of illness have varied across studies (Mishel, 1997b). Among patients in the acute or treatment phase of illnesses such as cardiovascular disease (Christman et al., 1988), cancer (Galloway & Graydon, 1996; Hilton, 1994), fibromyalgia (Johnson, Zautra, & Davis, 2006), and severe pediatric illness and cancer (Tomlinson, Kirschbaum, Harbaugh, & Anderson, 1996; Santacroce, 2002), severity of illness was positively associated with uncertainty in patients and/or family members. Thus, according to the UIT, the nature of the severity presents difficulty delineating a symptom pattern about the extent of the disease, resulting in uncertainty.

## Stimuli Frame: Symptom Pattern

Studies that address the process of identifying symptoms of a disease or condition and reaching a diagnosis are classified as addressing symptom pattern. The process of receiving a diagnosis requires that a symptom pattern exists and can be labeled as an illness or a condition. In the UIT, absence of the symptom pattern is associated with uncertainty. Uncertainty levels have been reported to be highest in those without a diagnosis and undergoing diagnostic examinations (Hilton, 1993; Mishel, 1981). In studies where patients' symptoms are not clearly distinguishable from those of other comorbid conditions, or where symptoms of recurrence can be confused with signs of aging or other natural processes and not recognizable as signs of disease, such as in lupus, breast cancer, and cardiac disease, symptoms are associated with uncertainty (Hilton, 1988; Mishel & Murdaugh, 1987; Nelson, 1996; Winters, 1999). In a study of long-term breast cancer survivors, it was not the symptoms that elicited uncertainty but events that triggered thoughts of recurrence or the meaning of physical symptoms from long-term treatment side effects (Gil et al., 2004). High levels of symptoms such as pain are associated with uncertainty when one does not know how to manage the symptoms (Johnson et al., 2006). Additionally, fatigue, insomnia, and affect changes were associated with elevated cancer-related uncertainty among young breast cancer survivors (Hall, Mishel, & Germino, 2014). Researchers investigating Korean breast cancer survivors' uncertainty across the trajectory of their treatment found women undergoing treatment experienced higher levels of uncertainty than after treatment, and the majority of the symptoms women experienced during radiation and chemotherapy treatment were correlated with uncertainty (Kim, Lee, & Lee, 2012). Other research has focused on understanding the ambiguity of symptom experience associated with preterm labor (Weiss, Saks, & Harris, 2002). Even previous experience with preterm labor did not reduce the ambiguity associated with this condition.

The erratic nature of symptom onset and disease progression is a major antecedent of uncertainty in chronic illness (Mishel, 1999). Symptoms that occur unpredictably fit the description of the stimuli frame component of event incongruence because there is no congruity between the cue and the outcome. The timing and nature of symptom onset, duration, intensity, and location are unforeseeable, characterized by periods of stability, erratic flares of exacerbation, or unpredictable recurrence resulting in uncertainty (Brown & Powell-Cope, 1991; Mast, 1998; Mishel & Braden, 1988; Sexton, Calcasola, Bottomley, & Funk, 1999). For example, research has demonstrated the association between uncertainty and physical symptoms of breast cancer survivors, demonstrating that unpredictable physical symptoms that come and go, such as fatigue and arm problems, can create uncertainty about breast cancer recurrence (Clayton et al., 2006; Wonghongkul et al., 2006). Similarly, difficulty being aware of physical symptoms and determining their meaning in acute heart failure patients has also been found to be related to greater uncertainty (Jurgens, 2006). Among parents of ill children, unpredictable trajectories with few markers of illness are positively associated with uncertainty (Cohen, 1993b). Difficulty in determining cause of illness has been found to be associated with uncertainty (Cohen, 1993a; Sharkey, 1995; Turner, Tomlinson, & Harbaugh, 1990). Recent work on patients with endometriosis found that because no cure exists and treatment effectiveness varies, patients experience uncertainty surrounding the relationship of diagnosis to treatment outcomes (Lemaire, 2004). In young adults with asthma, uncertainty has been proposed to occur due to episode severity and/or frequency, which is not contingent upon the person's attempt to manage the illness (Mullins, Chaney, Balderson, & Hommel, 2000).

## Stimuli Frame: Event Familiarity

Studies that focus on the healthcare or home environment for treatment of illness fit under the stimuli frame component of event familiarity. Although fewer studies have addressed this component of stimuli frame, the studies that have been conducted support that unfamiliarity with healthcare environment, organization, and expectations is associated with uncertainty. Healthcare environments characterized by novelty and confusion where the rules and routines are unknown and equipment and treatments are unfamiliar are associated with uncertainty (Horner, 1997; Stewart & Mishel, 2000; Turner et al., 1990). A synthesis and critique of the healthcare environment and uncertainty theories, including UIT, across disciplines can be found in the work of Han, Klein, and Arora (2011).

## Structure Providers: Social Support

In the UIT, social support from friends, family, and those with similar experiences are proposed to reduce uncertainty directly and indirectly by influencing the stimuli frame. Those with similar experience have been found to influence the stimuli frame by providing information about illness-related events and symptom pattern (Van Riper & Selder, 1989; White & Frasure-Smith, 1995). There are a number of studies that support the role of social support in reducing uncertainty among parents of ill children, adult and adolescent patients, and their care providers (Bennett, 1993; Davis, 1990; Mishel & Braden, 1987; Neville, 1998; Tomlinson et al., 1996). For example, research with Taiwanese older cancer patients identified family members and healthcare providers as key sources of social support where family members such as spouses provided emotional support and healthcare providers offered information support (Lien, Lin, Kuo, & Chen, 2009).

However, when the illness is stigmatized, the questionable acceptance by others limits the use of social support to manage uncertainty (Brown & Powell-Cope, 1991; Weitz, 1989). Social interaction also may not always be supportive. Unsupportive interactions serve to heighten uncertainty (Wineman, 1990). The dual impact of social support has also been investigated in men with HIV/AIDS. Brashers et al. (2004) reported that other individuals help HIV patients manage uncertainty by providing instrumental support, facilitating skill development, giving acceptance or validation, allowing ventilation, and encouraging a perspective shift. They also report that there are problems associated with social support and uncertainty management including a lack of coordination in managing uncertainty, the addition of relational uncertainty, and the burden of caregiver uncertainty. Other investigators have found that family members experience high levels of uncertainty, which may impair their ability to provide support for the patient (Brown & Powell-Cope, 1991; Mishel & Murdaugh, 1987; Wineman, O'Brien, Nealon, & Kaskel, 1993). In a study of uncertainty in African American and White family members of men with localized prostate cancer, uncertainty was associated with family members feeling less positive about treatments and patient recovery, feeling more psychological distress, and engaging in less active problem solving (Germino et al., 1998).

These findings bring into question the ability of family members to be sup-portive of the patient when family members are trying to deal with their own uncertainties. Among younger breast cancer survivors, both social support and uncertainty together explained 27% of the variance in quality of life, with higher levels of social support functioning to reduce uncertainty (Sammarco, 2001). Current research supports the theoretical relationship between social support and uncertainty and provides information on factors that influence effective social support.

## Structure Providers: Credible Authority

Credible authority refers to healthcare providers who are seen as credible information givers by the patient or family member. As experts, healthcare providers have been proposed to reduce uncertainty by providing informa-tion and promoting confidence in their clinical judgment and performance. Trust and confidence in the healthcare provider's ability to make a diagnosis, to control the illness, and to provide adequate treatment has been reported to be related to less uncertainty across a variety of acute and chronic illnesses (Mishel & Braden, 1988; Santacroce, 2000). On the other hand, patients' lack of confidence in the provider's abilities increases uncertainty (Becker, Janson-Bjerklie, Benner, Slobin, & Ferdetich, 1993; Smeltzer, 1994). Uncertainty has also been found to increase when patients report that they are not receiving adequate information from healthcare providers (Galloway & Graydon, 1996; Hilton, 1988; Nyhlin, 1990; Small & Graydon, 1993; Weems & Patterson, 1989).

## Appraisal of Uncertainty

According to the UIT, appraisal of uncertainty involves personality disposi-tions, attitudes, and beliefs, which influence whether uncertainty is appraised as a danger or an opportunity. There is support for the impact of uncertainty on reducing personality dispositions such as optimism, sense of coherence, and level of resourcefulness (Christman, 1990; Hilton, 1989; Mishel et al., 1984). Certain dispositions such as generalized negative outcome expectan-cies interact with uncertainty to predict psychological distress (Mullins et al., 1995). However, selected cognitive and personality factors have been reported to mediate the relationship between uncertainty and danger or opportunity. Mediators that decrease the impact of uncertainty on danger and adjustment include higher enabling skill, self-efficacy, mastery, hope, challenge, and existen-tial well-being (Braden, Mishel, Longman, & Burns, 1998; Landis, 1996; Mishel, Padilla, Grant, & Sorenson, 1991; Mishel & Sorenson, 1991; Wonghongkul et al., 2006; Wonghongkul, Moore, Musil, Schneider, & Deimling, 2000). Some studies where appraisals were found to be positive are of populations that are a num-ber of years posttreatment. Others have reported that positive appraisals of uncertainty can be found along with negative appraisals, enabling both to exist simultaneously. This has been reported for patients awaiting coronary artery bypass surgery where uncertainty can be seen as a source for hope (McCormick et al., 2006). However, work by Kang (2006) with a sample of patients with atrial fibrillation reported that appraisal of uncertainty as an opportunity had a negative relationship with depression, and appraisal of uncertainty as a danger was positively associated with depression. As uncertainty increased, so did the danger appraisal, which was related to a decrease in mental health (Kang, 2005).

## Coping With Uncertainty

Numerous investigators who have studied the management of uncertainty have found that higher uncertainty is associated with danger and resultant emotion-focused coping strategies such as wishful thinking, avoidance, and fatalism (Christman, 1990; Hilton, 1989; Mishel & Sorenson, 1991; Mishel et al., 1991; Redeker, 1992; Webster & Christman, 1988). Severe symptoms such as high levels of pain in interaction with uncertainty have been reported to reduce one's ability to cope with symptoms (Johnson et al., 2006). Others report more varied coping strategies for managing uncertainty including cognitive strategies such as downward comparison, constructing a personal scenario for the illness, use of faith or religion, and identifying markers and triggers (Baier, 1995; Mishel & Murdaugh, 1987; Wiener & Dodd, 1993). Mishel (1993) offered a review of major uncertainty management methods; however, there is little evidence for the use of any of these coping strategies mediating the relationship between uncertainty and emotional distress (Mast, 1998; Mishel & Sorenson, 1991; Mishel et al., 1991). Although there has not been much study of the role of hopefulness in managing uncertainty, findings from a study of participation in a clinical drug trial revealed that uncertainty was related to a decrease in hope during time in the trial. Those with more uncertainty and less hopefulness reported more negative moods (Wineman, Schwetz, Zeller, & Cyphert, 2003). Research with Thai patients being treated for head and neck cancer used the UIT as a framework to study factors that contribute to quality of life as a way to address coping approaches for this population. Findings indicated that symptom experience had a positive impact on uncertainty and uncertainty had a negative impact on quality of life (Detprapon, Sirapo-ngam, Sitthimongkol, Mishel, & Vorapongsathorn, 2009), leading the authors to suggest that coping with symptoms and uncertainty is critical to optimizing quality of life. In the area of uncertainty in children, Stewart (2003) reported that children emphasized the routine and ordinariness of their lives despite their cancer diagnosis and treatment as a way of coping.

## Uncertainty and Adjustment

According to the UIT, adjustment refers to returning to the individual's level of pre-illness functioning. However, most of the research has interpreted this as emotional stability or quality of life. Few studies have tested the complete outcome portion of the theory, including uncertainty, appraisal, coping strategies, and adjustment. Most studies examine the relationship between uncertainty and an outcome and relate these findings to the theory. The findings from these studies have consistently shown positive relationships between uncertainty and negative emotional outcomes (Bennett, 1993; Mast, 1998; Mishel, 1984; Mullins et al., 2001; Sanders-Dewey, Mullins, & Chaney, 2001; Small & Graydon, 1993; Taylor-Piliae & Molassiotis, 2001; Wineman, Schwetz, Goodkin, & Rudick, 1996). Further evidence for the significant effect of uncertainty on depression was reported by Mullins et al. (2000) in young adults with asthma. The effect of uncertainty on depression was at its maximum under conditions of increased illness severity. Uncertainty has also been related to poorer psychosocial adjustment in the areas of less life satisfaction (Hilton, 1994), negative attitudes toward healthcare, family relationships, recreation and employment (Mishel et al., 1984; Mishel & Braden, 1987), less satisfaction with healthcare services (Green & Murton, 1996), poor decision making (Mishel, 1999; Politi & Street, 2011), and poorer quality of life (D. Carroll, Hamilton, & McGovern, 1999; Padilla, Mishel, & Grant, 1992). Santacroce (2003) identified the linkage between uncertainty and negative outcomes in her literature review on parental uncertainty and posttraumatic stress in serious childhood illness.

There has been extensive study of uncertainty in illness based on the UIT, and most of the research supports components of the theory. Overall, the UIT has been very useful in guiding research with a variety of clinical populations and caregivers.

## ■ RESEARCH USING THE RUIT

Less attention has been given to the study of the RUIT, possibly due to difficulty in studying a process that evolves over time. Support for the RUIT has been found in qualitative studies that favor a transition through uncertainty to a new orientation toward life with acceptance of uncertainty as a part of life (Mishel, 1999). The samples for these studies included long-term diabetic patients (Nyhlin, 1990), chronically ill men (Charmaz, 1994), HIV patients (Brashers et al., 2003; Katz, 1996), persons with schizophrenia (Baier, 1995), spouses of heart transplant patients (Mishel & Murdaugh, 1987), family caregivers of AIDS patients (Brown & Powell-Cope, 1991), breast cancer survivors (Mishel et al., 2005; Nelson, 1996; Pelusi, 1997), women who are genetically predisposed to hereditary breast and ovarian cancer but have not been diagnosed (DiMillo et al., 2013), adolescent survivors of childhood cancer (Parry, 2003), and women recovering from cardiac disease (Fleury, Kimbrell, & Kruszewski, 1995). For example, Bailey, Wallace, and Mishel (2007), using the RUIT as an organizing framework, interviewed men who were undergoing watchful waiting during their treatment for prostate cancer. Although the findings were not totally supportive of the RUIT, men did express that they had generated options, created opportunities for themselves, and remained hopeful of a positive outcome. Parry's (2003) study of childhood cancer survivors suggests that uncertainty can be a catalyst for growth, for a greater appreciation for life, and for greater awareness of life purpose. However, in another study of survivors of childhood cancer, findings showed that uncertainty mediated the relationship between posttraumatic stress disorder and health promotion behaviors, indicating that uncertainty exists over time and reduces health promotion activities (Santacroce & Lee, 2006).

Results supporting the RUIT seem to differ by subject population and methodology, where more qualitative studies—compared with quantitative studies—support the RUIT. The transition through uncertainty toward a new view of life was framed differently by each investigator and included themes such as a revised life perspective, new ways of being in the world, growth through uncertainty, new levels of self-organization, new goals for living, devaluating what is worthwhile, redefining what is normal, and building new dreams (Bailey & Stewart, 2001). All the investigators described the gradual acceptance of uncertainty and the restructuring of reality as major components of the process, both of which are consistent with the RUIT.

Recently, the RUIT scale has been adapted to examine uncertainty among breast cancer patients and survivors (Farren, 2010; Hagen et al., 2015; Hall et al., 2014) including Korean breast cancer survivors (Kim, Lee, & Lee, 2012), Taiwanese breast cancer patients (Liao et al., 2008), and Taiwanese parents of children with cancer (Lin et al., 2010). The scale addresses growth through uncertainty toward a new view of life and was developed to address the discrepancy noted earlier between qualitative and quantitative approaches to study the RUIT. Initial use of the scale was reported by Mast (1998). The Growth Through Uncertainty Scale (GTUS) has been used in a few clinical investigations. In an intervention study guided by the RUIT, baseline analysis of the data included use of the GTUS. The analysis was to identify variables that would predict either negative mood state or personal growth (GTUS) in older African American and White long-term breast cancer survivors. Of the variables found to be significant predictors, negative cognitive state, which included uncertainty, was a significant predictor of both outcomes. The overall findings were supportive of the RUIT because cognitive reappraisal, defined as the tendency to address concerns from a positive point of view, predicted 40% of the variance in personal growth (GTUS; Porter et al., 2006). Also, in findings from this intervention study, at 10 months and 20 months postintervention, older long-term African American breast cancer survivors in the treatment group maintained or increased scores on the GTUS over time, while scores for subjects in the control group declined over time (Gil, Mishel, Belyea, Germino, Porter, & Clayton, 2006; Mishel et al., 2005).

## ◼ INTERVENTIONS TO MANAGE UNCERTAINTY

An uncertainty management intervention has been developed and tested in four clinical trials for breast cancer patients and patients with localized or advanced prostate cancer (Braden et al., 1998; Mishel, 1997a; Mitchell, Courtney, & Coyer, 2003; Mishel et al., 2002). The intervention was structured to follow the UIT and was delivered by weekly phone calls to cancer patients. All studies included equal numbers of White and minority samples. The intervention was effective in teaching patients skills to manage uncertainty including improvements in problem solving, cognitive reframing, treatment-related side effects, and patient–provider communication. Improvement was also found in the ability to manage the uncertainty related to side effects from cancer treatment. Religious participation and education were found to be moderators of the treatment outcomes of cancer knowledge and patient–provider communication in the intervention trial for men with localized prostate cancer. Education was a covariate in the study of older women during treatment for breast cancer. Using the UIT and RUIT as frameworks for study of an intervention for older long-term African American and White breast cancer survivors, a self-delivered uncertainty management intervention with nurse assistance was tested and results indicated that the intervention at 10-month and 20-month follow-up produced significant differences in experimental and control groups in cognitive reframing, cancer knowledge, patient–provider communication, and a variety of coping skills. The most important results were the improvement in the treatment groups' pursuit of further information along with declines in uncertainty and stable effects in personal growth over time (Gil et al., 2006; Mishel et al., 2005).

Further intervention work based on the UIT and the RUIT has been expanded to prostate cancer. Bailey, Mishel, Belyea, Stewart, and Mohler (2004) tested an intervention for men selecting watchful waiting for prostate cancer, finding it assisted the men in cognitively reframing and thus effectively managing their uncertainty. Specifically, the results from this clinical trial showed that men in the intervention improved on the GTUS on the subscale of living life in a new light and believing that their future would be improved. In another study with the same population, a pilot study with nine participants (Kazer, Baily, Sanda, Colberg, & Kelly, 2011) supported use of an Internet intervention to improve quality of life while uncertainty remained consistent. Additionally, Mishel et al. (2009) developed and tested a decision-making uncertainty management intervention for recently diagnosed prostate cancer patients. They found the intervention improved patients' knowledge, communication skills, problem solving, and resource management. In similar work, Song and colleagues used the UIT to guide a study evaluating a decision aid designed to improve information giving and questions asking during prostate cancer treatment consultations (Song et al., 2016). Findings showed that enhanced communication with providers empowered men and their family members.

In a study of an intervention program that incorporated uncertainty reduction for women with recurrent breast cancer and their family members, factual information about cancer recurrence and treatments encouraged assertive approaches with healthcare providers; participants focused on learning to live with uncertainty in preference to negative certainty (Northouse et al., 2002). An intervention trial for newly diagnosed breast cancer patients in Taiwan used the UIT framework and provided information to questions raised by patients. This continual supportive care was given at four points during treatment. The findings indicated that support was increased and uncertainty was decreased 1 month after surgery and 4 months after diagnosis (Liu, Li, Tang, Huang, & Chiou, 2006). Other intervention studies included uncertainty as a variable but did not use either the UIT or RUIT as a framework for the study or intervention (Kreulen & Braden, 2004; McCain et al., 2003; Taylor-Piliae & Chair, 2002). The number of intervention studies using one of the uncertainty theories or including interventions to address uncertainty is continually increasing in the literature.

## ■ USE OF THE THEORIES IN NURSING PRACTICE

Nurses are included in the UIT as part of the antecedent variable of structure providers. The clinical literature supports delivery of information as the major method to help patients manage uncertainty. Nurses provide information that helps patients develop meaning from the illness experience by providing structure to the stimuli frame. When considering the RUIT, nurses help patients manage chronic uncertainty by assisting with patients' reappraisal of uncertainty from stressful to hopeful in addition to providing relevant information.

Understanding the sources of patient uncertainty can help nurses plan for effective information giving and may greatly assist nurses to help patients manage or reduce their uncertainty. In one of the few articles to address the environmental component of the stimuli frame, Sharkey (1995) discussed how family coping could be enhanced by home care nurses normalizing healthcare into the familiar routines of families caring for a terminally ill child at home. Among cardiac patients, White and Frasure-Smith (1995) suggested that nurses promote the use of patient-solicited social support to manage uncertainty in percutaneous transluminal coronary angioplasty (PTCA) patients. These researchers suggested that the benefit from the social support received by PTCA patients was due to direct requests tailored to specific needs versus unsolicited social support due to simply being ill. In addition, information from nurses about the potential long-term success of this procedure might help reduce the higher uncertainty found in PTCA patients 3 months after surgery. Among breast cancer survivors, Gil et al. (2004, 2005) suggested that nurses can help women identify their personal triggers of uncertainty about recurrence and then teach coping skills such as breathing relaxation, pleasant imagery, calming self-talk, and distraction to help survivors manage their uncertainty.

The RUIT has also been used to inform clinical practice and help nurses understand sources of patient uncertainty. An example of how mental health nurses can assist patients by understanding sources of uncertainty is found in research by Brashers et al. (2003) describing the medical, social, and personal forms of uncertainty for persons living with HIV/AIDS. Further, this research suggests nurses should be aware that subgroups of the population such as women, drug users, gay and lesbian persons, transgender persons, and parents can experience different sources of uncertainty based on social stigma, role and/or identity confusion, and lack of familiarity with the medical system. Other research using the RUIT indicates that childhood cancer survivors often have late emerging side effects that impact quality of life and the experience of uncertainty similar to other long-term cancer survivors (Lee, 2006; Santacroce & Lee, 2006). These studies suggest that childhood cancer survivors who lack effective coping and uncertainty management skills may be unable to reappraise uncertainty and are at risk for the development of posttraumatic stress symptoms (PTSS) as a way of avoiding uncertainty when life demands become excessive (Lee, 2006). Health professionals who are aware of the increased risk of PTSS created by an inability to reappraise uncertainty can offer developmentally appropriate information, thereby clarifying the ambiguity of future survivorship and helping childhood cancer survivors manage the continual uncertainty in their lives (Santacroce & Lee, 2006).

Recognizing uncertainty and then providing contextual cues to reduce ambiguity and increase understanding is one approach that nurses can use when communicating with patients to decrease uncertainty. Contextual cues provide explanations of what patients will see, hear, and feel during procedures and tests, as well as what signs and symptoms they will experience at various points in their illness trajectory. Providing information and explanations about treatments and medications has been proposed to be the most important and frequent approach to reducing patient uncertainty (Mishel et al., 2002; Wineman et al., 1996). Galloway and Graydon (1996), who based their findings on recently discharged colon cancer patients, noted that nurses could provide information to alleviate the uncertainty of being discharged to the home environment. Correspondingly, Mitchell, Courtney, and Coyer (2003) found that nurses provide beneficial contextual cues and information to both families and patients on transfer from the intensive care unit to a general hospital floor. Families of patients who received clear information were more able to make decisions for patients, reported less anxiety, and were better able to provide emotional and physical patient support. Other effective methods for reducing patient uncertainty can include encouraging communication with patients who have successfully managed their uncertainties. Weems and Patterson (1989) suggest sharing the uncertainties of waiting for a renal transplant with someone who has already received a transplant, or sharing uncertainties of how to live with chronic obstructive pulmonary disease with someone who is successfully managing this chronic disease (Small & Graydon, 1993). This type of communication provides information to patients for structuring the stimuli and also functions as a source of social support.

Offering comprehensive information allows the nurse to function as a credible authority, strengthening the stimuli frame by enhancing disease predictability and reducing symptom ambiguity. Righter (1995) used the UIT to describe the role of an enterostomal therapy (ET) nurse as a credible authority for the ostomy patient. She describes the ET nurse as providing structure and order to the experience of the new ostomy patient through clinical expertise and experience. The ET nurse reduces the ambiguity of the ostomy experience by providing information, counseling, and support. This facilitates ostomy patients' adaptation to their newly altered perception of themselves and helps them regain a sense of control and mastery by creating order and predictability. Other ideas on changing clinical practice to reduce patient uncertainty include educational interventions delivered in person, by telephone, or by individualized patient information packets delivered through the mail (Calvin & Lane, 1999; Mishel et al., 2002). Research by Bailey et al. (2004) found that nurses can clarify information about treatment options that create confusion for men who have selected watchful waiting as their treatment choice for prostate cancer. Nurses can answer patient questions about variations in prostate-specific antigen values, thus reducing uncertainty about both disease progression and future events. Understanding the meaning of laboratory values helped men sort out the confusion associated with mixed messages given to them by family who promoted aggressive treatment and urologists who promoted watchful waiting. Mishel et al. (2002) found that prostate cancer patients immediately postsurgery or during radiation therapy felt reassured when their questions were answered by a nurse, resulting in reduced anxiety and uncertainty. These men also expressed appreciation for the concern of a health professional and subsequently reported feeling less alone in their battle with cancer.

When considering the predictability of illness trajectories, Sexton et al. (1999) found that advanced practice nurses helped patients manage a diagnosis of asthma by implementing nursing actions that helped patients predict and manage their asthma attacks. Similarly, among breast cancer survivors, unpredictable physical symptoms such as fatigue and arm problems, which may come and go, can create uncertainty about cancer recurrence (Clayton et al., 2006; Wonghongkul et al., 2006). Thus, providers—including advanced practice nurses—should try to communicate in a manner that fully explains existing symptoms and their relationship or lack thereof to cancer recurrence (Clayton, Dudley, & Musters, 2008).

Clinical journals are increasingly identifying patient uncertainty as an important part of the illness experience and provide suggestions for nursing actions to reduce patient uncertainty or facilitate a new outlook by focusing on choices and alternatives. Suggestions for managing uncertainty in clinical practice include work by Crigger (1996), who suggests that nurses can help women adapt positively to multiple sclerosis by shifting the emphasis from the management of physical disability to the management of uncertainty, thereby helping women achieve mastery over their daily lives. Similarly, Calvin and Lane (1999) suggested incorporating preoperative psychoeducational interventions to reduce uncertainty as part of orthopedic preadmission visits. Other examples of using the UIT to develop and implement nursing interventions to reduce uncertainty and regain control in clinical settings are suggested by Allan (1990) for HIV-positive men; Sterken (1996) for fathers of pediatric cancer patients; Northouse, Mood, Templin, Mellon, and George (2000) for patients with colon cancer; and Sharkey (1995) for homebound pediatric oncology patients. Ritz et al. (2000) report another nursing intervention to manage uncertainty in clinical practice. These clinicians investigated the effect of follow-up nursing care by the advanced practice nurse after discharge of newly treated breast cancer patients. Six months after diagnosis, uncertainty was reduced and quality of life was improved. Despite this early work and subsequent recommendations, uncertainty is not regularly assessed during routine nursing practice (Shaha et al., 2008). On the basis of the antecedent variables of UIT, Northouse et al. (2000) suggested that health professionals keep in mind individual characteristics of patients, social environments, and methods of illness appraisal when caring for patients with colon cancer. They suggested that nurses provide patients with a framework of expectations about the physical and emotional illness trajectory associated with the first year of managing this diagnosis. Thus, use of the UIT can help nurses recognize groups of patients and/or caregivers that may be at risk for increased uncertainty. For example, Sterken (1996) found that younger fathers did not understand the information given to them about their child's treatment and disease patterns as well as older fathers, illustrating how cognitive capacity influences uncertainty. Santacroce (2002) found that African American parents of children newly diagnosed with cancer experienced greater uncertainty than White parents. She posits that past experiences with the healthcare system can impact parental uncertainty. These studies illustrate the difficulty as well as the potential benefit in using demographic characteristics to identify persons at risk for heightened uncertainty.

Other investigators have explained how the theory can be applied to understanding a clinical situation, clinical diagnosis, or clinical practice. For example, it is important to realize when increased uncertainty can place patients at risk for additional illnesses, such as recognizing that uncertainty is a major factor contributing to depression in patients with hepatitis C (Saunders & Cookman, 2005). Some clinical areas such as women's health and cardiovascular disease have been studied in depth. In the area of women's health, Sorenson (1990) discusses the concepts of symptom pattern, event familiarity and congruency, cognitive capacity, structure providers, and credible authority, using examples from normal pregnancy to help nurses relate the theory to women who are experiencing difficulty adapting to the uncertainties of pregnancy. For women experiencing high-risk pregnancy, they preferred the coping strategy of avoidance as a means for managing uncertainty and preserving their sense of well-being (Giurgescu, Penckofer, Maurer, & Bryant, 2006). Suggestions are made about how perinatal nurses can help women accept impending motherhood and utilize more effective coping mechanisms to reduce uncertainty and improve psychological well-being. Lemaire and Lenz (1995) applied the UIT to the condition of menopause. The stimuli frame for menopause was defined as the symptoms that indicate approaching menopause, including mood swings, hot flashes, dry skin, and memory changes. If women received factual information from a source deemed credible, such as nurses and healthcare providers, it was thought that familiarity with the event of menopause would be increased and uncertainty about this normal life event would be decreased. Consistent with predictions of UIT, uncertainty declined after receipt of understandable information delivered by a credible source, allowing women to construct meaning from the ambiguity and unpredictability of their symptoms surrounding the normal process of menopause. Similarly, Lemaire (2004) suggests that nurses who understand the uncertainty associated with the symptoms of endometriosis are better able to care for women experiencing this condition. Nursing actions such as providing informational material, offering referrals to support groups, and sharing electronic resources can help women better understand and manage the ambiguity and unpredictability of symptoms such as cramping, nonmenstrual pain, and fatigue. Other research has focused on understanding the ambiguity of symptoms associated with preterm labor (Weiss et al., 2002). Weiss et al. found that women lacked familiarity with the symptom pattern of preterm labor. They suggest that language used by women in describing preterm labor be incorporated into educational materials available to all pregnant women to help them recognize preterm labor as differentiated from term labor. They stress that every expectant woman needs education about the cues to use in recognizing preterm labor.

In patients diagnosed with atrial fibrillation, the UIT can help nurses identify patients at risk for increased uncertainty (Kang et al., 2004). Focusing on the antecedents of uncertainty, findings showed that patients with more severe symptoms and those with less education experienced greater uncertainty, helping nurses to be more aware of which patients may be at risk. Other research has found that those patients who receive an implantable cardioverter defibrillator experience great uncertainty, never knowing when their arrhythmias may recur and when the device may "fire" (Flemme et al., 2005). S. L. Carroll and Arthur (2010) studied uncertainty, optimism, and anxiety in patients receiving their first implantable defibrillator. Further, hospital nurses may have little time to prepare these patients for discharge as there is no need for further hospitalization postimplantation of the device. Therefore, out-patient clinic and office nurses can provide key information and support to these patients, recognizing that the high levels of uncertainty frequently experienced by these patients put them at risk for poorer quality of life. In another study Rydström

Dalheim-Englund, Segesten, and Rasmussen (2004) note the uncertainty that affects the whole family when a child has asthma, suggesting education for both parents and siblings about asthma as well as the impact of asthma on family dynamics. Further, these authors stress the importance of communicating to families that their nurse is approachable about both disease issues and family dynamics issues as part of holistic disease management. Similarly, for women diagnosed with fibromyalgia, a recent study using the UIT as a guiding framework suggested that the information provided by health professionals helps reduce patient anxiety and uncertainty (Trivino Martinez, Solano Ruiz, & Siles Gonzalez, 2016).

Another approach to improving patient care is recognizing the importance of professional education on uncertainty to effect change in clinical practice. Wunderlich, Perry, Lavin, and Katz (1999) suggested that critical care nurses would benefit from staff development sessions on how to address the uncertainty that patients experience during the process of weaning from mechanical ventilation. Dombeck (1996) commented that healthcare professionals need to increase their own tolerance for ambiguity and uncertainty to effectively listen to clients who are experiencing ambiguity and uncertainty. Similarly, Light (1979) noted that healthcare providers have been socialized to minimize uncertainty; this socialization may make it difficult to effectively address patient uncertainty until healthcare workers learn more about it (Baier, 1995). Recognizing the importance of integrating UIT into a management strategy for asthma patients, the American Nurses Credentialing Center's Commission on Accreditation offered three credit hours for successful completion of a continuing education unit (CEU) quiz following the published article (Sexton et al., 1999) about coping with uncertainty. Other CEU offerings incorporating uncertainty theory have been offered following a case study on spiritual disequilibrium (Dombeck, 1996) and an article on weaning a patient from mechanical ventilation (Wunderlich et al., 1999).

## ■ CONCLUSION

The Uncertainty in Illness theories have been used in multiple ways to inform clinician understanding of patients, families, and illness situations. Because uncertainty is an inherent aspect of illness-related experiences (Babrow & Kline, 2000), it is not surprising it has evolved and moved to other disciplines such as the fields of medicine and health communication. Yet with such adaption comes different conceptualizations of uncertainty. In this chapter, uncertainty has been defined as the inability to determine the meaning of an illness-related event (Mishel, 1988). In medicine, uncertainty is defined as an individual's subjective, perceived ignorance that encompasses sources, issues, and loci, which influence actions and produce psychological responses (Han, Klein, & Arora, 2011; Han, Klein, Lehman, et al., 2011). Furthermore, in the health communication literature, uncertainty is seen as feeling unsure about possible choices, decisions, and/or actions due to incomplete, inaccurate, or complex information (Dean, & Street, 2015; Shaha et al., 2008). While different, underlying each of these definitions is a lack of understanding of one's situation due to an illness event or complex health experience.

Clinical research guided by both the original UIT (1988) and the RUIT (1990) for those coping with both acute and chronic illnesses will continue to help identify appropriate nursing interventions for many types of illnesses and patients. Ultimately, the recognition of the importance of uncertainty can change clinical practice, allowing the development of nursing interventions that facilitate a positive patient adaptation to the illness experience.

# ■ REFERENCES

Allan, J. D. (1990). Focusing on living, not dying: A naturalistic study of self-care among seropositive gay men. *Holistic Nursing Practice*, 4(2), 56–63.

Allen, D. G. (1985). Nursing research and social control: Alternative models of science that emphasize understanding and emancipation. *Image: Journal of Nursing Scholarship*, 17, 58–64.

Antonovsky, A. (1987). *Unraveling the mystery of health: How people manage stress and stay well*. San Francisco, CA: Jossey-Bass.

Babrow, A. S., & Kline, K. N. (2000). From 'reducing' to 'coping with' uncertainty: Reconceptualizing the central challenge in breast self-exams. *Social Science & Medicine*, 51, 1805–1816.

Baier, M. (1995). Uncertainty of illness for persons with schizophrenia. *Issues in Mental Health Nursing*, 16, 201–212.

Bailey, D. E., Mishel, M. H., Belyea, M., Stewart, J. L., & Mohler, J. (2004). Uncertainty intervention for watchful waiting in prostate cancer. *Cancer Nursing*, 27(5), 339–346.

Bailey, D. E., & Stewart, J. L. (2001). Mishel's theory of uncertainty in illness. In A. M. Mariner-Tomey & M. R. Alligood (Eds.), *Nursing theorists and their work* (5th ed., pp. 560–583). St. Louis, MO: Mosby.

Bailey, D. E., Wallace, M., Latini, D. M., Hegarty, J., Carroll, P. R., Klein, E. A., & Albertsen, P. C. (2011). Measuring illness uncertainty in men undergoing active surveillance for prostate cancer. *Applied Nursing Research*, 24, 193–199.

Bailey, D. E., Wallace, M., & Mishel, M. H. (2007). Watching, waiting and uncertainty in prostate cancer. *Journal of Clinical Nursing*, 16(4), 734–741.

Barron, C. R. (2000). Stress, uncertainty, and health. In V. H. Rice (Ed.), *Handbook of stress, coping and health: Implications for nursing research, theory, and practice* (pp. 517–539). Thousand Oaks, CA: Sage.

Becker, G., Janson-Bjerklie, S., Benner, P., Slobin, K., & Ferdetich, S. (1993). The dilemma of seeking urgent care: Asthma episodes and emergency service use. *Social Science & Medicine*, 37, 305–313.

Bennett, S. J. (1993). Relationships among selected antecedent variables and coping effectiveness in postmyocardial infarction patients. *Research in Nursing and Health, 16*, 131–139.

Bower, G. H. (1978). *The psychology of learning and motivation: Advances in research and theory.* New York, NY: Academic Press.

Braden, C. J., Mishel, M. H., Longman, A. J., & Burns, L. (1998). Self-help intervention project: Women receiving breast cancer treatment. *Cancer Practice, 6*(2), 87–98.

Brashers, D. E., Neidig, J. L., & Goldsmith, D. J. (2004). Social support and the management of uncertainty for people living with HIV. *Health Communication, 16*, 305–331.

Brashers, D. E., Neidig, J. L., Haas, S. M., Dobbs, L. K., Cardillo, L., & Russell, J. A. (2000). Communication in the management of uncertainty: The case of persons living with HIV or AIDS. *Communication Monographs, 67*(1), 63–84.

Brashers, D. E., Neidig, J. L., Russell, J. A., Cardillo, L. W., Haas, S. M., Dobbs, L. K., . . . Nemeth, S. (2003). The medical, personal, and social causes of uncertainty in HIV illness. *Issues in Mental Health Nursing, 24*(5), 497–522.

Brown, M. A., & Powell-Cope, G. M. (1991). AIDS family caregiving: Transitions through uncertainty. *Nursing Research, 40*, 337–345.

Budner, S. (1962). Intolerance of ambiguity as a personality variable. *Journal of Personality, 30*, 29–50.

Calvin, R., & Lane, P. (1999). Perioperative uncertainty and state anxiety of orthopaedic surgical patients. *Orthopedic Nursing, 18*(6), 61–66.

Carroll, D., Hamilton, G., & McGovern, B. (1999). Changes in health status and quality of life and the impact of uncertainty in patients who survive life-threatening arrhythmias. *Heart and Lung, 28*(4), 251–260.

Carroll, S. L., & Arthur, H. M. (2010). A comparative study of uncertainty, optimism and anxiety in patients receiving their first implantable defibrillator for primary and secondary prevention of sudden cardiac death. *International Journal of Nursing Studies, 47*, 836–845.

Charmaz, K. (1994). Identity dilemmas of chronically ill men. *The Sociological Quarterly, 35*(2), 269–288.

Christman, N. J. (1990). Uncertainty and adjustment during radiotherapy. *Nursing Research, 39*(1), 17–20.

Christman, N. J., McConnell, E. A., Pfeiffer, C., Webster, K. K., Schmitt, M., & Ries, J. (1988). Uncertainty, coping, and distress following myocardial infarction: Transition from home to hospital. *Research in Nursing and Health, 11*, 71–82.

Clayton, M. F., & Dudley, W. (2009). Patient-centered communication during oncology follow-up visits for breast cancer survivors: content and temporal structure. *Oncology Nursing Forum, 36*(2), E68–E79.

Clayton, M. F., Dudley, W. N., & Musters, A. (2008). Communication with breast cancer survivors. *Health Communication, 39*, 175.

Clayton, M. F., Mishel, M. H., & Belyea, M. (2006). Testing a model of symptoms, communication, uncertainty, and well-being, in older breast cancer survivors. *Research in Nursing and Health, 29*(1), 18–39.

Cohen, M. H. (1993a). Diagnostic closure and the spread of uncertainty. *Issues in Comprehensive Pediatric Nursing, 16*, 135–146.

Cohen, M. H. (1993b). The unknown and the unknowable: Managing sustained uncertainty. *Western Journal of Nursing Research, 15*(1), 77–96.

Crigger, N. J. (1996). Testing an uncertainty model for women with multiple sclerosis. *Advances in Nursing Science, 18*(3), 37–47.

Davis, L. L. (1990). Illness uncertainty, social support, and stress in recovering individuals and family caregivers. *Applied Nursing Research, 3*(2), 69–71.

Dean, M., & Street, R. L., Jr. (2015). Managing uncertainty in clinical encounters. In A. Hannawa & B. Spitzberg (Eds.), *Communication Competence* (pp. 477–501). Berlin, Germany: de Gruyter Mouton.

Detprapon, M., Sirapo-ngam, Y., Mishel, M. H., Sitthimongkol, Y., & Vorapongsathorn, T. (2009). Testing uncertainty in illness theory to predict quality of life among Thais with head and neck cancer. *Thai Journal of Nursing Research, 13*(1), 1–15. Retrieved from https://www.tci-thaijo.org/index.php/PRIJNR/article/view/6366

Dimillo, J., Samson, A., Thériault, A., Lowry, S., Corsini, L., Verma, S., & Tomiak, E. (2013). Living with the BRCA genetic mutation: An uncertain conclusion to an unending process. *Psychology, Health & Medicine, 18*(2), 125–134.

Dombeck, M. (1996). Chaos and self-organization as a consequence of spiritual disequilibrium. *Clinical Nurse Specialist, 10*(2), 69–73; quiz 74–75.

Farren, A. T. (2010). Power, uncertainty, self-transcendence, and quality of life in breast cancer survivors. *Nursing Science Quarterly, 23*(1), 63–71.

Flemme, I., Edvardsson, N., Hinic, H., Jinhage, B. M., Dalman, M., & Fridlund, B. (2005). Long-term quality of life and uncertainty in patients living with an implantable cardioverter defibrillator. *Heart & Lung, 34*(6), 386–392.

Fleury, J., Kimbrell, L. C., & Kruszewski, M. A. (1995). Life after a cardiac event: Women's experience in healing. *Heart & Lung, 24*, 474–482.

Galloway, S., & Graydon, J. (1996). Uncertainty, symptom distress, and information needs after surgery for cancer of the colon. *Cancer Nursing, 19*(2), 112–117.

Germino, B. B., Mishel, M. H., Belyea, M., Harris, L., Ware, A., & Mohler, J. (1998). Uncertainty in prostate cancer, ethnic and family patterns. *Cancer Practice, 6*(2), 102–113.

Gil, K. M., Mishel, M. H., Belyea, M., Germino, B., Porter, L., & Clayton, M. (2006). Benefits of the uncertainty management intervention for African American and White older breast cancer survivors: 20-month outcomes. *International Journal of Behavioral Medicine, 13*(4), 285–294.

Gil, K. M., Mishel, M. H., Belyea, M., Germino, B., Porter, L. S., LeNey, I. C., . . . Stewart, J. (2004). Triggers of uncertainty about recurrence and treatment side effects in long-term older breast African American and Caucasian cancer survivors. *Oncology Nursing Forum, 31*(3), 633–639.

Gil, K. M., Mishel, M. H., Germino, B., Porter, L. S., Carlton-LaNey, I., & Belyea, M. (2005). Uncertainty management intervention for older African American and Caucasian long-term breast cancer survivors. *Journal of Psychosocial Oncology, 23*(2–3), 3–21.

Giurgescu, C., Penckofer, S., Maurer, M. C., & Bryant, F. B. (2006). Impact of uncertainty, social support, and prenatal coping on the psychological well-being of high-risk pregnant women. *Nursing Research, 55*(5), 356–365.

Green, J., & Murton, F. (1996). Diagnosis of Duchenne muscular dystrophy: Parents' experiences and satisfaction. *Child: Care, Health & Development, 22*, 113–128.

Hagen, K. B., Aas, T., Lode, K., Gjerde, J., Lien, E., Kvaløy, J. T., . . . Lind, R. (2015). Illness uncertainty in breast cancer patients: Validation of the 5-item short form of the Mishel Uncertainty in Illness Scale. *European Journal of Oncology Nursing, 19*(2), 113–119.

Han, P. K. J., Klein, W. M. P., & Arora, N. K. (2011). Varieties of uncertainty in health care: A conceptual taxonomy. *Medical Decision Making, 31*(6), 828–838.

Han, P. K. J., Klein, W. M. P., Lehman, T., Killam, B., Massett, H., & Freedman, A. N. (2011). Communication of uncertainty regarding individualized cancer risk estimates: Effects and influential factors. *Medical Decision Making, 31*(6), 354–366.

Hall, D. L., Mishel, M. H., & Germino, B. B. (2014). Living with cancer-related uncertainty: Associations with fatigue, insomnia, and affect in younger breast cancer survivors. *Support Care Cancer Supportive Care in Cancer, 22*(9), 2489–2495.

Hebdon, M., Foli, K., & Mccomb, S. (2015). Survivor in the cancer context: A concept analysis. *Journal of Advanced Nursing, 71*(8), 1774–1786.

Hilton, B. A. (1988). The phenomenon of uncertainty in women with breast cancer. *Issues in Mental Health Nursing, 9*, 217–238.

Hilton, B. A. (1989). The relationship of uncertainty, control, commitment, and threat of recurrence to coping strategies used by women diagnosed with breast cancer. *Journal of Behavioral Medicine, 12*(1), 39–54.

Hilton, B. A. (1993). Issues, problems, and challenges for families coping with breast cancer. *Seminars in Oncology Nursing, 9*(2), 88–100.

Hilton, B. A. (1994). The uncertainty stress scale: Its development and psychometric properties. *Canadian Journal of Nursing Research, 26*(3), 15–30.

Horner, S. (1997). Uncertainty in mothers' care for their ill children. *Journal of Advanced Nursing, 26*, 658–663.

Johnson, L. M., Zautra, A. J., & Davis, M. C. (2006). The role of illness uncertainty on coping with fibromyalgia symptoms. *Health Psychology, 25*(6), 696–703.

Jurgens, C. Y. (2006). Somatic awareness, uncertainty, and delay in care-seeking in acute heart failure. *Research in Nursing and Health, 29*(2), 74–86.

Kang, Y. (2005). Effects of uncertainty on perceived health status in patients with atrial fibrillation. *British Association of Critical Care Nurses, Nursing in Critical Care, 10*(4), 184–191.

Kang, Y. (2006). Effect of uncertainty on depression in patients with newly diagnosed atrial fibrillation. *Progress in Cardiology Nursing, 21*(2), 83–88.

Kang, Y. (2011). The relationships between uncertainty and its antecedents in Korean patients with atrial fibrillation. *Journal of Clinical Nursing, 20*, 1880–1886.

Kang, Y., Daly, B. J., & Kim, J. S. (2004). Uncertainty and its antecedents in patients with atrial fibrillation. *Western Journal of Nursing Research, 26*(7), 770–783.

Katz, A. (1996). Gaining a new perspective on life as a consequence of uncertainty in HIV infection. *Journal of the Association of Nurses in AIDS Care, 7*(11), 51–60.

Kazer, M. W., Bailey, D. E., Sanda, M., Colberg, J., & Kelly, K. (2011). An internet intervention for management of uncertainty during active surveillance for prostate cancer. *Oncology Nursing Forum, 38*(5), 561–568.

Kim, S. H., Lee, R., & Lee, K. S. (2012). Symptoms and uncertainty in breast cancer survivors in Korea: Differences by treatment trajectory. *Journal of Clinical Nursing, 21*(7–8), 1014.

Kreulen, G. L., & Braden, C. J. (2004). Model test of the relationship between self-help promoting nursing interventions and self-care and health status outcomes. *Research in Nursing & Health, 27*, 97–101.

Landis, B. J. (1996). Uncertainty, spirituality, well-being, and psychosocial adjustment to chronic illness. *Issues in Mental Health Nursing, 17*, 217–231.

Lazarus, R. S. (1974). Psychological stress and coping in adaptation and illness. *International Journal of Psychiatry in Medicine, 5*, 321–333.

Lee, Y. L. (2006). The relationships between uncertainty and posttraumatic stress in survivors of childhood cancer. *Journal of Nursing Research, 14*(2), 133–142.

Lemaire, G. S. (2004). More than just menstrual cramps: Symptoms and uncertainty among women with endometriosis. *Journal of Obstetric, Gynecologic, and Neonatal Nursing, 33*(1), 71–79.

Lemaire, G. S., & Lenz, E. R. (1995). Perceived uncertainty about menopause in women attending an educational program. *International Journal of Nursing Studies, 32*(1), 39–48.

Liao, M., Chen, M., Chen, S., & Chen, P. (2008). Uncertainty and anxiety during the diagnostic period for women with suspected breast cancer. *Cancer Nursing, 31*(4), 274–283.

Lien, C., Lin, H., Kuo, I., & Chen, M. (2009). Perceived uncertainty, social support and psychological adjustment in older patients with cancer being treated with surgery. *Journal of Clinical Nursing, 18*(16), 2311–2319.

Light, D. (1979). Uncertainty and control in professional training. *Journal of Health and Social Behavior, 20*, 310–322.

Lin, L., Yeh, C., & Mishel, M. H. (2010). Evaluation of a conceptual model based on Mishel's theories of uncertainty in illness in a sample of Taiwanese parents of children with cancer: A cross-sectional questionnaire survey. *International Journal of Nursing Studies, 47*(12), 1510–1524.

Liu, L., Li, C. Y., Tang, S., Huang, C., & Chiou, A. (2006). Role of continuing supportive cares in increasing social support and reducing perceived uncertainty among women with newly diagnosed breast cancer in Taiwan. *Cancer Nursing, 29*(4), 273–282.

Mandler, G. (1979). Thought processes, consciousness and stress. In V. Hamilton & D. M. Warburton (Eds.), *Human stress and cognition: An information processing approach* (pp. 179–201). New York, NY: Wiley.

Mast, M. E. (1995). Adult uncertainty in illness: A critical review of research. *Scholarly Inquiry for Nursing Practice, 9*(1), 3–24.

Mast, M. E. (1998). Survivors of breast cancer: Illness uncertainty, positive reappraisal, and emotional distress. *Oncology Nursing Forum, 25*(3), 555–562.

McCain, N. L., Munjas, B. A., Munro, C. L., Elswick, R. K., Jr., Robins, J. L., Ferreira-Gonzalez, A., . . . Cochran, K. L. (2003). Effects of stress management on PNI-based outcomes in persons with HIV disease. *Research in Nursing & Health, 26*, 102–117.

McCormick, K. M. (2002). A concept analysis of uncertainty in illness. *Journal of Nursing Scholarship, 34*(2), 127–131.

McCormick, K. M., Naimark, B. J., & Tate, R. B. (2006). Uncertainty, symptom distress, anxiety, and functional status in patients awaiting coronary artery bypass surgery. *Heart & Lung, 35*(1), 34–44.

Middleton, A. V., LaVoie, N. R., & Brown, L. E. (2012). Sources of uncertainty in type 2 diabetes: Explication and implications for health communication theory and clinical practice. *Health Communication, 27*, 591–601.

Miller, L. E. (2014). Uncertainty management and information seeking in cancer survivorship. *Health Communication, 29*(3), 233–243.

Mishel, M. H. (1981). The measurement of uncertainty in illness. *Nursing Research, 30*, 258–263.

Mishel, M. H. (1983a). Adjusting the fit: Development of uncertainty scales for specific clinical populations. *Western Journal of Nursing Research, 5*(4), 355–370.

Mishel, M. H. (1983b). Parents' perception of uncertainty concerning their hospitalized child. *Nursing Research, 32*, 324–330.

Mishel, M. H. (1984). Perceived uncertainty and stress in illness. *Research in Nursing and Health, 7*, 163–171.

Mishel, M. H. (1988). Uncertainty in illness. *Journal of Nursing Scholarship, 20*, 225–231.

Mishel, M. H. (1990). Reconceptualization of the uncertainty in illness theory. *Image: Journal of Nursing Scholarship, 22*, 256–262.

Mishel, M. H. (1993). Living with chronic illness: Living with uncertainty. In S. G. Funk, E. M. Tornquist, M. T. Champagne, & R. A. Wiese (Eds.), *Key aspects of caring for the chronically ill: Hospital and home* (pp. 46–58). New York, NY: Springer Publishing.

Mishel, M. H. (1997a). *The efficacy of the uncertainty management intervention for older White and African American women with breast cancer.* Paper presented at the 11th Annual Conference of the Southern Nursing Research Society, Norfolk, VA.

Mishel, M. H. (1997b). Uncertainty in acute illness. *Annual Review of Nursing Research, 15*, 57–80.

Mishel, M. H. (1997c). *Uncertainty in illness scales manual.* Chapel Hill: School of Nursing, University of North Carolina. Retrieved from https://nursing.unc.edu/files/2012/12/mishel_uncertainty_scales.pdf

Mishel, M. H. (1999). Uncertainty in chronic illness. *Annual Review of Nursing Research, 17*, 269–294.

Mishel, M. H., Belyea, M., Germino, B. B., Stewart, J. L., Bailey, D. E., Robertson, C., & Mohler, J. (2002). Helping patients with localized prostate carcinoma manage uncertainty and treatment side effects: Nurse-delivered psychoeducational intervention over the telephone. *Cancer, 94*(6), 1854–1866.

Mishel, M. H., & Braden, C. J. (1987). Uncertainty: A mediator between support and adjustment. *Western Journal of Nursing Research, 9*, 43–57.

Mishel, M. H., & Braden, C. J. (1988). Finding meaning: Antecedents of uncertainty in illness. *Nursing Research, 37*, 98–127.

Mishel, M. H., & Clayton, M. F. (2003). Uncertainty in illness theories. In M. J. Smith & P. Liehr (Eds.), *Middle range theory in advanced practice nursing* (pp. 25–48). New York, NY: Springer Publishing.

Mishel, M. H., & Clayton, M. F. (2008). Theories of uncertainty in illness. In M. J. Smith & P. Liehr (Eds.), *Middle range theory for nursing* (2nd ed., pp. 55–84). New York, NY: Springer Publishing.

Mishel, M. H., Germino, B. B., Belyea, M., Stewart, J. L., Bailey, D. E., Mohler, J., & Robertson, C. (2003). Moderators of an uncertainty management intervention, for men with localized prostate cancer. *Nursing Research, 52*(2), 89–97.

Mishel, M. H., Germino, B. B., Gill, K. M., Belyea, M., Laney, I. C., Stewart, J., . . . Clayton, M. (2005). Benefits from an uncertainty management intervention for African-American and Caucasian older long-term breast cancer survivors. *Psycho-Oncology, 14*, 962–978.

Mishel, M. H., Germino, B. B., Lin, L., Pruthi, R. S., Wallen, E. M., Crandell, J., & Blyler, D. (2009). Managing uncertainty about treatment decision making in early stage prostate cancer: A randomized clinical trial. *Patient Education and Counseling, 77*(3), 349–359.

Mishel, M. H., Hostetter, T., King, B., & Graham, V. (1984). Predictors of psychosocial adjustment in patients newly diagnosed with gynecological cancer. *Cancer Nursing, 7*, 291–299.

Mishel, M. H., & Murdaugh, C. L. (1987). Family adjustment to heart transplantation: Redesigning the dream. *Nursing Research, 36*, 332–336.

Mishel, M. H., Padilla, G., Grant, M., & Sorenson, D. S. (1991). Uncertainty in illness theory: A replication of the mediating effects of mastery and coping. *Nursing Research, 40*, 236–240.

Mishel, M. H., & Sorenson, D. S. (1991). Uncertainty in gynecological cancer: A test of the mediating functions of mastery and coping. *Nursing Research, 40*, 167–171.

Mitchell, M. L., Courtney, M., & Coyer, F. (2003). Understanding uncertainty and minimizing families' anxiety at the time of transfer from intensive care. *Nursing & Health Sciences, 5*(3), 207–217.

Moos, R., & Tsu, V. (1977). The crisis of physical illness: An overview. In R. Moos (Ed.), *Coping with physical illness* (pp. 3–25). New York, NY: Plenum.

Mullins, L. L., Cheney, J. M., Balderson, B., & Hommel, K. A. (2000). The relationship of illness uncertainty, illness intrusiveness, and asthma severity to depression in young adults with long-standing asthma. *International Journal of Rehabilitation and Health, 5*(3), 177–185.

Mullins, L. L., Cheney, J. M., Hartman, V. L., Albin, K., Miles, B., & Roberson, S. (1995). Cognitive and affective features of postpolio syndrome: Illness uncertainty, attributional style, and adaptation. *International Journal of Rehabilitation and Health, 1*, 211–222.

Mullins, L. L., Cote, M. P., Fuemmeler, B. F., Jean, V. M., Beatty, W. W., & Paul, R. H. (2001). Illness intrusiveness, uncertainty, and distress in individuals with multiple sclerosis. *Rehabilitation Psychology, 46*(2), 139–153.

Nelson, J. P. (1996). Struggling to gain meaning: Living with the uncertainty of breast cancer. *Advances in Nursing Science, 18*(3), 59–76.

Neville, K. L. (1998). The relationships among uncertainty, social support, and psychological distress in adolescents recently diagnosed with cancer. *Journal of Pediatric Oncology Nursing, 15*(1), 37–46.

Neville, K. L. (2003). Uncertainty in illness: An integrative review. *Orthopaedic Nursing, 22*(3), 206–214.

Northouse, L., Mood, D., Templin, T., Mellon, S., & George, T. (2000). Couples' patterns of adjustment to colon cancer. *Social Science and Medicine, 50*(2), 271–284.

Northouse, L., Walker, J., Schafenacker, A., Mood, D., Mellon, S., Galvin, E., . . . Freeman-Gibb, L. (2002). A family-based program of care for women with recurrent breast cancer and their family members. *Oncology Nursing Forum, 29*(10), 1411–1419.

Norton, R. (1975). Measurement of ambiguity tolerance. *Journal of Personal Assessment, 39*, 607–619.

Nyhlin, K. T. (1990). Diabetic patients facing long-term complications: Coping with uncertainty. *Journal of Advanced Nursing, 15*, 1021–1029.

Padilla, G., Mishel, M., & Grant, M. (1992). Uncertainty, appraisal and quality of life. *Quality of Life Research, 1*, 155–165.

Parry, C. (2003). Embracing uncertainty: An exploration of the experiences of childhood cancer survivors. *Qualitative Health Research, 13*(2), 227–246.

Pelusi, J. (1997). The lived experience of surviving breast cancer. *Oncology Nursing Forum, 24*(8), 1343–1353.

Penrod, J. (2001). Refinement of the concept of uncertainty. *Journal of Advanced Nursing, 34*(2), 238–245.

Politi, M., & Street Jr., R. L. (2011). Patient-centered communication during collaborative decision-making. In T. L. Thompson, R. Parrott & J. F. Nussbaum (Eds.), *The Routledge handbook of health communication* (2nd ed., pp. 399–413). New York, NY: Routledge.

Porter, L. S., Clayton, M. F., Belyea, J., Mishel, M., Gil, K. M., & Germino, B. B. (2006). Predicting negative mood state and personal growth in African American and White long-term breast cancer survivors. *Annals of Behavioral Medicine, 31*(3), 195–204.

Prigogine, I., & Stengers, I. (1984). *Order out of chaos: Man's new dialogue with nature*. New York, NY: Bantam Books.

Redeker, N. S. (1992). The relationship between uncertainty and coping after coronary bypass surgery. *Western Journal of Nursing Research, 14*, 48–68.

Righter, B. (1995). Ostomy care. Uncertainty and the role of the credible authority during an ostomy experience. *Journal of Wound and Ostomy Care Nursing, 22*(2), 100–104.

Ritz, L., Nissen, M., Swenson, K., Farrell, J., Sperduto, P., Sladek, M., . . . Schroeder, L. M. (2000). Effects of advanced nursing care on quality of life and cost outcomes of women diagnosed with breast cancer. *Oncology Nursing Forum*, 27(6), 923–932.

Rydström, I., Dalheim-Englund, A.-C., Segesten, K., & Rasmussen, B. H. (2004). Relations governed by uncertainty: Part of life of families of a child with asthma. *Journal of Pediatric Nursing*, 19(2), 85–94.

Sammarco, A. (2001). Perceived social support, uncertainty, and quality of life of younger breast cancer survivors. *Cancer Nursing*, 24(3), 212–219.

Sammarco, A., & Konecny, L. M. (2010). Quality of life, social support and uncertainty among Latina and Caucasian breast cancer survivors: A comparative study. *Oncology Nursing Forum*, 37(1), 93–99.

Sanders-Dewey, N., Mullins, L., & Chaney, J. (2001). Coping style, perceived uncertainty in illness, and distress in individuals with Parkinson's disease and their caregivers. *Rehabilitation Psychology*, 46(4), 363–381.

Santacroce, S. J. (2000). Support from health care providers and parental uncertainty during the diagnosis phase of perinatally acquired HIV infection. *Journal of the Association of Nurses in AIDS Care*, 11(2), 63–75.

Santacroce, S. J. (2001). Measuring parental uncertainty during the diagnosis phase of serious illness in a child. *Journal of Pediatric Nursing*, 16(1), 3–12.

Santacroce, S. J. (2002). Uncertainty, anxiety, and symptoms of posttraumatic stress in parents of children recently diagnosed with cancer. *Journal of Pediatric Oncology Nursing*, 19(3), 104–111.

Santacroce, S. J. (2003). Parental uncertainty and posttraumatic stress in serious childhood illness. *Journal of Nursing Scholarship*, 35(1), 45–51.

Santacroce, S. J., & Lee, Y. L. (2006). Uncertainty, posttraumatic stress, and health behavior in young adult childhood cancer survivors. *Nursing Research*, 55(4), 259–266.

Saunders, J. C., & Cookman, C. A. (2005). A clarified conceptual meaning of hepatitis Crelated depression. *Gastroenterology Nursing*, 28(2), 123–129; quiz 120–121.

Sexton, D. L., Calcasola, S. L., Bottomley, S. R., & Funk, M. (1999). Adults' experience with asthma and their reported uncertainty and coping strategies. *Clinical Nurse Specialist*, 13(1), 8–17.

Shaha, M., Cox, C. L., Talman, K., & Kelly, D. (2008). Uncertainty in breast, prostate, and colorectal cancer: Implications for supportive care. *Journal of Nursing Scholarship*, 40(1), 60–67.

Shalit, B. (1977). Structural ambiguity and limits to coping. *Journal of Human Stress, 3*, 32–45.

Sharkey, T. (1995). The effects of uncertainty in families with children who are chronically ill. *Home Healthcare Nurse*, 13(4), 37–42.

Small, S. P., & Graydon, J. E. (1993). Uncertainty in hospitalized patients with chronic obstructive pulmonary disease. *International Journal of Nursing Studies, 30*, 239–246.

Smeltzer, S. C. (1994). The concerns of pregnant women with multiple sclerosis. *Qualitative Health Research, 4*, 497–501.

Song, L., Tyler, C., Clayton, M. F., Rodgiriguez-Rassi, E., Hill, L., Bai, J., . . . Bailey, D. E., Jr. (2016). Patient and family communication during consultation visits: The effects of a decision aid for treatment decision-making for localized prostate cancer. *Patient Education and Counseling, 100*(2), 267–275.

Sorenson, D. L. S. (1990). Uncertainty in pregnancy. *NAACOG's Clinical Issues in Perinatal and Women's Health Nursing, 1*(3), 289–296.

Sterken, D. J. (1996). Uncertainty and coping of fathers of children with cancer. *Journal of Pediatric Oncology Nursing, 13*, 81–90.

Stewart, J. L. (2003). "Getting used to it": Children finding the ordinary and routine in the uncertain context of cancer. *Qualitative Health Research, 13*(3), 394–407.

Stewart, J. L., Lynn, M. R., & Mishel, M. H. (2010). Psychometric evaluation of a new instrument to measure uncertainty in children and adolescents with cancer. *Nursing Research, 59*, 119–126.

Stewart, J. L., & Mishel, M. H. (2000). Uncertainty in childhood illness: A synthesis of the parent and child literature. *Scholarly Inquiry for Nursing Practice, 17*, 299–319.

Stewart, J. L., Mishel, M. H., Lynn, M. R., & Terhorst, L. (2010). Test of a conceptual model of uncertainty in children and adolescents with cancer. *Research in Nursing and Health, 33*, 179–191.

Taylor-Piliae, R. E., & Chair, S. Y. (2002). The effect of nursing intervention utilizing music theory or sensory information on Chinese patients' anxiety prior to cardiac catherization: A pilot study. *European Journal of Cardiovascular Nursing, 1*, 203–311.

Taylor-Piliae, R. E., & Molassiotis, A. (2001). An exploration of the relationships between uncertainty, psychological distress and type of coping strategy among Chinese men after cardiac catheterization. *Journal of Advanced Nursing, 33*(1), 79–88.

Tomlinson, P., Kirschbaum, M., Harbaugh, B., & Anderson, K. (1996). The influence of illness severity and family resources on maternal uncertainty during critical pediatric hospitalization. *American Journal of Critical Care, 5*, 140–146.

Trivino Martinez, A., Solano Ruiz, M. C., & Siles Gonzalez, J. (2016). Application of an uncertainty model for fibromyalgia. *Atencion Primaria, 48*(4), 219–225.

Turner, M., Tomlinson, P., & Harbaugh, B. (1990). Parental uncertainty in critical care hospitalization of children. *Maternal-Child Nursing Journal, 19*, 45–62.

Van Riper, M., & Selder, F. E. (1989). Parental responses to birth of a child with Down syndrome. *Loss, Grief and Care: A Journal of Professional Practice, 3*(3–4), 59–76.

Walker, L. O., & Avant, K. C. (1989). *Strategies for theory construction in nursing.* Norwalk, CT: Appleton-Century-Crofts.

Webster, K. K., & Christman, N. J. (1988). Perceived uncertainty and coping post myocardial infarction. *Western Journal of Nursing Research, 10*(4), 384–400.

Weems, J., & Patterson, E. T. (1989). Coping with uncertainty and ambivalence while awaiting a cadaveric renal transplant. *ANNA Journal, 16*(1), 27–32.

Weiss, M. E., Saks, N. P., & Harris, S. (2002). Resolving the uncertainty of preterm symptoms: Women's experiences with the onset of preterm labor. *Journal of Obstetric, Gynecologic, and Neonatal Nursing, 31*(1), 66–76.

Weitz, R. (1989). Uncertainty and the lives of persons with AIDS. *Journal of Health and Social Behavior, 30*, 270–281.

White, R. E., & Frasure-Smith, N. (1995). Uncertainty and psychologic stress after coronary angioplasty and coronary bypass surgery. *Heart & Lung, 24*(1), 19–27.

Wiener, C. L., & Dodd, M. J. (1993). Coping amid uncertainty: An illness trajectory perspective. *Scholarly Inquiry for Nursing Practice, 7*(1), 17–31.

Wineman, N. M. (1990). Adaptation to multiple sclerosis: The role of social support, functional disability, and perceived uncertainty. *Nursing Research, 39,* 294–299.

Wineman, N. M., O'Brien, R. A., Nealon, N. R., & Kaskel, B. (1993). Congruence in uncertainty between individuals with multiple sclerosis and their spouses. *Journal of Neuroscience Nursing, 25,* 356–361.

Wineman, N. M., Schwetz, K. M., Goodkin, D. E., & Rudick, R. A. (1996). Relationships among illness uncertainty, stress, coping, and emotional well-being at entry into a clinical drug trial. *Applied Nursing Research, 9*(2), 53–60.

Wineman, N. M., Schwetz, K. M., Zeller, R., & Cyphert, J. (2003). Longitudinal analysis of illness uncertainty, coping, hopefulness, and mood during participation in a clinical drug trial. *Journal of Neuroscience Nursing, 35*(2), 100–106.

Winters, C. A. (1999). Heart failure: Living with uncertainty. *Progress in Cardiovascular Nursing, 14,* 85–91.

Wonghongkul, T., Dechaprom, N., Phumivichuvate, L., & Losawatkul, S. (2006). Uncertainty appraisal coping and quality of life in breast cancer survivors. *Cancer Nursing, 29*(3), 250–257.

Wonghongkul, T., Moore, S., Musil, C., Schneider, S., & Deimling, G. (2000). The influence of uncertainty in illness, stress appraisal, and hope on coping in survivors of breast cancer. *Cancer Nursing, 23*(6), 422–429.

Wunderlich, R., Perry, A., Lavin, M., & Katz, B. (1999). Patients' perceptions of uncertainty and stress during weaning from mechanical ventilation. *Dimensions of Critical Care Nursing, 18*(1), 8–12.

# CHAPTER 5

## Theory of Meaning

### Teresa Daniel Ritchie, Suzy Mascaro Walter, and Patricia Starck

One of the greatest challenges faced by nurses and other health professionals—whether providing care to those with acute, life-threatening illnesses, chronic conditions, or seeking to remain healthy—is to find the key to human motivation. What keeps a person from hanging on versus giving up, from struggling to overcome versus giving in, and from making sacrificial changes now for a better tomorrow? A young man is injured in a diving accident and is suddenly and irrevocably changed with the resulting spinal cord injury. What can the nurse do to promote that fighting spirit to be the best of what can now be? Such were the ponderings that led Dr. Patricia Starck, the original author of this chapter, to search for answers.

Motivation and human behavior are usually thought to be the purview of psychology/psychiatry. Sigmund Freud believed that seeking pleasure was the primary factor in human behavior. Alfred Adler had a different theory—the chief force was the seeking of power—with the concepts of birth order position, inferiority complex, and so on. The philosophy most resonating with Patricia Starck was that of Viktor Frankl, who believed that the primary human motivation was to seek meaning and purpose in life.

Frankl laid the foundational concepts on what has been developed into the Theory of Meaning. Frankl's application was originally with patients with psychiatric or psychological disorders. It has been expanded to help patients with various health problems, including disabilities and catastrophic, life-changing events, as well as to help the average human being cope with the everyday stresses of life. The theory and its application has also evolved beyond the individual level to groups and to the community/society.

### ■ PURPOSE OF THE THEORY AND HOW IT WAS DEVELOPED

In Europe during Frankl's professional era, a precise set of assumptions and philosophy was called a school of thought. Thus, Frankl—as a Viennese psychiatrist and neurologist—was trained in the first school of Viennese psychiatry, known as the Will to Pleasure, espoused by Sigmund Freud, and later, the second school, or the Will to Power, developed by Alfred Adler.

Frankl (1978) acknowledged the worth of Freud and Adler, as well as behaviorists who followed, but based on his own practice and experiences came to believe that humans cannot be seen as beings whose basic concerns are to satisfy drives and gratify instincts or, for that matter, to reconcile id, ego, and superego; nor can the human reality be understood merely as the outcome of conditioning processes or conditioned reflexes. Rather, the human is revealed as a being in search of meaning, and when this search is thwarted, various physical, mental, and spiritual problems become manifest.

Frankl called his concept the Will to Meaning, and it became known as the third school of Viennese psychiatry. He postulated that human beings are motivated to seek answers to such questions as: Why am I here? He went on to develop a treatment, which he termed *logotherapy*, the practice of helping people with psychiatric problems find meaning and purpose in life, no matter what their life circumstances.

There is a common misperception that Frankl's theory emerged as a result of his internment in German concentration camps during World War II. This misperception was a source of great irritation to Frankl as he clarified that in actuality he formulated his ideas about meaning in life when he was a young child, with his first clear understanding at age 5. After his medical education, he planned to write a book about the theory. However, the plan was interrupted when he was seized by the Nazis in Germany and imprisoned (Fabry, 1991). During the concentration camp experience, observing the behavior of prisoners and guards, he validated the premise of the vital importance of humans seeking meaning in life experiences.

He found that in spite of great suffering, survival behaviors were more evident in those who had a strong reason to live than in those who did not. Frankl preserved the theory by recreating a manuscript he had lost when he was imprisoned. During his internment at four different concentration camps over a 2.5-year period, he wrote on scraps of paper to keep his mind focused on his reason to survive. After his release at the end of World War II, he published the book that was later titled *Man's Search for Meaning*, under the previous title *From Death Camp to Existentialism*. In the book, he described his experience in prison, detailing the unimaginable sufferings of the imprisoned. He began to develop his concept of human suffering by defining suffering as a challenge. In the experience of suffering, the challenge to the individual is to decide how to respond to unavoidable, deplorable life circumstances. It is an opportunity to show courage and to behave decently in spite of circumstances. He coined the term *logotherapy* from the Greek word, *logos*, denoting meaning. Logotherapy is the practice of the theory, which is intended to assist individuals to find purpose in life regardless of circumstances.

Starck (1985) examined Frankl's work in light of Kerlinger's (1973) criteria for a theory that describes, explains, and predicts human behavior. The postulates are the central core of the theory and are generalized statements of truth that serve as essential underpinnings for this body of knowledge. The postulates follow.

- A person's search for meaning is the primary motivation of life. This meaning is unique and specific in that it must and can be fulfilled by the person alone (Frankl, 1984, p. 121).
- A person is free to be responsible and is responsible for the realization of the meaning of life, the *logos* of existence (Frankl, 1961, p. 9).
- A person may find meaning in life even when confronted with a hopeless situation, when facing a fate that cannot be changed (Frankl, 1984, p. 135).
- A person's life offers meaning in every moment and in every situation (Fabry, 1991, p. 130).

The Theory of Meaning is a framework that lends itself to interdisciplinary endeavors. Frankl's work has been used as the basis for research and practice in many fields, including medicine, psychology, counseling, education, ministry, and nursing. Travelbee (1966, 1969, 1972) was the first nurse to use Frankl's work in practice. She used parables and other stories to help psychiatric patients realize that human suffering comes to all and that we have the means to combat life problems no matter the circumstances.

Starck had the privilege of knowing Viktor E. Frankl over a 20-year period beginning when she was a doctoral student seeking ways to promote rehabilitation of patients with spinal cord injuries. She came upon Frankl's work and wrote to him. He responded and encouraged her, saying she would be the first to apply his theory and practice to physically disabled individuals.

Starck met Frankl in 1979 when she presented her dissertation—including the logotherapeutic nursing intervention she had designed to the first World Congress of Logotherapy. Frankl quoted her work in his publications and presentations. Starck received further training in logotherapy from Frankl's protégé, Elizabeth Lukas, a logotherapist from Munich, Germany.

When Patricia Starck retired as the Dean of the University of Texas, Health Science Center—Houston, School of Nursing, she enthusiastically encouraged that the work be continued by emerging scholars. The current chapter authors, Teresa Ritchie and Suzy Mascaro Walter, learned the theory during doctoral study and began applying it to their practice and research. Ritchie is prepared with a doctorate of nursing practice and she serves as a family nurse practitioner in the primary care setting. Walter is prepared with a doctorate of philosophy in nursing and does research focused on the care of adolescents suffering with migraines. Together, Teresa Ritchie and Suzy Mascaro Walter have updated Starck's chapter.

## ■ CONCEPTS OF THE THEORY

Three major concepts from Frankl's works are the building blocks of the theory: life purpose, freedom to choose, and human suffering. These concepts are supported by three human dimensions: the physical or soma, the mental or psyche, and the spiritual or noos (Frankl, 1969). The physical and the mental dimensions can become ill but the spiritual dimension cannot. It can only become blocked or frustrated.

Frankl indicates that while we have these three dimensions of soma, psyche, and noos, at any point in time, from different points of view, different impressions and, therefore, different meanings reveal themselves. He called attention to the fact that a problem in one dimension may show up as a symptom in another. For example, spiritual emptiness may manifest in a physical symptom such as intense headaches. An important understanding when considering dimensional ontology is Frankl's emphasis on the human spirit, the noos, and the "defiant" power of the noos. Fabry (1991) interpreted this conceptualization as, "You *have* a body and a psyche, but you *are* your noos (spirit)" (p. 127). The human spirit can defy the odds and rise above the other dimensions.

Examples of the power of the noos are provided throughout this chapter as vignettes are shared and stories are told about people who excelled beyond expectations to accomplish extraordinary feats. The noos is essential to the pursuit of life purpose.

### Life Purpose

Life purpose is the central concept of the Theory of Meaning. It is the summary of reasons for one's existence, answering the questions: Who am I? and Why am I here? A sense of life purpose brings satisfaction with one's place in the world. Life purpose is that to which one may feel called and to which one is dedicated. There is a theme to one's life purpose—making a contribution, leaving the world a better place. The major premise of Frankl's theory is that the search for meaning in one's life is an overriding search for purpose. Life purpose flows from the "uniqueness of the person and the singularity of the situation" (Frankl, 1973, p. 63). Every person is "indispensable and irreplaceable" (Frankl, 1973, p. 117).

Fabry (1991) explained meaning from various existential viewpoints. The French existentialists, Sartre and Camus, believed that life itself had no meaning other than the meaning that humans gave to it. In contrast, the German existentialists, including Frankl, maintained that meaning exists and the task is to discover it, and in discovering meaning one also discovers life purpose. Fabry emphasized that our human spirits are the instruments for finding a purpose in life through tapping the spiritual treasure in each of us.

Frankl asserts that each person must discover his or her own meaning. It cannot be prescribed by another. A professional caregiver working with a person who has recently suffered a loss cannot tell the person how to look for meaning in another dimension of life, but the caregiver can help guide the person to find new avenues of meaning through shifting views of soma, psyche, and noos. "And meaning is something to be found rather than to be given, discovered rather than invented" (Frankl, 1969, p. 62).

Frankl (1984) postulated that meaning in life always changes but never ceases to be. He specified three different ways to find meaning on the path to uncovering life purpose: (a) creating a work or doing a deed that moves beyond self, (b) experiencing something or encountering someone, and (c) choosing our attitude toward our own fate. In the first way, a strong sense of purpose or meaning in life may be seen when a terminally ill person hangs on tenaciously until the achievement of some goal such as that person's child graduating from college. This will to meaning is a strong life force that can defy the odds given by the most expert clinician. Fabry (1980) distinguished between "meaning of the moment" in everyday choices we make and "universal meaning" or the bigger picture that we may not completely understand at the time. Meaning of the moment is the everyday situation where one has a chance to act in a meaningful way through action, experiences, and the stand one takes. Ultimate meaning is the trust that there is order in the universe and that humans are part of that order. It is the opposite of seeing the world as chaotic and humans as the victims of whim.

A second way to find meaning and enable life purpose is through experiences like loving or encountering another human being. Frankl believed that love goes beyond an individual and is long-lasting. "Love is so little directed toward the body of the beloved that it can easily outlast the other's death, can exist in the lover's heart until his own death" (Frankl, 1973, p. 138).

The third way to find meaning on the path of life purpose is by choosing one's own attitude to whatever life presents. Choosing to remain positive, brave, or optimistic in spite of difficult circumstances illustrates this way of finding meaning. Purpose in life can come when a choice is made to deliberately change one's attitude and view the situation in a different way.

Frankl identified two states that describe a lack of meaning: existential frustration and existential vacuum. Existential frustration is searching for meaning in which there is a state of being unsettled, of wanting more from life (Frankl, 1969). Existential vacuum is a sense of utter despair, of hopelessness, that life has no meaning and all is of no use (Frankl, 1969). This is an inner emptiness where one feels trapped in unhappiness. Times of transition may lead to an existential vacuum, such as when a person is dissatisfied with work but is afraid of risking change. Existential vacuum may also occur during times of loss, such as the sudden, unexpected death of a child, when one does not trust values that have formerly been a guide. Fabry (1980) believed that lack of meaning can surface as a life crisis, leading to unhealthy ways that people cope including drugs, workaholism, thrill-seeking, and overeating. This crisis experience may also serve as a stimulus to find a more meaningful existence.

A poignant example of finding meaning and accomplishing life purpose, even at the end of life, is a story that will live in history as one in which individuals transcended self for the good of others. On September 11, 2001, passengers on United Airlines flight 93 found that fate had placed them on a plane hijacked by terrorists intent on a suicide mission to destroy innocent lives and symbols of American democracy. With the aid of cell phone technology, some passengers learned there had already been terrorist attacks occurring through the hijack of other commercial flights that morning and there was no doubt what their fate was to be. Many talked to family members about the things that gave meaning to their lives—the love they had, and they expressed wish for the family to go on to complete meaningful lives. Yet, in the face of their own death, they had freedom of choice. They had a chance to transcend their own fears, one last chance to do something good for humanity. In the last moments of their lives, they could and did perform a selfless act—they made sure the plane did not reach its intended target but rather crashed in a nonpopulated area in Pennsylvania. In accomplishing this unexpected life purpose, they gave meaning to their lives and left a legacy of heroism, not only for their loved ones but also for every American citizen and many others around the world. If among this group there were one person whose life had been meaningless, when that person exercised freedom to act and to transcend his or her own needs, by this one act in the final moments, life was flooded with meaning and purpose.

## Freedom to Choose

Freedom to choose is the second concept of the Theory of Meaning. It is the process of selecting among options over which one has control. In enduring the most intense imaginable hardship, that of the Holocaust, Frankl (1973) pointed out that there is value to be found in a person's attitude toward the limiting factors of life. Being confronted by an unalterable destiny where one can act only by acceptance provides a unique opportunity to choose one's attitude. "The way in which he accepts, the way in which he bears his cross, what courage he manifests in suffering, what dignity he displays in doom and disaster, is the measure of his human fulfillment" (Frankl, 1973, p. 44). One can be subjected to torture, humiliation, and worse, and yet retain the attitude to face one's fate with courage. It is the attitude of the sufferer that drives the behavior, not the actions of the persecutor. The right to choose one's own attitude may be thought of as spiritual freedom or independence of mind.

> We who lived in concentration camps can remember the men who walked through the huts comforting others, giving away their last piece of bread. They may have been few in number, but they offer sufficient proof that everything can be taken from a man but one thing: the last of the human

freedoms—to choose one's attitude in any given set of circumstances, to choose one's own way. (Frankl, 1984, p. 86)

Fabry (1991) offered practical guidelines for modifying attitudes by considering that something positive can be found in all situations. Some sample questions to stimulate one's attitude change are: "What am I still able to do that would benefit someone? Whom do I love and wish to protect in this situation?" (p. 43). By asking these questions, one shifts the attention away from what has been lost and from self to others. Fabry (1991) suggested that one's attitude can begin to change by "acting as if" one has the attribute. For example, if a person wanted to be courageous, then to act "as if" would be to get a change in attitude.

Lukas (1984, 1986) introduced several ideas that are important to Frankl's work. She expanded understanding of freedom to choose by indicating that life events can be classified as either fate or freedom. Fate is when we cannot change the situation, whereas freedom includes what one can do, including choosing what attitude to adopt. When confronting a problem, the person should ask: Where are my areas of freedom? Which possible choices do I have? Which one do I want to actualize?

## Human Suffering

Human suffering is the third concept of the Theory of Meaning. It is a subjective experience that is unique to an individual and varies from simple transitory discomfort to extreme anguish and despair (Starck & McGovern, 1992). Frankl did not define suffering but rather described it as a subjective, all-consuming human experience. He believed that "the meaning of suffering . . . is the deepest possible meaning" (Frankl, 1969, p. 75) and the ultimate meaning of life or human suffering can never be found.

Frankl was clear that there is no meaning *in* suffering. For example, there is no meaning in cancer. However, one can find meaning *in spite of* having cancer. Suffering is a part of the human experience. Things happen to us that are undeserved, unexplainable, and unavoidable. We do not need to look for meaning in these events; rather, meaning comes from stances we take toward the suffering, for example, the courageous way a person chooses to live with the cancer. Frankl (1975) described the worst kind of suffering as "despair, suffering without meaning" (p. 137).

## ■ RELATIONSHIPS AMONG THE CONCEPTS: THE MODEL

The relationships among the concepts of the theory are depicted in Figure 5.1. This illustration suggests that meaning is a journey toward life purpose with the freedom to choose one's path in spite of inevitable suffering.

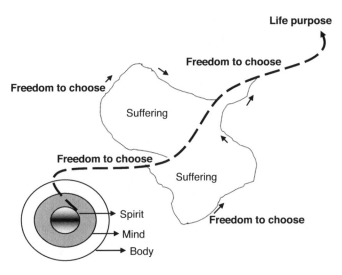

**FIGURE 5.1** The Theory of Meaning.

## ■ USE OF THE THEORY IN NURSING RESEARCH

### Instruments

Instruments, which empirically measure the concepts related to meaning, can serve as guides to optimize care in clinical practice. The following describes some of the more widely known instruments: the Purpose in Life measure (PIL); Seeking of Noetic Goals measure (SONG); the Schedule for Meaning in Life Evaluation (SMiLE); and the nurse-derived Meaning in Suffering Test (MIST).

The PIL is a 20-item self-report that evaluates whether the respondent has a perceived sense of meaning and purpose in life or alternatively experiences an existential frustration or existential vacuum (Crumbaugh, 1968; Crumbaugh & Maholick, 1964). Responses consist of a 7-point Likert scale (ranging from 1 "never" to 7 "constantly") with the sum of scores ranging from 20 to 140, which represents the degree to which meaning has been found (scores ≥113 represent definite purpose in life, 92–112 represent feelings of indecisiveness, and scores ≤92 demonstrate a lack of clear meaning and purpose in life, respectively; Hedberg, Gustafson, & Brulin, 2010). Sample items read:

- In life I have: no goals or aims versus clear goals and aims.
- In achieving life goals I have: made no progress whatsoever versus progressed to complete fulfillment.
- I have discovered: no mission or purpose in life versus a satisfying life purpose.

The SONG was developed to complement the PIL. As described earlier, the PIL indicates the degree of meaning found by the respondent whereas the SONG represents the degree of motivation to find meaning (Crumbaugh,

1977). The SONG consists of a 20-item self-report with responses based upon a 7-point Likert scale (ranging from 1 "never" to 7 "constantly") with the sum of scores ranging from 20 to 140 and the higher scores representing a stronger degree of motivation to find meaning (Crumbaugh, 1977). Sample items read:

- I feel the lack of (and the need to find) a real meaning and purpose in my life.
- Over my lifetime I have felt a strong urge to find myself.

The SMiLE was developed to assess individual meaning in life (Fegg, Kramer, L'hoste, & Borasio, 2008). The SMiLE consists of three questions with the first asking respondents to note a minimum of three to a maximum of seven areas that give meaning to living in their current situation. Second, respondents are to rate the level of satisfaction in the present with each of the noted areas on a 7-point Likert scale ranging from −3 (very unsatisfied) to +3 (very satisfied). Third, the respondents are asked to rate the importance of each area to overall meaning in life using an 8-point scale, ranging from 0 (not important) to 7 (extremely important). Three indices are then calculated. The Index of Weighting (IoW) represents the mean level of importance of the meaning in life areas; the Index of Satisfaction (IoS) represents the mean satisfaction or dissatisfaction in the individual meaning in life areas; and the total SMiLE index (or Index of Weighted Satisfaction [IoWS]) is a combination of the ratings for importance and satisfaction. Scores for the aforementioned indices range from 0 to 100 with the higher scores indicating higher meaning in life.

The MIST was developed by Starck (1983). This measure consists of two parts (MIST 1; MIST 2). MIST 1 is a 20-item self-report querying the meaning found in suffering. Responses are scored using a 7-point Likert scale, ranging from "never" to "constantly." Sample items from MIST 1 read:

- I believe I have the spiritual help (not necessarily religious) to overcome the burdens of my suffering.
- I believe suffering causes a person to find new and more worthwhile life goals.
- I believe I understand life better because of the suffering I have experienced.

MIST 2 is a 17-item measure that queries responses to suffering. Sample items from MIST 2 include:

- What do you think suffering teaches if anything? (name 3 if possible)
- What "good" or positive aspects resulted from your suffering? (name 3 if possible)
- How has your suffering affected your body, mind, and spirit? (name 3 ways, if possible)

Although these four measures provide an avenue for quantifying meaning in life, the complexity of the phenomenon defies simplistic quantification.

Detailed reviews of meaning in life assessments have been reported and offer an extensive list of the published instruments as well as descriptions and psychometric properties of the instruments (Brandstatter, Baumann, Borasio, & Fegg, 2012; Fjelland, Barron, & Foxall, 2008; White, 2004). Another important resource for meaning in life instruments and research studies is the Viktor Frankl Institute of Logotherapy website (http://logotherapyinstitute.org/Home.html), which provides information for membership, the biannual World Congress, and the institute's official journal entitled *The International Forum for Logotherapy: Journal of Search for Meaning*.

## ■ RESEARCH IN NURSING AND OTHER DISCIPLINES

Since the turn of the century, research on the role of meaning in healthcare has greatly expanded—internationally as well as across disciplines. Patient conditions where the role of meaning has been explored include myocardial infarction (MI), cancer, rheumatoid arthritis, addictions, bereavement, battered women, and HIV-positive individuals.

Health professionals from various disciplines have contributed to research in the significance of meaning and purpose. Prior to the 1970s, much of the research was in the domain of psychology/psychiatry professionals and related to mental health views. Starck (1979) developed and tested a nursing intervention model for a population of individuals in the community with permanent spinal cord injury. Other disciplines have evaluated spinal cord injury in terms of psychological resources and how purpose in life impacts participation (Peter et al., 2014) and depressive symptoms (Peter et al., 2015).

Nursing researchers (Coward, 1991, 1994, 1995, 1996, 1998; Coward & Dickerson, 2003; Coward & Kahn, 2004, 2005; Coward & Lewis, 1993; Coward & Reed, 1996) have studied meaning and purpose in life in a healthy population as well as patients with breast cancer, AIDS, and at the end of life. Coward emphasized self-transcendence, combining the work of Frankl and others in helping patients overcome spiritual disequilibrium. Starck, Ulrich, and Duffy (2009) reported that the most intense suffering was reported by hospitalized psychiatric patients as compared with hospitalized patients with either a medical–surgical or high-risk prenatal diagnosis.

In the 1980s and 1990s, Steeves and Kahn (1987), Kahn and Steeves (1995), and Steeves (1992, 1996) studied the concept of suffering in various populations including hospice patients and their families and patients undergoing bone marrow transplantations. Steeves, Kahn, and Benoliel (1990) studied how nurses experience and react to a person's suffering. Researchers in palliative care have evaluated the extent to which bereaved informal caregivers of palliative care patients experience meaning in their lives (Brandstatter et al., 2014) as well as the feasibility and validity of using a Hindi version of SMiLE for hospice patients experiencing end of life (Kudla et al., 2015).

Several nursing studies have evaluated meaning in life in nursing home patients (Haugan, 2014; Haugan & Moksnes, 2013; Haugan, Moksnes, & Lohre, 2016). Haugan and Moksnes (2013) performed a validation study of the purpose in life for evaluating meaning in life in nursing home patients. The PIL showed good interitem consistency (Cronbach's alpha), good composite reliability, and good construct validity (Haugan & Moksnes, 2013). Haugan (2014) also investigated the association between meaning in life and physical, emotional, functional and social well-being in a nursing home population. Meaning in life was found to be associated with all dimensions of well-being. Thus, facilitating perceived meaning in life for the cognitively intact elderly nursing home resident may result in improved well-being (Haugan, 2014). In a third study, associations were investigated between meaning in life, hope, self-transcendence, and perceived nurse–patient interaction with quality of life (Haugan et al., 2016). Meaning in life, as well as self-transcendence and nurse–patient interaction, demonstrated strong associations with quality of life.

There are several studies addressing life meaning and purpose for populations with chronic disease including MI, congestive heart failure (CHF), progressive supranuclear palsy (PSP), and rheumatoid arthritis. In a 5-year longitudinal study of patients with MI, Baldacchino (2011) documented that by finding meaning in the illness experiences and by clarifying values and purpose in life, MI patients were motivated to make lifestyle change, particularly in the immediate aftermath of their MI. However, by the third year onward, compliance with lifestyle modification was inconsistent (Baldacchino, 2010). In a cross-sectional study of patients hospitalized with CHF, researchers evaluated factors that gave meaning in life using the SMiLE tool (Mello & Ashcraft, 2014). Subjects reported that family was an area important for meaning in life; thus, providers need to understand family relationships when discussing advanced planning decision making at end of life (Mello & Ashcraft, 2014).

An exploratory study using the SMiLE investigated meaning in patients with PSP (Fegg, Kogler, Abright, Hensler, & Lorenzl, 2014). When compared with healthy people, those with PSP were less likely to list health and more likely to list partner, leisure, home/garden, and pleasure as areas important for meaning in life. These areas provide the framework for which individuals with PSP find meaning and are important to consider when developing psychosocial interventions and plans of care to maintain and enhance meaning in life in this population (Fegg et al., 2014). In a study with 156 patients diagnosed with rheumatoid arthritis, Verduin et al. (2008) documented the independent contribution of life purpose to the mental health component of quality of life. In the exploration of the relationship between spirituality, purpose in life and well-being in HIV-positive people, Litwinczuk and Groh (2007) found a significant relationship between spirituality and purpose in life in 46 HIV-positive men and women. The researchers recommended the design of nursing interventions to help HIV-positive people redefine themselves and find meaning in life.

Studies of life meaning and purpose with cancer patients have been reported. For instance, in longitudinal work with more than 500 cancer survivors, Jim and Anderson (2007) found that loss of life meaning contributed to poor social and physical functioning. In other research where investigators accepted the premise that many newly diagnosed cancer patients experience existential distress, Lee (2008) and Lee, Cohen, Edgar, Laizner, and Gagnon (2006) studied a meaning-making intervention, using a Lifeline exercise. The Lifeline exercise engaged participants in marking important life events in the past, and noting plans to achieve important life goals in the future. Use of the Lifeline exercise resulted in improved self-esteem, optimism, and self-efficacy in this randomized controlled trial.

Studies in both psychology and nursing examined cancer using the PIL and SONG (Brunelli et al., 2012; Scrignaro et al., 2015) as well as the SMiLE (Tomas-Sabado et al., 2015) instruments. Brunelli et al. (2012) demonstrated validation of the Italian versions of the PIL and SONG in cancer patients. Those who had high PIL scores (meaning in life attainment) had lower SONG scores (will to meaning), which demonstrates that participants with a well-defined existential meaning did not have meaning seeking needs. Those with low meaning in life attainment scores (PIL) had high seeking meaning scores (SONG). Scrignaro et al. (2015) also evaluated the search for meaning (SONG) and presence of meaning (PIL) in cancer patients. This study demonstrated that higher levels of a search for meaning were significantly associated with lower levels of meaning in cancer patients. Tomas-Sabado et al. (2015) evaluated meaning in life in patients with advanced cancer admitted to an acute care unit. The areas most frequently reported contributing to meaning in life derived from the SMiLE measure included family, partner, well-being, and friends. Only one of the patients reported financial situation as a contributor to life meaning. Thus, implementing plans of care to ensure access to family and friends may be key to enhancing life meaning for cancer patients facing end of life (Tomas-Sabado et al., 2015).

Life meaning and purpose has also been studied in populations with addictive disorders. In research on Hungarian men and women, meaning in life as measured with the PIL differentiated nonsmokers from daily smokers. Life meaning had a significant negative impact on smoking intensity for females (Thege, Bachner, Martos, & Kushnir, 2009). In another study of cocaine abusers in treatment, PIL significantly predicted relapse to cocaine and to alcohol use, as well as the number of days of use, 6 months after treatment (Martin, MacKinnon, Johnson, & Rohsenow, 2011). Martin et al. (2011) suggest that increasing one's sense of purpose in life may be an important component of treatment for cocaine-addicted patients.

Korean researchers (Kang & Kim, 2011) reported a study of life purpose and resilience in a group of 110 battered women. Greater life purpose was positively associated with higher resilience, measured as self-efficacy, communication efficiency, and optimism. Findings led the researchers to conclude that practitioners can help battered women to clarify their values and meaning in life and thereby improve their resilience.

Meaning and purpose in life play a significant role in health outcomes for a broad range of patients. The most often used measures are the PIL (Crumbaugh, 1968) and the SONG (Crumbaugh, 1977). Nurse researchers are now positioned to develop and test meaning-making interventions (Lee, 2008; Lee et al., 2006) and the move to intervention research to examine change in life purpose and health outcomes for people with chronic illness. This research can be accommodated with guidance from the Theory of Meaning.

## ■ USE OF THE THEORY IN NURSING PRACTICE

Fabry (1980) has described logotherapy as "guiding people toward understanding themselves as they are and could be and their place in the totality of living" (p. xiii). When contrasted with traditional psychotherapy, it is less retrospective and introspective (Frankl, 1984). Other comparisons between psychotherapy and logotherapy are found in Table 5.1.

The goal of logotherapy is to help persons separate themselves from their symptoms, to tap into the resources of their noetic dimension, and to arouse the dynamic power of the human spirit. Helping another find meaning may be described as promoting an unfolding of what is already there. It is helping the other discover his or her values and facilitating awareness of subconscious beliefs and commitments.

Frankl does not advocate techniques in a routine procedural sense but rather encourages creativity based on the situation at hand. Frankl (1969) has described *three* logotherapeutic approaches. These approaches are dereflection, paradoxical intention, and Socratic dialogue. Both dereflection and paradoxical intention "rest on two essential qualities of human existence, namely, man's capacities of self-transcendence and self-detachment" (Frankl, 1969, p. 99).

**TABLE 5.1** Contrast of Psychotherapy and Logotherapy

| Psychotherapy | Logotherapy |
| --- | --- |
| Sees life in terms of problems | Sees life in terms of solutions |
| Focuses on obstacles | Focuses on goals |
| Reductionistic | Holistic |
| Emphasis on uncovering | Emphasis on discovering |
| Analytical style | Uniqueness and improvisational style |

## Dereflection

Dereflection is a technique of logotherapy developed by Frankl following World War II, based on the concept of self-transcendence and moving beyond oneself (Ameli & Dattilio, 2013). Dereflection is the act of de-emphasizing or ceasing to focus on a troublesome phenomenon, issue, or problem; it is putting this issue aside. Dereflection strengthens the capacity for self-transcendence.

Obsessions are recognized as hyperreflection or excess attention, described as the "compulsion to self-observation" (Frankl, 1973, p. 253). The urge for better sexual performance is an example. "Sexual performance or experience is strangled to the extent to which it is made either an object of attention or an objective of intention" (Frankl, 1969, p. 101).

Complaining is an example of hyperreflection, as an excessive amount of attention is given to the self. Dereflection counteracts hyperreflection, shifts attention away from the problem, and redirects attention to a more meaningful area (Ameli & Dattilio, 2013; Frankl, 2004). Dereflection helps the person stop fighting an anxiety, a neurosis, or a psychosis, and spares the person the reinforcement of additional suffering. If a person is depressed, dereflection can help achieve distance between the person and the depression, "to see himself—not as a person who is depressed but—as a full human being who has depressions with the capacity to find meaning despite the depressions" (Fabry, 1991, p. 136). The main objective of dereflection is to encourage an awareness of a person's meaningful values, meaningful goals and then align the two to help the person define precise and purposeful goals (Ameli & Dattilio, 2013, p. 389).

## Paradoxical Intention

Paradoxical intention is purposefully acting the opposite to one's desired ends, thereby confronting one's fears and anxieties. Paradoxical intention strengthens the capacity for self-distancing. By distancing from the triggers of problems, these triggers become ineffective. Paradoxical intention is helpful in dealing with the problem of anticipatory anxiety. The object of the person's fear is fear itself. The underlying dynamic is apprehension about the potential effects of the anxiety attacks. And, of course, the fear of the fear increases the fear, producing precisely what the person is afraid of. The person is caught in a restricting cycle. The aim of therapy is to break the cycle, to interfere with the feedback mechanism. In logotherapy, one is asked to replace fear with a paradoxical wish, to wish for the very thing one fears. By this treatment, Frankl said, "the wind is taken out of the sails of the anxiety" (1984, p. 147).

This approach makes use of the specific human capacity for self-detachment. For example, in sleep disturbances when a person worries that he or she will not be able to get to sleep and focuses on trying to go to sleep, sleep will not come. The fear of sleeplessness results in the hyperintention to fall asleep, which inevitably leads to sleeplessness. Applying paradoxical intention requires instruction for the person who has difficulty initiating sleep, to intentionally avoid any attempts to try to fall asleep and remain passively awake. This process may decrease performance anxiety and lead to the onset of sleep (Morgenthaler et al., 2006).

Paradoxical intention can be used to change unwanted behavior patterns. This does not depend upon understanding how and why the behavior started. It simply breaks the cycle of fear. Ascher and Schotte (1999) demonstrated that individuals with public speaking phobia complicated by recursive anxiety—for example, fear of loss of bladder control, vomiting, and so on—showed greater improvement when paradoxical intention was included in treatment.

Similarly, another example of paradoxical intention is adding exaggerated humor by wishing for the worst fear or anxiety-provoking event to occur. For example, for a person whose greatest fear is having a heart attack, the individual is advised to tell himself or herself that he or she looks forward to having a heart attack, falling to the ground, and making a spectacle of himself or herself (Ameli & Dattilio, 2013). Paradoxical intention counteracts the anticipated anxiety of having a heart attack by having a reciprocal impact on the symptoms, which in turn breaks the anxiety cycle (Ameli & Dattilio, 2013).

Based on the finding that 55% of patients with a psychiatric disorder who presented in the emergency department were diagnosed with conversion disorders, Ataoglu, Ozcetin, Icmeli, and Ozbulut (2003) conducted a study and concluded that paradoxical intention therapy provided greater improvement than diazepam therapy.

## Socratic Dialogue

Socratic dialogue is a conversation of questions and answers, probing deeply into existential issues such as one's values. It is rhetorical debate to trigger a change in attitude, behavior, or both. Socratic dialogue is self-discovery discourse and seeks to get rid of masks that have been put on to please or to be accepted. The therapist poses questions so that patients become aware of their unconscious decisions, their repressed hopes, and their unadmitted self-knowledge. In Socratic dialogue, experiences of the past are explored as well as fantasies for the future to modulate attitude (Fabry, 1980). Socratic dialogue requires improvisation and intuition and asks probing questions like the following:

- Was there a time when life had meaning?
- Who do you know who leads a meaningful life? What keeps you from living like this person?
- Who are the people who need you?
- Tell me about an experience that made you see things differently.
- Tell me something you said you couldn't do but you did it.

As an example, Lukas (1984), working with a patient who strongly valued physical ability and who had undergone a leg amputation, asked the question, "Does the value of human existence depend on the use of two legs?" (p. 47).

When engaging in Socratic dialogue with a patient in the clinical setting, it is important for the clinician to be totally present. This requires attentive listening in order to understand the patient's concerns, values, and cultural beliefs. As an example, Dattilio and Hannah (2012) used Socratic questioning as one approach to aid in gaining trust and respect in the care of a physician assistant who began having panic attacks after experiencing the loss of a young patient near his age in the emergency department (p. 157).

Fabry (1991) proposed five guideposts to probe areas of meaning. These are self-discovery, choice, uniqueness, responsibility, and self-transcendence. Fabry also identified a number of creative methods and exercises to illustrate choice, where family members act out the role of others in the way they wish the others had responded. The flashlight technique can be useful in self-discovery and in aggressive discussion. The facilitator shines the flashlight on the partner who says something offensive to the other, indicating that the person must rephrase what has been said without hostility or sarcasm, thus helping reshape attitudes and behaviors. Fabry (1991) also has guidelines for groups, wherein the Socratic dialogue becomes a multilogue.

A family who was experiencing problems thought to be caused by one child who had a physical condition requiring most of the mother's attention, making her less available to her other children and to her husband, sought logotherapy. The therapist asked the "identified patient" this question in the presence of the entire family—"If you could give your condition to anyone else in the family, who would you give it to?" The mother quickly spoke and said, "I would take it." The therapist specified that the child was the one to answer the question. After looking at each member of his family, the child responded, "I would keep it myself because I think I am the best one to handle it." This attitude changed the family dynamic; the child was seen as a hero and not a burden to others.

## Other Practices Using Logotherapy

Pearce (2005), a parish nurse, declared that Frankl was a forerunner to integrative medicine and holistic nursing, contrasting this with today's fragmented system of healers specializing in healing only a part of the whole. Patients with a complex interaction of physical, psychological, and spiritual suffering often find their way to logotherapy after being disappointed with the existing healthcare system. Logotherapy provides tools to tap into inner resources for the individual to emerge as a stronger and more joyous self.

Winters and Schulenberg (2006) pointed out that diagnosis is a necessary evil in practice. Diagnosis is inherently reductionistic and focuses on defeats. To address this problem, the authors developed a holistic, logotherapeutic model of diagnosis. The diagnostic process is a bio-psychosocial–spiritual one and incorporates an assessment of one's inner strength. For example, the provider might include a positive history of emotional balance and a history of making it through previous difficult times as noetic resources. Logotherapy is aimed at empowering the patient by emphasizing choice, responsibility, and hope.

Practice applications of meaning theory, both patient-related and provider-related, have been developed. Cho (2008) introduced the logo-autobiography program, which focused on improving meaning in life and mental health in wives of alcoholics. The logo-autobiography program incorporates autobiography, writing and sharing of life stories, with logotherapy (Cho, 2008). Wong (2010) developed two approaches to meaning therapy including the PURE strategy (purpose, understanding, responsible action, and evaluation) and the ABCDE strategy (accept, believe, commit, discover, and evaluate).

The central ideas of the Theory of Meaning are proving useful for a range of life-altering illnesses and significant lifetime points. For instance, there is perhaps no greater challenge than finding meaning when confronting end of life. There is a growing recognition that symptoms of psychological distress and existential concerns are ever more prevalent and problematic than pain and other physical concerns when facing imminent death (Breitbart, Gibson, Poppito, & Berg, 2004).

Finding meaning in the traumatic experience of cardiac disease is used by psychotherapists to help patients reconstruct basic assumptions about self and others and to reestablish predictability in their lives (Sheikh & Marotta, 2008). An education-based intervention using the concepts of logotherapy was found to have a significant effect on quality of life after coronary artery bypass grafting surgery (Mahdizadeh, Alavi, & Ghazavi, 2016). A meaning-centered intervention has also been used in treating veterans with chronic combat-related posttraumatic stress disorder (Southwick, Gilmartin, McDonough, & Morrissey, 2006).

Significant effects of group logotherapy in populations experiencing infertility, breast cancer, and depression, as well as parents of children with disabilities have also been documented (Faramarzi & Bavali, 2017; Mohabbat-Bahar, Golzari, Moradi-Joo, & Akbari, 2014; Mosalanejad & Khodabakshi, 2013; Robatmili et al., 2015). Mosalanejad and Khodabakshi (2013) studied the effect of group logotherapy on stress in infertile women. Findings demonstrated that the logotherapy intervention resulted in a significant decrease in worry and stress leading to an increased likelihood to find meaning in life in spite of infertility. In a second report, Mohabbat-Bahar et al. (2014) studied the efficacy of group logotherapy on decreasing anxiety in women with breast cancer. The results of this study indicated that logotherapy significantly reduced anxiety in women with breast cancer. In a third study, Robatmili et al. (2014) reported on the effect of group therapy on meaning in life and depression level of Iranian students. The experimental group received 10 sessions of group logotherapy. The mean scores for the experimental group were lower for depression and higher in regard to meaning in life (PIL scores) when compared to the control group (Robatmili et al., 2014). Last, Faramarzi and Bavali (2017) studied the effectiveness of group logotherapy to improve psychological well-being of mothers with intellectually disabled children. The group logotherapy consisted of eight weekly sessions lasting 90 minutes. The researchers reported that group logotherapy led to increased psychological well-being including positive relationships with others, personal growth, autonomy, and environmental mastery (p. 45).

Not only do patients benefit from a sense of meaning and life purpose, care providers also benefit. Taubman-Ben-Ari and Weintroub (2008) studied physicians and nurses frequently exposed to terminally ill children in Israel. A higher level of exposure to patient death, higher optimism and professional self-esteem, and lower secondary traumatization (being close to someone who experienced trauma) predicted the sense of meaning in life. Fillion and colleagues have studied nurses who work in a palliative care setting. They designed a meaning-centered intervention consisting of group therapy in four sessions plus a closing session (Fillion, Dupuis, Tremblay, De Grace, & Breitbart, 2006). In the intervention, enhancing meaning in palliative care, the focus of each session was (a) search for and sources of meaning, (b) historical perspective and sense of accomplishment as creative values, (c) meaning and suffering through attitudinal change, and (d) affective experiences and humor in experiential values. Each session consisted of didactic content, exercises, and group discussion, plus home assignments. In a follow-up study, the researchers sought to ameliorate stress and improve job satisfaction and quality of life for nurses working in palliative care. The four-session meaning-centered intervention was conducted (Fillion et al., 2009) using a wait list design. Outcome measures included personal and job-related measures. Even though spiritual and emotional quality of life remained unchanged, nurses who received the intervention reported greater job benefits associated with working in the palliative care setting.

The influence of working environment on palliative care versus maternity ward healthcare professional's (HCP's) meaning in life has also been studied (Fegg, L'hoste, Brandstatter, & Borasio, 2014). This cross-sectional study evaluated personal values (Schwartz Value Survey), meaning in life (SMiLE), and private religiousness (Idler Index of Religiosity) for HCPs working in a palliative care setting (confronted with death) versus those working in a maternity ward. The maternity ward HCPs listed family more often than the palliative care HCPs as an area for finding meaning in life and were more satisfied with meaning in life if they found meaning in the area of family. Palliative care workers listed spirituality and nature experiences more often as areas where they found life meaning compared to the maternity ward HCPs (Fegg et al., 2014). These findings indicate the importance of family for finding life meaning for maternity ward HCPs and religion/nature experiences for the palliative care HCPs (Fegg et al., 2014). Palliative care HCPs seemed to find meaning in life in three key areas: creativity and self-direction; experiences that generated excitement, curiosity, and adventurous attitudes toward life; and attitudinal values exhibited by a focus on spirituality (Fegg et al., 2014). The authors concede that it is unknown whether the differences in responses between the groups are due to the consequences of the working environment and that a longitudinal study is needed to fully evaluate working environment influences on meaning in life. However, findings may be applied to health promotion/prevention programs for palliative care workers, including therapies that promote mindfulness through meditation and enhance experience values through time away from work (Fegg et al., 2014). Optimizing opportunities for accessing areas that support life meaning for HCPs may not only influence care of patients and families but also may play an important role in the mental hygiene of HCPs working in demanding areas of healthcare (Fegg et al., 2014; Fillion et al., 2009).

## ■ CONCLUSION

The Theory of Meaning can be a useful guide in research and practice. The theory focuses on discovering meaning when facing life challenges that threaten one's purpose in relation to unique circumstances. Nurse researchers and practitioners can draw on the theory to understand ordinary life stresses, as well as life-changing events and human suffering.

## ■ REFERENCES

Ameli, M., & Dattilio, F. M. (2013). Enhancing cognitive behavior therapy with logotherapy: techniques for clinical practice. *Psychotherapy.(Chic.)*, *50*, 387–391.

Ascher, L. M., & Schotte, D. E. (1999). Paradoxical intention and recursive anxiety. *Journal of Behavior Therapy and Experimental Psychiatry*, *30*, 71–79.

Ataoglu, A., Ozcetin, A., Icmeli, C., & Ozbulut, O. (2003). Paradoxical therapy in conversion reaction. *Journal of Korean medical science*, *18*, 581–584.

Baldacchino, D. (2010). Long-term causal meaning of myocardial infarction. *British Journal of Nursing*, *19*(12), 774–781.

Baldacchino, D. (2011). Myocardial infarction: A turning point in meaning in life over time. *British Journal of Nursing*, *20*(2), 107–114.

Brandstatter, M., Baumann, U., Borasio, G. D., & Fegg, M. J. (2012). Systematic review of meaning in life assessment instruments. *Psychooncology*, *21*, 1034–1052.

Brandstatter, M., Kogler, M., Baumann, U., Fensterer, V., Kuchenhoff, H., Borasio, G. D., & Fegg, M. J. (2014). Experience of meaning in life in bereaved informal caregivers of palliative care patients. *Supportive Care in Cancer*, *22*, 1391–1399.

Breitbart, W., Gibson, C., Poppito, S. R., & Berg, A. (2004). Psychotherapeutic interventions at the end of life: A focus on meaning and spirituality. *Canadian Journal of Psychiatry*, *49*(6), 366–372.

Brunelli, C., Bianchi, E., Murru, L., Monformoso, P., Bosisio, M., Gangeri, L., . . . Borreani, C. (2012). Italian validation of the Purpose in life (PIL) test and the Seeking Of Noetic Goals (SONG) test in a population of cancer patients. *Supportive Care in Cancer, 20,* 2775–2783.

Cho, S. (2008). Effects of Logo-autobiography Program on Meaning in Life and Mental Health in the Wives of Alcoholics. *Asian Nursing Research, 2,* 129–139.

Coward, D. D. (1991). Self-transcendence and emotional well-being in women with advanced breast cancer. *Oncology Nursing Forum, 18,* 857–863.

Coward, D. D. (1994). Meaning and purpose in the lives of persons with AIDS. *Public Health Nursing, 11,* 331–336.

Coward, D. D. (1995). The lived experience of self-transcendence in women with AIDS. *Journal of Obstetric, Gynecologic and Neonatal Nursing, 24,* 314–318.

Coward, D. D. (1996). Self-transcendence and correlates in a health population. *Nursing Research, 45*(2), 116–121.

Coward, D. D. (1998). Facilitation of self-transcendence in a breast cancer support group. *Oncology Nursing Forum, 25*(1), 75–84.

Coward, D. D., & Dickerson, D. (2003). Facilitation of self-transcendence in breast cancer support group: II. *Oncology Nursing Forum, 30*(2), 291–300.

Coward, D. D., & Kahn, D. L. (2004). Resolution of spiritual disequilibrium by women newly diagnosed with breast cancer. *Oncology Nursing Forum, 31*(2), 24–31.

Coward, D. D., & Kahn, D. L. (2005). Transcending breast cancer: Making meaning from diagnosis and treatment. *Journal of Holistic Nursing, 23*(3), 264–283.

Coward, D. D., & Lewis, F. M. (1993). The lived experience of self-transcendence in gay men with AIDS. *Oncology Nursing Forum, 20,* 1363–1368.

Coward, D. D., & Reed, P. G. (1996). Self-transcendence: A resource for healing at the end of life. *Issues in Mental Health Nursing, 17,* 275–288.

Crumbaugh, J. C. (1968). Cross-validation of purpose in life test based on Frankl's concepts. *Journal of Individual Psychology, 24,* 74–81.

Crumbaugh, J. C. (1977). The Seeking of Noetic Goals test (SONG): A complementary scale to the purpose in life test (PIL). *Journal of Clinical Psychology, 33,* 900–907.

Crumbaugh, J. C., & Maholick, L. T. (1964). An experimental study in existentialism: The psychometric approach to Frankl's concept of noogenic neurosis. *Journal of Clinical Psychology, 20,* 200–207.

Dattilio, F., & Hanna, M., (2012). Collaboration in cognitive-behavioral therapy. *Journal of Clinical Psychology:In session, 68*(2), 146–158.

Faramarzi, S., & Bavali, F. (2017). The effectiveness of group logotherapy to improve psychological well-being of mothers with intellectually disabled children. *International Journal of Developmental Disabilities, 63*(1), 45–51. doi:10.1080/2047386 9.2016.1144298

Fabry, J. B. (1980). *The pursuit of meaning.* New York, NY: Harper & Row.

Fabry, J. B. (1991). *Guideposts to meaning: Discovering what really matters.* Oakland, CA: New Harbinger.

Fegg, M. J., Kogler, M., Abright, C., Hensler, M., & Lorenzl, S. (2014). Meaning in life in patients with progressive supranuclear palsy. *American Journal of Hospice and Palliative Medicine, 31,* 543–547.

Fegg, M. J., Kramer, M., L'hoste, S., & Borasio, G. D. (2008). The Schedule for Meaning in Life Evaluation (SMiLE): Validation of a new instrument for meaning-in-life research. *Journal of Pain and Symptom Management, 35,* 356–364.

Fegg, M. J., L'hoste, S., Brandstatter, M., & Borasio, G. D. (2014). Does the working environment influence health care professionals' values, meaning in life and religiousness? Palliative care units compared with maternity wards. *Journal of Pain and Symptom Management, 48,* 915–923.

Fillion, L., Dupuis, R., Tremblay, I., De Grace, G. R., & Breitbart, W. (2006). Enhancing meaning in palliative care practice: A meaning-centered intervention to promote job satisfaction. *Palliative and Supportive Care, 4,* 333–344.

Fillion, L., Duval, S., Dumont, S., Gagnon, P., Tremblay, I., Bairati, I., & Breitbart, W. S. (2009). Impact of a meaning-centered intervention on job satisfaction and on quality of life among palliative care nurses. *Psycho-Oncology, 18,* 1300–1310.

Fjelland, J. E., Barron, C. R., & Foxall, M. (2008). A review of instruments measuring two aspects of meaning: Search for meaning and meaning in illness. *Journal of Advanced Nursing, 62*(4), 394–406.

Frankl, V. E. (1961). Dynamics, existence, and values. *Journal of Existential Psychiatry, 11*(5), 5–16.

Frankl, V. E. (1969). *The will to meaning.* New York, NY: New American Library.

Frankl, V. E. (1973). *The doctor and the soul.* New York, NY: Vintage.

Frankl, V. E. (1975). *The unconscious God.* New York, NY: Simon & Schuster.

Frankl, V. E. (1978). *The unheard cry for meaning.* New York, NY: Simon & Schuster.

Frankl, V. E. (1984). *Man's search for meaning: An introduction to logotherapy.* Boston, MA: Beacon.

Frankl, V. E. (2004). *On the theory and therapy of mental disorders (J. M. Dubois, Trans.).* New York, NY: Brunner-Routledge.

Haugan, G. (2014). Meaning-in-life in nursing-home patients: a valuable approach for enhancing psychological and physical well-being? *Journal of Clinical Nursing, 23,* 1830–1844.

Haugan, G., & Moksnes, U. K. (2013). Meaning-in-life in nursing home patients: A validation study of the Purpose-in-Life test. *Journal of Nursing Measurement, 21,* 296–319.

Haugan, G., Moksnes, U. K., & Lohre, A. (2016). Intrapersonal self-transcendence, meaning-in-life and nurse-patient interaction: Powerful assets for quality of life in cognitively intact nursing-home patients. *Scandinavian Journal of Caring Sciences, 30,* 790–801.

Hedberg, P., Gustafson, Y., & Brulin, C. (2010). Purpose in life among men and women aged 85 years and older. *The International Journal of Aging and Human Development, 70,* 213–229.

Jim, H. S., & Andersen, B. L. (2007). Meaning in life mediates the relationship between social and physical functioning and distress in cancer survivors. *British Journal of Health Psychology, 12,* 363–381.

Kahn, D. L., & Steeves, R. H. (1995). The significance of suffering in cancer care. *Seminars in Oncology Nursing, 11*(1), 9–16.

Kang, S. K., & Kim, W. (2011). A study of battered women's purpose of life and resilience in South Korea. *Asian Social Work and Policy Review, 5*, 145–159.

Kudla, D., Kujur, J., Tigga, S., Tirkey, P., Rai, P., & Fegg, M. J. (2015). Meaning in life experience at the end of life: Validation of the Hindi version of the Schedule for Meaning in Life Evaluation and a cross-cultural comparison between Indian and German palliative care patients. *Journal of Pain and Symptom Management, 49*, 79–88.

Kerlinger, F. H. (1973). *Foundations of research* (2nd ed.). New York, NY: Holt, Rinehart, and Winston.

Lee, V. (2008). The existential plight of cancer: Meaning making as a concrete approach to the intangible search for meaning. *Supportive Care in Cancer, 16*, 779–785.

Lee, V., Cohen, S. R., Edgar, L., Laizner, A. M., & Gagnon, A. J. (2006). Meaning-making and psychological adjustment to cancer: Development of an intervention and pilot results. *Oncology Nursing Forum, 33*(2), 291–302.

Litwinczuk, K. M., & Groh, C. J. (2007). The relationship between spirituality, purpose in life, and well-being in HIV-positive persons. *Journal of the Association of Nurses in Aids Care, 18*(3), 13–22.

Lukas, E. (1984). *Meaningful living: A logotherapeutic guide to health*. Cambridge, MA: Schenkman.

Lukas, E. (1986). *Meaning in suffering: Comfort in crisis through logotherapy*. Berkeley, CA: Institute of Logotherapy Press.

Mahdizadeh, M., Alavi, M., & Ghazavi, Z. (2016). The effect of education based on the main concepts of logotherapy approach on the quality of life in patients after coronary artery bypass grafting surgery. *Iranian Journal of Nursing and Midwifery Research, 21*, 14–19.

Martin, R. A., MacKinnon, S., Johnson, J., & Rohsenow, D. (2011). Purpose in life predicts treatment outcome among adult cocaine abusers in treatment. *Journal of Substance Abuse Treatment, 40*, 183–188.

Mello, I. T., & Ashcraft, A. S. (2014). The meaning in life for patients recently hospitalized with congestive heart failure. *Journal of the American Association of Nurse Practitioners, 26*, 70–76.

Mohabbat-Bahar, S., Golzari, M., Moradi-Joo, M., & Akbari, M. E. (2014). Efficacy of group logotherapy on decreasing anxiety in women with breast cancer. *Iranian Journal of Cancer Prevention, 7*, 165–170.

Morgenthaler, T., Kramer, M., Alessi, C., Friedman, L., Boehlecke, B., Brown, T., . . . Swick, T. (2006). Practice parameters for the psychological and behavioral treatment of insomnia: An update. An American Academy of Sleep Medicine report. *Sleep, 29*(11), 1415–1419.

Mosalanejad, L., & Khodabakshi, K. A. (2013). Looking at infertility treatment through the lens of the meaning of life: the effect of Group Logotherapy on psychological distress in infertile women. *International Journal of Sterility and Fertility, 6*, 224–231.

Pearce, M. (2005). Appeal and application of logotherapy in parish nursing practice. *The International Forum of Logotherapy: Journal of Search for Meaning, 28*(1), 26–30.

Peter, C., Muller, R., Post, M. W., van Leeuwen, C. M., Werner, C. S., & Geyh, S. (2014). Psychological resources, appraisals, and coping and their relationship to participation in spinal cord injury: A path analysis. *Archives of Physical Medicine and Rehabilitation, 95,* 1662–1671.

Peter, C., Muller, R., Post, M. W., van Leeuwen, C. M., Werner, C. S., & Geyh, S. (2015). Depression in spinal cord injury: Assessing the role of psychological resources. *Rehabilitation Psychology, 60,* 67–80.

Robatmili, S., Sohrabi, F., Shahrak, M. A., Talepasand, S., Nokani, M., & Hasani, M. (2015). The effect of group logotherapy on meaning in life and depression levels of Iranian students. *International Journal for the Advancement of Counselling, 37,* 54–62.

Scrignaro, M., Bianchi, E., Brunelli, C., Miccinesi, G., Ripamonti, C. I., Magrin, M. E., . . . Borreani, C. (2015). Seeking and experiencing meaning: exploring the role of meaning in promoting mental adjustment and eudaimonic well-being in cancer patients. *Palliative and Supportive Care, 13,* 673–681.

Sheikh, A. I., & Marotta, S. A. (2008). Best practices for counseling in cardiac rehabilitation settings. *Journal of Counseling & Development, 86,* 111–120.

Southwick, S. M., Gilmartin, R., McDonough, P., & Morrissey, P. (2006). Logotherapy as an adjunctive treatment for chronic combat-related PTSD: A meaning-based intervention. *American Journal of Psychotherapy, 60*(2), 161–174.

Starck, P. L. (1979). Spinal cord injured clients' perception of meaning and purpose in life, measurement before and after nursing intervention. *Dissertation Abstracts International, 40*(10), 4741. (UMI No. 8007891)

Starck, P. L. (1983). Patient's perceptions of the meaning of suffering. *International Forum for Logotherapy, 6,* 110–116.

Starck, P. L. (1985). Logotherapy comes of age: Birth of a theory. *The International Forum of Logotherapy: Journal of Search for Meaning, 8*(2), 71–75.

Starck, P. L., & McGovern, J. P. (1992). The meaning in suffering. In P. L. Starck & J. P. McGovern (Eds.), *The hidden dimension of illness: Human suffering* (pp. 25–42). New York, NY: National League for Nursing Press.

Starck, P. L., Ulrich, E., & Duffy, M. E. (2009). The meaning of suffering experiences. In Batthyany & Levinson (Eds), *Existential psychotherapy of meaning: A handbook of logotherapy and existential analysis.* Phoenix, AZ: Zeis, Tucker & Theisen.

Steeves, R. H. (1992). Patients who have undergone bone marrow transplantation: Their quest for meaning. *Oncology Nursing Forum, 19,* 899–905.

Steeves, R. H. (1996). Loss, grief, and the search for meaning. *Oncology Nursing Society, 23,* 897–903.

Steeves, R. H., & Kahn, D. L. (1987). Experience of meaning in suffering. *Journal of Nursing Scholarship, 19*(3), 114–116.

Steeves, R. H., Kahn, D. L., & Benoliel, J. Q. (1990). Nurses' interpretation of the suffering of their patients. *Western Journal of Nursing Research, 12*(6), 715–731.

Taubman-Ben-Ari, O., & Weintraub, A. (2008). Meaning in life and personal growth among pediatric physicians and nurses. *Death Studies, 32,* 621–645.

Thege, B. K., Bachner, Y. G., Martos, T., & Kushnir, T. (2009). Meaning in life: Does it play a role in smoking? *Substance Use & Misuse, 44,* 1566–1577.

Tomas-Sabado, J., Villavicencio-Chavez, C., Monforte-Royo, C., Guerrero-Torrelles, M., Fegg, M. J., & Balaguer, A. (2015). What gives meaning in life to patients with advanced cancer? A comparison between Spanish, German, and Swiss patients. *Journal of Pain and Symptom Management, 50,* 861–866.

Travelbee, J. (1966). *Interpersonal aspects of nursing.* Philadelphia, PA: F. A. Davis.

Travelbee, J. (1969). *Intervention in psychiatric nursing: Process in the one-to-one relationship.* Philadelphia, PA: F. A. Davis.

Travelbee, J. (1972). To find meaning in illness. *Nursing, 72*(2), 6–7.

Verduin, P. J. M., de Bock, G. H., Vliet Vlieland, T. P. M., Peeters, A. J., Verhoef, J., & Otten, W. (2008). Purpose in life in patients with rheumatoid arthritis. *Clinical Rheumatology, 27,* 899–908.

Winters, M., & Schulenberg, S. (2006). Diagnosis in logotherapy: Overuse and suggestions for appropriate use. *The International Forum of Logotherapy: Journal of Search for Meaning, 29*(1), 16–24.

White, C. A. (2004). Meaning and its measurement in psychosocial oncology. *Psychooncology, 13,* 468–481.

Wong, P. T. P. (2010). Meaning therapy: An integrative and positive existential psychotherapy. *Journal of Contemporary Psychotherapy, 40,* 85–93.

# CHAPTER 6

## Theory of Bureaucratic Caring

**Marilyn A. Ray**

In 1977, Leininger declared that "caring: [is] the essence and central focus of nursing" (p. 1). From an anthropological perspective, caring is one of the oldest and most universal expectations for human development and survival throughout human history. Caring is claimed by archeologists (besides the evolution of the brain) as paramount in human development (Ray, 1981b). Based on a philosophical analysis related to meaningfulness and understanding, I determined that, for nursing, caring and love are synonymous (Ray, 1981a, p. 32). Four decades ago, as a doctoral student researcher, my passion was the study of caring within hospitals as a way of knowing caring in nursing in practice. I wanted to learn about the meaning of care and caring in the hospital culture, and embarked on a study focusing on the *meaning and action* of caring. My dissertation was a qualitative study that laid the foundation for the Theory of Bureaucratic Caring. This chapter about the Theory of Bureaucratic Caring includes: explication of the purpose of the theory; description of processes undertaken to generate the middle range theory; definition of the theoretical concepts; and identification of uses of the theory in research and practice.

### ■ PURPOSE OF THE THEORY AND HOW IT WAS DEVELOPED

The middle range Theory of Bureaucratic Caring was discovered through description, analysis, and interpretation of the meaning of the phenomenon of caring in the complex institutional culture of the hospital. Interview data were analyzed from over 192 diverse healthcare professionals including nurses, physicians, and allied health personnel as well as patients. Also included were field notes or memos from participant observation of the nursing/social process in the hospital culture. This analysis prompted deep reflective thinking about the meaning of the lived experience of caring and interpretation of patterns of culture or the organizational context from which the meaning was derived. The initial analysis led to the integration of data into a classification system of institutional caring—psychological, practical, interactional, and philosophical (Ray, 1981b, 1984). Subsequently, substantive and formal grounded theories were discovered to articulate the fullness of the meaning of caring in the organizational context. Qualitative data illuminated a paradox, juxtaposing the meaning of caring as humanistic, spiritual, and ethical with the bureaucratic system as political, economic, technological, legal, educational, and social–cultural. Through the use of Hegelian dialectical analysis of the thesis (caring) and antithesis (bureaucracy), a synthesis was articulated as the Theory of Bureaucratic Caring (Ray, 1981b, 1984, 2010a).

## ■ EVOLUTION OF THE THEORY OF BUREAUCRATIC CARING

Over three decades, with the research expertise of Dr. Marian Turkel and federally funded grants using research approaches that drew on our growing understanding of complexity sciences, testing of the Theory of Bureaucratic Caring was ongoing. We accomplished tool development using mixed methods to create valid and reliable professional and patient questionnaires, focusing on economic caring. Further data collection and analysis of the meaning of caring in organizational cultures in public, private, and military hospitals led to the determination that the Theory of Bureaucratic Caring demanded holographic expression with *spiritual–ethical caring* as the central essence. Many publications validated the theory as a middle range theory with strong potential for guiding practice and research (Coffman, 2014, 2018; Davidson, Ray, & Turkel, 2011; Gibson, 2008; Ray, 1987a, 1987b, 1989, 1997, 1998a, 1998b, 2010a, 2010b, 2010c, 2010d, 2010e, 2011, 2013a, 2013b, 2016; Ray & Turkel, 2010, 2012, 2014, 2015; Ray, Turkel, & Marino, 2002; Ray, Morris, & McFarland, 2013; Turkel, 2007; Turkel & Ray, 2000, 2001, 2004).

*ask students – give example of each*

## ■ CONCEPTS OF THE THEORY

**Bureaucratic Caring** is spiritual–ethical caring emerging in bureaucracies. Bureaucracies are complex systems with political, legal, economic, technological, physical, educational and social–cultural dimensions. The central concept of the Theory of Bureaucratic Caring is spiritual–ethical caring. Spiritual–ethical caring interconnects with the dimensional concepts gleaned and interpreted from data. Each of the concepts of the theory is briefly defined.

**Spiritual–Ethical Caring** is defined as creativity, loyalty, faithfulness to spiritual or religious traditions and is revealed in patterns of love, compassion, empathy, respect, and communication to facilitate moral choices for the good of self, persons, things, and the environment.

The **Social–Cultural** dimension is defined as values, beliefs, and attitudes regarding ethnicity, patterns of identity, or diverse social structures, such as family and communities that impact social structures, political, economic, legal, and technological factors in complex national or international systems.

The **Physical** dimension is defined as factors related to the physical, mental, and emotional states of being, health/illness, healing, and dying (or peaceful death) of patients or persons in organizational healthcare contexts.

The **Educational** dimension is defined as both formal and informal teaching–learning communicating caring processes and programs to improve the health, healing, and well-being of persons, families, communities, and organizations.

The **Political** dimension is defined as the energy patterns and communicative action associated with power, control, and authoritative behaviors, usually of leaders, administrators, and staff. Political relates to hierarchical systems, roles and their differentiation or stratification, unions, and governmental influences that facilitate competition and cooperation in complex organizations.

The **Economic** dimension is defined as the exchange of goods, money, services, insurance systems, and healthcare laws, including an understanding of caring as interpersonal resources to appreciate and manage budgets and to maintain the financial viability and fiscal management of an organization that interfaces with the larger community or social structure.

The **Technological** dimension is defined as nonhuman resources, such as machines and diagnostic instruments, pharmacologic agents, computers, electronic health records (EHRs), smartphones, social media in the virtual world, and robots, and the ethical caring knowledge and skill needed to support persons, families, communities, organizations, and cultures.

The **Legal** dimension is defined as factors related to responsibility and accountability for rules, regulations, standards of practice, procedures, informed consent, rights to privacy, professional behaviors, insurance systems or laws, and issues that endeavor to facilitate social justice and stability in complex systems.

## ■ RELATIONSHIP AMONG THE CONCEPTS: THE MODEL

The model of the Theory of Bureaucratic Caring (Figure 6.1) is represented by a circle that shows the interrelationship among the central and surrounding concepts. The theory model is intended to be holographic in the sense that the part and the whole are interconnected, "…everything is a whole in one context and a part in another—each part being in the whole and the whole being in the part" (Ray & Turkel, 2015, pp. 464–465). Spiritual–ethical caring is central to the model and relates to and with dimensional concepts (economic, political, legal, technological, educational, physical, social–cultural) at the periphery of the circle. Data revealed that the meaning of caring was not only spiritual and ethical but also was expressed by participants in the research and interpreted by the researcher as contextual—the interrelationship of caring with structural phenomena of complex organizations, the bureaucracy. "Caring [spiritual–ethical caring] is a relational pattern; it is the

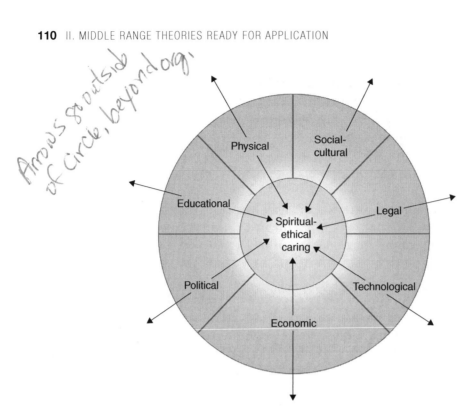

*Arrows go outside of circle, beyond org.*

**FIGURE 6.1** Holographic theory of bureaucratic caring.

*Source:* With permission from Parker, M., & Smith, M. (2015). *Nursing theories and nursing practice* (4th ed.). Philadelphia, PA: F. A. Davis.

flow of nurses' and others own experiences in the structural context of the organization [the bureaucracy]" (Ray & Turkel, 2015, p. 464). The arrows in the model extend outward from each of the dimensional concepts to show that Bureaucratic Caring connects beyond the organization, to the environment or the social world or culture at large.

Bureaucracies are cultures; they are cocreated through the interactions of people within them, each with their specific cultural orientations, goals, norms, patterns of behaviors, rituals, professional practices, and languages. Spiritual–ethical caring thus is in relationship with the dimensional concepts descriptive of the organization—economic, political, technological, legal, physical, educational, and social–cultural (Ray & Turkel, 2015). As a living system, the bureaucratic organization manifests in different ways depending on the processes that are valued. Bureaucratic organizations thus are "complex, dynamic, relational, integral, informational, computational and emergent, and open to sets of possibilities" (Ray & Turkel, 2015. p. 465). Decisions are made in networks of relationships that represent a simultaneous patterning of interacting parts. The Theory of Bureaucratic Caring (Coffman, 2014, 2018; Davidson, Ray, & Turkel, 2011; Ray & Turkel, 2015) emerges to reflect the reality of what it means to care for persons in an organization in the contemporary Western and developing world.

# ■ USE OF THE THEORY IN NURSING RESEARCH

The following presentation illuminates the diverse ways in which the Theory of Bureaucratic Caring was tested or used to guide research. Classification systems, conceptual models, or further middle range theories emerged from this theory-guided research. For example, a classification system, called an Institutional Caring Classification System, was developed by Ray (1984). A conceptual model of Technological Caring, called Experiential and Principle-Based Ethics in Critical Care, was intuited from a phenomenological study of patients and nurses in the intensive care unit (Ray, 1987b). Clarification of the ethical principles of beneficence, justice, and autonomy emerged from this study. A theory of Reflective Ethics emerged from a study in a critical care step-down unit (Ray, 1998a). Technological Caring was reinforced in the research of Wu and colleagues on the use of virtual technologies in a study of patients with cardiac disease comorbid with diabetes (Wu & Ray, 2016). From knowledge on economic caring reported by Ray (1981b, 1989), Turkel (1997) discovered *Struggling to Find a Balance: A Grounded Theory of the Nurse-Patient Relationship Within an Economic Context*. Ray and Turkel conducted research from 1995 to 2004 using Grounded Theory, phenomenological methods, and other mixed methods for the study of caring and the economics of caring in diverse public, private, and military hospitals (Davidson, Ray, & Turkel, 2011; Ray & Turkel, 2009; 2012; Turkel & Ray, 2000, 2001). Political caring was identified in a study of reservists in the U.S. Air Force (USAF) regarding the expansion of the military TriCare health system (Ray & Turkel, 2001; Turkel & Ray, 2003). All of the research of Ray and Turkel led to further grounded theories: the Theory of Relational Complexity, the Theory of Relational Caring Complexity; and a Theory of Workplace Redevelopment (Ray, Turkel, & Marino, 2002). The economic caring research of Ray and Turkel was enhanced by theoretical testing and tool development to understand more fully the meaning and the statistical significance of the economics and politics of caring.

Many researchers were interested in theory-guided research and practice using the Theory of Bureaucratic Caring. In 1997, Valentine applied the theory in her study of economics and caring. Prestia (2016a) followed through with an application of Ray's ideas (1997) emerging from a phenomenological study of caring in nursing administration; Prestia studied caring strategies for living leadership presence in nursing administration. Nyberg (1990) applied the Theory of Bureaucratic Caring to facilitate understanding, research and development of nursing economics with nurse administrators and in the organizational culture. Eggenberger (2011) used the theory to guide a qualitative research related to charge nurses on the front line of practice. Conroy (2013) applied the Theory of Bureaucratic Caring in a study of the effect of the organizational culture on implementation of evidence-based practice and how the staff assigns a value to improvements in nursing practice. The Theory of Bureaucratic Caring was incorporated by Prestia (2016b) into her dissertation research, a phenomenological study of chief nursing officers in the continued practice of nursing leadership. In the USAF Medical Service, a research study was conducted by Potter (2015) using the Theory for Nurse-Directed Primary Care of patients with type 2 diabetes resulting in quality improvements in clinical health and healing and sizable economic outcomes. In the Veterans Administration, Lusk (2015) conducted a mixed method study using the Theory of Bureaucratic Caring to compare the knowledge, skills, and attitudes of newly hired nursing staff before and after the implementation of a quality and safety competency-based nursing orientation program.

Overall, the Theory of Bureaucratic Caring has provided substantive guidance for researchers wishing to focus on systems of care and those who are employed in those systems. It is a middle range theory that shifts attention to macrosystem perspectives, linking institutional culture, while considering the interplay of macrosystems with microsystems, like caring. The theory provides a structure for researchers to study the meaning of caring in institutional nursing and healthcare practice.

## ■ USE OF THE THEORY IN NURSING PRACTICE AND EDUCATION

Nursing practice addresses the needs of patients, nurses, and administrators as well as an understanding of the context within which nursing practice occurs. The challenge in nursing practice is the integration of knowledge gleaned from nursing education and experience, which should align with the philosophy, vision, and values that nursing has adopted. The Magnet Recognition Program® has been established to achieve nursing excellence by incorporating theory-guided or conceptual professional practice models to transform nursing and healthcare (Turkel, 2004). Theory-guided practice encompasses the why of nursing through ways in which practitioners of nursing have integrated their knowledge and understanding of what makes things work—the pedagogy, philosophy of caring, health, and social–cultural sciences to inform the art of nursing. The philosopher Hans-Georg Gadamer remarked that we, as human beings are always *theorizing*—we are meaning-making people who are always seeking to understand—trying to make sense out of relationships and things of this world (van Manen, 2014). The art of practice, thus ". . . serves to foster and strengthen the embodied ontology [way of being], epistemology [ways of knowing], and axiology [ways of valuing what is valuable or ethical] of thoughtful and tactful action" (van Manen, 2014, p. 15). The following highlights ways in which the Theory of Bureaucratic Caring is being used to guide nursing education as well as nursing, healthcare, and organizational practice.

O'Brien (2008) incorporated the core principles of the Theory of Bureaucratic Caring in her project to orient new public health nursing consultants in a major state public health nursing system (Personal communication, 2008). In a correctional facility for adolescents in Georgia, McCray-Stewart used the theory to improve the care of young detainees and reduce recidivism (Personal communication, 2008). In 2012, Iowa Health (three hospitals), in Des Moines, Iowa, adopted the Theory of Bureaucratic Caring to guide interprofessional practice (Iowa Health) and as the theoretical foundation for Magnet recognition status to become a center of excellence.

Elevating a successful innovation of an interprofessional practice model is focused on a commitment by leaders to all stakeholders. Leaders must be cognizant of how a system can continue to form or enhance relationships with its members in current and projected environments. A significant goal of achieving the status of a Magnet facility employs both the spread or horizontal diffusion of an idea, such as a nursing theory or model of caring, and scale or centralized action to implement a single system of excellence for nursing and other disciplinary practices across a whole organization (Bar-Yam, 2004; Martin, 2017; Turkel, 2004). Collaboration of this magnitude for policy development takes knowledge of theory, and a theory-guided effort to determine its impact on a complex organization and multidisciplinary practice. The collaboration takes a deep understanding of relationships and caring communication, especially in a complex bureaucratic culture and with people who may continue to embrace an individualized professional culture or belief system. The process of developing a model using the middle range Theory of Bureaucratic Caring in the Iowa Health System took a commitment by nurse leaders and others to make things work (Bar-Yam, 2004). Inspiring a collection of diverse healthcare providers from varying disciplines to undertake whole system change focused on unified healthcare is a challenge but the Iowa Health System embraced the challenge.

Within nursing education, the Nevada State College under the leadership of Dr. Sherrilyn Coffman (2014) from 2007 to 2014, applied, in part, the Theory of Bureaucratic Caring for the development of a curriculum model for the Bachelor of Science in Nursing program. In the nursing administration program at the Capital University in Ohio, Burkett (2016) used the theory to guide administrative course development. Johnson (2015) developed a conceptual framework applying the Theory of Bureaucratic Caring for advanced practice nurses as primary care providers using a new approach—making house calls with the homebound population to meet their healthcare needs. The Theory of Bureaucratic Caring is currently being used in nursing education at the National University in Bogota, Colombia, and the University of Santiago in Santiago, Chile.

The Theory of Bureaucratic Caring is being applied in primary nursing practice by the USAF Nurse Corps to improve the care of patients with type 2 diabetes (Potter, 2015). Creation of an Interdisciplinary Professional Person-Centered Practice Model in the USAF is in process.

# ■ CONCLUSION

The Theory of Bureaucratic Caring originated from qualitative research focused on caring in a complex organizational culture. It was published first as a dissertation (Ray, 1981b) and appeared in the literature in 1989 and in subsequent publications noted throughout this chapter (Coffman, 2014, 2018; Ray, 2001, 2010a, 2010e; Ray & Turkel, 2010, 2012, 2014, 2015). The theory symbolizes a dynamic structure of caring that was synthesized from the dialectic of caring as humanistic, social, educational, ethical, and religious/spiritual (elements of humanism and caring), and the antithesis of caring as economic, political, legal, and technological (elements of bureaucracy) into a new synthesis—the Theory of Bureaucratic Caring (Ray, 1989, 2010a, 2010b, 2010c, 2010d, 2010e). The interplay between and among the dimensions highlighting spiritual–ethical caring and the bureaucratic system as holographic or emergent showed that the whole is in the part and the part is in the whole; everything is an unbroken whole (Bohm, 2002; Coffman, 2014). Humanistic caring and the elements of the bureaucracy are value-added. Interactions and symbolic meaning systems are formed and reproduced from the construction of dominant values held within nursing and indeed, other professions, including patients, *and* the organization. A hospital, community health, or a healthcare system is a *living* organization. By understanding and incorporating the Theory of Bureaucratic Caring, nurses bring caring into being that makes a human community and an organization edifying to our spiritual well-being and intellectual lives.

# ■ REFERENCES

Bar-Yam, Y. (2004). *Making things work: Solving complex problems in a complex world.* Boston, MA: NECSI, Knowledge Press.

Bohm, D. (2002). *Wholeness and the implicate order.* London, UK: Routledge.

Burkett, M. (2016). *Nursing administration curriculum.* Columbus, OH: Capital University.

Coffman, S. (2014). Marilyn Anne Ray's theory of bureaucratic caring. In M. Alligood (Ed.), *Nursing theorists and their work* (8th ed., pp. 98–119). St. Louis, MO: Mosby/ Elsevier.

Coffman, S. (2018). Marilyn Anne Ray: Theory of bureaucratic caring. In M. Alligood (Ed.), *Nursing theorists and their work* (9th ed., pp. 80–97). St. Louis, MO: Elsevier.

Conroy, C. (2013). *The effect of organizational culture on the implementation and uptake of evidence-based practice: How staff ascribe value to practice innovation.* Doctor of Nursing Practice Project. Boston, MA: Regis College.

Davidson, A., Ray, M., & Turkel, M. (Eds.). (2011). *Nursing, caring and complexity science: For human-environment well-being.* New York, NY: Springer Publishing.

Eggenberger, T. (2011). *Holding the frontline: The experience of being a charge nurses in an acute care setting* (Dissertation). The Christine E. Lynn College of Nursing, Florida Atlantic University, Boca Raton, FL.

Gibson, S. (2008). Legal caring: Preventing retraumatization of abused children through the caring nursing interview using Roach's six Cs. *International Association for Human Caring*, *12*(4), 32–37.

Johnson, P. (2015). Ray's theory of bureaucratic caring: A conceptual framework for APRN primary care providers and the homebound population. *International Journal for Human Caring*, *19*(2), 41–44.

Leininger, M. (1977). The phenomenon of caring. Part V. Caring: The essence and central focus of nursing. *Nursing Research Report*, *1*, 2, 4.

Lusk, D. (2015). *Comparing the knowledge, skills and attitudes of newly hired nursing staff before and after implementation of a quality and safety competency-based nursing orientation program*. Doctor of Nursing Practice Project, Denver, CO: Regis University.

Martin, D. (2017). *Better now: Six big ideas to improve health care for all Canadians*. Toronto, Canada: Penguin Books.

Nyberg, J. (1990). The effects of caring and economics on nursing practice. *Nursing Administration Quarterly*, *20*(5), 13–18.

O'Brien, K. (2008). *Application of bureaucratic caring theory in public health nursing*. Director of Public Health Nursing, State of Colorado, Denver CO.

Potter, M. (2015). *Using theory-guided practice to improve diabetes health outcomes in primary care*. Doctor of Nursing Practice Project. Chicago, IL: Chamberlain University.

Prestia, A. (2016a). Existential authenticity: Caring strategies for living leadership presence. *International Journal for Human Caring*, *10*(1), 8–11.

Prestia, A. (2016b). *Chief nursing officer sustainment in the continued practice of nursing leadership: A phenomenological inquiry* (Unpublished doctoral dissertation). Retrieved from ProQuest dissertations database (UMI No. 3691821).

Ray, M. (1981a). A philosophical analysis of caring within nursing. In M. Leininger (Ed.), *Caring: An essential human need*. Thorofare, NJ: Slack.

Ray, M. (1981b). *A study of caring within the institutional culture*. Doctor of Philosophy. University of Utah, Salt Lake City, UT. Dissertation Abstracts International, *42*(06) (University Microfilms No. 8127787).

Ray, M. (1984). The development of a nursing classification system of caring. In M. Leininger (Ed.), *Care: The essence of nursing and health* (pp. 93–112). Thorofare, NJ: Charles B. Slack.

Ray, M. (1987a). Health care economics and human caring: Why the moral conflict must be resolved. *Family and Community Health*, *10*(1), 35–43.

Ray, M. (1987b). Technological caring: A new model in critical care. *Dimensions in Critical Care*, *6*(3), 166–173.

Ray, M. (1989). The theory of bureaucratic caring for nursing practice in the organizational culture. *Nursing Administration Quarterly*, *13*(2), 31–42.

Ray, M. (1997). The ethical theory of existential authenticity: The lived experience of the art of caring in nursing administration. *Canadian Journal of Nursing Research*, *29*(1), 111–126.

Ray, M. (1998a). A phenomenologic study of the interface of caring and technology: A new reflective ethics in intermediate care. *Holistic Nursing Practice, 12*(4), 71–79.

Ray, M. (1998b). Complexity and nursing science. *Nursing Science Quarterly, 11*, 91–93.

Ray, M. (2001). Marilyn Anne Ray, the theory of bureaucratic caring. In M. Parker (Ed.), *Nursing theories and nursing practice* (pp. 431–431). Philadelphia, PA: F. A. Davis.

Ray, M. (2010a). *A study of caring within an institutional culture: The discovery of the theory of bureaucratic caring.* Saarbrücken, Germany: Lambert Academic Publishing.

Ray, M. (2010b). Creating caring organizations and cultures through communitarian ethics. *World Universities Forum Journal, 3*(5), 41–52.

Ray, M. (2010c). Grounded theory method for the study of transcultural nursing. In M. Douglas & D. Pacquiao (Eds.), *Core curriculum for transcultural nursing and health care.* Thousand Oaks, CA: Sage.

Ray, M. (2010d). Phenomenological-hermeneutical research method for the study of transcultural nursing. In M. Douglas & D. Pacquiao (Eds.), *Core curriculum for transcultural nursing and health care.* Thousand Oaks, CA: Sage.

Ray, M. (2010e). *Transcultural caring dynamics in nursing and health care.* Philadelphia, PA: F. A. Davis.

Ray, M. (2011). Complex caring dynamics: A unifying model of nursing inquiry. In A. Davidson, M. Ray, & M. Turkel. (Eds.), *Nursing, caring, and complexity science: For human-environment well-being* (pp. 31–52). New York, NY: Springer Publishing.

Ray, M. (2013a). Caring inquiry: The esthetic process in the way of compassion. In In M. Smith, M. Turkel, & Z. Wolf (Eds.), *Caring classics in nursing* (pp. 339–345). New York, NY: Springer Publishing.

Ray, M. (2013b). The theory of bureaucratic caring. In M. Smith, M. Turkel, & Z. Wolf (Eds.), *Caring classics in nursing* (pp. 309–320). New York, NY: Springer Publishing.

Ray, M. (2016). *Transcultural caring dynamics in nursing and health care* (2nd ed.). Philadelphia, PA: F. A. Davis.

Ray, M., Morris, E., & McFarland, M. (2013). Ethnonursing method of Dr. Madeleine Leininger. In C. Beck (Ed.), *The Routledge international handbook of qualitative nursing research* (pp. 213–229). New York, NY: Routledge.

Ray, M., & Turkel, M. (2001). Impact of TRICARE/managed care on total force readiness. *Military Medicine, 166*(4), 281–289.

Ray, M., & Turkel, M. (2009). Relational caring questionnaires. In J. Watson (Ed.), *Assessing and measuring caring in nursing and health sciences* (2nd ed. pp. 209–218). New York, NY: Springer Publishing.

Ray, M., & Turkel, M. (2010). The theory of bureaucratic caring. In M. Parker & M. Smith (Eds.), *Nursing theory and nursing practice* (3rd ed., pp. 472–494). Philadelphia, PA: F. A. Davis.

Ray, M., & Turkel, M. (2012). A transtheoretical evolution of caring science within complex systems. *International Journal for Human Caring, 16*(2), 28–49. (Includes Patient and Professional questionnaires)

Ray, M., & Turkel. M. (2014). Caring as emancipatory nursing praxis: The theory of Relational Caring Complexity. *Advances in Nursing Science, 37*(2), 137–146.

Ray, M., & Turkel, M. (2015). The theory of bureaucratic caring. In M. Smith & M. Parker (Eds.), *Nursing theory and nursing practice* (4th ed., pp. 461–482). Philadelphia, PA: F. A. Davis.

Ray, M., Turkel, M., & Marino, F. (2002). The transformative process for nursing in workforce redevelopment. *Nursing Administration Quarterly, 26*(2), 1–14.

Turkel, M. (1997). *Struggling to find balance: A grounded theory of the nurse-patient relationship within an economic context* (Doctoral dissertation). University of Miami, Miami, FL.

Turkel, M. (2004). *Magnet status: Assessing, pursuing, and achieving nursing excellence.* Marblehead, MA: HCPro.

Turkel, M. (2007). Dr. Marilyn Ray's theory of bureaucratic caring. *International Journal for Human Caring, 11*(4), 57–74.

Turkel, M., & Ray, M. (2000). Relational complexity: A theory of the nurse-patient relationship within an economic context. *Nursing Science Quarterly, 13*(4), 307–313.

Turkel, M., & Ray, M. (2001). Relational complexity: From grounded theory to instrument development and theoretical testing. *Nursing Science Quarterly, 14*(4), 281–287.

Turkel, M., & Ray, M. (2003). A process model for policy analysis within the context of political caring. *International Journal for Human Caring, 7*(3), 17–25.

Turkel, M., & Ray, M. (2004). Creating a caring practice environment through self-renewal. *Nursing Administration Quarterly, 28*(4), 249–254.

Valentine, K. (1997). Exploration of the relationship between caring and cost. *Holistic Nursing Practice, 11*(4), 71–81.

van Manen, M. (2014). *Phenomenology of practice: Meaning-giving methods in phenomenological research and writing.* Walnut Creek, CA: Left Coast Press.

Wu, C.-J., & Ray, M. (2016). Technological caring for complexities of patient with cardiac disease comorbid with diabetes. *International Journal for Human Caring, 21*(2), 83–87.

# CHAPTER 7

## Theory of Self-Transcendence

**Pamela G. Reed**

A central focus of nursing is in understanding and facilitating the human capacity for well-being in the context of difficult health-related experiences. The nursing Theory of Self-Transcendence was created from a developmental perspective of human–environment processes of health. The word *developmental* is used in the theory to emphasize inherent change processes that are ongoing, innovative, and context-related while also acknowledging inevitable changes that are random or decremental. Self-Transcendence Theory originated from an interest in understanding how people transcend adversity and the relationship among psychosocial development, mental health, and well-being. The theory is applicable to individuals across the life span regarding challenging life experiences, with supporting empirical findings from research with those in adolescence, adulthood, aging, and end of life.

### ■ PURPOSE OF THE THEORY AND HOW IT WAS DEVELOPED

According to the intermodern philosophy of nursing science (Reed, 2011), nursing theories most broadly are open systems of knowledge that incorporate various ways of knowing including empirical, ethical, and practice-based sources. Middle range theory in particular is a structure and process for building nursing knowledge through inquiry and practice. Knowledge from research and practice is organized into theories for creative applications with people who need nursing care. The purpose of the middle range Theory of Self-Transcendence is to provide a framework for inquiry and practice regarding the promotion of well-being in the midst of difficult life situations. Research and practice using Self-Transcendence Theory may generate new discoveries about the processes by which people attain well-being.

The idea for a Theory of Self-Transcendence was influenced by three major events in the history of science, the history of nursing, and my own professional history. First, the 1970s life-span movement in developmental psychology provided philosophical perspective and empirical evidence that the potential for developmental change exists across the life span, beyond childhood and adolescence, into adulthood, and throughout the processes of aging and dying (Reed, 1983). Research findings indicated that developmental change was influenced less by chronological age or passage of time and more by normative and non-normative life events and the accruement of life experiences.

Second, postulations by the scholar Martha Rogers (1970) about the nature of change in human beings provided further inspiration for development of the theory (Reed, 1997b). Rogerian ideas were congruent with life-span principles of development. Philosophical views include the pandimensionality of human beings and the human potential for healing and well-being. Pandimensionality refers in part to various dimensions, known and as yet unknown, about human beings and their environment, and to the capacity to expand personal boundaries in various ways. Several nursing theories were also foundational to the Theory of Self-Transcendence.

Third, this theory was motivated by my clinical nurse specialist practice experiences in applying developmental theories in child and adolescent psychiatric–mental healthcare. Successful approaches to fostering mental health and well-being required in-depth understanding of patients' biopsychosocial developmental processes and the strengths they may obtain through development.

A detailed explanation of how these elements came together in the development of Self-Transcendence Theory is described in Reed (1991b). The predominant approach was deductive reformulation, which incorporated various strategies of theory development from philosophical, theoretical, empirical, and practice-based sources. The underlying assumptions, concepts, and relationships among the concepts involved in the theory development are described in the next two sections. Research and practice, presented in later sections, also influence development and ongoing refinement of the theory.

## ■ CONCEPTS OF THE THEORY

The concept of the Theory of Self-Transcendence derived in part from two major assumptions. First, it is assumed that people are integral with their environment and are pandimensional, as postulated in Rogers's (1980, 1994) Science of Unitary Human Beings. This suggests that human beings may be capable of an awareness that extends beyond physical and temporal dimensions (Reed, 1997a). Using current scientific methods, this is measurable in reference to everyday experiences of expanding one's boundaries by reaching deeper within the self and reaching out to others, to nature, to one's god, or other sources of transcendence. An important point is that *boundaries* not dimensions are transcended. Contrary to views of self-transcendence as meaning a *separation* from self, others, and the environment, in this theory self-transcendence refers to *connections with* self, others, and the environment.

The second assumption is that self-transcendence is a developmental imperative, meaning that it is a human resource that demands expression as do other developmental processes such as walking in toddlers, abstract reasoning in adolescents, and grieving in those who have suffered a loss. These resources are a part of being human and facilitate potential for well-being. As such, the person's participation in self-transcendence is integral to well-being, and nursing has a role in facilitating this process.

## Self-Transcendence

Self-transcendence is the central concept of the theory. It refers to the capacity to expand personal boundaries in many ways, examples of which are as follows: intrapersonally (toward greater awareness of one's philosophy, values, and dreams), interpersonally (to relate to others and one's environment), temporally (to integrate one's past and future in a way that has meaning for the present), and transpersonally (to connect with dimensions beyond the typically observable world). Self-transcendence is a characteristic of developmental maturity in terms of an enhanced awareness of the environment and an orientation toward broadened perspectives about life. It is expressed and measured through life perspectives and behaviors that reflect expansion of personal boundaries.

## Developmental Theories

Neo-Piagetian theories about development in adulthood and later life were influential in formulating the concept of self-transcendence. Beginning in the 1970s, life-span development researchers discovered *postformal* patterns of thinking in older adults that extended beyond Piaget's formal operations, once thought to be the final stage of cognitive development. Life-span developmental theories on social–cognitive development extended Piaget's original theory on reasoning, which had identified *formal operations* (abstract and symbolic reasoning) in youth and young adulthood as the apex of cognitive development. Researchers identified *postformal* stages from older adults' continued social and cognitive development well into later life beyond the phase of formal operations, for example, Arlin's (1975) problem-finding stage, Riegel's (1976) and Basseches's (1984) dialectic operations, and Koplowitz's (1984) unitary stage. Researchers found that this mature reasoning was more contextual, more pragmatic, more spiritual, and more tolerant of ambiguity and paradoxes in life than was the reasoning of earlier developmental phases (e.g., Commons, Demick, & Goldberg, 1996; Sinnott, 1998, 2011). The person using this mature form of reasoning does not seek absolute answers to questions in life but rather seeks meaning from perspectives beyond the immediate situation that integrate moral, social, and historical dimensions. A perspective of relativism from seeing multiple, sometimes conflicting views is balanced by the ability to make a commitment to one's beliefs.

Self-transcendence was conceptualized in reference to these views, with goals more in line with Erikson's generativity and ego integrity than with self-absorbed strivings for identity and intimacy characteristic of earlier developmental phases (Sheldon & Kasser, 2001). Self-transcendence is expressed through various behaviors and perspectives such as sharing wisdom with others, integrating the physical changes of aging, accepting death as a part of life, having an interest in helping others and learning about the world, letting go of losses, and finding spiritual meaning in life.

## Nursing Theories

Self-transcendence is a concept relevant to nursing. Themes of self-transcendence are evident in other nursing *theories*. For example, in Parse's (1992, 2015) paradigm of human becoming, cotranscending is a major theme underlying the philosophical assumptions of her theory and "inspiring transcendence" is an exemplary nursing practice. Newman's (1994) theory of health as expanding consciousness postulates a transcendence of time and space as one reaches beyond illness to develop an awareness of one's patterns, self-identity, and higher level of consciousness. Although all of these theorists present unique views of transcendence, they generally share the idea of expanded awareness beyond the immediate or constricted views of oneself and the world to transform life experiences into healing (Reed, 1996). More recently, developmental psychologists studying self-transcendence suggested it is a universal concept related to well-being in adulthood and aging, as a way of extending personal boundaries outward to others and the community (Hofer et al., 2016).

## Nursing Philosophy

Self-transcendence is also congruent with *philosophical* views of nursing. Sarter (1988) identified the term as one of the central themes in the philosophical foundations of nursing. Newman's (1992) unitary–transformative paradigm presents human beings as embedded in an ongoing developmental process of changing complexity and organization, a process integrally related to well-being. Furthermore, self-transcendence is an example of Reed's (1997a) ontology of nursing, where nursing most basically is defined as a self-organizing process inherent among human systems that is related to well-being. Maslow (1969) is frequently cited for his concept of self-transcendence, but his conceptualization diverges from nursing by his view of self-transcendence as an elevation or a separation of self from the environment. It is an awareness of person–environment connections when fragmentation threatens one's well-being (Reed, 1997b).

## Well-Being

A second major concept of the theory is well-being. Well-being is a sense of feeling whole and healthy, in accord with one's own criteria for wholeness and health. Well-being may be defined in many ways, depending upon the individual or patient population. Indicators of well-being are as diverse as human perceptions of health and wellness, for example, life satisfaction, positive self-concept, hopefulness, happiness, morale, self-care, and sense of meaning in life.

Self-transcendence, as a basic human pattern of development, is logically linked with positive, health-promoting experiences and is therefore a correlate if not a predictor and resource for well-being. Well-being is a correlate and outcome of self-transcendence. Theoretical analyses and empirical studies have consistently supported this conceptualization of self-transcendence as a contributor to well-being (Lundman et al., 2010; McCarthy, 2011; Reed, 2009; Teixeira, 2008).

## Vulnerability

Another key concept of the theory is vulnerability. Vulnerability involves awareness of personal mortality or risk to one's well-being. It is theorized that self-transcendence, as a developmental capacity (and perhaps as a survival mechanism), emerges naturally in health-related experiences and life events that confront a person with issues of mortality and immortality. Life events that heighten one's sense of mortality, inadequacy, or vulnerability can—if they do not crush the individual's inner self—motivate developmental progress toward a renewed sense of identity and expanded self-boundaries (Corless, Germino, & Pittman, 1994; Erikson, 1986; Frankl, 1963; Marshall, 1980). Examples of these life events include serious or chronic illness, disability, aging, parenting, child rearing, family caregiving, loss of a loved one, career, and other life crises. Self-transcendence is evoked through such events and may enhance well-being by transforming losses and difficulties into growth experiences (Reed, 1996).

## ■ RELATIONSHIPS AMONG THE CONCEPTS: THE MODEL

The model of the Theory of Self-Transcendence is presented in Figure 7.1. Four basic sets of relationships among the concepts are proposed by the theory. First, there is a relationship between the experience of vulnerability and self-transcendence such that increased levels of vulnerability, as brought on by health events, for example, motivate increased levels of self-transcendence. Further, this relationship may be moderated by personal and contextual factors, particularly at high levels of vulnerability.

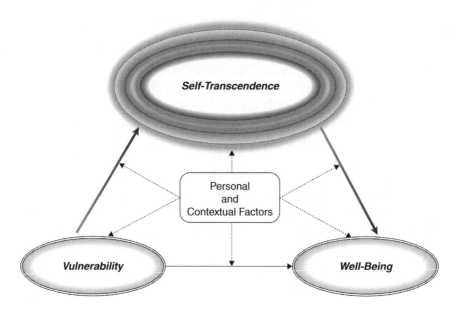

**FIGURE 7.1** Self-Transcendence Theory.

A second relationship exists between self-transcendence and well-being. This relationship is direct and positive. For example, self-transcendence relates positively to sense of well-being and morale, and self-transcendence relates negatively to depression as a "negative" indicator of well-being. This relationship represents more than a coping process; it is the integration or transcending of a current situation to move forward toward a changed life rather than simply a return to previous perspectives and behaviors (Willis & Grace, 2011).

Third, self-transcendence functions as a mediator between experiences of vulnerability and well-being. Research findings indicate that self-transcendence is a mechanism that helps explain the relationship between vulnerability and well-being. Self-transcendence may mediate the effects of vulnerability on well-being, with vulnerability experienced as, for example, illness distress; lack of optimism, hope, or power; uncertainty; death anxiety. Without self-transcendence, vulnerability could result in diminishing rather than sustaining well-being. Several studies discussed later provide empirical support for this mediator hypothesis. Self-transcendence, then, may be an underlying process that explains how well-being is possible in difficult or life-threatening situations that people endure.

Fourth, personal and contextual factors may also have a role in this healing process. A wide variety of personal and contextual factors and their interactions may moderate or otherwise influence the process of self-transcendence as it relates to well-being. Examples of these factors are age, gender, cognitive ability, health status, past significant life events, personal beliefs, family support, and sociopolitical environment. These factors can enhance or diminish the strength of the three key variables and their relationships. For example, advanced age or education may potentiate the relationship between self-transcendence and well-being. The idea that personal and contextual factors have a role in the theory derives from Rogers's (1980) integrality principle about the ongoing person–environment process over the life span.

The relationships posited by Self-Transcendence Theory identify areas for research and, with adequate empirical support, for nursing interventions to facilitate well-being in situations of increased vulnerability. From my nursing perspective, which focuses on understanding inherent resources that foster human well-being, I conceptualized self-transcendence as an *independent* variable—a contributor to and predictor of well-being outcomes—rather than as the dependent or outcome variable. Therefore, nursing interventions that support the person's inner resource for self-transcendence may focus directly on facilitating self-transcendence as it mediates the relationship between vulnerability and well-being, or as it directly relates to well-being. Interventions may also address influential personal or contextual factors that directly relate to vulnerability or to self-transcendence, or that moderate the relationships between vulnerability and self-transcendence, and between self-transcendence and well-being (Figure 7.1).

## ■ USE OF THE THEORY IN NURSING RESEARCH

Research results to date indicate that self-transcendence is a resource that accompanies serious life experiences that intensify one's sense of vulnerability or mortality. Self-transcendence is a process of expanding personal boundaries that helps people attain some sense of well-being in the context of difficult health situations. Findings also support the theorized direct relationship between self-transcendence and many indicators of well-being across groups of study participants facing a wide variety of health experiences.

### The Self-Transcendence Scale

The *Self-Transcendence Scale* (STS; Reed, 2009) has been used in much of the research concerning the theory. However, other measures may be used—and, in fact, qualitative approaches have been used—to study self-transcendence. The STS is a unidimensional instrument with 15 items measured on 4-point Likert-type scaling. It originated from a 36-item instrument, the *Developmental Resources of Later Adulthood* (DRLA) scale (Reed, 1986, 1989), which measured the level of developmentally based psychosocial resources reflective of developmental maturity. The DRLA was constructed from an extensive review of theoretical and empirical literatures on adult development and aging, selected nursing conceptual models and life-span theories, and clinical practice in psychiatric–mental health nursing.

The STS was developed around a self-transcendence factor that explained half of the variance in the DRLA with good internal consistency. The STS factor consisted of items describing various behaviors and perspectives by which an individual may expand personal boundaries inward and outward, and temporally. The STS has demonstrated reliability (internal consistency) and validity (content, construct) across studies of various populations and health experiences. It is brief and easy to administer either as a questionnaire or in an interview format. Many researchers and graduate students have used the instrument in studying self-transcendence as it relates to various health experiences and outcomes.

## Initial Research

The initial research used to build the Theory of Self-Transcendence focused on older adults, both well and those hospitalized for psychiatric treatment of depression, as a group more likely to be facing vulnerability or end-of-life issues than younger adults. Correlational and longitudinal studies (Reed, 1986, 1989) were designed to examine the nature and significance of the relationship between self-transcendence and mental health outcomes, particularly an inverse relationship between self-transcendence and depression. Quantitative and qualitative findings in a study of oldest-old adults, aged 80 to 100 years, also produced the same results (Reed, 1991a). In addition, four conceptual clusters representing different aspects of self-transcendence were generated from a content analysis: generativity, introjectivity, temporal integration, and body transcendence. Elders who scored high on depression reflected weak patterns in these four areas, particularly in body transcendence, inner-directed activities, and positive integration of present and future.

Similar results were generated later, in research by Haugan, Hannssen, and Moksnes (2013) in a study of self-transcendence in 202 nursing home older adult residents. Their STS results could be empirically organized into two factors, intrapersonal and interpersonal, which also included temporal and transpersonal items, providing further support for Self-Transcendence Theory that posited expanding personal boundaries as a correlate of well-being in later adulthood.

## Basic and Practice-Based Research by Coward

Doris Coward, who as a doctoral student studied with Reed, continued research into self-transcendence with a focus on middle-aged adults confronting their mortality through serious illness, advanced cancer, and AIDS. Coward (1990, 1995) initially studied the lived experience of self-transcendence in women with advanced breast cancer. Results from her phenomenological study were consistent with findings from quantitative studies. Self-transcendence perspectives were salient in this group, which had a heightened awareness of personal mortality. Self-transcendence was expressed in terms of reaching out beyond self to help others, to permit others to help them, and to accept the present, unchangeable events in time. This research validated Reed's (1989) quantitative measure of self-transcendence. In subsequent phenomenological research, Coward and Lewis (1993) explored self-transcendence in women and men with AIDS. Despite increased fear and sadness at the prospect of death, all participants indicated self-transcendence perspectives, which in turn helped them find meaning and achieve emotional well-being. Findings from a study of 107 women with stages III and IV breast cancer, in which structural equation modeling was used to analyze responses, indicated that self-transcendence had a significant and direct positive effect on emotional well-being by mediating the effect of illness distress on well-being (Coward, 1991).

Coward (1996) also studied healthy adults, who ranged in age from 19 to 85 years. She was interested in extending the Theory of Self-Transcendence by examining its salience in a group of adults who were not as actively confronted with end-of-life issues as other seriously ill populations. Self-transcendence was again found to be a significant and strong correlate of well-being indicators, namely coherence, self-esteem, hope, and other variables assessing emotional well-being. Coward concluded that while her research supported the hypothesized relationship between self-transcendence and mental health variables, the findings from her sample of healthy adults suggested that self-transcendence may surface at times in the life span other than end of life, as proposed by Victor Frankl (1969). Coward's work helped expand the scope of the theory to other age groups where self-transcendence may be salient. Nevertheless, her results do not necessarily dispute the idea that some awareness of human mortality is integral to self-transcendence. Awareness of mortality is a basic characteristic of the human condition among both healthy and ill adults, and may emerge slowly from the accumulation of life experiences as well as suddenly by a health crisis event.

Intervention research by Coward and Kahn (2004, 2005) focused on the experiences and functions of self-transcendence in women newly diagnosed with breast cancer. Self-transcendence practices and perspectives were particularly effective in helping women to resolve spiritual disequilibrium often experienced after diagnosis of breast cancer (Coward & Kahn, 2004). In their 2005 study, the investigators compared a traditional community cancer support group with a Self-Transcendence Theory–based group on outcomes regarding the experiences of self-transcendence and physical and emotional well-being. Women in the self-transcendence treatment group were able to attain a better sense of community with their support group. However, the most striking finding was that women in both groups had self-transcendence experiences that sustained them through the diagnosis and treatment of their illness. They expressed themes of outward, inward, and temporal expansion of self-boundaries such as reaching out for support and information, finding inner strength to endure, and constructing meaning out of past experiences and future hopes. The authors interpreted this finding as support for Reed's theoretical idea that the capacity for transcending an adverse event is a universal trait that motivates expansion of one's conceptual boundaries in multiple and beneficial ways.

## Research by Reed and Colleagues

In an attempt to examine the theory in a group of adults that was healthy and younger than the elders typically studied, Ellermann and Reed (2001) found evidence of self-transcendence in middle-aged adults in the forms of parenting, self-acceptance, and spirituality as expressions of expanding self-boundaries related to mental health. Their results indicated a strong inverse relationship between self-transcendence and level of depression in middle-aged adults, particularly among women.

Decker and Reed (2005) studied self-transcendence and moral reasoning within the context of several contextual and developmental factors to better understand end-of-life treatment preferences among older adults. Self-transcendence was found to be significantly and positively related to a higher level of reasoning called *integrated* moral reasoning, which includes both the autonomous and social domains of moral decision making. This finding was expected based on life-span developmental theory on adult cognition. Self-transcendence did not relate significantly to the desired level of aggressiveness of end-of-life treatment, although investigators argued that more research is needed into the role of self-transcendence and end-of-life decisions. The results help explain why reasoning about end-of-life treatment options may involve a complex and integrated approach.

Runquist and Reed (2007) studied correlates of well-being in 61 homeless men and women. Self-transcendence coupled with positive physical health status were identified as independent correlates of well-being, explaining a significant 60% of the variance in well-being in this sample. Self-transcendence held the larger and more significant correlation with well-being. These findings suggest that interventions to foster well-being among homeless persons include those that support self-transcendence as well as physical health.

## Research by Other Investigators

Other research conducted over the past 25 years has provided support for the Theory of Self-Transcendence. In most but not all of the quantitative studies reported here, researchers measured self-transcendence with Reed's (2009) STS. In the case of qualitative studies, researchers worked from a conceptualization of self-transcendence congruent with Reed's theory. Research has focused on various populations and health events.

## Chronic Physical Illness, Mental Health, and Aging

Several researchers in addition to Reed have studied self-transcendence in older adults in reference to chronic and serious illness and mental health and well-being. The various indicators of well-being found to be associated with self-transcendence, are **bolded** in the following research descriptions.

Walton, Shultz, Beck, and Walls (1991) explored self-transcendence using a 58-item scale based on Peck's (1968) developmental stages of old age. They identified a significant inverse relationship between self-transcendence and **loneliness** among 107 healthy older adults.

Billard (2001) examined the role of self-transcendence in the well-being of aging Catholic sisters for her doctoral research. Specifically, she combined Reed's (1987) *Spiritual Perspective Scale* with Reed's (1991a) STS to measure the concept of spiritual transcendence and found that spiritual transcendence, along with selected personality and demographic factors, contributed significantly to explaining **emotional intelligence** in a sample of 377 elder Catholic sisters.

In **suicide** research with 35 older adults hospitalized for depression, Buchanan, Farran, and Clark (1995) found that self-transcendence was integral to older adults coping with the changes in later life. Desire for death and self-transcendence (as measured by the STS) were significantly and inversely related. Klaas (1998) studied self-transcendence and **depression** in 77 depressed and nondepressed elders, finding self-transcendence was negatively correlated with depressive feelings and positively correlated with meaning in life in these groups. Similarly, in a study of Taiwanese older adults residing in nursing homes, self-transcendence was negatively correlated with depressive symptoms (Hsu, Badger, Reed, & Jones, 2013).

The **capacity to engage in activities of daily living** and self-transcendence was found to be significantly positively related in two studies, one with 88 chronically ill elders (Upchurch, 1999) and another with older African Americans where Upchurch and Mueller (2005) found that self-transcendence was significantly and positively related to the ability to carry out *instrumental activities of daily living* (IADLs). Self-transcendence was interpreted as a developmental strength influential in explaining why some elders continued to remain independent while others did not, regardless of health status. Related to IADLs, investigators Upchurch and Mueller (2005) recommended that caregivers can support older adults' **self-care** capacity by approaches that promote self-transcendence. On a similar theme, other investigators suggest continued research into the possible relationship between self-transcendence and medication adherence (N. F. Thomas & Dunn, 2014).

Walker (2002) measured self-transcendence and **mastery of stress** in testing his theory of transformative aging. He proposed that stressful events can bring about transformative change that enables the person to deal with the losses and challenges that accompany aging. Self-transcendence was found to be significantly and positively related to mastery of stress and significantly inversely related to stress of aging. His findings have implications for engaging the resource of self-transcendence to assist middle-aged and older adults in mastering stress and existential anxiety over the aging process.

Self-transcendence was found to be related to mediate and **reduce stresses of progressive diseases** of multiple sclerosis and systemic lupus erythematosus, prostate cancer, and oral cancer, respectively (H.-C. Chen 2012; Chin-A-Loy & Fernsler, 1998; Iwamoto, Yamawaki, & Sato, 2011). Similarly, in a study of older women living with rheumatoid arthritis, Neill (2002) found that transcendence of self-boundaries and personal transformation represented a process of **living successfully** with a chronic illness.

In a correlational study of oldest-old adults, Swedish researchers (Nygren et al., 2005) found significant, positive relationships of moderate magnitude between self-transcendence and several mental and physical health outcomes including **resilience, sense of coherence, and purpose in life.** Their results overall indicated that oldest-old adults were capable of experiencing levels of self-transcendence and other positive factors comparable to those in younger adults, although this capacity may differ between men and women, indicating the need for further research into gender differences. Several researchers have studied **inner strength** as a variable very similar to self-transcendence in its definition and in a way it is proposed to promote well-being in oldest-old men and women, that is, in terms of increased resilience, purpose in life, and sense of coherence (Lundman et al., 2010; Viglund, Jonsén, Strandberg, Lundman, & Nygren, 2014). One major conclusion was that while oldest-old individuals are more vulnerable to illness than are younger people, they also may have increased inner strength to help them not only cope but find joy in later life (Moe, Hellzen, Ekker, & Enmarker, 2013).

## Life-Threatening Illness in Adults

Considerable research on self-transcendence has focused on people who have life-threatening or life-limiting illness. Results from these studies provide consistent support for Self-Transcendence Theory. Examples of this research include individuals with cancer, HIV/AIDS, and other life-threatening illnesses.

### CANCER

In a phenomenological study of eight women who had completed breast cancer therapy, Pelusi (1997) found that surviving breast cancer very much involved self-transcendence, expressed as setting life priorities, finding meaning in life, and looking within self. Similar findings occurred in a study by Kinney (1996), who reported on her own journey through breast cancer. A process of listening to and trusting one's inner voice facilitated transcendence. Self-transcendence in turn was central to the reconstruction of self. Self-transcendence also was significant in adjusting to recurrence of breast cancer (Sarenmalm, Thorén-Jönsson, Gaston-Hohansson, & Öhlén, 2009).

In its mediating role, self-transcendence alone partially mediated the relationship between optimism and the outcome of emotional well-being in a group of 93 women receiving radiation treatment for breast cancer (Matthews & Cook, 2009). Farren's (2010) study of 104 breast cancer survivors produced findings that self-transcendence was a significant mediator in two relationships—between power (knowing participation) and quality of life and between uncertainty and quality of life. Uncertainty reduces quality of life by reducing self-transcendence. Farren used Reed's theory to describe self-transcendence as a profound awareness of one's wholeness while having awareness of fluctuations in one's human–environmental field patterns.

## HIV/AIDS

Self-transcendence and quality of life were studied in 46 HIV-positive adults by Mellors, Riley, and Erlen (1997). Data analysis revealed a significant moderate positive relationship between self-transcendence and quality of life for the group, particularly for those who were the most seriously ill. Similarly, Stevens (1999) found self-transcendence and depression to be significantly and inversely related in young adults with AIDS.

Results from other research also attest to the capacity for seriously ill individuals to transcend their illness. Persons with AIDS were able to transcend the suffering associated with their illness in a study by Mellors, Erlen, Coontz, and Lucke (2001). The participants demonstrated three dominant patterns indicative of self-transcendence: creating a meaningful life pattern, achieving a sense of connectedness, and engaging in self-care.

A group of investigators (Ramer, Johnson, Chan, & Barrett, 2006) interested in quality of life among persons with HIV/AIDS studied 420 mostly Hispanic, male patients. Among the findings was a significant positive relationship between self-transcendence and level of energy in the patients. In addition, researchers found that levels of acculturation and self-transcendence were significantly related, suggesting that the meaning of self-transcendence may be influenced by cultural factors. Their study not only provided support for the relevance of self-transcendence among these patients but also suggested that acculturation may moderate the relationship between self-transcendence and health outcome variables in people with HIV/AIDS.

## OTHER LIFE-THREATENING ILLNESSES

In a study of liver transplant recipients, Wright (2003) found self-transcendence to be positively related to quality of life and negatively related to fatigue, with further research needed to identify potential causal direction in these relationships. Bean and Wagner (2006) also studied liver transplant recipients (N = 471) with results indicating that self-transcendence becomes salient following the experience of liver transplant and was related significantly to higher quality of life and also may function as a mediator to decrease the effects of illness distress on quality of life.

In a phenomenological study of individuals with spinal muscular atrophy (SMA), self-transcendence was central to living with a sense of integrity, hope, and meaning amid the physical limitations experienced by individuals with these individuals (Ho, Tseng, Hsin, Chao, & Lin, 2016). Williams (2012) conducted a phenomenological study of eight men and women who had received a stem cell translation the previous year. Analyses showed that self-transcendence is brought about by the intense suffering, as lived through the physical effects of the treatment, facing death, and eventually drawing strength from within themselves and from spiritual support. The findings suggested that effects of vulnerability on well-being were mediated by self-transcendence.

## Research on Nurses and Other Caregivers

Self-transcendence is studied as it occurs in family caregivers, nurses, and others providing care to patients. This area of research has increased over the years to reveal the significance of self-transcendence in the well-being of caregivers.

Enyert and Burman (1999) found caregivers' self-transcendence behaviors, such as being with and doing for their loved one as death approached, facilitated personal growth and new meaning, and they were able to reach out to help others besides their family member. Poole's (1999) research revealed that self-transcendence was an important phase in being a caregiver in Grounded Theory research with 19 family caregivers in the process of being a caregiver for frail older adults at home. Three phases of caregiving—connecting, discovering self, and transcending self—were identified by which the caregiver became able to work with healthcare personnel as a partner instead of perpetuating conflict in the relationship.

Acton and Wright (2000) and Acton (2002) addressed self-transcendence in family caregivers of adults with dementia, proposing self-transcendence to be a relevant and potentially therapeutic experience for family caregivers. However, when Acton (2002) conducted a naturalistic field study of family caregivers, she found that caregivers of adults with dementia had little opportunity to nurture self-transcendence and instead experienced social isolation, ambivalence, emotional fragility, and burden of caring for their family member. She concluded that some of these negative experiences associated with caregiving may inhibit development of self-transcendence in caregivers and interfere with their continued growth and well-being. Kim et al. (2011) demonstrated significant positive links between self-transcendence and emotional well-being among family caregivers of chronically ill elders.

From interviews with 16 African American and White groups of great-grandmothers, Reese and Murray (1996) identified five domains of self-transcendence: connectedness, religion, being wise, values, and stories. The authors considered great-grandparents vital in facilitating self-transcendence and good relationships among family members.

As part of her study of spiritual growth in nurses, Kilpatrick (2002) studied the relationships among self-transcendence, spiritual perspective, and spiritual well-being in female nursing students and faculty. She found positive correlations among those variables in students and faculty. Nursing students and faculty differed significantly on level of self-transcendence and spiritual well-being, suggesting that self-transcendence may increase with development. Wasner, Longaker, Fegg, and Borasio (2005) found that spiritual care intervention training with 48 palliative care professionals increased their self-transcendence, spiritual well-being, and positive attitude toward work with dying patients.

McGee (2004) employed the method of interpretive phenomenology to examine self-transcendence and its impact on nurses' practice. Among results from the moving stories of nurses, McGee found self-transcendence to be an important mechanism of healing for nurses who have experienced difficult and traumatic personal life experiences. Her work highlighted the role of self-transcendence in healing the *nurse* and in enriching the practice of nurses for the mutual benefit of both patient and nurse.

Along a similar line of thinking, Hunnibell, Reed, Quinn-Griffin, and Fitzpatrick (2008) conducted dissertation research based on Self-Transcendence Theory. They studied self-transcendence as related to burnout syndrome in hospice and oncology nurses. Both groups of nurses face death and life-threatening illness through their work with patients. However, they hypothesized that because of the philosophy of their healthcare setting and opportunities to process loss, hospice nurses would demonstrate higher levels of self-transcendence and lower levels of burnout than oncology nurses. Their findings also provided empirical support for the hypothesis and for an inverse relationship between self-transcendence and three types of burnout. Hunnibell et al. concluded that self-transcendence is a resource for nurses and may protect them against burnout.

Significant, positive relationships between work engagement (measured as vigor, dedication, and absorption) and self-transcendence were found by Palmer, Quinn Griffin, Reed, and Fitzpatrick (2010) in their study of 84 acute care staff registered nurses. Through self-transcendence, the nurses increased self-awareness and inner strength and made sense of challenging work situations.

In summary, nurses and caregivers experience vulnerability and related health experiences through the challenges of their work as well as in their personal lives. Overall, research findings provide consistent evidence of the significance of self-transcendence in the well-being of nurses and other caregivers.

## ■ USE OF THE THEORY IN NURSING PRACTICE

### Theory-Informed Strategies for Practice

Research results indicate that a variety of strategies derived from Self-Transcendence Theory have been successful in promoting well-being and in diminishing negative outcomes in practice settings. The following sections are loosely organized by various strategies of expanding personal boundaries intrapersonally, interpersonally, and transpersonally.

### INTRAPERSONAL STRATEGIES

Intrapersonal strategies may help a person expand personal boundaries inward to clarify knowledge about self and find or create meaning and purpose in a difficult life experience. Meditation, prayer, visualization, life review, structured reminiscence, self-reflection, and journaling are the techniques of self-transcendence that nurses may facilitate in patients to help them recognize patterns of their own healing.

Nurses may use cognitive strategies to support self-transcendence in helping patients integrate a difficult health event into their lives. Targeting information about the illness, using positive self-talk, and engaging in meaningful and challenging activities are techniques that can help a person integrate and grow from the illness experience (Coward & Reed, 1996).

The personal narrative was tested in a randomized, clinical trial as an intervention for enhancing self-transcendence in women with HIV, multiple sclerosis, and systemic lupus erythematosus (Diener, 2003). STS scores increased significantly in the intervention groups, suggesting that the intervention was successful in helping the women address issues related to having a life-threatening or life-altering illness.

McCarthy, Jiying, and Carini (2013) and McCarthy, Jiying, Bowland, Hall, and Connelly (2015) developed and tested a "Psychoeducational Approach to Transcendence and Health" (PATH) program to facilitate self-transcendence in promoting well-being in older adults. Strategies that promote self-transcendence may even be helpful with individuals with Alzheimer's disease, as demonstrated in a case study of a family with a family member having this disease (Vitale, Shaffer, & Fenton, 2014).

### INTERPERSONAL STRATEGIES

Interpersonal strategies for facilitating self-transcendence focus on connecting the person to others through formal or informal means, ranging from face to face or telephone to connecting on the Internet. Nurse visits, peer counseling, informal networks, and formal support groups are examples of interpersonal strategies that the nurse may arrange for the person (Acton & Wright, 2000). Maintaining meaningful relationships and strengthening affiliations with civic groups or a faith community are strategies that the nurse can facilitate (McCormick, Holder, Wetsel, & Cawthon, 2001). A computer-mediated self-help intervention was designed to facilitate connections among lesbian, gay, bisexual, and transgender (LGBT) persons who shared similar interests (DiNapoli, Garcia-Dia, Garcia-One, O'Flaherty, & Siller, 2014).

Support groups are often cited as an effective way to connect people facing a difficult life situation. Groups that bring together people of similar health experiences can facilitate self-transcendence by connecting the person to others who can share the loss and exchange information and wisdom about coping with the experience and by providing an opportunity to reach beyond the self to help another. Joffrion and Douglas (1994) reported that nurses can facilitate self-transcendence during bereavement by helping the person participate in church or civic groups, develop or resume a hobby, share personal experiences of grief with others, and support others who have experienced loss.

In a series of pre-experimental and quasi-experimental studies, Coward (1998, 2003) developed and refined a series of support group sessions to facilitate self-transcendence. These sessions provided a variety of activities designed to support self-transcendence in women facing breast cancer: orientation and information sessions, sharing cancer stories, problem solving, assertive communication training, relaxation training, values clarification, ongoing educational components, constructive thinking and self-instructional training, feelings management, and pleasant activity planning. In another quasi-experimental study with individuals with multiple sclerosis, peer support groups facilitated self-transcendence and physical well-being (JadidMilani, Ashktorab, Aben-Saeedi, & AlaviMaid, 2014). Similarly, Norberg et al. (2015) suggested that self-transcendence facilitated social contact, outdoor activities, and other functions that can increase longevity in elders with life-limiting medical conditions.

Group psychotherapy is another intervention strategy for enhancing self-transcendence. Young and Reed (1995) found that this intervention approach was effective in generating a variety of outcomes for a group of elders, for example, intrapersonally in terms of achieving self-enrichment, self-esteem, and self-affirmation; interpersonally in terms of bonding with and helping others, enabling self-disclosure, and overcoming self-absorption; and temporally in terms of gaining acceptance of one's past and feeling empowered about the future. A 6-week group reminiscing intervention showed an increase in self-transcendence and a nonsignificant decrease in depression for women in an assisted living facility (Stinson & Kirk, 2006). Self-transcendence and depression level were significantly, inversely related in this group.

Altruistic activities facilitate self-transcendence by providing a context for learning new things and expanding awareness about oneself and one's world (Coward & Reed, 1996). Altruism also enhances a person's inner sense of worth and purpose. McGee (2000) explained that practicing humility and providing service to others are tools of self-transcendence that can empower individuals to maintain a healthy lifestyle. Connections between people, whether to receive or provide support, are key strategies for enhancing self-transcendence. Chan and Chan (2011) tested interventions designed to expand boundaries toward others through participation in volunteer work and social activities. These activities promoted acceptance and finding meaning in spousal death by facilitating the passing of time among bereaved Hong Kong Chinese older adults.

In a study by Willis and Griffith (2010) of school-age boys victimized by bullying, altruistic views and practices were found to facilitate healing. The boys reached out to others in helping and seeking help, having an interest in learning and engaging in fun hobbies, and feeling empathy toward others. The authors emphasized to practitioners the importance of planning activities and interactions that can foster self-transcendence.

Elderly nursing home residents were studied for their perceptions on what personal qualities allowed them to rise above the difficulties of advanced age (Bickerstaff, Grasser, & McCabe, 2003). Results from this qualitative study were consistent with patterns of self-transcendence identified earlier by Reed (1991a) in her study of community-dwelling oldest-old adults: generativity, introjectivity, temporal integration, body transcendence, and one not previously identified, "relationship with self/others/higher being." Many participants exhibited more than one pattern of self-transcendence. The researchers concluded that caregivers of older adults in long-term care facilities and at home should look beyond custodial care to incorporate activities that build upon the residents' capacity for self-transcendence that can help them cope with the losses of later life. Results from several studies support self-transcendence as clinically important in nurse–patient interactions to promote mental health among older adults in long-term care (Haugan, 2014; Haugan, Hanssen, & Mokenes, 2013; Haugan, Rannestad, Hammervold, Garasen, & Espnes, 2013, 2014).

## TRANSPERSONAL STRATEGIES

Transpersonal strategies of self-transcendence are designed to help the person connect with a power or purpose greater than self. The nurse's role in this process is often one of creating an environment in which transpersonal exploration can occur. It is worth noting here that several of the intervention strategies that foster intrapersonal growth can also foster a sense of transpersonal connection, such as meditation, prayer, visualization, artistic expression, and journaling.

Spiritual perspective or spiritual well-being, rather than religion per se, has been found to relate to self-transcendence by several researchers over the years, including Haase, Britt, Coward, Leidy, and Penn (1992), J. C. Thomas, Burton, Quinn Griffin, and Fitzpatrick (2010), and Sharpnack, Quinn Griffin, Benders, and Fitzpatrick (2010, 2011) in their two studies on the Amish community's use of spiritual and alternative healthcare practices to foster well-being. Religious activities and prayer are also identified as significant to the well-being of persons facing life crises. McGee (2000) explained the need for the nurse to provide an environment in which patients can look beyond themselves toward a higher power for help and be inspired to help others.

Schumann (1999) found that self-transcendence enhanced well-being in ventilated patients. Spiritual connections enabled patients to use temporal perspectives of past and future to empower themselves; they synchronized their lives with the realities of being on a ventilator and anticipating extubation and were then better able to manage this life-threatening health experience.

Artistic modalities such as art-making activities, creative bonding practice, memorial quilt making, and watching a therapeutic music video were based on Self-Transcendence Theory. These artistic modalities expand personal boundaries and facilitate transcendence, which in turn increase well-being (Burns, Robb, & Haase, 2009; S. Chen & Walsh, 2009; Kausch & Amer, 2007; Walsh, Radcliffe, Castillo, Kumar, & Broschard, 2007). Robb et al. (2014) used Haase's *Resilience in Illness* model to study a music video intervention with adolescents and young adults undergoing hematopoietic stem cell transplantation. They found this intervention facilitated self-transcendence and resilience along with factors relevant to well-being in these young individuals.

Other researchers found that poetry writing was an expressive therapy for facilitating self-transcendence in caregivers facing difficult life situations, and subsequently leading to positive outcomes of self-affirmation, sense of achievement, catharsis, and acceptance among dementia caregivers (Kidd, Zauszniewski, & Morris, 2011). However, caregivers may need pragmatic assistance before they can engage in activities that support self-transcendence; for example, to foster self-transcendence in family caregivers of adults with dementia, Acton and Wright (2000) identified the importance of helping arrange for in-home assistance or day care so that the family members have the time and energy to engage in activities that promote transpersonal awareness.

## ■ SUMMARY

Research findings have shown that self-transcendence is integral to well-being across a diversity of health experiences that nurses address in practice. Nursing practices that facilitate self-transcendence result in healing outcomes during these health events, as in, for example, diminished depression and loneliness among depressed elders; increased hopefulness and self-care among chronically ill elders; and increased meaning in life among persons with advanced breast cancer and other life-threatening illnesses; and increased well-being and self-affirmation in family and professional caregiving.

## ■ CONCLUSION

### Adequacy of the Theory

Professional nurses are defined in large part by their ability to engage human capacities for healing and well-being. Self-transcendence was presented as a resource for well-being. It represents "both a human capacity and a human struggle that can be facilitated by nursing" (Reed, 1996, p. 3). A goal in developing the theory was to gain better understanding of the dynamics of self-transcendence as it relates to health and well-being. This knowledge, in addition to that acquired through personal and ethical knowing and practice experience, can be used by nurses to foster well-being through strategies of self-transcendence.

There is **internal consistency** among the elements within the theory—the concepts, their definitions, and proposed relationships. Positive relationships were identified between vulnerability and self-transcendence and between self-transcendence and well-being. Self-transcendence functions as a resource, correlate, or facilitator of specific indicators of well-being. Self-transcendence is often found to be a mediator between vulnerability experiences and well-being outcomes. Self-transcendence has also been conceptualized as an outcome or a process of well-being in its own right. Finally, in addition to the three key concepts in the theory, research findings provide evidence on the role of various moderators in the process of self-transcendence.

The **scope** of Self-Transcendence Theory now reaches beyond the initial focus on older adults to include children, adolescents, and adults of all ages who experience vulnerability. The theory is being studied across cultures around the world. Research findings are broadening applications of the theory to include a variety of normative life transitions and developmental events where processes of self-transcendence have yet to be explored in depth.

The theory provides a perspective **relevant to nursing practice** in proposing self-transcendence as a process by which human beings may sustain well-being in times of vulnerability. That is, self-transcendence is a process of expanding one's boundaries to gain new insights for organizing and tackling health-related events. This process has **empirical support**. Findings from research consistently indicate that self-transcendence is associated with a wide variety of well-being indicators, from successful aging and meaning in life, to specific outcomes such as decreased fatigue or increased self-care activities of daily living. In addition, the scholarship of advanced practice nurses, graduate students, and researchers continues to build knowledge about personal, contextual, and cultural factors that influence the process of self-transcendence.

Self-Transcendence Theory has **social congruence**. Self-transcendence has emerged as a foundational process in promoting societal welfare, as a developmental imperative across the life span for a wide variety of health-related events. As such, nursing must be there to develop the knowledge and provide the expert support that facilitates this cost-effective and holistic process of well-being for society.

# ■ REFERENCES

Acton, G. J. (2002). Self-transcendent views and behaviors: Exploring growth in caregivers of adults with dementia. *Journal of Gerontological Nursing, 28*(12), 22–30.

Acton, G. J., & Wright, K. B. (2000). Self-transcendence and family caregivers of adults with dementia. *Journal of Holistic Nursing, 18*, 143–158.

Arlin, P. K. (1975). Cognitive development in adulthood: A fifth stage? *Developmental Psychology, 11*, 602–606.

Basseches, M. (1984). *Dialectical thinking and adult development*. Norwood, NJ: Ablex.

Bean, K. B., & Wagner, K. (2006). Self-transcendence, illness distress, and quality of life among liver transplant recipients. *Journal of Theory Construction & Testing, 10*(2), 47–53.

Bickerstaff, K. A., Grasser, C. M., & McCabe, B. (2003). How elderly nursing home residents transcend losses of later life. *Holistic Nursing Practice, 17*(3), 159–165.

Billard, A. (2001). *The impact of spiritual transcendence on the well-being of aging Catholic sisters* (Unpublished doctoral dissertation). Loyola College, Baltimore, MD.

Buchanan, D., Farran, C., & Clark, D. (1995). Suicidal thought and self-transcendence in older adults. *Journal of Psychosocial Nursing, 33*(10), 31–34.

Burns, D. S., Robb, S. L., & Haase, J. E. (2009). Exploring the feasibility of a therapeutic music video intervention in adolescents and young adults during stem cell transplantation. *Cancer Nursing, 32*(5), 8–16.

Chan, W. C., & Chan, C. L. W. (2011). Acceptance of spousal death: The factor of time in bereaved older adults' search for meaning. *Death Studies, 35*, 147–162.

Chen, H.-C. (2012). *Self-transcendence, illness perception, and depression in Taiwanese men with oral cancer* (Unpublished doctoral dissertation). The University of Arizona, Tucson, AZ. Retrieved from http://arizona.openrepository.com/arizona/bitstream/10150/228132/3/azu_etd_12083_sip1_m.pdf

Chen, S., & Walsh, S. M. (2009). Effect of a creative-bonding intervention on Taiwanese nursing students' self-transcendence and attitudes toward elders. *Research in Nursing & Health, 32*, 204–216.

Chin-A-Loy, S. S., & Fernsler, J. I. (1998). Self-transcendence in older men attending a prostate cancer support group. *Cancer Nursing, 21*, 358–363.

Commons, M., Demick, J., & Goldberg, C. (1996). *Clinical approaches to adult development*. Norwood, NJ: Ablex.

Corless, I. B., Germino, B. B., & Pittman, M. (1994). *Dying, death, and bereavement: Theoretical perspectives and other ways of knowing*. Boston, MA: Jones & Bartlett.

Coward, D. D. (1990). The lived experience of self-transcendence in women with advanced breast cancer. *Nursing Science Quarterly, 3*, 162–169.

Coward, D. D. (1991). Self-transcendence and emotional well-being in women with advanced breast cancer. *Oncology Nursing Forum, 18*, 857–863.

Coward, D. D. (1995). Lived experience of self-transcendence in women with AIDS. *Journal of Obstetric, Gynecologic, and Neonatal Nursing, 24*, 314–318.

Coward, D. D. (1996). Self-transcendence and correlates in a healthy population. *Nursing Research, 45*, 116–122.

Coward, D. D. (1998). Facilitation of self-transcendence in a breast cancer support group. *Oncology Nursing Forum, 25*, 75–84.

Coward, D. D. (2003). Facilitation of self-transcendence in a breast cancer support group: Part II. *Oncology Nursing Forum, 30*(2), 291–300.

Coward, D. D., & Kahn, D. L. (2004). Resolution of spiritual disequilibrium by women newly diagnosed with breast cancer. *Oncology Nursing Forum, 31*(2), E1–E8.

Coward, D. D., & Kahn, D. L. (2005). Transcending breast cancer: Making meaning from diagnosis and treatment. *Journal of Holistic Nursing, 23*(3), 264–283.

Coward, D. D., & Lewis, F. M. (1993). The lived experience of self-transcendence in gay men with AIDS. *Oncology Nursing Forum, 20,* 1363–1369.

Coward, D. D., & Reed, P. G. (1996). Self-transcendence: A resource for healing at the end of life. *Issues in Mental Health Nursing, 17,* 275–288.

Decker, I. M., & Reed, P. G. (2005). Developmental and contextual correlates of elders' anticipated end-of-life treatment decisions. *Death Studies, 29,* 827–846.

Diener, J. E. S. (2003). *Personal narrative as an intervention to enhance self-transcendence in women with chronic illness* (Unpublished doctoral dissertation). University of Missouri, St. Louis, MO.

DiNapoli, J. M., Garcia-Dia, M. J., Garcia-Ona, L., O'Flaherty, D., & Siller, J. (2014). A theory-based computer mediated communication intervention to promote mental health and reduce high-risk behaviors in the LGBT population. *Applied Nursing Research, 27*(1), 91–93.

Ellermann, C. R., & Reed, P. G. (2001). Self-transcendence and depression in middle-aged adults. *Western Journal of Nursing Research, 23,* 698–713.

Enyert, G., & Burman, M. E. (1999). A qualitative study of self-transcendence in caregivers of terminally ill patients. *American Journal of Hospice and Palliative Care, 16*(2), 455–462.

Erikson, E. H. (1986). *Vital involvement in old age.* New York, NY: Norton.

Farren, A. T. (2010). Power, uncertainty, self-transcendence, and quality of life in breast cancer survivors. *Nursing Science Quarterly, 23*(1), 63–71.

Frankl, V. E. (1963). *Man's search for meaning.* New York, NY: Pocket Books.

Frankl, V. E. (1969). *The will to meaning.* New York, NY: New American Library.

Haase, J. E., Britt, T., Coward, D. D., Leidy, N. K., & Penn, P. E. (1992). Simultaneous concept analysis of spiritual perspective, hope, acceptance and self-transcendence. *Image: Journal of Nursing Scholarship, 24,* 141–147.

Haugan, G. (2014). Nurse-patient interaction as a resource for hope, meaning in life and self-transcendence in nursing home patients. *Scandinavian Journal of Caring Sciences, 28*(1), 74–88.

Haugan, G., Hannssen, B., & Moksnes, U. K. (2013). Self-transcendence, nurse-patient interaction, and the outcome of multidimensional well-being in cognitively intact nursing home patients. *Scandinavian Journal of Caring Sciences, 27*(4), 882–893.

Haugan, G. Rannestad, T., Hammervold, R., Garåsen, H., & Espnes, G. A. (2013). Self-transcendence in cognitively intact nursing-home patients: A resource for well-being. *Journal of Advanced Nursing, 69*(5), 1147–1160.

Haugan, G., Rannestad, T., Hammervold, R., Garåsen, H., & Espnes, G. A. (2014). The relationships between self-transcendence and spiritual well-being in cognitively intact nursing home patients. *International Journal of Older People Nursing, 9,* 65–78.

Ho, H.-M., Tseng, Y.-H., Hsin, Y.-M., Chou, F.-H., & Lin, W.-T. (2016). Living with illness and self-transcendence: The lived experience of patients with spinal muscular atrophy. *Journal of Advanced Nursing, 72*(11), 2695–2705.

Hofer, J., Busch, H., Au, A., Šolcová, I. P., Tavel, P., & Tsien Wong, T. (2016). Generativity does not necessarily satisfy all your needs: Associations among cultural demand for generativity, generative concern, generative action, and need satisfaction in the elderly in four cultures. *Developmental Psychology, 52*(3), 509–519.

Hsu, Y. C., Badger, T., Reed, P., & Jones, E. (2013). Factors associated with depressive symptoms in older Taiwanese adults in a long-term care community. *International Psychogeriatrics, 25*(6), 1013–1021.

Hunnibell, L. S., Reed, P. G., Quinn-Griffin, M. Q., & Fitzpatrick, J. J. (2008). Self-transcendence and burnout in hospice and oncology nurses. *Journal of Hospice and Palliative Nursing, 10*(3), 172–179.

Iwamoto, R., Yamawaki, N., & Sato, T. (2011). Increased self-transcendence in patients with intractable diseases. *Psychiatry and Clinical Neuroscience, 65,* 638–647.

JadidMilani, M., Ashktorab, T., AbedSaeedi, Z., & AlayiMaid, H. (2015). The impact of self-transcendence on physical health status promotion in multiple sclerosis patients attending peer support groups. *International Journal of Nursing Practice, 2*(6), 725–732.

Joffrion, L. P., & Douglas, D. (1994). Grief resolution: Facilitating self-transcendence in the bereaved. *Journal of Psychosocial Nursing, 32*(3), 13–19.

Kausch, K. D., & Amer, K. (2007). Self-transcendence and depression among AIDS memorial quilt panel makers. *Journal of Psychosocial Nursing, 45*(6), 45–53.

Kidd, L. I., Zauszniewski, J. A., & Morris, D. L. (2011). Benefits of a poetry writing intervention for family caregivers of elders with dementia. *Issues in Mental Health Nursing, 32,* 598–604.

Kilpatrick, J. A. W. (2002). *Spiritual perspective, self-transcendence, and spiritual wellbeing in female nursing students and female nursing faculty* (Unpublished doctoral dissertation). Widener University, Wilmington, DE.

Kim, S., Reed, P. G., Hayward, R. D., Kang, Y., & Koenig, H. G. (2011). Spirituality and psychological well-being: Testing a theory of family interdependence among family caregivers and their elders. *Research in Nursing and Health, 34,* 103–115.

Kinney, C. K. (1996). Transcending breast cancer: Reconstructing one's self. *Issues in Mental Health Nursing, 17*(3), 201–216.

Klaas, D. (1998). Testing two elements of spirituality in depressed and non-depressed elders. *The International Journal of Psychiatric Nursing Research, 4,* 452–462.

Koplowitz, H. (1984). A projection beyond Piaget's formal operational stage: A general systems stage and a unitary stage. In M. L. Commons, F. A. Richards, & C. Armon (Eds.), *Beyond formal operations: Late adolescence and adult cognitive development* (pp. 272–296). New York, NY: Praeger.

Lundman, B., Aléx, L., Jonsén, E., Norberg, A., Nygren, B., Santamäki, R., & Strandberg, G. (2010). Inner strength—A theoretical analysis of salutogenic concepts. *International Journal of Nursing Studies, 47*(2), 251–260.

Marshall, V. M. (1980). *Last chapter: A sociology of aging and dying.* Monterey, CA: Brooks-Cole.

Maslow, A. H. (1969). Various meanings of transcendence. *Journal of Transpersonal Psychology, 1,* 56–66.

Matthews, E. E., & Cook, P. F. (2009). Relationships among optimism, well-being, self-transcendence, coping, and social support in women during treatment for breast cancer. *Psycho-Oncology, 18,* 716–726.

McCarthy, V. L. (2011). A new look at successful aging: Exploring a mid-range nursing theory among older adults in a low-income retirement community. *The Journal of Theory Construction & Testing, 15*(1), 17–23.

McCarthy, V. L., Jiying, L., Bowland, S., Hall, L. A., & Connelly, J. (2015). Promoting self-transcendence and well-being in community-dwelling older adults: A pilot study of a psychoeducational intervention. *Geriatric Nursing, 26*(6), 431–437.

McCarthy, V. L., Jiying, L., & Carini, R. M. (2013). The role of self-transcendence: A missing variable in the pursuit of successful aging? *Research in Gerontological Nursing, 6*, 178–186.

McCormick, D. P., Holder, B., Wetsel, M. A., & Cawthon, T. W. (2001). Spirituality and HIV disease: An integrated perspective. *Journal of the Association of Nurses in AIDS Care, 12*(3), 58–65.

McGee, E. M. (2000). Alcoholics anonymous and nursing. *Journal of Holistic Nursing, 18*(1), 11–26.

McGee, E. M. (2004). *I'm better for having known you: An exploration of self-transcendence in nurses* (Unpublished doctoral dissertation). Boston College, Boston, MA.

Mellors, M. P., Erlen, J. A., Coontz, P. D., & Lucke, K. T. (2001). Transcending the suffering of AIDS. *Journal of Community Health Nursing, 18*(4), 235–246.

Mellors, M. P., Riley, T. A., & Erlen, J. A. (1997). HIV, self-transcendence, and quality of life. *Journal of the Association of Nurses in AIDS Care, 2*, 59–69.

Moe, A., Hellzen, O., Ekker, K., & Enmarker, I. (2013). Inner strength in relation to perceived physical and mental health among the oldest old people with chronic illness. *Aging & Mental Health, 17*(2), 189–196.

Neill, J. (2002). Transcendence and transformation in the life patterns of women living with rheumatoid arthritis. *Advances in Nursing Science, 24*(4), 27–47.

Newman, M. (1992). Prevailing paradigms in nursing. *Nursing Outlook, 40*, 10–13.

Newman, M. (1994). *Health as expanding consciousness* (2nd ed.). New York, NY: National League for Nursing.

Norberg, A., Lundman, B., Gustafson, Y., Norberg, C., Fischer, R. S., & Lövheim, H. (2015). Self-transcendence (ST) among very old people: Its associations to social and medical factors and development over five years. *Archives of Gerontology & Geriatrics, 61*(2), 247–253.

Nygren, B., Aléx, L., Jonsén, E., Gustafson, Y., Norberg, A., & Lundman, B. (2005). Resilience, sense of coherence, purpose in life and self-transcendence in relation to perceived physical and mental health among the oldest old. *Aging & Mental Health, 9*(4), 354–362.

Palmer, B., Quinn Griffin, M. T., Reed, P., & Fitzpatrick, J. J. (2010). Self-transcendence and work engagement in acute care staff registered nurses. *Critical Care Nursing Quarterly, 33*(2), 138–147.

Parse, R. R. (1992). Human becoming: Parse's theory of nursing. *Nursing Science Quarterly, 5*, 35–42.

Parse, R. R. (2015). Rosemarie Rizzo Parse's humanbecoming paradigm. In M. C. Smith & M. E. Parker (Eds.), *Nursing theories and nursing practice* (4th ed., pp. 263–277). Philadelphia, PA: F. A. Davis.

Peck, R. C. (1968). Psychological development in the second half of life. In B. L. Neugarten (Ed.), *Middle age and aging* (pp. 88–92). Chicago, IL: University of Chicago Press.

Pelusi, J. (1997). The lived experience of surviving breast cancer. *Oncology Nursing Forum, 24*(8), 1343–1353.

Poole, D. K. (1999). *Partnering with a formal program: Expanding the boundaries of family caregiving for frail older adults* (Unpublished doctoral dissertation). Medical College of Georgia, Augusta, GA.

Ramer, L., Johnson, D., Chan, L., & Barrett, M. T. (2006). The effect of HIV/AIDS disease progression on spirituality and self-transcendence in a multi-cultural population. *Journal of Transcultural Nursing, 17*(3), 280–289.

Reed, P. G. (1983). Implications of the life-span developmental framework for well-being in adulthood and aging. *Advances in Nursing Science, 6,* 18–25.

Reed, P. G. (1986). Developmental resources and depression in the elderly: A longitudinal study. *Nursing Research, 35,* 368–374.

Reed, P. G. (1987). Spirituality and well-being in terminally ill hospitalized adults. *Research in Nursing and Health, 10*(5), 335–344.

Reed, P. G. (1989). Mental health of older adults. *Western Journal of Nursing Research, 11*(2), 143–163.

Reed, P. G. (1991a). Self-transcendence and mental health in oldest-old adults. *Nursing Research, 40,* 7–11.

Reed, P. G. (1991b). Toward a nursing theory of self-transcendence: Deductive reformulation using developmental theories. *Advances in Nursing Science, 13*(4), 64–77.

Reed, P. G. (1996). Transcendence: Formulating nursing perspectives. *Nursing Science Quarterly, 9*(1), 2–4.

Reed, P. G. (1997a). Nursing: The ontology of the discipline. *Nursing Science Quarterly, 10*(2), 76–79.

Reed, P. G. (1997b). The place of transcendence in nursing's science of unitary human beings: Theory and research. In M. Madrid (Ed.), *Patterns of Rogerian knowing* (pp. 187–196). New York, NY: National League for Nursing.

Reed, P. G. (2009). Demystifying self-transcendence for mental health nursing practice and research. *Archives of Psychiatric Nursing, 23*(5), 397–400.

Reed, P. G. (2011). The spiral path of nursing knowledge. In P. G. Reed & N. B. C. Shearer (Eds.), *Nursing knowledge and theory innovation: Advancing the science of nursing practice* (pp. 1–35). New York, NY: Springer Publishing.

Reese, C. G., & Murray, R. B. (1996). Transcendence: The meaning of great-grandmothering. *Archives of Psychiatric Nursing, 10*(4), 245–251.

Riegel, K. F. (1976). The dialectics of human development. *American Psychologist, 31,* 631–647.

Robb, S. L., Burns, D. S., Stegenga, K. A., Haut, P. R., Monahan, P. O., Meza, J., . . . Haase, J. E. (2014). Randomized clinical trial of therapeutic music video intervention for resilience outcomes in adolescents/young adults undergoing hematopoietic stem cell transplant: A report from the Children's Oncology Group. *Cancer, 120*(6), 909–917.

Rogers, M. E. (1970). *Introduction to the theoretical basis of nursing.* Philadelphia, PA: F. A. Davis.

Rogers, M. E. (1980). A science of unitary man. In J. P. Riehl & C. Roy (Eds.), *Conceptual modes for nursing practice* (2nd ed., pp. 329–337). New York, NY: Appleton-Century-Crofts.

Rogers, M. E. (1994). The science of unitary human beings: Current perspectives. *Nursing Science Quarterly, 7*(1), 33–35.

Runquist, J. J., & Reed, P. G. (2007). Self-transcendence and well-being in homeless adults. *Journal of Holistic Nursing, 25*(1), 5–13; discussion, 14–15.

Sarenmalm, E. K., Thorén-Jönsson, A., Gaston-Hohansson, F., & Öhlén, J. (2009). Making sense of living under the shadow of death: Adjusting to a recurrent breast cancer illness. *Qualitative Health Research, 19*(8), 1116–1130.

Sarter, B. (1988). Philosophical sources of nursing theory. *Nursing Science Quarterly, 1*(2), 52–59.

Schumann, R. R. (1999). *Intensive care patients' perceptions of the experience of mechanical ventilation* (Unpublished doctoral dissertation). Texas Women's University, Denton, TX.

Sharpnack, P. A., Quinn Griffin, M. T., Benders, A. M., & Fitzpatrick, J. J. (2010). Spiritual and alternative healthcare practices of the Amish. *Holistic Nursing Practice, 24,* 64–72.

Sharpnack, P. A., Quinn Griffin, M. T., Benders, A. M., & Fitzpatrick, J. J. (2011). Self-transcendence and spiritual well-being in the Amish. *Journal of Holistic Nursing, 29*(2), 91–97.

Sheldon, K. M., & Kasser, T. (2001). Getting older, getting better? Personal strivings and psychological maturity across the life span. *Developmental Psychology, 37,* 491–501.

Sinnott, J. D. (1998). *The development of logic in adulthood: Postformal thought and its applications.* New York, NY: Plenum.

Sinnott, J. D. (2011). Constructing the self in the face of aging and death: Complex thought and learning. In C. Hoare (Ed.), *Oxford handbook of adult development and learning* (2nd ed., pp. 248–264). New York, NY: Oxford University Press.

Stevens, D. D. (1999). *Spirituality, self-transcendence and depression in young adults with AIDS* (Unpublished doctoral dissertation). University of Miami, Coral Gables, FL.

Stinson, C. K., & Kirk, E. (2006). Structured reminiscence: An intervention to decrease depression and increase self-transcendence in older women. *Journal of Clinical Nursing, 15*(2), 208–218.

Teixeira, M. E. (2008). Self-transcendence: A concept analysis for nursing praxis. *Holistic Nursing Practice, 22*(1), 25–31.

Thomas, J. C., Burton, M., Quinn Griffin, M. T., & Fitzpatrick, J. J. (2010). Self-transcendence, spiritual well-being, and spiritual practices of women with breast cancer. *Journal of Holistic Nursing, 28*(2), 115–122.

Thomas, N. F., & Dunn, K. S. (2014). Self-transcendence and medication adherence in older adults with hypertension. *Journal of Holistic Nursing, 32*(4), 316–326.

Upchurch, S. (1999). Self-transcendence and activities of daily living: The woman with the pink slippers. *Journal of Holistic Nursing, 17,* 251–266.

Upchurch, S., & Mueller, W. H. (2005). Spiritual influences on ability to engage in self-care activities among older African Americans. *International Journal of Aging and Human Development*, 60(1), 77–94.

Viglund, K., Jonsén, E., Strandberg, G., Luncman, B., & Hygren, B. (2014). Inner strength as a mediator of the relationship between disease and self-rated health among old people. *Journal of Advanced Nursing*, 70(1), 144–152.

Vitale, S. A., Shaffer, C. M., & Fenton, H. R. A. (2014). Self-transcendence in Alzheimer's disease: The application of theory in practice. *Journal of Holistic Nursing*, 23(4), 347–355.

Walker, C. A. (2002). Transformative aging: How mature adults respond to growing older. *Journal of Theory Construction & Testing*, 6(2), 109–116.

Walsh, S. M., Radcliffe, R. S., Castillo, L. C., Kumar, A. M., & Broschard, D. M. (2007). A pilot study to test the effect of art-making classes for family caregivers of patients with cancer. *Oncology Nursing Forum*, 34(1), E9–E16. doi:10.1188/07.ONF. E9-E16

Walton, C. G., Shultz, C., Beck, C. M., & Walls, R. C. (1991). Psychological correlates of loneliness in the older adult. *Archives of Psychiatric Nursing*, 5(3), 165–170.

Wasner, M., Longaker, C., Fegg, J. J., & Borasio, G. D. (2005). Effects of spiritual care training for palliative care professionals. *Palliative Medicine*, 19, 99–104.

Williams, B. J. (2012). Self-transcendence in stem cell transplantation recipients: A phenomenologic inquiry. *Oncology Nursing Forum*, 39(4), E41–E48. doi:10.1188/12. ONF.E41-E48

Willis, D. G., & Grace, P. J. (2011). The applied philosopher-scientist: Intersections among phenomenological research, nursing science, and theory as a basis for practice aimed at facilitating boys' healing from being bullied. *Advances in Nursing Science*, 34(1), 19–28.

Willis, D. G., & Griffith, C. A. (2010). Healing patterns revealed in middle school boys' experiences of being bullied using Rogers' Science of Unitary Human Beings. *Journal of Child and Adolescent Psychiatric Nursing*, 23(3), 125–132.

Wright, K. B. (2003). *Quality of life, self-transcendence, illness distress, and fatigue in liver transplant recipients* (Unpublished doctoral dissertation). University of Texas at Austin.

Young, C., & Reed, P. G. (1995). Elders' perceptions of the effectiveness of group psychotherapy in fostering self-transcendence. *Archives of Psychiatric Nursing*, 9, 338–347.

# CHAPTER 8

## Theory of Symptom Management

Melinda S. Bender, Susan L. Janson, Linda S. Franck, and Kathryn Aldrich Lee

A symptom is defined as a subjective experience reflecting changes in the bio-psychosocial functioning, sensations, or cognition of an individual. In contrast, a sign is defined as any abnormality indicative of disease that is detectable by the individual or others (Dodd et al., 2001). Signs and symptoms are important aspects of health and illness that disrupt physical, mental, and social functioning. An acute or unrelenting symptom is often what brings the patient into the healthcare system, particularly after self-care management strategies have failed. The presence of a symptom or a cluster of symptoms may be the first indication to the patient or clinician of a developing illness. Symptoms can also be brought on by prescribed pharmacologic or medical therapy. Whether the goal is to eliminate the symptom or to minimize the distress of the symptom experience, the Symptom Management Theory (SMT) provides a useful framework for organizing the relevant concepts for research and practice. This middle range theory serves to guide symptom assessment and treatment in nursing practice and to suggest questions and hypotheses for nursing research.

## ■ PURPOSE OF THE THEORY AND HOW IT WAS DEVELOPED

The faculty at the University of California, San Francisco (UCSF) School of Nursing first introduced the Symptom Management Model in 1994 (Larson et al., 1994). That original model provided a framework to allow faculty involved in symptom research and clinical practice to improve collaboration and move forward in a more organized way of thinking about the symptom experience, management strategies, and outcomes of symptom management. The conceptualization at that time was based on models that had been developed by nurses, such as Orem's Self-Care Model (1985) and Sorofman, Tripp-Reimer, Lauer, and Martin's (1990) Model of Symptoms of Self-Care, and other related models from anthropology, sociology, and psychology. The UCSF faculty concluded that none of these frameworks adequately addressed the patient's role in self-care *and* the "patient's experience, his or her tested management strategies, or the desired outcomes" (Larson et al., 1994, p. 273). With further testing of the model and its components, and ongoing discussion among the UCSF faculty and students, the UCSF Symptom

Management Model was revised in 2001 (Dodd et al., 2001). Selected published research studies were used to build an evidence-based foundation and to compare and contrast the concepts across symptoms. In the 2001 revision, the concept labels and nature of the relationships among the concepts were slightly altered. In addition, the influence of person, environment, and health and illness domains were made explicit by situating the entire model within these spheres. With this chapter, we have updated the growing body of research that uses the SMT as a theoretical basis. As depicted in Figure 8.1, the three concepts of symptom experience, management strategies, and outcomes continue to form the conceptual basis of the SMT for research and practice. The SMT addresses specific phenomena but does not necessarily limit application to one narrow patient population. The SMT also proposes explicit and testable relationships among three concepts, provides a structure for understanding the connections among these concepts, and provides a framework for considering interventions and outcomes. As shown later in this chapter, the SMT continues to provide a strong basis for research and has also begun to inform practice and education in nursing.

## ■ CONCEPTS OF THE THEORY

The three essential concepts of the SMT are symptom experience, symptom management strategies, and outcomes, with a change in the status of the

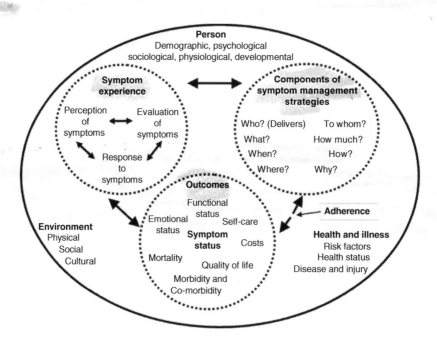

**FIGURE 8.1**  Symptom Management Theory.

*Source:* Adapted from Dodd, M., Janson, S., Facione, N., Faucett, J., Froelicher, E. S., Humphreys, J., . . . Taylor, D. (2001). Advancing the science of symptom management. *Journal of Advanced Nursing*, *33*, 668–676.

symptom (its frequency, severity, or distress) being the key outcome of interest. These concepts are nested within three domains of nursing science (person, environment, and heath/illness) to serve as a reminder of the contextual considerations for nursing research. For instance, a woman's symptom experience will vary by age and reproductive status as well as by her genetic risk factors (person domain), her cultural beliefs about the meaning of a symptom or whether she is assessed in the laboratory, clinic, home, or job (environmental domain), and her current state of health or diagnosis (health/illness domain).

Symptom experience is a simultaneous perception, evaluation, and response to a change in one's usual feeling. The change can be in frequency (how often) or severity (how bad). Further, frequency or severity may not change, but distress associated with the symptom could be altered by an intervention strategy. For example, a woman may suddenly feel hot and diaphoretic. In response to her awareness of these symptoms, she begins to evaluate and consider potential responses that may include taking no action. This symptom perception and response differs depending on whether it occurs during an important meeting or during the night while asleep. If it continues with sufficient frequency and severity over time and is perceived as distressing and interfering with her life, her response is likely to include seeking help and more effective strategies to eliminate or minimize the symptom.

The symptom experience may include not just one but several synergistic symptoms. Some of the investigators who developed the SMT have explored this phenomenon by studying individuals who experience clusters of symptoms (Dodd, Miaskowski, & Lee, 2004; Dodd, Miaskowski, & Paul, 2001; Voss, Portillo, Holzemer, & Dodd, 2007). In fact, this approach has been one of the more rapidly developing aspects of the SMT (Dodd, Cho, Cooper, & Miaskowski, 2010; E. Kim et al., 2009; K. A. Lee et al., 2009; Miaskowski, 2006; Miaskowski, Aouizerat, Dodd, & Cooper, 2007; Miaskowski, Paul, et al., 2011; Voss et al., 2007; C. Xiao, 2010).

Symptom management strategies are efforts to avert, delay, or minimize the symptom experience. The strategy can be effective in three ways: (a) reducing the frequency of the symptom experience, (b) decreasing the severity of the symptom, or (c) relieving the distress associated with the symptom (Portenoy et al., 1994). A framework for the study and development of management strategies includes the specifications of who, how, where, when, and what the intervention strategy entails. To continue again with the woman who suddenly feels hot and diaphoretic—to cool her body temperature down to relieve the symptom at one moment in time—she might either remove some clothing or begin to fan herself. Her circumstances (environment), personal characteristics (person), and health status (health/illness) continue over time to influence her symptom management strategies as do the frequency and severity of the symptoms.

Increasing attention is being given to self-management strategies used by patients (Koller, Miaskowski, De Geest, Opitz, & Spichiger, 2013; Landers, McCarthy, & Savage, 2011; Zimmerman et al., 2011). An outcome of this effort is to shift more of the responsibility of managing symptoms to the individual, particularly in the setting of a chronic illness. Patients essentially become their own primary caregivers and manage their own symptoms, perhaps with the help of an informal family caregiver, on a day-to-day basis. The location where an intervention strategy is tested or used, such as in the laboratory or home, can impact or modulate the symptom. For example, an intervention for insomnia may have a different effect when tested in the home compared with a sleep laboratory.

The "what" is viewed as the strategy itself; one strategy might be a medical therapy that also needs clinician input (e.g., adjusting a daily diuretic dosage to manage symptoms of dyspnea and orthopnea), whereas another may involve a complementary therapy or relaxation technique that the patient or family can carry out on a daily basis. Yet another strategy may involve alteration of the hospital room, home, or work environment. Patients and providers may also attempt more than one strategy and use a combination of interventions that have a greater effect on the symptom or cluster of symptoms. Tailoring the management strategy to the person or the family has been shown to be important in bringing about behavior change (Committee on Quality of Health Care in America, 2001; Leeman, Skelly, Burns, Carlson, & Soward, 2008; Skelly, Carlson, Leeman, Soward, & Burns, 2009) and symptom reduction.

The dose (i.e., how much) and the timing (i.e., when) aspects of intervention strategies are also important to modulate symptoms in nursing practice and research. The dose is an important consideration, particularly when implementing a behavioral intervention. Dose could include the actual time spent exercising, number of times a stress reduction session was attended, or hours spent in an education session. The dose of time spent by the healthcare provider or family member administering the intervention is also critical to consider in terms of how much time and support is actually provided to the person experiencing the symptom. One example of dose related to environmental management may be the degree of job improvement or disability accommodation that a workplace provides (Faucett & McCarthy, 2003). Donesky-Cuenco, Janson, Neuhaus, Neilands, and Carrieri-Kohlman (2007) found that when reporting dose and timing, the use of intuitively understood units of measurement improved comparisons across interventions and programs of research. In their study, "minutes per session" and "number of sessions per week" were units of exercise measurement that were easily understood as a dose of intervention; in contrast, cumulative minutes during a 6-month study were less useful as a measurement unit of comparison.

Symptom outcomes are clear and measurable outcomes to assess before and after implementing an intervention strategy. Outcomes include the obvious change in symptom status, whereby the symptom is less frequent, less intense, or less distressing. This improvement in symptoms can lead to better physical and mental functioning, improved quality of life, shorter hospital stay, quicker return to work, and greater productivity, all with less cost to the individual, family, healthcare system, or employer.

## ■ RELATIONSHIPS AMONG THE CONCEPTS: THE MODEL

The SMT has three major concepts: symptom experience, symptom management strategies, and symptom outcomes. The bidirectional arrows within the model are meant to indicate a simultaneous interaction among all three concepts. The symptom experience is conceptualized as influencing and being influenced by both symptom management strategies and outcomes. As individuals become aware of symptoms, initiate strategies, and assess outcomes, their symptom perception is affected. This interaction can take place in a matter of moments as is often the case in common symptom self-care management (e.g., minor colds, rashes, stomach upset). However, when symptoms are more pronounced (in frequency or severity) or distressing, other strategies may be sought and symptom outcomes may be assessed in a more formal fashion. This iterative process continues until symptoms resolve or stabilize.

The process of managing symptoms to achieve an outcome goes amiss when adherence becomes a problem. (Adherence in the SMT considers whether the intended recipient of the strategy actually receives or uses the strategy in the prescribed dose.) This breakdown is illustrated by the broken arrow between the symptom management strategies and symptom outcomes concept of the SMT. Placement of adherence in the model is supported by numerous studies of asthma and chronic obstructive pulmonary disease (COPD; Donesky-Cuenco, Janson, Neuhaus, Neilands, & Carrieri-Kohlman, 2007; Janson, McGrath, Covington, Baron, & Lazarus, 2010; Janson, McGrath, Covington, Cheng, & Boushey, 2009; Janson et al., 2003, 2015). Within the SMT, nonadherence may occur when interventions are too demanding, are not applied in the correct dose, or are applied inconsistently. In addition, factors situated in the person, environment, and heath/illness domains may contribute to nonadherence in managing symptoms. For example, in a recent study of adherence to a biologic therapy for allergic asthma requiring injection in a clinic setting, adherence was related to age, lung function, and frequency of dosing required (Janson et al., 2015). In another study, concern about adherence to antiretroviral therapy was related to variance in quality of life in people living with HIV (Corless et al., 2013).

## ■ USE OF THE THEORY IN NURSING RESEARCH

The SMT has evolved as more research studies have contributed to the understanding and development of relationships among the three concepts and three domains of the theoretical framework. Likewise, the study of symptom experience—both with individual and clusters of symptoms—has continued to flourish using the SMT as a conceptual guide. The works of Carrieri-Kohlman, Janson-Bjerklie, and colleagues provide an illustration of the systematic development of knowledge for clinical practice that has been possible with the SMT. Their initial research sought to explore patient symptom experience and responses to dyspnea (Carrieri-Kohlman, Demir-Deviren, Cuenco, Eiser, & Stulbarg, 2000; Carrieri-Kohlman, Gormley, Douglas, Paul, & Stulbarg, 1996; Carrieri-Kohlman et al., 2001; Carrieri-Kohlman & Janson-Bjerklie, 1986; Carrieri-Kohlman, Kieckhefer, Janson-Bjerklie, & Souza, 1991; Janson-Bjerklie, Carrieri-Kohlman, & Hudes, 1986; Janson-Bjerklie, Ferketich, Benner, & Becker, 1992). Their research uncovered the diverse symptom experience of individuals and the variety of terms patients used to describe their experience. They produced some of the earliest evidence for the affective distress dimension of dyspnea and have continued to explore dyspnea-related distress in the clinical setting (Carrieri-Kohlman et al., 2010).

Subsequent testing of the effect of management strategies on symptom experience and other multivariate outcomes, such as exercise performance, depression, self-efficacy for managing dyspnea, health-related quality of life, adherence, and healthcare utilization, has provided an understanding of how patients manage their symptoms and how those symptoms and their management affect outcomes such as functional status (Carrieri-Kohlman et al., 2005; A. H. Davis, Carrieri-Kohlman, Janson, Gold, & Stulbarg, 2006; Donesky et al., 2011; Nguyen & Carrieri-Kohlman, 2005). For example, the dyspnea self-management program developed from the work of Carrieri-Kohlman et al. has been transferred to an Internet platform to improve accessibility of self-management support outside the traditional time and space of a clinic (Nguyen et al., 2008, 2011). Adoption of alternative modalities of exercise, such as yoga, has also shown promise as a dyspnea management strategy (Donesky-Cuenco, Nguyen, Paul, & Carrieri-Kohlman, 2009).

Similarly, application of the SMT to research on asthma revealed the distinct role of monitoring symptoms for asthma control. Increasing chronic asthma symptoms or the sudden onset of acute symptoms signals loss of asthma control and requires actions to preserve life, yet many adults delay seeking urgent medical care when asthma worsens (Janson & Becker, 1998). Interventions designed to increase self-management skills for responding to acute episodes and controlling chronic asthma have produced improved adherence to anti-inflammatory therapy and control of asthma (Janson et al., 2003). A refinement of the self-management intervention tailored to the severity of asthma, inhaler technique, and skin test allergy profile was further tested in a randomized controlled trial in which training in self-management skills significantly improved adherence to inhaled corticosteroid therapy, nighttime asthma symptoms, and perception of asthma control in the intervention group compared to attention controls (Janson et al., 2009). Building on the importance of symptom recognition as a warning sign of worsening asthma, a cluster randomized controlled trial was also conducted to test the effect of providing asthmatic adults with monthly written interpretations of their graphed peak flow data based on zones of reduction matching their symptom reports (Janson et al., 2010). This feedback intervention resulted in significant improvement in self-management during winter (physical environment), typically a period of vulnerability related to colds and flu. Outcomes were evidenced by significantly fewer episodes of worsening symptoms, fewer courses of oral steroids, and fewer urgent care visits in the intervention group compared with controls. All these studies show effects of self-monitoring on asthma symptoms. Moreover, the results provide a growing body of evidence to support the SMT.

The SMT has seen increasing use in other areas of research. A search of both research and practice-focused literature from 2007 to 2013 produced 40 additional publications that explicitly address the theory and 64 additional publications that cite the SMT in support of the study of symptoms. Among these documents, 35 reported on research that used SMT as the conceptual basis. Two articles discussed SMT as part of a focused review of the literature on acute coronary syndromes (Arslanian-Engoren & Engoren, 2010) and symptom clusters (C. Xiao, 2010). Another article used SMT as a basis for developing and testing a tailored intervention (Skelly, Leeman, Carlson, Soward, & Burns, 2008; Skelly et al., 2009). Linder (2010) conducted a theoretical analysis and Brant, Beck, and Miaskowski (2010) compared the SMT with another theory and suggested directions for new theory development.

Since the 2014 revisions of this chapter, another literature search was performed to identify publications from 2013 through 2016 that explicitly used or applied the SMT in research, resulting in 83 new publications. Among these publications, 73 met the inclusion criteria: 19 addressed the symptom experience, 12 were related to SMT domains, 7 discussed symptom management strategies, 2 focused on adherence to management strategies, 4 used SMT in studies involving children and families, 15 focused on clinical practice and instrument development (e.g., questionnaires), and 4 centered on the overall SMT itself. Moreover, four studies used the SMT to guide systematic reviews of the literature involving nursing research. Finally, with the ever expanding body of science, this middle range theory has been gaining international prominence, with six international publications on SMT. The following sections include and highlight these additional publications.

## SMT as a Theoretical Framework

Previously identified studies have used the SMT as a framework in a variety of ways, including guiding the study design to illustrate the symptom experience (Ahlberg, Ekman, & Gaston-Johansson, 2005) or integrating SMT with other theories to formulate conceptual models (Maag, Buccheri, Capella, & Jennings, 2006). Since 2013 several studies have used similar applications of the SMT. Conchon,

Nascimento, Fonseca, and Aroni (2015) used SMT as a framework to analyze existing literature on the symptom experience of perioperative thirst. Brant, Dudley, Beck, and Miaskowski (2016) contrasted SMT with a variety of symptom models and theories to propose a new Dynamic Symptoms Model addressing the complex nature of symptoms that co-occur, interact, and change over time. Further innovative applications of the SMT were used by Landers, McCarthy, and Savage (2013) comparing the SMT with other symptom theories to describe the process of choosing a theoretical framework to guide their study on bowel symptoms and self-care strategies. Two book chapters also by Landers (2014, 2016) outlined the SMT and expounded on the theory's evolution, the model components, concepts, and interrelation between concepts and domains. The Landers chapter (2016), subsequently provides an analysis of self-care strategies.

## Systematic Reviews

Another use of SMT has been to guide systematic reviews and analysis of specific symptoms and management strategies. Three recent articles used SMT to guide reviews in oncology nursing (L. L. Davis, Carpenter, & Otte, 2016; Hammer et al., 2015; W. Xiao, Chow, So, Leung, & Chan, 2016). Another review focused on analysis of instruments to measure the symptom of thirst in people with congestive heart failure (Allida, Inglis, Davidson, Hayward, & Newton, 2014). Arslanian-Engoren and Engoren (2010) used symptom experience as a framework for reviewing the available research on acute coronary syndromes.

## Global Reach

The global influence of the SMT is evident from new publications in several international settings, including Brazil, France, China, Korea, and Germany. In Brazil, nurses used SMT to guide an analysis of the symptom of perioperative thirst (Conchon et al., 2014). A team in France developed a French version of the SMT and applied it to research and practice (Eicher, Delmas, Cohen, Baeriswyl, & Python, 2013). SMT was used in Korea to develop a disability intervention for older adults with arthritis (Shin, 2014). In China, theoretical extensions and applications of SMT were developed (Fangming & Jianhua, 2012) and used to guide the design of survey studies (W. Xiao et al., 2016). A unique use of SMT in Germany guided multiprofessional teams in treatment of oncology-related symptoms (Titzer, 2016).

## Research Studies Using the SMT

Research has varied in the extent to which SMT has been used as a conceptual basis, but has continued to develop over time. In fact, the body of knowledge grounded in SMT for cancer, dyspnea, and diabetes mellitus patient populations has progressed to the point where researchers have described symptom experiences, developed symptom management strategies, and conducted tests of their effectiveness. SMT research has expanded to include instrument development, such as questionnaires and checklists to validate and characterize patients' symptom experiences that can be used in research and practice. Moreover, research methods used to test the overall SMT or its components have diversified and become more sophisticated. Findings from these research studies remain remarkably similar and supportive of SMT across diverse populations using varied methods. In particular, the patients' varied symptom experiences, diverse management strategies, and the influence of person, environment, and health/illness domains were confirmed in every study included in the following sections.

## SYMPTOM EXPERIENCE

The symptom experience component remains the most researched aspect of the SMT. There were 19 studies published between 2013 and 2016 that specifically focused on the symptom experience within SMT. Seven of the 19 studies (37%) involved cancer patients and their symptom experiences (Astrup, Rustoen, Miaskowski, Paul, & Bjordal, 2015; Kyranou et al., 2014; Landers, McCarthy, Livingstone, & Savage, 2014; Lindviksmoen, Hofso, Paul, Miaskowski, & Rustoen, 2013; Oksholm et al., 2015; Wang et al., 2013; Wu, Natavio, Davis, & Yarandi, 2013). In contrast, for an entire 10-year period prior to 2013 (2002–2012) there were only seven studies focused on cancer patients that referenced the SMT (Dodd et al., 2010; Johnson, Moore, and Fortner, 2007; Miaskowski, Lee, et al., 2011; Miaskowski, Paul, et al., 2011; Merriman et al., 2011; Van Onselen et al., 2010) and one study focused on family caregivers of cancer patients (Fletcher, Dodd, Schumacher, & Miaskowski, 2008). While the seven prior studies only included patients in Northern California, the most recent studies include cancer patients from more diverse areas such as Indiana (Wang et al., 2013) and Michigan (Wu et al., 2013), as well as Ireland (Landers et al., 2014) and Norway (Astrup et al., 2015; Lindviksmoen et al., 2013; Oksholm et al., 2015). For the current seven studies involving cancer patients, symptoms ranged from depression and anxiety (Astrup et al., 2015; Kyranou et al., 2014; Lindviksmoen et al., 2013) to preoperative and postoperative symptoms of lack of energy in lung cancer patients (Oksholm et al., 2015) and pain in breast cancer or head and neck cancer patients (Wang et al., 2013; Wu et al., 2013).

Three of the 19 studies (16%) involved menopausal-related symptom experiences and focused on either bladder symptoms (Jones, Huang, Subak, Brown, & Lee, 2016) or psychological symptoms (Im, Kim, Chee, & Chee, 2016; Sternberg and Lee, 2013). These three studies are notable for their attention to ethnic and racial differences in symptom experiences of women living in California or Pennsylvania. Prior to 2013, the only study that reported using the SMT for research with a sample of healthy women was published by Yuan et al. (2011) and involved the fatigue experience of nurses in Taiwan who worked different shift schedules.

The remaining nine studies published between 2013 and 2016 involved acute and chronic illness populations. Only two of the nine studies involved acute illness: acute brain injury symptoms over time in a sample of patients in Michigan (Bergman et al., 2013) and symptom of thirst after surgery (daSilva, Aroni, & Fonseca, 2016). The remaining seven studies involved a chronic illness. Chronic illnesses included HIV infection and experience with lack of energy as distinct from fatigue (Aouizerat, Gay, Lerdal, Portillo, & Lee, 2013), COPD (Bentsen, Gundersen, Assmus, Bringsvor, & Berland, 2013), osteoarthritis (Jenkins & McCoy, 2015), the thirst experience in hemodialysis patients (Kara, 2016), schizophrenia (Leutwyler et al., 2014a, 2014b), multiple sclerosis (Newland, Flick, Thomas, & Shannon, 2014), and symptom side effects associated with treatment for hepatitis C virus (Rasi et al., 2014).

The 19 studies published between 2013 and 2016 utilized a variety of symptom measures. The most common measure for depressive symptoms was the Center for Epidemiologic Studies Depression Scale (CES-D) (Astrup, et al., 2015; Jones et al., 2016; Lindviksmoen et al., 2013; Sternberg and Lee, 2013). The CES-D addresses the frequency with which 20 symptoms occurred over the past week. In contrast, other depressive symptom measures may focus on severity or distress associated with the symptom and time frames may vary. Other frequently used measures were the Memorial Symptom Assessment Scale (MSAS) (Aouizerat et al., 2013; Oksholm et al., 2015) to assess frequency, severity, and distress associated with a variety of symptoms, and the Brief Pain Inventory (Wang et al., 2013; Wu et al., 2013), with 0 to 10 numeric scales for intensity, distress, and interference associated with the pain experience. Of note was the publication of results from a Thirst Distress Scale (Kara, 2016) in which hemodialysis patients were also asked about the timing (season of the year, time of day) of their thirst experience.

There were only two qualitative studies that used the SMT. One involved side effects experienced with therapy for hepatitis C virus (Rasi et al., 2014). The other qualitative study used a measure of thirst severity on a numeric rating scale of 0 to 10. If the thirst severity score was greater than 5, the patient was asked to participate in the qualitative component of the study to better understand their thirst experience (daSilva et al., 2016). Other measures were illness-specific and included a breathing problem questionnaire for COPD patient symptoms (Bentsen et al., 2013), severity and extent of being bothered by brain symptom (Bergman et al., 2013), frequency of bladder symptoms (Jones et al., 2016), severity of menopausal symptoms (Im, Kim, Chee, & Chee, 2016), frequency and interference of bowel symptoms (Lander et al., 2014), severity of schizophrenia symptoms (Leutwyler, Hubbard, Jeste, Miller, & Vinogradov, 2014a, 2014b), and frequency of multiple sclerosis symptoms (Newland et al., 2014).

An intriguing and rapidly growing area of interest is the study of symptom clusters. Although the original SMT focused on how a single symptom can be studied (as noted in earlier sections of this chapter), the symptom experience is likely to involve more than one symptom. Dodd et al. (2004) define symptom clusters as two or more symptoms that are both related to one another and occur concurrently. Commonly occurring symptom clusters include: (a) nausea, vomiting, and poor appetite; (b) pain, depression, disturbed sleep, and fatigue; or (c) wheezing, chest tightness, and shortness of breath. In asthma, symptom clusters commonly occur: chest tightness, shortness of breath, wheeze, and cough often occur together when asthma flares. These symptoms have been measured together on separate visual analog or numerical rating scales (Janson, Hardie, Fahy, & Boushey, 2001; Janson et al., 2003). Although there is a developing body of research that addresses symptom clusters (Dodd et al., 2010; E. Kim et al., 2009; Voss et al., 2007; C. Xiao, 2010), there are still considerable methodological issues to resolve (Miaskowski et al., 2007). Miaskowski (2006) suggests that research into symptom clusters may provide new insights into the underlying mechanisms. "If common biological mechanisms are found for specific symptom clusters, this knowledge may lead to the development of novel symptoms management strategies" (p. 793).

## ■ SYMPTOM EXPERIENCE WITHIN THE DOMAINS OF NURSING SCIENCE

More common were studies that describe the symptom experience and also sought to explore the relationship between this concept and one or more of the three domains of nursing science (person, environment, health/illness). Doorenbos, Given, Given, and Verbitsky (2006) conducted a secondary analysis from their three prospective, descriptive longitudinal studies to determine whether end-of-life symptom experiences changed with proximity to death or differed by gender, cancer site, or age. Nosek et al. (2010) found that the environmental factors influenced women's menopausal symptom experience. K. H. Kim and Lee (2009) compared the sleep and fatigue experiences of women before and at two time points after a hysterectomy according to procedure and contextual factors. Voss et al. (2007) found that fatigue severity was related to the health/illness domain; however, demographic and environmental variables influenced symptom experience more than the health/illness domain. Bay and Bergman (2006) examined the symptom experience of individuals with mild-to-moderate traumatic brain injury and found that postinjury symptoms varied by age and gender. Borge, Wahl, and Moum (2010) were among the several researchers who studied symptom experience of people with COPD. They found that individuals with COPD suffered a wide array of symptoms that were greatly affected by personal, environmental, and health/illness factors. They concluded that the healthcare providers who work with people with COPD need to expand their focus beyond single-item measure of symptoms. Possibly due to cultural differences, Korean immigrants identified "problems with urination" and "numbness and tingling" as frequent, distressing symptoms (Park, Stotts, Douglas, Donesky-Cuenco, & Carrieri-Kohlman,

2011) and were less likely to report sadness, feeling irritable, or nervousness compared with the Western samples of adults living with COPD.

The role of genetics in human disease can encompass the environment and health/illness domains as well as the person domain of the SMT. Identifying genetic predictors of symptoms that may account for personal or interindividual variation in symptom experience can be either disease-specific (e.g., cancer, HIV disease) or general determinants of symptoms that operate across chronic diseases (Baggott, 2012; Bentsen, Rustoen, & Miaskowski, 2011; Miaskowski et al., 2007).

More recent research applying SMT has centered on associations between symptom experiences and sociodemographics that are components of the three domains of nursing science (person, environment, and health/illness), specifically race/ethnicity, gender, age, and environmental factors. Budhrani Lengacher, Kip, Tofthagen, and Jim (2014) examined racial/ethnic differences in sleep disturbance among breast cancer survivors; White women slept longer than diverse minority women, and race/ethnicity modified the effect of depression and fatigue on their sleep disturbance. Im and colleagues conducted secondary analyses on midlife women from diverse racial/ethnic groups and reported on differences in cardiovascular symptoms (Im, Ham, Chee, & Chee, 2015b), depressive symptoms (Im, Ham, Chee, & Chee, 2015a), and factors influencing quality of life in cancer patients (Im, Chang, & Chee, 2014). Chang, Chee, & Im (2013) examined racial/ethnic groups of midlife women and the effects of physical activities on menopausal symptoms. Wright et al. (2015) assessed whether sociodemographic and clinical characteristics and symptoms were associated with trajectories of fatigue. Most recently, Matura, McDonough, and Carroll, (2016) examined sociodemographic and clinical factors influencing symptoms and quality of life.

Among studies focused on person (older age adults) and health/illness dimensions of the symptom experience, Byma, Given, and Given (2013b) studied cancer diagnosis and pain among older adults participating in a Home and Community Based Waiver Program. Leutwyler and associates studied older adults with schizophrenia and their symptoms associated with neurocognition (Leutwyler et al., 2014a) and mobility (Leutwyler et al., 2014b).

The environmental domain has received less attention from researchers than person or health/illness domains, yet research shows these three domains to be intrinsically related and difficult to parse into research components. Corless et al. (2013) examined how stressful life events, in addition to symptom experience and adherence concerns, contributed to quality of life among people living with HIV. Samuels and Eckardt (2014) examined postoperative pain and found that pain severity was influenced by the hospital setting, the surgical procedure, and repeated assessments of pain. Findings from these more recent studies provide important evidence to guide policies to improve symptom management and alleviate distressing symptoms.

## ■ SYMPTOM EXPERIENCE OF CHILDREN AND FAMILIES

The SMT has provided a conceptual framework for nursing-led pediatric research over the past decade, with a focus on children with cancer and their families (Baggott, Cooper, Marina, Matthay, & Miaskowski, 2011; Gedaly-Duff, Lee, Nail, Nicholson, & Johnson, 2006; Linder, 2010; Rodgers et al., 2008; van Cleve et al., 2004). SMT continues to be a useful framework for more recent research extending knowledge related to symptom reporting, symptom prevalence, and intervention effectiveness. Using SMT as a framework, Baggott, Cooper, Marina, Matthay, and Miaskowski (2014) compared child and parent symptom reports during chemotherapy in children and adolescents (ages 10–18 years) and Linder and Seitz (2016) described symptom "bother" in children and adolescents (ages 7–18 years) during hospitalization. Rodgers, Krance, Street, and Hockenberry (2014) examined symptom prevalence, distress, and physiologic parameters after a mobile application intervention designed to promote eating and manage gastrointestinal symptoms in adolescents after hematopoietic stem cell transplant. However, relatively few publications on children's symptoms reference SMT compared with the adult literature and the application of SMT has focused exclusively on children with cancer with the exception of one publication on pediatric asthma (Newcomb, 2010). There are no references to SMT in research focused on other family members of children with health conditions, such as parents or siblings.

The dearth of literature on SMT with respect to children and families may relate to the predominance of other theoretical frameworks for research in these populations, such as developmental theories or symptom-specific theories (e.g., pain). However, these theories may not be sufficiently comprehensive to adequately guide nursing research and practice with these populations. SMT suggests ways in which the symptom experience, management, and outcomes in children and their families may be influenced by personal characteristics—particularly developmental, health/illness, and environment. We encourage future research and theoretical work to explore SMT as a framework for theory, research, and clinical practice with children and families.

## ■ SYMPTOM MANAGEMENT STRATEGIES

From 2013 to 2016, there have been five new studies (Eller et al., 2013; Koller, Miaskowski, De Geest, Opitz, & Spichiger, 2013; Taylor & Holston, 2014; Yang, Lee, Lo, & Beckstead, 2015; Yeager et al., 2016) and two new protocols published (Eaton et al., 2014; Klainin-Yobas et al., 2015) guided by the SMT that tested, or are testing, symptom management strategies. Two of the five newly published studies focused on managing symptoms of cancer or cancer treatment–related symptoms.

Using a qualitative approach, Yeager et al. (2016) studied a sample of African Americans living in poverty with advanced cancer to learn how they relieve and manage daily symptoms. They found that participants used two major symptom management strategies: making continual adjustments to medications and lifestyle behaviors, and finding stability through spirituality with faith and prayer. Focusing on self-management of cancer-related pain, Koller et al. (2013) used the PRO-SELF Plus Pain Control Program in a small randomized controlled pilot study of German oncology outpatients with persistent pain. The intervention consisted of six visits and four phone calls delivered by a trained nurse that focused on education, skill building, and nurse coaching. The intervention group had statistically significant gains in knowledge but no significant difference in pain scores compared to controls. The small sample size and high attrition rate in this study may have caused it to be underpowered.

Three additional new studies focused on management of depressive symptoms in people with HIV/AIDS (Eller et al., 2005), management of auditory hallucination symptoms in people with schizophrenia (Yang et al., 2015), and management of symptoms experienced by incarcerated and formerly incarcerated woman victims of intimate partner violence (IPV; Taylor & Holston, 2014). In a subsample of people living with HIV, Eller et al. (2013) conducted a secondary analysis of data from their original larger randomized clinical trial to identify the effect of a symptom management manual on depressive symptoms. In this highly diverse sample from multiple countries, they found the most used self-care strategies were distraction techniques and prayer. In the second study, using a nonrandomized experimental design, Yang et al. (2015) evaluated the effectiveness of an auditory hallucinatory symptom management intervention delivered in 60-minute weekly group sessions for 10 weeks to the experimental group. The comparison control group received routine care. The sessions included sharing hallucinatory experiences, teaching management strategies, and opportunity to practice these skills. The intervention group showed a nonsignificant improvement in anxiety symptoms over time compared to controls. The third study investigated the efficacy of a group psychoeducation music intervention on symptoms experienced by woman survivors of IPV using a repeated measures design. The purpose of this pilot study was to change symptoms related to IPV, such as depressive symptoms, anxiety, low self-esteem, and social isolation, among both incarcerated and formerly incarcerated women. Using the Music and Account-Making for Behavioral-Related Adaptation program, the intervention included participatory CD music design and psychoeducation to explore experiences of violence and recovery over four theme-focused sessions. They reported a sustained decrease in symptoms and sustained increase in self-esteem over time.

Two papers described protocols of ongoing clinical trials. Using a cluster randomized clinical trial design, Eaton et al. (2014) developed and is testing a telehealth-enhanced intervention for chronic pain management in patients of community health providers across multiple geographic locations. The intervention uses low-cost, commercially available technology to deliver the three components of the intervention: video case conferences between providers and pain experts, weekly reports of patients' symptoms, and weekly graphs of patients' pain experience. The study aims are to evaluate the efficacy and cost-effectiveness of the intervention compared to usual care. In the second ongoing study protocol using a randomized single-blind controlled trial, Klainin-Yobas et al. (2015) are testing a symptom management program for hospitalized patients with acute myocardial infarction. The self-management intervention targets both physiological and psychological symptoms experienced by these hospitalized patients and includes individualized symptom management sessions delivered through a virtual reality device followed by phone calls and booster sessions postdischarge.

Prior to 2013, seven studies focused on symptom management strategies documented that patients and others use a variety of approaches to manage their symptoms (Faucett, Meyers, Miles, Janowitz, & Fathallah, 2007; Landers et al., 2011; K. A. Lee & Gay, 2011; Suwanno, Petpichetchian, Riegel, & Issaramalai, 2009; Webel & Holzemer, 2009; Wells et al., 2007; Zimmerman et al., 2011). Using qualitative methods, Landers, McCarthy, and Savage (2011) found that even 2 years after sphincter-saving surgery for rectal cancer, patients struggled to manage an array of symptoms with varying success. Zimmerman et al. (2011) found gender-based differences in their test of the effectiveness of a symptom management intervention with women reporting fewer symptoms and better outcomes postcoronary artery bypass surgery compared with men. Suwanno et al. (2009) noted that person, health/ illness, and environment domains influenced symptom management strategies in heart failure patients. Faucett et al. (2007) tested a symptom management strategy to reduce the musculoskeletal pain and fatigue associated with strenuous fieldwork in the agricultural industry. They added four brief rest breaks to the usual shift pattern and productivity was relatively unchanged. The success of this intervention was most clearly demonstrated when the managers and workers agreed to retain the intervention after the research was completed. Webel and Holzemer (2009) found that urban, HIV-infected women were very interested in participating in a community-based, peer-led intervention to facilitate symptom management. A randomized clinical trial to change the bedroom environment improved the sleep of parents and, in fact, worked best for parents with low socioeconomic status (K. A. Lee & Gay, 2011). These studies on symptom management strategies indicate strong evidence that healthcare providers need to foster open communication with patients if they are to learn self-care strategies and increase patient awareness of the most beneficial approach for their unique situation.

In total, 16 studies included measures of all three key concepts: symptom experience, symptom management strategies, and outcomes (Chou, Dodd,

Abrams, & Padilla, 2007; Eaton et al., 2014; Eller et al., 2013, 2005; Fuller et al., 2005; Hearson, 2006; Henoch et al., 2008; Janson et al., 2003, 2009, 2010; Klainin-Yorbas et al., 2015; Koller et al., 2013; Taylor & Holston, 2014; Tsai, Holzemer, & Leu, 2005; Yang et al., 2015; Yeager et al., 2016). Yeager et al. (2016) and Henoch et al. (2008) used qualitative methods to uncover the full range of patients' symptom experiences, management strategies, and outcomes. Of note, both studies found that the patients' symptom experiences also included an existential impact involving faith, hope, hopelessness, and thoughts of death, areas of the symptom experience not previously reported. Chou et al. (2007) explored the cancer symptom experience, self-care strategies, and quality of life among Chinese Americans during outpatient chemotherapy. Participants reported approximately 14 symptoms weekly and averaged two self-care strategies per symptom that were of low-to-moderate effectiveness.

Five studies reported on interventions to reduce symptoms in patients with cancer (Koller et al., 2013; J. Lee, Dodd, Dibble, & Abrams, 2008; Ruegg, Curran, & Lamb, 2009; Skrutkowski et al., 2008; Yeager et al., 2016). Skelly and colleagues (Leeman et al., 2008; Skelly et al., 2008, 2009) used the SMT to develop a conceptual model of symptom-focused diabetes care for African Americans. They then conducted a randomized controlled trial of their nursing intervention to improve outcomes among older African American women with type 2 diabetes, and pilot-tested a tailored diabetes self-care intervention with older rural African American women. Both studies demonstrated the success of well-conceptualized and tailored interventions to reduce symptoms in diabetes.

■ USE OF THE THEORY IN NURSING PRACTICE

There has been a proliferation in research applying SMT to support nursing practice. Prior to 2013, there were only five publications using SMT related to practice. Jablonski and Wyatt (2005) examined end-of-life care as a way to better understand the needs of dying patients and environmental barriers preventing them from getting care. Ahlberg, Ekman, and Gaston-Johansson (2005) used SMT as a framework for cancer-related fatigue. Maag et al. (2006) synthesized SMT with other theories to form a conceptual framework for a clinical nurse leader education program. They include SMT to ensure that the clinical nurse leader graduate will effectively evaluate patient symptoms and develop and implement effective management strategies to achieve optimal outcomes. Johnson et al. (2007) and Carpenter et al. (2008) noted that symptom assessments can be computerized, but unless such systems are seamlessly integrated into electronic health records, symptoms are unlikely to be assessed.

Most recently (2013–2016), 12 published reports regarding implementing SMT in nursing practice were found related to symptom assessments, management strategies, and outcome evaluations for interdisciplinary patient care teams. Four of these studies centered on nursing assessments of symptom experience to guide development of a symptom management plan for patients with cancer (Lynch, 2014), postoperative pain (Samuels and Manworren, 2014), patients with COPD (Srirat, Hanucharurnkul, Aree-Ue, Viwatwongkasem, & Junda, 2014), or patients in intensive care units on a ventilator (Randen, Lerdal, & Bjork, 2013). Four other studies focused on symptom assessment tools that nurses can use for patients with cancer (Swenson et al., 2013), pulmonary hypertension (Matura, McDonough, Hanlon, & Carroll, 2015), and auditory hallucinations (Trygstad, Buccheri, Buffum, Ju, & Dowling, 2015).

Two publications offered practice tools to improve nursing symptom assessments to tailor a patient's symptom management plan. Buccheri, Trygstad, Buffum, Birmingham, & Dowling (2013) offered the Unpleasant Auditory Hallucinations Practice Model to help mental health nurses. Yoshioka, Moriyama, and Ohno (2014) described continuing education programs for nurses specializing in end-of-life patient care, and Rosen, Bergh, Schwartz-Barcott, and Martensson (2014) discussed the need for nursing outcome evaluations of postoperative patient self-care management strategies to further tailor a more effective management plan for symptom relief.

Finally, two other recent publications referencing SMT offered innovative symptom management strategies to support nursing practice. Beebe (2014) highlighted hypnotherapy as an option to help women during childbirth. Titzer (2016) used the SMT as a framework to outline a comprehensive multi-professional management care plan for patients with cancer.

An emerging area of research using SMT related to nursing practice is the development of instruments, questionnaires, interview guides, and checklists to help the clinician better characterize a patient's symptom experience. Several psychometric studies have identified instrument properties and tested the reliability and validity of such tools that can be used in clinical practice. Prior to 2013, only one publication was identified focused on instrument development using SMT. Nieveen, Zimmerman, Barnason, and Yates (2008) used the symptom experience concept as the basis for developing the Cardiac Symptom Survey.

Since 2013, six additional studies were identified that used the SMT for instrument development: (a) Byma, Given, and Given (2013a) validated the Depression Rating Scale as a tool to identify depressive symptoms in older adults; (b) Hirai, Kanda, Takagai, and Hosokawa (2015) described the Hirai Cancer Fatigue Scale to assess fatigue experiences among cancer patients; (c) Kara (2013) reported on the Turkish version of the Thirst Distress Scale to assess thirst in patients on hemodialysis; (d) Trygstad et al. (2015) described the Auditory Hallucinations Interview Guide to assess auditory hallucination in mental health patients; (e) Matura et al. (2015) reported on the Pulmonary Arterial Hypertension Symptom Scale to assess symptom clusters in patients with pulmonary arterial hypertension; and finally (f) Swenson et al. (2013)

compared several available measures to evaluate the best tool to assess changes in musculosketal symptoms and physical functioning in women with breast cancer.

Further research is needed to validate these tools for symptom measurement. Nevertheless, these instruments provide important options for valid and reliable measures of a patient's symptom experience to further the underpinnings of the SMT. Findings from these studies would help to inform practice related to symptom management strategies, to evaluate the success of these strategies with outcome-specific measures, and ultimately to identify effective strategies for individualized symptom relief.

## ■ CONCLUSION

The body of knowledge acquired from research using the SMT is growing. Across multiple studies with diverse samples and methods, the results are remarkably similar. Patients experience a wide range of symptoms and use a variety of terms and phrases to describe these sensations. They largely attempt to manage symptoms themselves using strategies without evidence-based support and strategies of questionable value. Clinicians are seen as an important source of information about symptoms, but so are family, friends, employers, the media, and the Internet including chat rooms. There is clear evidence that providers must have good patient–provider communication if they are to understand and accept their patient's symptom experience, and implement effective management strategies to achieve the outcome of interest for the patient. It is also essential for providers to consider the strengths and limitations imposed on patients within the person, environment, and health/illness dimensions. When symptoms are not adequately addressed within the context of one's environment and health status, patients continue to suffer with a poor quality of life at high costs to the individual, family, healthcare system, workplace, and society.

The National Institutes of Health Symptom Science Model is a nursing science driven model that provides an investigative guide for symptom research to reduce symptoms and improve patient outcomes (Cashion, Gill, Hawes, Henderson, & Saligan, 2016). From a more multidisciplinary and futuristic perspective, three key developments are already in place: the national Patient-Centered Outcomes Research Initiative (PCORI), use of common data elements with similar coding for symptom(s) of interest, and more sophisticated analyses of big data and epigenetics in symptom science research. These three areas will no doubt test all symptom-related theories and lead to future modifications of SMT as well. Corwin et al. (2014) have outlined several specific research and policy suggestions in these areas that would advance symptom science in the future. These suggestions are all supported by the National Institute of Nursing Research (K. A. Lee, Meek, & Grady, 2014).

The SMT may continue to evolve and may need future revisions. The time, or temporal dimension, is missing from the model. A reference to time only appears in the management strategies' concept circle as "when" a strategy is initiated or administered. More sophisticated studies use longitudinal designs to document the natural history of symptoms as well as the effect of repeated doses of interventions on symptom status. The need to consider changes in symptom status over time is also important because change in the status of symptoms may influence adherence to a prescribed strategy. For the highest possible benefit from symptom management strategies, researchers and clinicians must be able to determine when management strategies are best received and when outcomes, including a change in the status of the symptom, are best measured. Recent technological advances, such as electronic symptom diaries or wearable monitoring sensors, have facilitated the collection of patient-reported outcomes in real time. Likewise, researchers can now collect patients' daily reports of their use of self-care strategies. How symptom severity or distress changes with symptom management patterns over time may lead to important discoveries regarding the efficacy of the intervention. Henly, Kallas, Klatt, and Swenson (2003) attempted to address this limitation by positing a new theory that includes four temporal dimensions of symptoms. However in doing so, they created a more linear framework that fails to consider the multidimensional nature of symptoms. Nonetheless, their efforts provide insight into future versions of SMT.

The prior depiction of the SMT model within three suspended circles representing the three dimensions of nursing science may work for a three-dimensional holographic representation but was difficult to depict in a two-dimensional representation on paper. In this current modification of the SMT, one suspended circle around the three concepts provides more clarity with respect to the dimensions of nursing science (see Figure 8.1).

The SMT assumes that a symptom is reported from the perspective of the individual who is experiencing it. Data from family caregivers' perspectives of the symptom experience remain ubiquitous in pediatrics and commonplace in the care of most adults with chronic conditions. The family caregivers' perspectives are not always congruent with the patient's self-report, adding complexity to the evaluation of symptom experiences. Revision of the SMT to make it clearer, more parsimonious, and more representative of "real life" may also increase its usefulness to researchers and clinicians.

In almost two decades since the SMT was originally introduced, it has gained acceptance as a valuable theory for organizing knowledge for research and clinical practice, especially for the symptom experience concept within the person, environment, and health/illness domains of nursing science. The symptom management concept provides guidance in evaluating self-management strategies in addition to clinician-prescribed strategies, and the factors within the outcomes concept underscore the importance of evaluating changes in the status of the symptom itself (frequency, severity, and distress). The key outcomes related to the symptom experience have always been patient-oriented and remain a strength of the SMT. The SMT has brought together researchers and clinicians from diverse backgrounds and countries around a shared interest in managing symptoms. The many perspectives have expanded knowledge in the areas of symptom clusters, and knowledge gained in one symptom area has been extrapolated to similarities in assessment of the experience, formulation of testable management strategies, and evaluation of many relevant outcomes. Research and practice within the SMT concepts and domains support its current value and continuing efforts to refine the theory are encouraged for ongoing research and application to clinical practice.

## ■ REFERENCES

Ahlberg, K., Ekman, T., & Gaston-Johansson, F. (2005). Fatigue, psychological distress, coping resources, and functional status during radiotherapy for uterine cancer. *Oncology Nursing Forum*, *32*(3), 633–640.

Allida, S. M., Inglis, S. C., Davidson, P. M., Hayward, C. S., & Newton, P. J. (2014). Measurement of thirst in chronic heart failure–A review. *Contemporary Nurse*, *48*(1), 2–9. doi:10.5172/conu.2014.48.1.2

Aouizerat, B. E., Gay, C. L., Lerdal, A., Portillo, C. J., & Lee, K. A. (2013). Lack of energy: An important and distinct component of HIV-related fatigue and daytime function. *Journal of Pain and Symptom Management*, *45*(2), 191–201. doi:10.1016/j.jpainsymman.2012.01.011

Arslanian-Engoren, C., & Engoren, M. (2010). Physiological and anatomical bases for sex differences in pain and nausea as presenting symptoms of acute coronary syndromes. *Heart & Lung: The Journal of Acute and Critical Care*, *39*(5), 386–393.

Astrup, G. L., Rustoen, T., Miaskowski, C., Paul, S. M., & Bjordal, K. (2015). A longitudinal study of depressive symptoms in patients with head and neck cancer undergoing radiotherapy. *Cancer Nursing*, *38*(6), 436–446. doi:10.1097/NCC.0000000000000225

Baggott, C. (2012). *Evaluation of candidate genes for chemotherapy-induced nausea and vomiting* (Mentored Research Scholar Grant ed.). New York, NY: American Cancer Society. MRSG-12-01-PCSM.

Baggott, C., Cooper, B. A., Marina, N., Matthay, K. K., & Miaskowski, C. (2011). Symptom cluster analyses based on symptom occurrence and severity ratings among pediatric oncology patients during myelosuppressive chemotherapy. *Cancer Nursing*, *35*(1), 19–28.

Baggott, C., Cooper, B. A., Marina, N., Matthay, K. K., & Miaskowski, C. (2014). Symptom assessment in pediatric oncology: How should concordance between children's and parents' reports be evaluated? *Cancer Nursing*, *37*(4), 252–262. doi:10.1097/NCC.0000000000000111

Bay, E., & Bergman, K. (2006). Symptom experience and emotional distress after traumatic brain injury. *Care Management Journals: Journal of Case Management; The Journal of Long Term Home Health Care, 7*(1), 3–9.

Beebe, K. (2014). Hypnotherapy for labor and birth. *Nursing for Women's Health, 18*(1), 48–59. doi:10.1111/1751-486X.12093

Bentsen, S. B., Gundersen, D., Assmus, J., Bringsvor, H., & Berland, A. (2013). Multiple symptoms in patients with chronic obstructive pulmonary disease in Norway. *Nursing & Health Sciences, 15*(3), 292–299. doi:10.1111/nhs.12031

Bentsen, S. B., Rustoen, T., & Miaskowski, C. (2011). Prevalence and characteristics of pain in patients with chronic obstructive pulmonary disease compared to the Norwegian general population. *The Journal of Pain: Official Journal of the American Pain Society, 12*(5), 539–545.

Bergman, K., Given, B., Fabiano, R., Schutte, D., von Eye, A., & Davidson, S. (2013). Symptoms associated with mild traumatic brain injury/concussion: The role of bother. *Journal of Neuroscience Nursing, 45*(3), 124–132. doi:10.1097/JNN.0b013e31828a418b

Borge, C. R., Wahl, A. K., & Moum, T. (2010). Association of breathlessness with multiple symptoms in chronic obstructive pulmonary disease. *Journal of Advanced Nursing, 66*(12), 2688–2700.

Brant, J. M., Beck, S., & Miaskowski, C. (2010). Building dynamic models and theories to advance the science of symptom management research. *Journal of Advanced Nursing, 66*(1), 228–240.

Brant, J. M., Dudley, W. N., Beck, S., & Miaskowski, C. (2016). Evolution of the dynamic symptoms model. *Oncology Nursing Forum, 43*(5), 651–654. doi:10.1188/16.ONF.651-654

Buccheri, R. K., Trygstad, L. N., Buffum, M. D., Birmingham, P., & Dowling, G. A. (2013). Self-management of unpleasant auditory hallucinations: a tested practice model. *Journal of Psychosocial Nursing and Mental Health Services, 51*(11), 26–34. doi:10.3928/02793695-20130731-02

Budhrani, P. H., Lengacher, C. A., Kip, K. E., Tofthagen, C., & Jim, H (2014). Minority breast cancer survivors: The association between race/ethnicity, objective sleep disturbances, and physical and psychological symptoms. *Nursing Research and Practice, 2014*, 858403. doi:10.1155/2014/858403

Byma, E. A., Given, C. W., & Given, B. A. (2013a). Associations among indicators of depression in Medicaid-eligible community-dwelling older adults. *Gerontologist, 53*(4), 608–617. doi:10.1093/geront/gns130

Byma, E. A., Given, B. A., & Given, C. W. (2013b). Longitudinal differences in pain among older adult Home and Community Based Waiver Program participants in relation to diagnosis of cancer. *Home Health Care Services Quarterly, 32*(4), 249–266. doi:10.1080/01621424.2013.851051

Carpenter, J. S., Rawl, S., Porter, J., Schmidt, K., Tornatta, J., Ojewole, F., . . . Giesler, R. B. (2008). Oncology outpatient and provider responses to a computerized symptom assessment system. *Oncology Nursing Forum, 35*(4), 661–669.

Carrieri-Kohlman, V., Demir-Deviren, S., Cuenco, D., Eiser, S., & Stulbarg, M. S. (2000). Effect of exercise dose on affective response to dyspnea in COPD. *American Journal of Respiratory and Critical Care Medicine, 161 (Suppl.),* A705.

Carrieri-Kohlman, V., Donesky-Cuenco, D., Park, S. K., Mackin, L., Nguyen, H. Q., & Paul, S. M. (2010). Additional evidence for the affective dimension of dyspnea in patients with COPD. *Research in Nursing & Health, 33*(1), 4–19.

Carrieri-Kohlman, V., Gormley, J. M., Douglas, M. K., Paul, S. M., & Stulbarg, M. S. (1996). Differentiation between dyspnea and its affective components. *Western Journal of Nursing Research, 18*(6), 626–642.

Carrieri-Kohlman, V., Gormley, J. M., Eiser, S., Demir-Deviren, S., Nguyen, H., Paul, S. M., & Stulbarg, M. S. (2001). Dyspnea and the affective response during exercise training in obstructive pulmonary disease. *Nursing Research, 50*(3), 136–146.

Carrieri-Kohlman, V., & Janson-Bjerklie, S. (1986). Strategies patients use to manage the sensation of dyspnea. *Western Journal of Nursing Research, 8*(3), 284–305.

Carrieri-Kohlman, V., Kieckhefer, G., Janson-Bjerklie, S., & Souza, J. (1991). The sensation of pulmonary dyspnea in school-age children. *Nursing Research, 40*(2), 81–85.

Carrieri-Kohlman, V., Nguyen, H. Q., Donesky-Cuenco, D., Demir-Deviren, S., Neuhaus, J., & Stulbarg, M. S. (2005). Impact of brief or extended exercise training on the benefit of a dyspnea self-management program in COPD. *Journal of Cardiopulmonary Rehabilitation, 25*(5), 275–284.

Cashion, A. K., Gill, J., Hawes, R., Henderson, W. A., & Saligan, L. (2016). National Institutes of Health Symptom Science Model sheds light on patient symptoms. *Nursing Outlook, 64*(5), 499–506.

Chang, S. J., Chee, W., & Im, E.-O. (2013). Menopausal symptoms and physical activity in multiethnic groups of midlife women: a secondary analysis. *Journal of Advanced Nursing, 69*(9), 1953–1965. doi:10.1111/jan.12056

Chou, F.-Y., Dodd, M., Abrams, D., & Padilla, G. (2007). Symptoms, self-care, and quality of life of Chinese American patients with cancer. *Oncology Nursing Forum, 34*(6), 1162–1167.

Committee on Quality of Health Care in America. (2001). *Crossing the quality chasm.* Washington, DC: National Academies Press.

Conchon, M. F., Nascimento, L. A., Fonseca, L. F., & Aroni, P. (2015). Perioperative thirst: an analysis from the perspective of the Symptom Management Theory. *Revista da Escola de Enfermagem da USP, 49*(1), 122–128. doi:10.1590/S0080-623420150000100016

Corless, I. B., Voss, J., Guarino, A. J., Wantland, D., Holzemer, W., Hamilton, M. J., . . . Cuca, Y. (2013). The impact of stressful life events, symptom status, and adherence concerns on quality of life in people living with HIV. *Journal of the Association of Nurses in AIDS Care, 24*(6), 478–490. doi:10.1016/j.jana.2012.11.005

Corwin, E. J., Berg, J. A., Armstrong, T. S., DeVito Dabbs, A., Lee, K. A., Meek, P., & Redeker, N. (2014). Envisioning the future in symptom science. *Nursing Outlook, 62*(5), 346–351.

daSilva, L., Aroni, P., & Fonseca, L. (2016). I am thirsty! Experience of the surgical patient in the perioperative period. *Revista SOBECC, 21*(2), 75–81. doi:10.5327/Z1414-4425201600020003

Davis, A. H., Carrieri-Kohlman, V., Janson, S. L., Gold, W. M., & Stulbarg, M. S. (2006). Effects of treatment on two types of self-efficacy in people with chronic obstructive pulmonary disease. *Journal of Pain and Symptom Management, 32*(1), 60–70.

Davis, L. L., Carpenter, J. S., & Otte, J. L. (2016). State of the science: Taxane-induced musculoskeletal pain. *Cancer Nursing, 39*(3), 187–196. doi:10.1097/NCC.0000000000000273

Dodd, M. J., Cho, M. H., Cooper, B. A., & Miaskowski, C. (2010). The effect of symptom clusters on functional status and quality of life in women with breast cancer. *European Journal of Oncology Nursing: The Official Journal of European Oncology Nursing Society, 14*(2), 101–110.

Dodd, M. J., Janson, S., Facione, N., Faucett, J., Froelicher, E. S., Humphreys, J., . . . Taylor, D. (2001). Advancing the science of symptom management. *Journal of Advanced Nursing, 33*(5), 668–676.

Dodd, M. J., Miaskowski, C., & Lee, K. A. (2004). Occurrence of symptom clusters. *Journal of the National Cancer Institute. Monographs,* (32), 76–78.

Dodd, M. J., Miaskowski, C., & Paul, S. M. (2001). Symptom clusters and their effect on the functional status of patients with cancer. *Oncology Nursing Forum, 28*(3), 465–470.

Donesky, D., Janson, S. L., Nguyen, H. Q., Neuhaus, J., Neilands, T. B., & Carrieri-Kohlman, V. (2011). Determinants of frequency, duration, and continuity of home walking in patients with COPD. *Geriatric Nursing, 32*(3), 178–187.

Donesky-Cuenco, D., Janson, S., Neuhaus, J., Neilands, T. B., & Carrieri-Kohlman, V. (2007). Adherence to a home-walking prescription in patients with chronic obstructive pulmonary disease. *Heart & Lung: The Journal of Critical Care, 36*(5), 348–363.

Donesky-Cuenco, D., Nguyen, H. Q., Paul, S., & Carrieri-Kohlman, V. (2009). Yoga therapy decreases dyspnea-related distress and improves functional performance in people with chronic obstructive pulmonary disease: A pilot study. *Journal of Alternative and Complementary Medicine, 15*(3), 225–234.

Doorenbos, A. Z., Given, C. W., Given, B., & Verbitsky, N. (2006). Symptom experience in the last year of life among individuals with cancer. *Journal of Pain and Symptom Management, 32*(5), 403–412.

Eaton, L. H., Gordon, D. B., Wyant, S., Theodore, B. R., Meins, A. R., Rue, T., . . . Doorenbos, A. Z. (2014). Development and implementation of a telehealth-enhanced intervention for pain and symptom management. *Contemporary Clinical Trials, 38*(2), 213–220. doi:10.1016/j.cct.2014.05.005

Eicher, M., Delmas, P., Cohen, C., Baeriswyl, C., & Python, N. V. (2013). The French version of Symptom Management Theory and its application. *Recherche en soins infirmiers,* (112), 14–25.

Eller, L. S., Corless, I., Bunch, E. H., Kemppainen, J., Holzemer, W., Nokes, K., . . . Nicholas, P. (2005). Self-care strategies for depressive symptoms in people with HIV disease. *Journal of Advanced Nursing, 51*(2), 119–130.

Eller, L. S., Kirksey, K. M., Nicholas, P. K., Corless, I. B., Holzemer, W. L., Wantland, D. J., . . . Human, S. (2013). A randomized controlled trial of an HIV/AIDS symptom management manual for depressive symptoms. *AIDS Care, 25*(4), 391–399. doi:10.1080/09540121.2012.712662

Fangming, F., & Jianhua, L. (2012). Development on symptom management theory. *Chinese Nursing Research*, 26(4A), 874–876.

Faucett, J., & McCarthy, D. (2003). Chronic pain in the workplace. *The Nursing Clinics of North America*, 38(3), 509–523.

Faucett, J., Meyers, J., Miles, J., Janowitz, I., & Fathallah, F. (2007). Rest break interventions in stoop labor tasks. *Applied Ergonomics*, 38(2), 219–226.

Fletcher, B. A. S., Dodd, M. J., Schumacher, K. L., & Miaskowski, C. (2008). Symptom experience of family caregivers of patients with cancer. *Oncology Nursing Forum*, 35(2), E23–E44; E23.

Fuller, E., Welch, J. L., Backer, J. H., & Rawl, S. M. (2005). Symptom experience of chronically constipated women with pelvic floor disorders. *Clinical Nurse Specialist*, 19, 34–40.

Gedaly-Duff, V., Lee, K. A., Nail, L., Nicholson, H. S., & Johnson, K. P. (2006). Pain, sleep disturbance, and fatigue in children with leukemia and their parents: A pilot study. *Oncology Nursing Forum*, 33(3), 641–646.

Hammer, M. J., Ercolano, E. A., Wright, F., Dickson, V. V., Chyun, D., & Melkus, G. D. (2015). Self-management for adult patients with cancer: An integrative review. *Cancer Nursing*, 38(2), E10–E26. doi:10.1097/NCC.0000000000000122

Hearson, B. (2006). Sleep disturbance in family caregivers: Application of the revised symptom management model. *Journal of Palliative Care*, 22(3), 216.

Henly, S. J., Kallas, K. D., Klatt, C. M., & Swenson, K. K. (2003). The notion of time in symptom experiences. *Nursing Research*, 52(6), 410–417.

Henoch, I., Bergman, B., & Danielson, E. (2008). Dyspnea experience and management strategies in patients with lung cancer. *Psycho-Oncology*, 17(7), 709–715.

Hirai, K., Kanda, K., Takagai, J., & Hosokawa, M. (2015). Development of the Hirai Cancer Fatigue Scale: Testing its reliability and validity. *European Journal of Oncology Nursing*, 19(4), 427–432. doi:10.1016/j.ejon.2014.12.004

Hsu, M. C., & Tu, C. H. (2014). Improving quality-of-life outcomes for patients with cancer through mediating effects of depressive symptoms and functional status: A three-path mediation model. *Journal of Clinical Nursing*, 23(17–18), 2461–2472. doi:10.1111/jocn.12399

Im, E.-O., Chang, S. J., & Chee, E. (2014). Predictors of quality of life in cancer survivors: White and Asian American women. *Women & Therapy*, 37(3–4), 282–300. doi:10.1080/02703149.2014.897554

Im, E.-O., Ham, O. K., Chee, E., & Chee, W. (2015a). Physical activity and depressive symptoms in four ethnic groups of midlife women. *Western Journal of Nursing Research*, 37(6), 746–766. doi:10.1177/0193945914537123

Im, E.-O., Ham, O. K., Chee, E., & Chee, W. (2015b). Racial/ethnic differences in cardiovascular symptoms in four major racial/ethnic groups of midlife women: A secondary analysis. *Women Health*, 55(5), 525–547. doi:10.1080/03630242.2015.102 2813

Im, E.-O., Kim, J., Chee, E., & Chee, W. (2016). The relationships between psychological symptoms and cardiovascular symptoms experienced during the menopausal transition: Racial/ethnic differences. *Menopause*, 23(4), 396–402. doi:10.1097/GME.0000000000000545

Jablonski, A., & Wyatt, G. K. (2005). A model for identifying barriers to effective symptom management at the end of life. *Journal of Hospice & Palliative Nursing*, 7(1), 23–36.

Janson, S. L., & Becker, G. (1998). Reasons for delay in seeking treatment for acute asthma: The patient's perspective. *Journal of Asthma: Official Journal of the Association for the Care of Asthma*, 35(5), 427–435.

Janson, S. L., Fahy, J. V., Covington, J. K., Paul, S. M., Gold, W. M., & Boushey, H. A. (2003). Effects of individual self-management education on clinical, biological, and adherence outcomes in asthma. *The American Journal of Medicine*, 115(8), 620–626.

Janson, S. L., Hardie, G., Fahy, J., & Boushey, H. (2001). Use of biological markers of airway inflammation to detect the efficacy of nurse-delivered asthma education. *Heart & Lung: The Journal of Critical Care*, 30(1), 39–46.

Janson, S. L., McGrath, K. W., Covington, J. K., Baron, R. B., & Lazarus, S. C. (2010). Objective airway monitoring improves asthma control in the cold and flu season: A cluster randomized trial. *Chest*, 138(5), 1148–1155.

Janson, S. L., McGrath, K. W., Covington, J. K., Cheng, S. C., & Boushey, H. A. (2009). Individualized asthma self-management improves medication adherence and markers of asthma control. *Journal of Allergy and Clinical Immunology*, 123(4), 840–846.

Janson, S. L., Solari, P. G., Trzaskoma, B., Chen, H., Haselkorn, T., & Zazzali, J. L. (2015). Omalizumab adherence in an observational study of patients with moderate to severe allergic asthma. *Annals of Allergy, Asthma & Immunology*, 114(6), 516–521. doi:10.1016/j.anai.2015.04.010

Janson-Bjerklie, S., Carrieri-Kohlman, V., & Hudes, M. (1986). The sensations of pulmonary dyspnea. *Nursing Research*, 35(3), 154–159.

Janson-Bjerklie, S., Ferketich, S., Benner, P., & Becker, G. (1992). Clinical markers of asthma severity and risk: Importance of subjective as well as objective factors. *Heart & Lung: The Journal of Critical Care*, 21(3), 265–272.

Jenkins, J. B., & McCoy, T. P. (2015). Symptom clusters, functional status, and quality of life in older adults with osteoarthritis. *Orthopaedic Nursing*, 34(1), 36–42; quiz 43–34. doi:10.1097/NOR.0000000000000112

Johnson, G. D., Moore, K., & Fortner, B. (2007). Baseline evaluation of the AIM higher initiative: Establishing the mark from which to measure. *Oncology Nursing Forum*, 34(3), 729–734.

Jones, H. J., Huang, A. J., Subak, L. L., Brown, J. S., & Lee, K. A. (2016). Bladder symptoms in the early menopausal transition. *Journal of Women's Health (Larchmt)*, 25(5), 457–463. doi:10.1089/jwh.2015.5370

Kara, B. (2013). Validity and reliability of the Turkish version of the thirst distress scale in patients on hemodialysis. *Asian Nursing Research (Korean Soc Nurs Sci)*, 7(4), 212–218. doi:10.1016/j.anr.2013.10.001

Kara, B. (2016). Determinants of thirst distress in patients on hemodialysis. *International Urology and Nephrology*, 48(9), 1525–1532. doi:10.1007/s11255-016-1327-7

Kim, E., Jahan, T., Aouizerat, B. E., Dodd, M. J., Cooper, B. A., Paul, S. M., . . . Miaskowski, C. (2009). Changes in symptom clusters in patients undergoing radiation therapy. *Supportive Care in Cancer: Official Journal of the Multinational Association of Supportive Care in Cancer*, 17(11), 1383–1391.

Kim, K. H., & Lee, K. A. (2009). Sleep and fatigue symptoms in women before and 6 weeks after hysterectomy. *Journal of Obstetric, Gynecologic, and Neonatal Nursing, 38*(3), 344–352.

Klainin-Yobas, P., Koh, K. W., Ambhore, A. A., Chai, P., Chan, S. W., & He, H. G. (2015). A study protocol of a randomized controlled trial examining the efficacy of a symptom self-management programme for people with acute myocardial infarction. *Journal of Advanced Nursing, 71*(6), 1299–1309. doi:10.1111/jan.12594

Koller, A., Miaskowski, C., De Geest, S., Opitz, O., & Spichiger, E. (2013). Results of a randomized controlled pilot study of a self-management intervention for cancer pain. *European Journal of Oncology Nursing, 17*(3), 284–291. doi:10.1016/j.ejon.2012.08.002

Kyranou, M., Puntillo, K., Dunn, L. B., Aouizerat, B. E., Paul, S. M., Cooper, B. A., . . . Miaskowski, C. (2014). Predictors of initial levels and trajectories of anxiety in women before and for 6 months after breast cancer surgery. *Cancer Nursing, 37*(6), 406–417. doi:10.1097/NCC.0000000000000131

Landers, M. (2014). Symptom management theory. In J. Fitzpatrick & G. McCarthy (Eds.), *Theories guiding nursing research and practice: Making nursing knowledge development explicit* (pp. 35–50). New York, NY: Springer Publishing.

Landers, M. (2016). Self-care strategies. In J. J. Fitzpatrick & G. McCarthy (Eds.), *Nursing concept analysis: Applications to research and practice* (pp. 107–114). New York, NY: Springer Publishing.

Landers, M., McCarthy, G., Livingstone, V., & Savage, E. (2014). Patients' bowel symptom experiences and self-care strategies following sphincter-saving surgery for rectal cancer. *Journal of Clinical Nursing, 23*(15–16), 2343–2354. doi:10.1111/jocn.12516

Landers, M., McCarthy, G., & Savage, E. (2011). Bowel symptom experiences and management following sphincter saving surgery for rectal cancer: A qualitative perspective. *European Journal of Oncology Nursing: The Official Journal of European Oncology Nursing Society, 16*(3), 293–300.

Landers, M., McCarthy, G., & Savage, E. (2013). A theoretical framework to guide a study of patients' bowel symptoms and self-care strategies following sphincter-saving surgery for rectal cancer. *Applied Nursing Research, 26*(3), 157–159. doi:10.1016/j.apnr.2013.05.002

Larson, P. J., Carrieri-Kohlman, V., Dodd, M. J., Douglas, M., Faucett, J., Froelicher, E. S., . . . Underwood, P. R. (1994). A model for symptom management. *Journal of Nursing Scholarship, 26*(4), 272–276.

Lee, J., Dodd, M. J., Dibble, S. L., & Abrams, D. I. (2008). Nausea at the end of adjuvant cancer treatment in relation to exercise during treatment in patients with breast cancer. *Oncology Nursing Forum, 35*(5), 830–835.

Lee, K. A., & Gay, C. L. (2011). Can modifications to the bedroom environment improve the sleep of new parents? *Research in Nursing & Health, 34*, 7–19.

Lee, K. A., Gay, C. L., Portillo, C. J., Coggins, T., Davis, H., Pullinger, C. R., & Aouizerat, B. E. (2009). Symptom experience in HIV-infected adults: A function of demographic and clinical characteristics. *Journal of Pain and Symptom Management, 38*(6), 882–893.

Lee, K. A., Meek, P., & Grady, P. A. (2014). Advancing symptom science: nurse researchers lead the way. *Nursing Outlook*, *62*(5), 301–302. doi:10.1016/j.outlook.2014.05.010

Leeman, J., Skelly, A. H., Burns, D., Carlson, J., & Soward, A. (2008). Tailoring a diabetes self-care intervention for use with older, rural African American women. *Diabetes Educator*, *34*(2), 310–317.

Leutwyler, H., Hubbard, E., Jeste, D., Miller, B., & Vinogradov, S. (2014a). Association between schizophrenia symptoms and neurocognition on mobility in older adults with schizophrenia. *Aging & Mental Health*, *18*(8), 1006–1012. doi:10.1080/13607863.2014.903467

Leutwyler, H., Hubbard, E., Jeste, D., Miller, B., & Vinogradov, S. (2014b). Associations of schizophrenia symptoms and neurocognition with physical activity in older adults with schizophrenia. *Biological Research For Nursing*, *16*(1), 23–30. doi:10.1177/1099800413500845

Linder, L. A. (2010). Analysis of the UCSF symptom management theory: Implications for pediatric oncology nursing. *Journal of Pediatric Oncology Nursing: Official Journal of the Association of Pediatric Oncology Nurses*, *27*(6), 316–324.

Linder, L. A., & Seitz, M. (2016). Through their words: Sources of bother for hospitalized children and adolescents with cancer. *Journal of Pediatric Oncology Nursing*. doi:10.1177/1043454216631308

Lindviksmoen, G., Hofso, K. P., Paul, S. M., Miaskowski, C., & Rustoen, T. (2013). Predictors of initial levels and trajectories of depressive symptoms in women with breast cancer undergoing radiation therapy. *Cancer Nursing*, *36*(6), E34–E43. doi:10.1097/NCC.0b013e31826fc9cc

Lynch, M. T. (2014). Palliative care at the end of life. *Seminars in Oncology Nursing*, *30*(4), 268–279. doi:10.1016/j.soncn.2014.08.009

Maag, M. M., Buccheri, R., Capella, E., & Jennings, D. L. (2006). A conceptual framework for a clinical nurse leader program. *Journal of Professional Nursing: Official Journal of the American Association of Colleges of Nursing*, *22*(6), 367–372.

Matura, L. A., McDonough, A., & Carroll, D. L. (2016). Symptom interference severity and health-related quality of life in pulmonary arterial hypertension. *Journal of Pain and Symptom Management*, *51*(1), 25–32. doi:10.1016/j.jpainsymman.2015.07.012

Matura, L. A., McDonough, A., Hanlon, A. L., & Carroll, D. L. (2015). Development and initial psychometric properties of the Pulmonary Arterial Hypertension Symptom Scale (PAHSS). *Applied Nursing Research*, *28*(1), 42–47. doi:10.1016/j.apnr.2014.04.001

Merriman, J. D., Dodd, M., Lee, K., Paul, S. M., Cooper, B. A., Aouizerat, B. E., . . . Miaskowski, C. (2011). Differences in self-reported attentional fatigue between patients with breast and prostate cancer at the initiation of radiation therapy. *Cancer Nursing*, *34*(5), 345–353.

Miaskowski, C. (2006). Symptom clusters: Establishing the link between clinical practice and symptom management research. *Supportive Care in Cancer: Official Journal of the Multinational Association of Supportive Care in Cancer*, *14*(8), 792–794.

Miaskowski, C., Aouizerat, B. E., Dodd, M., & Cooper, B. (2007). Conceptual issues in symptom clusters research and their implications for quality-of-life assessment in patients with cancer. *Journal of the National Cancer Institute Monographs*, (37), 39–46.

Miaskowski, C., Lee, K., Dunn, L., Dodd, M., Aouizerat, B. E., West, C., . . . Swift, P. (2011). Sleep-wake circadian activity rhythm parameters and fatigue in oncology patients before the initiation of radiation therapy. *Cancer Nursing, 34*(4), 255–268.

Miaskowski, C., Paul, S. M., Cooper, B. A., Lee, K., Dodd, M., West, C., . . . Wara, W. (2011). Predictors of the trajectories of self-reported sleep disturbance in men with prostate cancer during and following radiation therapy. *Sleep, 34*(2), 171–179.

Newcomb, P. (2010). Using symptom management theory to explain how nurse practitioners care for children with asthma. *Journal of Theory Construction & Testing, 14*(2), 40–44.

Newland, P. K., Flick, L. H., Thomas, F. P., & Shannon, W. D. (2014). Identifying symptom co-occurrence in persons with multiple sclerosis. *Clinical Nursing Research, 23*(5), 529–543. doi:10.1177/1054773813497221

Nguyen, H. Q., & Carrieri-Kohlman, V. (2005). Dyspnea self-management in patients with chronic obstructive pulmonary disease: Moderating effects of depressed mood. *Psychosomatics, 46*(5), 402–410.

Nguyen, H. Q., Donesky-Cuenco, D., Wolpin, S., Benditt, J. O., Paul, S., & Carrieri-Kohlman, V. (2011). A randomized controlled trial of an internet-based dyspnea self-management program in patients with COPD. *American Journal of Respiratory and Critical Care Medicine, 183,* A5818.

Nguyen, H. Q., Donesky-Cuenco, D., Wolpin, S., Reinke, L. F., Benditt, J. O., Paul, S. M., & Carrieri-Kohlman, V. (2008). Randomized controlled trial of an internet-based versus face-to-face dyspnea self-management program for patients with chronic obstructive pulmonary disease: Pilot study. *Journal of Medical Internet Research, 10*(2), e9.

Nieveen, J. L., Zimmerman, L. M., Barnason, S. A., & Yates, B. C. (2008). Development and content validity testing of the cardiac symptom survey in patients after coronary artery bypass grafting. *Heart & Lung: The Journal of Acute and Critical Care, 37*(1), 17–27.

Nosek, M., Kennedy, H. P., Beyene, Y., Taylor, D., Gilliss, C., & Lee, K. (2010). The effects of perceived stress and attitudes toward menopause and aging on symptoms of menopause. *Journal of Midwifery & Women's Health, 55,* 328–334.

Oksholm, T., Miaskowski, C., Solberg, S., Lie, I. C., B., Paul, S. M., Kongerud, J. S., & Rustoen, T. (2015). Changes in symptom occurrence and severity before and after lung cancer surgery. *Cancer Nursing, 38*(5), 351–357. doi:10.1097/NCC.0000000000000198 14

Orem, D. E. (1985). *Nursing: Concepts of practice* (3rd ed.). New York, NY: McGraw-Hill.

Park, S. K., Stotts, N. A., Douglas, M. K., Donesky-Cuenco, D., & Carrieri-Kohlman, V. (2011). Symptoms and functional performance in Korean immigrants with asthma or chronic obstructive pulmonary disease. *Heart & Lung: The Journal of Critical Care, 41*(3), 226–237.

Portenoy, R. K., Thaler, H. T., Kornblith, A. B., Lepore, J. M., Friedlander-Klar, H., Kiyasu, E., & Norton, L. (1994). The memorial symptom assessment scale: An instrument for the evaluation of symptom prevalence, characteristics and distress. *European Journal of Cancer, 30A*(9), 1326–1336.

Randen, I., Lerdal, A., & Bjork, I. T. (2013). Nurses' perceptions of unpleasant symptoms and signs in ventilated and sedated patients. *Nursing in Critical Care, 18*(4), 176–186. doi:10.1111/nicc.12012

Rasi, M., Kunzler-Heule, P., Schmid, P., Semela, D., Bruggmann, P., Fehr, J., . . . Nicca, D. (2014). "Fighting an uphill battle": Experience with the HCV triple therapy: A qualitative thematic analysis. *BMC Infectious Diseases, 14*, 507. doi:10.1186/1471-2334-14-507

Rodgers, C., Wills-Alcoser, P., Monroe, R., McDonald, L., Trevino, M., & Hockenberry, M. (2008). Growth patterns and gastrointestinal symptoms in pediatric patients after hematopoietic stem cell transplantation. *Oncology Nursing Forum, 35*(3), 443–448.

Rodgers, C. C., Krance, R., Street, R. L., & Hockenberry, M. J. (2014). Symptom prevalence and physiologic biomarkers among adolescents using a mobile phone intervention following hematopoietic stem cell transplantation. *Oncology Nursing Forum, 41*(3), 229–236. doi:10.1188/14.ONF.229-236

Rosen, H. I., Bergh, I. H., Schwartz-Barcott, D., & Martensson, L. B. (2014). The recovery process after day surgery within the symptom management theory. *Nurs Forum, 49*(2), 100–109. doi:10.1111/nuf.12062

Ruegg, T. A., Curran, C. R., & Lamb, T. (2009). Use of buffered lidocaine in bone marrow biopsies: A randomized, controlled trial. *Oncology Nursing Forum, 36*(1), 52–60.

Samuels, J. G., & Eckardt, P. (2014). The impact of assessment and reassessment documentation on the trajectory of postoperative pain severity: A pilot study. *Pain Management Nursing, 15*(3), 652–663. doi:10.1016/j.pmn.2013.07.007

Samuels, J. G., & Manworren, R. C. (2014). Determining the value of postoperative pain management using timed electronic data. *Nursing Economic, 32*(2), 80–88, 98.

Shin, S. Y. (2014). Disability intervention model for older adults with arthritis: An integration of theory of symptom management and disablement process model. *Asian Nursing Research (Korean Soc Nurs Sci), 8*(4), 241–246. doi:10.1016/j.anr.2014.08.004

Skelly, A. H., Carlson, J., Leeman, J., Soward, A., & Burns, D. (2009). Controlled trial of nursing interventions to improve health outcomes of older African American women with type 2 diabetes. *Nursing Research, 58*(6), 410–418.

Skelly, A. H., Leeman, J., Carlson, J., Soward, A. C., & Burns, D. (2008). Conceptual model of symptom-focused diabetes care for African Americans. *Journal of Nursing Scholarship, 40*(3), 261–267.

Skrutkowski, M., Saucier, A., Eades, M., Swidzinski, M., Ritchie, J., Marchionni, C., & Ladouceur, M. (2008). Impact of a pivot nurse in oncology on patients with lung or breast cancer: Symptom distress, fatigue, quality of life, and use of healthcare resources. *Oncology Nursing Forum, 35*(6), 948–954.

Sorofman, B., Tripp-Reimer, T., Lauer, G. M., & Martin, M. E. (1990). Symptom self-care. *Holistic Nursing Practice, 4*(2), 45–55.

Srirat, C., Hanucharurnkul, S., Aree-Ue, S., Viwatwongkasem, C., & Junda, T. (2014). Symptom distress, cluster, and management in Thais with COPD. *Pacific Rim International Journal Nursing Research, 18*(3), 244–262.

Sternberg, R. M., & Lee, K. A. (2013). Depressive symptoms of midlife Latinas: effect of immigration and sociodemographic factors. *International Journal of Women's Health, 5*, 301–308. doi:10.2147/IJWH.S43132

Suwanno, J., Petpichetchian, W., Riegel, B., & Issaramalai, S. (2009). A model predicting health status of patients with heart failure. *Journal of Cardiovascular Nursing, 24*(2), 118–126.

Swenson, K. K., Nissen, M. J., Henly, S. J., Maybon, L., Pupkes, J., Zwicky, K., . . . Shapiro, A. C. (2013). Identification of tools to measure changes in musculoskeletal symptoms and physical functioning in women with breast cancer receiving aromatase inhibitors. *Oncology Nursing Forum, 40*(6), 549–557. doi:10.1188/13.ONF.549-557

Taylor, J. Y., & Holston, E. C. (2014). MAMBRA's impact on IPV symptoms of incarcerated and formerly incarcerated women. *Issues in Mental Health Nursing, 35*(5), 344–355. doi:10.3109/01612840.2013.868962

Titzer, H. (2016). Symptom management: Intergral-component of multiprofession treatment in oncology. *Onkologe, 22*(9), 645–650. doi:10.1007/s00761-016-0062-0

Trygstad, L. N., Buccheri, R. K., Buffum, M. D., Ju, D. S., & Dowling, G. A. (2015). Auditory hallucinations interview guide: promoting recovery with an interactive assessment tool. *Journal of Psychosocial Nursing and Mental Health Services, 53*(1), 20–28. doi:10.3928/02793695-20141203-01

Tsai, Y.-F., Holzemer, W. L., & Leu, H.-S. (2005). An evaluation of the effects of a manual on management of HIV/AIDS symptoms. *International Journal of STD & AIDS, 16*(9), 625–629.

Van Cleve, L., Bossert, E., Beecroft, P., Adlard, K., Alvarez, O., & Savedra, M. C. (2004). The pain experience of children with leukemia during the first year after diagnosis. *Nursing Research, 53*(1), 1–10.

Van Onselen, C., Dunn, L. B., Lee, K., Dodd, M., Koetters, T., West, C., . . . Miaskowski, C. (2010). Relationship between mood disturbance and sleep quality in oncology outpatients at the initiation of radiation therapy. *European Journal of Oncology Nursing, 14*(5), 373–379.

Voss, J., Portillo, C. J., Holzemer, W. L., & Dodd, M. J. (2007). Symptom cluster of fatigue and depression in HIV/AIDS. *Journal of Prevention & Intervention in the Community, 33*(1–2), 19–34.

Wang, H.-L., Keck, J. F., Weaver, M. T., Mikesky, A., Bunnell, K., Buelow, J. M., & Rawl, S. M. (2013). Shoulder pain, functional status, and health-related quality of life after head and neck cancer surgery. *Rehabilitation Research and Practice, 2013*, 601768. doi:10.1155/2013/601768

Webel, A. R., & Holzemer, W. L. (2009). Positive self-management program for women living with HIV: A descriptive analysis. *JANAC-Journal of the Association of Nurses in Aids Care, 20*(6), 458–467.

Wells, M., Sarna, L., Cooley, M. E., Brown, J. K., Chernecky, C., Williams, R. D., . . . Danao, L. L. (2007). Use of complementary and alternative medicine therapies to control symptoms in women living with lung cancer. *Cancer Nursing, 30*(1), 45–55.

Wright, F., D'Eramo Melkus, G., Hammer, M., Schmidt, B. L., Knobf, M. T., Paul, S. M., . . . Miaskowski, C. (2015). Trajectories of evening fatigue in oncology outpatients receiving chemotherapy. *Journal of Pain and Symptom Management*, *50*(2), 163–175. doi:10.1016/j.jpainsymman.2015.02.015

Wu, H.-S., Natavio, T., Davis, J. E., & Yarandi, H. N. (2013). Pain in outpatients treated for breast cancer: Prevalence, pharmacological treatment, and impact on quality of life. *Cancer Nursing*, *36*(3), 229–235. doi:10.1097/NCC.0b013e3182664c95

Xiao, C. (2010). The state of science in the study of cancer symptom clusters. *European Journal of Oncology Nursing*, *14*(5), 417–34.

Xiao, W., Chow, K., So, W., Leung, D., & Chan, C. (2016). The effectiveness of psychoeducation intervention on managing symptom clusters in patients with cancer: A systematic review of randomized controlled trials. *Cancer Nursing*, *39*(2), 279–291. doi:10.1097/NCC.0000000000000313

Yang, C.-Y., Lee, T.-H., Lo, S.-C., & Beckstead, J. W. (2015). The effects of auditory hallucination symptom management programme for people with schizophrenia: A quasi-experimental design. *Journal of Advanced Nursing*, *71*(12), 2886–2897. doi:10.1111/jan.12754

Yeager, K. A., Sterk, C. E., Quest, T. E., DiIorio, C., Vena, C., & Bauer-Wu, S. (2016). Managing one's symptoms: A qualitative study of low-income African Americans with advanced cancer. *Cancer Nursing*, *39*(4), 303–312. doi:10.1097/NCC.0000000000000284

Yoshioka, S., Moriyama, M., & Ohno, Y. (2014). Efficacy of the end-of-life nursing care continuing education program for nurses in general wards in Japan. *American Journal of Hospice and Palliative Medicine*, *31*(5), 513–520. doi:10.1177/1049909113491133

Yuan, S. C., Chou, M. C., Chen, C. J., Lin, Y. J., Chen, M.-C., Liu, H.-H., & Kuo, H.-W. (2011). Influences of shift work on fatigue among nurses. *Journal of Nursing Management*, *19*(3), 339–345.

Zimmerman, L., Barnason, S., Hertzog, M., Young, L., Niemen, J., Schulz, P., & Tu, C. (2011). Gender differences in recovery outcomes after an early recovery symptom management intervention. *Heart & Lung*, *40*(5), 429–439.

# CHAPTER 9

## Theory of Unpleasant Symptoms

**Elizabeth R. Lenz and Linda C. Pugh**

Symptom management has become increasingly central to nursing practice and continues to emerge as an important focus of nursing science. The National Institute of Nursing Research (NINR) has identified symptom science as one of the key investment areas in its strategic plan (NINR, 2016; see also Redeker et al., 2015), noting that "In promoting symptom and symptom management science, NINR supports research focused on understanding the biological and behavioral aspects of symptoms, with the goal of developing and testing new interventions to reduce the disabling effects of symptoms and improving patient health outcomes and quality of life" (NINR, 2016, p. 12). Cashion and Grady (2015) underscore the importance of symptom research, stating:

> The multitude of symptoms associated with a single illness; or, in many cases, occurring with co-morbid illnesses or conditions, often compromise or govern the lived experiences of individuals suffering from these conditions. Nursing science, with its foundational link to the lived experiences of individuals, provides a unique scientific perspective into both the clinical and biologic features of symptoms and sequelae. (p. 485)

As nurses assume more of the responsibility for managing care of patients with both acute and chronic illnesses, their interest in improving the management of symptoms has stimulated additional basic and translational research. An important and challenging development has been the growing body of literature revealing the complexity and pervasiveness of symptom clusters. In this chapter, we describe the middle range Theory of Unpleasant Symptoms (TOUS): its components, the process by which it was developed, examples and theoretical implications of its application in nursing research and practice, and plans for future development. Notable features of this theory are that it is applicable to multiple symptoms that can occur in conjunction with many different illnesses; it highlights the multidimensionality of symptoms; and it includes the reality that multiple symptoms often occur together. The latter characteristic has made it the theoretical foundation of choice for many investigators studying symptom clusters.

# ■ PURPOSE OF THE THEORY AND HOW IT WAS DEVELOPED

The TOUS was designed to integrate existing knowledge about a variety of symptoms. It was based on the premise that there are commonalities across different symptoms that are experienced by a variety of clinical populations in varied situations. A framework that highlights common elements and dimensions has the potential to be useful in both nursing practice and research. The purpose of the theory is to improve understanding of the symptom experience in various contexts and to provide information useful for designing effective interventions to prevent, ameliorate, or manage unpleasant symptoms and their negative effects. Because it is more general than a situation-specific theory describing or explaining a specific symptom, illness, or experience, the TOUS lacks some of the detail that may be useful in working with a particular symptom in a given clinical population. On the other hand, by highlighting dimensions and considerations that are common to many symptoms and illnesses, investigators and clinicians are encouraged to think about aspects that are not readily apparent and to consider symptoms both alone and in combination. It serves as a useful heuristic by providing an organizing scheme that encourages thought about the interplay among the many aspects of the symptom experience.

The TOUS also is useful for stimulating collaboration in both research and practice. It provides a framework within which multiple researchers can work simultaneously, ultimately combining the results of their many programs of research. It provides common definitions and dimensions for examining symptoms, ultimately enhancing the probability that the results from multiple studies can be combined to produce convincing evidence on which to base practice.

Because the symptom experience, by definition, occurs at the level of individual perception, the theory is applicable at the level of the individual. However, the theory does not consider the individual in isolation. Rather, it positions the individual within the context of his or her family, social and organizational networks, and community by taking into account situational factors in the environment that may influence the symptom experience. It embodies an inclusive perspective that is not limited to the physical domain of human experience, but also acknowledges the influence of psychological factors and situational or environmental factors, as well as their interplay, on symptoms. It also defines the outcome of the symptom experience in terms of performance, a concept that considers its impact on the individual's interactions with others and his or her short- and long-term physical, cognitive, and social functioning.

The TOUS was developed by four nurse researchers who shared interest in the nature and experience of different symptoms (specifically fatigue and dyspnea) and in the processes of concept and theory development. Audrey Gift, Renee Milligan, Linda Pugh, and Elizabeth Lenz had collaborated in dyads or triads on various empirical studies and theoretical articles. They shared geographic proximity, which facilitated collaboration. By virtue of their common association with the University of Maryland's PhD program in nursing, they also shared exposure to the same philosophical and metatheoretical perspectives regarding the development and substance of nursing science. They had access to an eminent philosopher of science colleague, Frederick Suppe, who played an important role in shaping their understanding of middle range theory and who assisted in the theory development process.

This is a theory that was developed inductively from specific to general and from concrete observation in the practice environment to theoretical ideas. That is, it had its beginnings at the relatively narrow scope of single symptoms; it is grounded in the reality of practice. Three of the theory developers—all with extensive clinical experience—had conducted dissertation research regarding a specific symptom: Gift studied dyspnea, and Milligan and Pugh studied fatigue. When their initial studies about individual symptoms were carried out, they had no intention of developing a theory. The opportunity to do so evolved over time, as they began to realize that their work on individual symptoms represented concept development activity. It became apparent—as they continued to identify and discuss the elements that were common across the experience of dyspnea and fatigue in both ill and healthy populations—that their thinking was moving to the level of middle range theory.

The initial collaboration took place between Pugh and Milligan; each was studying the symptom of fatigue during a different phase of the perinatal experience. Pugh (1990) studied correlates of fatigue during labor and delivery. Milligan (1989) had conducted qualitative and quantitative research about fatigue during the postpartum period and was also carrying out concept development and measurement studies (Milligan, Lenz, Parks, Pugh, & Kitzman, 1996). Pugh and Milligan (1993)—who were also engaged in clinical practice in labor and delivery and postpartum environments—combined their findings about the concept to develop a framework for the study of fatigue during childbearing. Milligan's inductive analysis of fatigue during the postpartum period included clinical observations, interviews with postpartum mothers, and data from a quantitative measure of fatigue. Her work pointed out the importance of differentiating fatigue from related concepts, such as depression, and the desirability of differentiating different types of fatigue. From Pugh's deductive work—which was based on existing models of fatigue—came the identification of physiological, psychological, and situational factors that influence fatigue during labor, and the recognition that fatigue is a multidimensional phenomenon. Pugh and Milligan (1995) recognized commonalities in their conceptualizations of and findings about fatigue at different stages in the childbearing process. They developed a framework that they then tested in a longitudinal study of pregnant women. Examples of the commonalities include the cumulative nature of the symptom experience and the importance of energy depletion. The framework that emerged from this collaboration incorporated a nursing diagnosis–based definition of fatigue and the results of empirical studies of fatigue from other disciplines, as well as theoretical models developed within nursing to explain fatigue in childbearing situations.

The second collaboration took place when Pugh began to discuss the model of fatigue with Gift (Gift, 1990; Gift & Cahill, 1990), who had conducted multiple studies of dyspnea in patients with chronic obstructive pulmonary disease (COPD) and asthma. They realized that their conceptualizations were similar and discovered a number of commonalities between the two symptoms. They developed a model combining elements of their previous work that was meant to be equally applicable to dyspnea and fatigue (Gift & Pugh, 1993).

Gift had carried out Wilsonian concept development activities, which clarified the nature and measurement of dyspnea as a subjective phenomenon. She used pain as an analog to develop a model depicting dyspnea with physiological and psychological components and as variable in intensity, duration, and the degree of distress experienced. Her conceptualization bore similarities to Pugh and Milligan's framework for studying fatigue: for example, the respective symptom having both acute and chronic manifestations, being influenced by the same categories of factors, and affecting performance or functional ability.

Having developed the multiple-concept dyspnea/fatigue model, which was also potentially applicable to pain, the investigators went on to reason that they could develop a more generic theory that was at an even higher level of abstraction and could be extended to encompass additional symptoms. Lenz had expertise in model and theory development, was familiar with the work of all three researchers, and had offered ongoing critique of their work. Collaboratively they decided to develop a middle range theory and began to meet regularly. Discussions revolved around resolving differences in the models for individual symptoms and agreeing on the elements of a more inclusive theory. The resulting TOUS was introduced and described briefly in an article advocating the development of middle range theories to guide nursing practice (Lenz, Suppe, Gift, Pugh, & Milligan, 1995). The call for papers about middle range nursing theory by *Advances in Nursing Science* (*ANS*) served as an important stimulus for this theory development activity.

The TOUS generated considerable interest in the nursing academic community, as indicated by correspondence received by the authors, much of which came from graduate students who sought clinically relevant theories on which to base their research. Its publication and more general exposure also pointed out some weaknesses of the theory and some aspects that were unclear. As a result, the authors continued to work on refining it, and an updated, improved version was subsequently published (Lenz, Pugh, Milligan, Gift, & Suppe, 1997). This second version added considerable complexity in the relationships among the theory components, and the potential for multiple symptoms to occur simultaneously Again, the prospect of an opportunity to publish the refinements in *ANS* served to stimulate the revision.

In considering the process by which the TOUS was developed, several observations are pertinent. First, it was not preplanned but occurred spontaneously, stimulated by shared interests and the opportunity for frequent communication. Proximity that allowed face-to-face meetings, a common background in philosophy and interest in theory development acquired during doctoral study, a tradition of scholarly and collegial interchange, and the ability to take the time required to debate difficult conceptual issues facilitated the collaborative efforts at all stages. Second, forward movement on the development of the theory has tended to occur in spurts of activity, undertaken in response to external stimuli, primarily publication opportunities, and explicit critiques. This seems to underscore the importance of nursing journal editors' willingness to publish the results of theoretical work and related research findings. It also reaffirms the value of scholarly dialogue and debate of ideas. Third, the development of the theory occurred in an inductive fashion, which contributed to its practice relevance. At every step, concept analysis and clarification were grounded in nursing practice and in practice-related research. The theory was not conceived from armchair musings but was based on real-world observations and attempts to study and solve problems encountered in practice.

## ■ CONCEPTS OF THE THEORY

The TOUS has three major concepts: the symptom(s), influencing factors, and performance outcomes. Literature supporting the structure of the theory was cited in the published descriptions of the original theory (Lenz et al., 1995) and the updated version (Lenz et al., 1997) and is also incorporated in the description of the theory components that follows.

### Symptoms

Symptoms were the starting point for conceptualizing the theory, and hence should be considered to be the central concept. Thus far, the TOUS has focused on subjectively perceived symptoms rather than on objectively observed signs. However, Hee-Ju Kim, McGuire, Tulman, and Barsevick (2005) argued in their discussion of "symptom clusters" that the term—by definition including multiple symptoms and often signs, and by extension including theories that address them—should be broad enough to include both self-reported symptoms and objective, observed signs. For purposes of the TOUS, symptoms are defined subjectively as "the perceived indicators of change in normal functioning as experienced by patients" (Rhodes & Watson, 1987, p. 242). Most but not all symptoms are experienced as unpleasant sensations. The perception-based definition assumes awareness by the individual and that the nature of a symptom can only be truly known and described by the individual experiencing it. The implication of this stance is that measurement of the theory's component concepts must be subjective. The extent to which objectively observable signs can be explained by the theory warrants systematic attention. Such exploration hypothetically would expand the applicability of the theory, particularly in light of the reality that many expressions of symptoms are nonverbal and easily observed by others. Unfortunately, clinicians tend to underestimate the severity, incidence, and/or distress of patients' symptoms (Xiao, Polomano, & Bruner, 2013).

The TOUS asserts that symptoms can occur either in isolation—one at a time—or in combination and potentially in interaction with other symptoms. Although the term is not used in the TOUS and the model does not depict clusters in the usual way, the TOUS has been recognized to be one of the few generic symptom theories to address and visually depict multiple symptoms experienced simultaneously (Brant, Beck, & Miaskowski, 2009; Jurgens et al., 2009). As a result, it has been the theoretical framework of choice for underpinning many studies of symptom clusters (e.g., Gift, Jablonski, Stommel, & Given, 2004; Herr et al., 2014; Hee-Ju Kim, Barsevick, & Tulman, 2009; Park, Stotts, Douglas, Donesky-Cuenco, & Carrieri-Kohlman, 2012; Phligbua et al., 2013; Roland & Hendrich, 2011; Wang & Fu, 2014; Wilmoth, Coleman, & Wahab, 2009). The concept of symptom cluster continues to receive much attention in the literature regarding cancer and other chronic illnesses (Ameringer, Erickson, Macpherson, Stegenga, & Linder, 2015; Atay, Conk & Bahar, 2012; Baggott, Cooper, Matthay, & Miaskowski, 2012; Barsevick, Whitmore, Nail, Beck, & Dudley, 2006; E. Chen et al., 2011; Cherwin, 2012; Chow & Merrick, 2010; Cleeland et al., 2013; Dodd, Miaskowski, & Lee, 2004; Dong et al., 2016; T.-Y. Huang et al., 2013, 2016; Jurgens et al., 2009; Lang et al., 2006; Laird et al., 2011; Miaskowski, Dodd, & Lee, 2004; Motl, Suh, & Weikert, 2010; Motl, Weikert, Suh, & Dlugonski, 2010; Shahrbanian, Duquette, Kuspinar, & Mayo, 2015; Wang & Fu, 2014).

In some situations, one symptom may precede and possibly give rise to another. For example, extreme fatigue may precipitate episodes of nausea, vertigo, and confusion. When more than one symptom is experienced at the same time, or even cumulatively as total symptom burden (a related concept; see Abbott, Baranson, & Zimmerman, 2010; Cleeland et al., 2013; Coolbrandt et al., 2014; Farrell & Savage, 2010; Rodgers, Hooke, & Hockenberry, 2013), the net effect can be multiplicative, often more powerful than a sum of the individual symptoms would suggest (Armstrong, 2003; Motl, Suh, & Weikert, 2010; Wilmoth, Coleman, Smith, & Davis, 2004). However, Motl et al. (2010) found that the addition of two more symptoms to the cluster of fatigue, depression, and pain made little difference in the magnitude of the cluster's effect on the performance outcome. Different levels of pain can also moderate the relationship of fatigue to psychological variables. For example, Francoeur (2005) found several interactions among symptoms in a study of cancer patients with recurrent disease, including the interaction of pain with fever, fatigue, and weight loss in predicting depressive affect. In longitudinal studies, Atay, Conk, and Bahar (2012), J. Huang et al. (2016), and Hee-Ju Kim, McDermott, and Barsevick (2014) found that symptom clusters changed over time, as did patients' ratings of the severity of specific symptoms within a cluster.

In the TOUS, symptoms are conceptualized as manifesting multiple variable and measurable dimensions. It is asserted that all symptoms vary in intensity or severity, degree of associated distress, timing, and quality. These dimensions are also related to one another (Jurgens et al., 2009); however, the relationships are not always consistent in that symptom intensity does not necessarily correlate positively with duration or distress (Jablonsky, 2007). Intensity is the dimension that quantifies the degree, strength, or severity of the symptom and is the frequently measured aspect of the symptom experience. It is part of the routine assessment of most hospitalized patients to ask them to express the intensity or severity of their pain in numeric terms or on a visual analog scale. Intensity is often the simplest characteristic for patients to rate. In pediatric practice, nonnumeric measures of pain are often used to capture children's ratings of its intensity (e.g., the Faces pain scale and the Oucher scale). Observational scales are also used to infer pain intensity. For example, Crosta, Ward, Walker, and Peters (2014) reviewed several pain measures that can be used for hospitalized children with cognitive impairment, and concluded that the revised Face, Leg, Activity, Cry, and Consolability scale was feasible. Keller (2004; Keller & Keck, 2006) developed an index to measure nausea based on observable indicators for use with preverbal children and those unable to self-report.

The distress dimension reflects an affective aspect of the symptom experience; it refers to the degree to which the individual experiencing the symptom is bothered by it. Kugler et al. (2009) defined symptom distress as the emotional burden caused by the symptom. Because of differences in pain threshold levels and cultural expectations, individuals exposed to the same intensity of pain-inducing stimuli can experience very different levels of distress. Generally the degree of distress experienced with a symptom is related to its intensity (e.g., Hsiao, Moore, Insel, & Merkle, 2014); however, it can also be influenced by other considerations. Examples include anxiety, type of surgery, coping strategies, and occupation after surgery (Wu et al., 2015). Distress can be affected by the degree of focused attention that the individual directs toward the symptom and by the extent of interference it causes in everyday life. Interference is an aspect of symptoms that is included in several symptom measures (Lenz, Pugh, Milligan, & Gift, 2017). However, caution is suggested by Eckhardt, DeVon, Piano, Ryan, and Zerwic (2014) who found that qualitative interviews elicited higher interference levels than standardized measures. Cherwin (2012) reported that the distress dimension was underreported in the literature about gastrointestinal cancer, although the symptoms are very distressing to patients.

One of the symptom management strategies designed to lessen distress is diverting attention from the symptom. For example, the breathing techniques during childbirth help divert attention from pain, and introduction of another stimulus can compete with pain for the individual's attention. One of the most important influences on the degree of distress that is associated with a given symptom is the meaning that the individual attaches to the symptom. For example, a woman who has been treated for infertility may perceive nausea associated with pregnancy as a very welcome symptom and not be bothered by it, whereas a cancer patient could perceive considerable distress associated with chemotherapy-induced nausea of the same severity because of its potentially negative connotations. Armstrong (2003), in her concept analysis–based model of the symptom experience, included meaning as a dimension that is separate from, and additional to, distress (Armstrong, Cohen, Eriksen, & Hickey, 2004). She determined that meaning is an important dimension to consider when the emotional consequences of the symptom experience are being examined.

The time dimension includes the way symptoms vary in duration, frequency, and pattern of occurrence. Duration is the length of time that a symptom continues; thus, it highlights the importance of the patient's experiential history. It is common to differentiate acute from chronic symptoms because they tend to be different in nature and to be treated differently. They also may hold very different meaning for the individual experiencing them. Chronic symptoms may be particularly distress-producing; moreover, the approaches to managing a symptom often change with duration. Strategies that are appropriate for acute pain, for example, are not necessarily useful in treating chronic pain (Badke & Boissonnault, 2006). The dimension of time also takes into account the frequency or rapidity with which symptoms occur and also the pattern with which they vary over time or recur. For example, symptoms that are intermittent can vary in regularity and periodicity. Likewise, persistent symptoms can vary in intensity over time (L.-H. Chen, Li, Shieh, Yin, & Chiou, 2010). Nausea that occurs every morning for 3 hours during the first trimester of pregnancy can be described, and hence measured, along several time-related dimensions.

The importance of time as a dimension of the symptom experience was emphasized by Henley, Kallas, Klatt, and Swenson (2003) in their Symptom Experience in Time Model. It underscores the value of examining intraindividual change over time. They also expanded the notion of time dimension, arguing that the analysis of time-related symptom patterns should take into consideration perceived, biological/social, and clock/calendar conceptions of time. They described the impact of time on the meaning the individual attaches to the symptom by virtue of its effect on the self-evaluation of the symptom experience and emotional response to it. In the TOUS, this would suggest acknowledging the relationship of symptom timing to the extent of distress.

The final dimension of the symptom incorporated in the TOUS is the quality of the symptom. This dimension refers to the nature of the symptom or the way in which it is manifested or experienced; that is, what it feels like to have the symptom. By including this dimension, the TOUS acknowledges that in addition to reflecting characteristics that are common across all symptoms, each symptom has unique characteristics. The descriptors that best characterize each symptom are highly specific. For example, pain is often characterized by the nature of the sensation, such as stinging, burning, stabbing, pounding, and so forth, and by its location. Changes in the nature of the pain may signal changes in disease progression; hence, they are incorporated in many of the widely used symptom-specific measures. Dyspnea can be characterized by the way the shortness of breath feels to the individual, for example, tight versus suffocating. These descriptors are important because they differ systematically from one disease state or stage of progression to another and even from one illness to another. Thus, symptom quality may provide valuable clues to assessment and effective management.

Describing and measuring the quality of specific symptoms (and symptom clusters) depends on the patient's ability to articulate what he or she is experiencing. Individuals differ in the descriptors that they use and also in their ability to communicate. Qualitative research with a variety of patient populations is often valuable in describing symptoms (Wilmoth, Hatmaker-Flannigan, LaLoggia, & Nixon, 2011). Qualitative methods are frequently appropriate in the early phases of a study to identify descriptors, which are then used as the basis for the subsequent development of quantitative measures (Lang et al., 2006; Waltz, Strickland, & Lenz, 2017). They are also useful in helping to analyze whether two different terms that are often used interchangeably actually name the same concept or two different concepts (Milligan, Lenz, et al., 1996). The measurement of the symptom(s) is most informative when all four characteristics are included. However, measuring one, two, or three characteristics is valid and helpful for healthcare providers in symptom management.

## Influencing Factors

Three categories of factors that influence symptoms (and can, in turn, be influenced by them and by one another) are identified in the TOUS: physiological factors, psychological factors, and situational factors. The specific factors that are most relevant in influencing a given symptom may be different from those that are most relevant for another. The combination and/or interaction of multiple influencing factors can impact the symptom experience differently from any single one. For example, the combination of a late-stage illness (physiological), depressive mood (psychological), and lack of social support (situational) is likely to result in a more intense and distressing symptom experience than one or even two of these factors alone. H. S. Kim, Oh, Lee, Kim, and Kim (2015) found that all three types of influencing factors were related to symptom severity and symptom interference with everyday life in a study of cancer patients undergoing chemotherapy. The psychological factors of depression and fighting spirit were the strongest predictors.

## PHYSIOLOGICAL FACTORS

Physiological factors include anatomical/structural, physiological, genetic, illness-related, and treatment-related variables. Examples of variables in this category include the presence of structural anomalies, existence of pathology or disease states including comorbidities, stage and duration of illness, inflammation due to infection or trauma, fluctuations in hormone or energy levels, adequacy of hydration and nutrition, level of consciousness, genetic makeup, race/ethnicity, age, developmental stage, pretreatment physical performance status, and—importantly—the type and duration of treatment. All may influence the occurrence of a symptom and how it is experienced. For example, Wu et al. (2015) found that the types of surgery and chemotherapy influenced symptom distress in patients with esophageal cancer.

The interplay among different physiological influencing factors can be quite complex, as is pointed out in the many studies of symptom clusters. For example, see the studies of symptom clusters in heart failure by Jurgens et al. (2009) and by Herr et al. (2014), as well as the concept analysis of symptom clusters in cancer populations by Hee-Ju Kim, McGuire, Tulman, and Barsevick (2005). Breastfeeding mothers' experiences of fatigue are influenced by many physiological factors, including the duration of labor, type of delivery, level of hydration, time since delivery, hormonal changes, maternal age, presence of infection, and the amount and quality of sleep (Pugh & Milligan, 1998). Lifestyle behaviors such as exercise, diet, and smoking can impact the symptom experience. In addition, treatments often give rise to unpleasant symptoms. The classic examples are chemotherapy and radiation treatments for cancer (e.g., Chan, Richardson, & Richardson, 2011; E. Chen et al., 2011; J. Huang et al., 2016; Hee-Ju Kim, Malone, & Barsevick, 2014; H.-S. Kim et al., 2015; Skerman, Yates, & Battistutta, 2012; So et al., 2013). Many medications used to treat illnesses or to prevent complications (e.g., immunosuppressant drugs following transplant surgery) produce side effects that are experienced as unpleasant symptoms (Francoeur, 2005; Kiser, Greer, Wilmoth, Dmochowski, & Naumann, 2010; Kugler et al., 2009; Lester & Bernhard, 2009; Wilmoth et al., 2004).

Symptoms are often the indicators that pathology exists and is either worsening or improving, but the relationship is not necessarily straightforward or simple. Jurgens et al. (2009) pointed out complications that advanced age may impose on individuals' perceptions and interpretations of the symptom experience. Their example was that heart failure patients experiencing dyspnea associated with that diagnosis may be unable to differentiate it from dyspnea associated with comorbid conditions. As a result, patients may ignore symptom changes that indicate worsening heart failure and delay seeking advice or initiating self-help measures, ultimately leading to further deterioration in their condition. This example demonstrates that there is a reciprocal relationship between physiologic factors and symptoms and that age, a physiological factor, can moderate that relationship.

## PSYCHOLOGICAL FACTORS

Psychological factors represent not only one of the more complex components of the model, but also one of the most important. They include both affective and cognitive variables. The individual's affective state or mood (e.g., level of anxiety, depression, or anger) during or preceding the time of the symptom experience—even if unrelated to the symptom—and the emotional response to the illness or the symptom itself can serve to intensify the symptom and associated distress (L.-H. Chen et al., 2010; Duncan, Bott, Thompson, & Gajewski, 2009; Eckhardt et al., 2014; Hee-Ju Kim, Malone, & Barsevick, 2014; Song, Chang, Park, Kim, & Nam, 2010; Tankumpuan, Utriyaprasit, Chayaput, & Itthimathin, 2015; Thompson, 2007; Wu et al., 2015). Cognitive variables that may impact the symptom experience include the degree of uncertainty surrounding it, the individual's level of knowledge about the illness or the symptom, the meaning of the symptom experience to the individual, his or her repertoire of cognitive coping skills, including a fighting spirit (H.-S. Kim et al., 2015), meaning in life (Thompson, 2007), and the perceived availability of coping resources. Self-efficacy was found by Motl, McAuley, and Sandoff (2013) to be the best predictor of declining physical activity over a 2.5-year period in multiple sclerosis patients, despite no longitudinal changes in pain, depression, or fatigue. As psychobiological research underscores the physiological basis for mood, it becomes increasingly evident that the psychological and physiological factors impacting the symptom experience may be difficult to separate.

## SITUATIONAL FACTORS

The third category of influencing factors is situational. It encompasses the individual's environment, both social and physical. For instance, the experience of symptoms can vary by culture because there is a learned component to interpreting and expressing symptoms (Spector, 2017). Other situational factors that can influence the experience of symptoms include those that are associated with the individual's experiential background and access to resources, including the availability of financial, emotional, and instrumental help in dealing with the symptom. Examples are socioeconomic status, marital and family status, religion, occupation, demands of work or family, access to and receipt of companionship and social support, access to healthcare, and adequacy of healthcare and support provided. For example, Jaremka et al. (2014) found that loneliness was a risk factor for developing pain, depression, and fatigue in both cancer survivors and caregivers of persons with dementia. Social support had large effects on functional and social well-being in So et al.'s (2013) study of Chinese women being treated for breast cancer. In addition to being a situational factor, social support can be considered a psychological influencing factor if it is conceptualized (and measured) to reflect the individual's perception about the potential availability of support, rather than the level of support that is actually available and/or received.

The characteristics of the setting in which the individual is receiving care—whether it be an institution (e.g., policies and procedures, staffing levels, certifications) or home (e.g., equipment available, caregiver knowledge and skill, proximity to healthcare facilities)—may also be important situational considerations. However, Duncan et al. (2009) found that situational variables describing the setting and the care provided were not strong predictors of symptoms in nursing home residents with cancer. The physical environment can also influence symptoms; it includes altitude, temperature, humidity, noise level, light, and presence of toxins, pollutants, or irritants in the air or water. The situational factors are contextual, that is, external to the individual.

## Performance Outcomes

The outcome concept in the TOUS is performance. It represents the consequences of the symptom experience. Simply stated, the theory asserts that the experience of symptoms can have an impact on the individual's ability to function or perform physically, cognitively, and in socially defined roles. Role performance is the ability to carry out personal care and social roles, including activities of daily living and employment-related expectations. Cognitive performance is the ability to carry out cognitive functions. It includes memory, comprehension, learning, concentration, and problem solving. Designation of performance as the key outcome of the TOUS reflects a pragmatic orientation and a desire for relatively straightforward measurability. It is also consistent with generation of the theory from practice-based observations in maternal–infant and adult health nursing domains.

Dong et al. (2016) found that several symptom clusters predicted physical, role, and social functioning in patients with advanced cancer. They acknowledged the TOUS as a framework that is appropriate for studying the impact of symptom clusters on functioning. In a study of elderly cancer patients receiving chemotherapy or radiotherapy, Cheng and Lee (2011) found that the symptom cluster of pain, fatigue, insomnia, and mood disturbance had a persistent effect on functional status and quality of life (QOL), even with the influence of age, gender, comorbidity, stage of illness, and treatment modality controlled. Similarly, Laird et al. (2011) and Motl and McAuley (2009) found that the three-symptom cluster of pain, depression, and fatigue had a strong relationship to physical functioning of patients with advanced cancer and multiple sclerosis, respectively. Thompson (2007) found that fatigue and other symptoms were related to physical and social performance in breast cancer survivors. In a population-based study of cancer patients in the year following diagnosis and in the last year of life, Sudradhar et al. (2014) found that fatigue, appetite, and well-being were related, albeit weakly, to performance status. Tankumpuan et al. (2015) found that pain, sleep disturbance, confusion, mood disturbance, fatigue, and vigor predicted physical functioning postoperatively in brain tumor patients; total mood disturbance was the strongest predictor of physical functioning, which included work-related functioning. Hsiao et al. (2014), in a study of men who had been treated for prostate cancer, found that the severity and frequency of symptoms were related to symptom self-management. Whereas symptom distress was related to self-management of urinary symptoms, this was not the case for bowel or sexual dysfunction symptoms. An unusual finding was that Crane (2005) found no relationship of fatigue to participation in physical activity in a sample of women following myocardial infarction.

A given symptom or set of symptoms may generate a number of different performance outcomes that may occur simultaneously but also can be time ordered. Performance outcomes that are proximal in time to the symptom experience can influence more distal outcomes, particularly if the symptom is sustained for a period of time. An example would be a person with COPD who suffers from extreme dyspnea. The symptom interferes with the ability to walk uphill, climb steps, and carry groceries. As a result of these more proximal functional limitations, the more distal performance outcomes might be the inability to carry out the demands of a job or to live independently. Another example would be that denying nicotine to smokers who are admitted to intensive care settings can result in a number of unpleasant symptoms of nicotine withdrawal that can affect cognitive functioning (e.g., delirium) and, in turn, result in increased length of hospital stay (Ely et al., 2001, 2004). The TOUS does not explicitly include QOL as an outcome, in part because of the high degree of overlap with functional status in many QOL measures.

Evidence indicates that symptoms influence not only the physical but also the affective aspects of QOL (Dabbs et al., 2003; Hsu & Tu, 2014; Jurgens et al., 2009; Motl, Suh, & Weikert, 2010; Motl, Weikert, et al., 2010; Wang & Fu, 2014) and that mood may both impact and be impacted by symptoms (Clayton, Mishel, & Belyea, 2006; Kugler et al., 2009), which suggest the need to consider adding affective outcomes and/or QOL to the TOUS. Some critiques of the TOUS have noted that failure to include QOL as an explicit outcome is a weakness (Brant, Beck, & Miaskowski, 2009). Although QOL is defined in many different ways, it is frequently investigated as an outcome in symptom research and is included in several existing and proposed models of symptom management. Currently, the influence of symptoms on affective variables is addressed in the TOUS by the feedback loop from the symptom experience to psychological factors and by the direct relationship of symptoms to cognitive performance.

## ■ RELATIONSHIPS AMONG CONCEPTS: THE MODEL

The overall structure of the theory, which is portrayed in Figure 9.1, asserts that three related categories of factors (physiological, psychological, and situational) influence predisposition to and manifestation of a given symptom or multiple symptoms and the nature of the symptom experience. The symptom, in turn, affects the individual's performance, which encompasses cognitive, physical, and social functioning. The performance outcomes can feed back to influence the symptom experience itself, as well as to modify the influencing factors. The current version of the TOUS (Figure 9.1) acknowledges the complexity of the symptom experience by depicting the relationships among the three major components (influencing factors, symptoms, and performance) as bidirectional or reciprocal. That is, the influencing factors are hypothesized to impact the nature of the symptom, which, in turn, impacts performance.

However, experiencing symptoms can also change the patient's psychological, physiological, and/or situational status (influencing factors). For example, experiencing the symptoms of severe pain and fatigue can negatively impact one's mood (a psychological influencing factor; Francoeur, 2005; Runquist, Morin, & Stetzer, 2009). Clayton, Mishel, and Belyea (2006) found that symptom bother (similar to the dimension of symptom distress) was related to mood both directly and indirectly, with the relationship mediated by uncertainty. Performance can have a reciprocal relationship to the experience of unpleasant symptoms and to influencing factors. For example, the experience of the multiple unpleasant symptoms stemming from use of some immunosuppressive drugs was associated with the performance outcome of increased nonadherence to the medication regimen, which, in turn, worsened other symptoms and ultimately increased the probability of organ rejection following solid organ transplantation (Kugler et al., 2009). Ensari, Adamson, and Motl (2015) found a reciprocal relationship between depressive symptoms and walking impairment

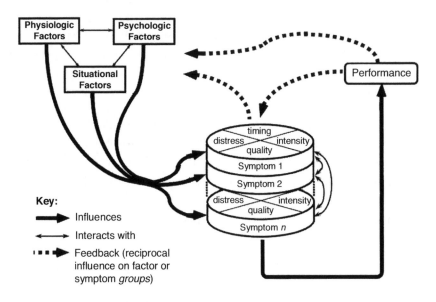

**FIGURE 9.1**  Unpleasant symptoms.

*Source:* Reprinted with permission from Lenz, E. R., Pugh, L.C., Milligan, R. A., Gift, A. G., & Suppe, F. (1997). The middle-range theory of unpleasant symptoms: An update. *Advances in Nursing Science, 19*(3), 17.

in persons with relapsing–remitting multiple sclerosis. In a study of breast cancer patients receiving chemotherapy postoperatively, Yang, Tsai, Huang, and Lin (2011) found that an experimental group of patients who participated in a moderate-intensity, home-based walking program (physical performance) reported lower symptom severity and mood disturbance than those in the control group throughout the 12-week follow-up period. Thus, performance was related reciprocally to both symptom severity and mood disturbance, a psychological influencing factor. Barsevick, Dudley, and Beck (2006) found that performance could also act as a mediator of the relationship between symptoms and influencing factors. They found that functional status mediated the relationship of fatigue to depression: As ability to perform everyday tasks (performance) became more difficult with increasing fatigue (symptom), patients reported higher levels of depressive symptoms (influencing factor).

Symptoms can serve as mediating or moderating variables between influencing factors and performance. A mediating relationship might be exemplified by the finding that symptoms among breast cancer survivors mediate the relationship of age to well-being, measured by mood state and troublesome thoughts about recurrence (Clayton, Mishel, & Belyea, 2006). Beck, Dudley, and Barsevick (2005) found that sleep disturbance mediated the relationship of pain to fatigue; pain also had a direct effect on fatigue. In a study of cancer patients, Hsu and Tu (2014) found that the relationship between fatigue and QOL, in addition to being direct, was mediated by depressive symptoms and functional status, the former explaining more of the variance than the latter. However, Redeker, Lev, and Ruggiero (2000) did not find fatigue and insomnia to be important mediators between psychological factors and QOL.

Consistent with a large body of literature supporting the moderating effect of social support on illness, E.-H. Lee, Chung, Park, and Chun (2004) found a moderating relationship between psychological factors and symptoms. Among Korean women with breast cancer, mood disturbances were related more strongly to symptoms when social support (a situational influencing factor) was low than when it was high. Psychosocial factors (depression, anxiety and perceived social support) were also important moderators of dyspnea in T.-Y. Huang et al.'s (2013) study of heart failure patients in Taiwan and the United States. In a study of fatigue across the transition to parenthood, gender moderated the relationship of infant characteristics (sleep duration and negativity) to postpartal fatigue, in that the relationships were stronger in mothers than in fathers (Loutzenhizer, McAuslan, & Sharpe, 2015).

The most recent version of the TOUS asserts that performance can have a feedback effect on the physiological, psychological, and situational factors. A breast cancer patient's severe pain (symptom) can impair the desire to interact with others, and hence decrease or increase the frequency of social interaction (performance). In turn, decreased interaction with others in the social network can result not only in decreased network size as others withdraw, but also in reduction of the social support available and received from the network (situational influencing factors).

The three categories of influencing factors are hypothesized to influence one another and to interact in their relation to the symptom experience. McCann and Boore (2000) found these relationships to be complex in renal failure patients requiring hemodialysis. In their sample, depression was related to physical health, sleep problems, and anxiety, as well as to symptoms and to physical functioning. A common finding is that in persons with chronic illnesses, psychological factors, such as depression, anxiety, and uncertainty, mediate the relationships of physiological or situational factors to symptoms. There is a positive impact of social support in mitigating the negative impact of physical illness or stress on the severity of symptoms (e.g., Yang et al., 2011), exemplifying the interaction of situational factors with physiological and psychological factors in their relationships to symptoms.

The three influencing factor categories are quite broad, encompassing many potential variables that can be measured in many different ways. Any given study can tap only a few of those variables and measures. Therefore, it is unlikely that all of the variables within a category will relate in the same way or with equal strength to the symptoms. It is also possible that the variables within a category relate to others in the same category in ways that mediate or moderate their effects. An example is that among postpartum women, the effects of childcare stress (a psychological factor) on postpartum fatigue were mediated by postpartum depression (also a psychological factor; Song et al., 2010).

The TOUS hypothesizes that when patients experience more than one symptom, the symptom experiences are related to one another. This hypothesis has been supported by multiple studies (e.g., Jurgens et al., 2009; Motl et al., 2010; Phligbua et al., 2013). It is at the heart of the concept of symptom cluster. The relationships among symptoms experienced simultaneously can be interactive, including multiplicative. That is, the experience of a given unpleasant symptom, such as pain, is exacerbated or fundamentally changed in other ways when it occurs simultaneously with another symptom, such as nausea. The relationships among symptoms experienced simultaneously can change over time (J. Huang et al., 2016; Phligbua et al., 2013).

It is likely that the cumulative effect of multiple symptoms on function is greater than the sum of the individual symptoms; however, this conjecture has not been tested thoroughly, so is not necessarily a straightforward conclusion. For example, Fox and Lyon (2006) found in a small sample of lung cancer survivors that fatigue and dyspnea were highly correlated. The cluster of the two symptoms explained 29% of the variance in QOL; however, when the impact of each symptom in the cluster was compared, dyspnea wielded much greater explanatory power than fatigue. Motl, McAuley, et al. (2010) predicted that the more numerous the symptoms in a cluster, the stronger the relationship of the cluster to the outcome of physical performance among persons with multiple sclerosis. However, they found that a three-symptom cluster (fatigue, pain, and depression) had a stronger relationship to physical activity than a five-symptom cluster that also included poor sleep quality and perceived cognitive dysfunction.

## ■ USE OF THE THEORY IN RESEARCH

An increasing number of investigators are using the TOUS as the conceptual framework on which to base their studies. S. E. Lee, Vincent, and Finnegan (2016) identified 31 studies published between 2000 and March 2016 that were guided by the TOUS. It is a middle range theory that effectively highlights important aspects of a phenomenon for examination (Barsevick, Whitmore, Nail, Beck, & Dudley, 2006; Eckhardt et al., 2014; Hyo-Jin Kim, Kim, Lee, & Oh, 2014), or is consistent with the conceptualization used in or findings of a symptom-related study (Franck et al., 2004; Kugler et al., 2009). The TOUS has also been used as the basis for instrument development (S.-H. Kim, Oh, & Lee, 2006; S.-H. Kim, Oh, Lee, et al., 2006; Lester, Bernhard, & Ryan-Wenger, 2012), for analyzing a concept (Farrell & Savage, 2010), or developing a more elaborate or more specific theory about one or more symptoms (Dabbs, Hoffman, Swigart, et al., 2004; Henley et al., 2003; Hoffman, 2013; McCann & Boore, 2000; Song et al., 2010). Clinical populations in which it has been applied for research include cancer survivors and cancer patients undergoing treatment, persons who have experienced a myocardial infarction or heart failure, patients with mitral valve prolapse syndrome, liver cirrhosis, hepatitis C, COPD, renal failure, and stroke; victims of intimate partner violence; and pregnant, postpartum, and breastfeeding women and their partners. The most frequent use has been in studies of persons with cancer and cancer survivors. A number of the studies based on the TOUS have been carried out in locations outside of the United States, for example, in Canada, Korea, Hong Kong, Mainland China, Taiwan, and Thailand. It should be noted that the theory is also being used as the theoretical framework guiding research in other fields, such as kinesiology and physical therapy (Motl, McAuley, et al., 2010). The TOUS authors receive multiple inquiries from master's and doctoral students and faculty who have found the theory to be extremely relevant to the phenomena they are studying, and either plan to use or are already using it as the theoretical framework for their research.

A review of the published research based on the TOUS has provided evidence to substantiate many of the conceptualizations and hypothesized relationships in the theory. Some examples of assertions in the TOUS that have been supported empirically are described in the following.

1. One of the most frequently validated assertions is that the symptom experience is individualized and highly variable. The TOUS delineation of variable dimensions of symptoms has been very useful and has been validated empirically (Jurgens et al., 2009; Kapella, Larson, Patel, Covey, & Berry, 2006; S.-H. Kim et al., 2006; Liu, 2006). Most commonly measured dimensions are intensity, distress, frequency, and duration. All of these dimensions have been measured successfully and their importance as predictors of outcomes substantiated. They have been found to vary independently; for example, a symptom that occurs infrequently can be very intense and distressing (S.-H. Kim, Oh, Lee, et al., 2006). Quality has been studied less often than the others, but when studied qualitatively, has yielded descriptors of the symptom experience that may be helpful in differentiating different types or stages of illness and/or have proven useful for incorporation in quantitative measures (Lang et al., 2006; Liu, 2006). As noted earlier, the meaning of the symptom(s) has been included in some models as an additional dimension of the symptom experience to examine (Armstrong, 2003). The TOUS incorporates meaning in the distress dimension. In an interesting departure from the TOUS model, L.-H. Chen et al. (2010) identified a concept they termed symptomatic distress and conceptualized it to be categorized as a physiological factor, rather than as a measure of the distress dimension of the symptom experience. They found it to be the strongest predictor of fatigue, which was the target symptom for their research. Regarding the dimension of time, Henley et al. (2003) have provided evidence of the complex nature of time in the symptom experience. They included time as the key component of their theory, which they identify as an extension of the TOUS. The relatedness of time with the other dimensions of the symptom experience has been demonstrated, for example, by Tzeng, Teng, Chou, and Tu (2009) in their study of expectant fathers. The degree of interference with everyday activities is another aspect of symptoms that has been used to describe the symptom experience (e.g., Eckhardt et al., 2014).

2. The revised version of the TOUS (Lenz et al., 1997) embodies the assertion that multiple symptoms can occur concurrently. As noted earlier, the current literature is replete with studies validating the existence of symptom clusters, which are defined in various ways in different disciplines, but all of which share the idea that the symptoms co-occur. The current literature documents that in many illness- or stress-related situations, multiple symptoms are experienced simultaneously (Dong et al., 2016; Hee-Ju Kim et al., 2009; H.-S. Kim et al., 2015; Jurgens et al., 2009; Laird et al., 2011; Park et al., 2012). For example, cancer patients with solid tumors and with nasopharyngeal cancer experienced an average of 11 to 13 and 8.3 to 19.5 concurrent symptoms, respectively (Armstrong et al., 2004; M. L. Chen & Huang,

2007). Patients who had undergone lung or heart–lung transplantations experienced as many as 29 symptoms (Dabbs et al., 2003). Dong et al. (2016) in a study of advanced cancer patients found four robust clusters: "tense-irritable-worry-depressed (emotional cluster); fatigue-pain cluster; nausea-vomiting cluster; and concentration-memory (cognitive cluster)" (p. 88). Herr et al. (2015) identified three symptom clusters in heart failure: sickness behavior (anxiety, depression, fatigue, daytime sleepiness, and cognitive dysfunction), discomforts of illness (shortness of breath, edema, and pain), and gastrointestinal (loss of appetite and reduced hunger). Park et al. (2012) found three symptom clusters in Korean immigrants with either asthma or COPD. Two of the three contained seven symptoms. One of the seven-symptom clusters (feeling nervous, numbness and tingling in the hands and feet, difficulty sleeping, shortness of breath, feeling sad, and worrying) was a predictor of functional performance. Lang et al. (2006) found that 62% of a sample of people living with a chronic hepatitis C infection reported symptom clustering. The TOUS does not depict symptoms as grape-like clusters, but rather as occurring simultaneously. Thus, it is consistent with, but differs somewhat from, some definitions and depictions of symptom clusters. For example, Hee-Ju Kim et al. (2005) stated that symptom clusters are ". . . composed of stable groups of symptoms, are relatively independent of other clusters, and may reveal specific underlying dimensions of symptoms" (p. 270).

The assertion that symptoms tend to occur in clusters is viewed as a critical consideration in conceptualizing the symptom experience (Dodd et al., 2004; Hee-Ju Kim et al., 2005). When a number of symptoms are experienced simultaneously, they may not all impact outcomes to the same degree. Instead, one or more symptoms may emerge as predictors while other clusters do not (Herr et al., 2015). A given symptom within a cluster may explain a higher proportion of the variance in outcomes, or be perceived as more distress-producing than any of the others in the cluster; and this pattern can change over the course of treatment (T.-Y. Huang et al., 2013). There can also be a pattern of sequencing in which one symptom can impact other symptoms (Carpenter et al., 2004).

3. The three categories of influencing factors (physiological, psychological, and situational) have varied in their importance as predictors or correlates of the symptom experience from one study to another. In some studies, a given category of factors was unrelated to the symptom experience; for example, situational factors, such as nursing home facility characteristics and staffing, were not related to symptoms in the study by Duncan et al. (2009). However, such patterns are not consistent, and there is considerable evidence that all three categories are meaningful in explaining the symptom experience.

The inconsistency can be attributed, at least in part, to the specific variables chosen as indicators of the category and other methodological considerations, such as sample size and instrumentation. For example, a given concept (e.g., insomnia or poor sleep quality) in some studies is set forth as a symptom and in others as a situational factor (Barsevick, 2007; Kapella et al., 2006; Pugh, Milligan, & Lenz, 2000). Liu (2006) categorized age and gender, and Carpenter et al. (2004) categorized nighttime hot flashes as situational variables; however, in the TOUS, age and gender are included in the physiological factors category, and nighttime hot flashes would be considered symptoms. Oh, Kim, Lee, and Kim (2004) categorized dyspnea as a physiological factor impacting the symptom of fatigue, whereas in most studies, it is considered a symptom. L.-H. Chen et al. (2010) categorized symptomatic distress as a physiological variable, and found it to be the strongest predictor of fatigue in a sample of Taiwanese patients with heart failure. However, the somatic distress instrument was a list of 17 symptoms for which patients reported frequency during the previous week. Duncan et al. (2009) categorized physical dependence as a physiological influencing factor that was related to pain, shortness of breath, and weight loss. In the TOUS it would be considered a performance outcome. Corwin, Brownstead, Barton, Heckar, and Morin (2005) pointed out the desirability of differentiating stable from variable predictors. Stable predictors (such as psychological traits and many social environmental variables) are difficult to change, and hence are less amenable to intervention than dynamic predictors.

4. The influencing factors category that was most often documented to be associated with the symptom experience was psychological factors. Common findings, for example, were the strong association of depression with symptoms such as fatigue, pain, and dyspnea (L.-H. Chen et al., 2010; Corwin et al., 2005; Hee-Ju Kim, Malone, & Barsevick, 2014; Motl, McAuley, et al., 2010; Song et al., 2010). Psychological factors were more important predictors than physiological factors in some studies (Kapella et al., 2006; K. Lee et al., 2010). Some issues remain to be clarified regarding the conceptualization and measurement of some of the frequently studied psychological factors, particularly depression. For example, fatigue is often included as an item on measures of depression; therefore, it is hardly surprising that the two variables have been found to be related quite strongly. Hutchinson and Wilson (1998) found the boundaries of the three influencing factor categories and symptom consequences/performance outcomes to be blurred and sometimes overlapping. For example, the psychological factor component of the model (anxiety, memory loss, and depression) was difficult to differentiate from some of the symptoms themselves. They

concluded that the components of the TOUS are not necessarily mutually exclusive when applied to patients with Alzheimer's disease but are better conceptualized as fluid and possibly interchangeable depending on the context in which they occur. Redeker et al. (2000) also noted that the redundancy among measures of psychological factors, symptoms, and QOL can obscure the nature of the relationships among the TOUS components.

5. In the revised version of the TOUS, relationships among the components of the model were hypothesized to be reciprocal and potentially to involve interactions. This assertion that the interplay among symptoms is often very complex has been substantiated as detailed previously.

6. The outcome of interest in the TOUS is performance, conceptualized to include physical, cognitive, and social functioning. This conceptualization has been criticized as too limited (Brant et al., 2009; Henely et al., 2003), but continues to have utility (e.g., Dong et al., 2016; Sudradhar et al., 2014). The most commonly studied outcome to date has been functional performance or functional status, measured by either disease-specific or general instruments. Other outcomes have included performance in occupational and caregiving roles (Scordo, 2005; Tyler & Pugh, 2009), care-seeking patterns (Jurgens, 2006; Liu, 2006), use of health resources (Scordo, 2005), health concerns (Scordo, 2005), and death/survival (Franck et al., 2004; K. Lee et al., 2010). Virtually all of the studies that included performance outcomes revealed relationships with symptoms. An exception is the finding by Michael, Allen, and Macko (2006) that fatigue in a sample of community-dwelling subjects with chronic hemiparetic stroke was not related to ambulatory activity.

## ■ USE OF THE THEORY IN NURSING PRACTICE

There continues to be limited published evidence of sustained application of the TOUS in clinical practice; however, several studies have tested TOUS-based clinical interventions. Pugh and Milligan (1995, 1998) conducted several experimental studies to test a positioning intervention based on the TOUS to minimize fatigue in nursing mothers, because fatigue was found to be a major barrier to breastfeeding success (Milligan, Flenniken, & Pugh, 1996). The multifaceted intervention addressed all three TOUS categories of influencing factors. It was found to be effective, in that the experimental group of mothers had lower fatigue at 2 weeks postpartum and sustained breastfeeding for an average of 6 weeks longer than the control group. In several additional studies, similar results were found (Pugh, Milligan, & Brown, 2001; Pugh, Milligan, Frick, Spatz, & Bronner, 2002; Pugh et al., 2010).

In an intervention study Jurgens, Lee, Reitano, and Riegel (2013) tested the effects of a training program designed to teach patients with heart failure to recognize and respond appropriately to changes in their symptoms. The experimental and control groups did not differ in 90-day event-free survival, but the experimental group had more improvement in self-care, maintenance, and confidence scores than those receiving usual care. Chan, Richardson, and Richardson (2011) also tested a TOUS-inspired educational program in late-stage cancer patients undergoing radiation therapy. Designed to help decrease breathlessness, anxiety, and fatigue, the intervention included discussions with a nurse about the symptoms, suggestions for self-care, and instruction in progressive muscle relaxation. Johnson and Robertson (2014) used the TOUS as a model to evaluate relaxation training and sleep hygiene instruction as complements to pharmacological interventions in depressed patients. Bekelman et al. (2016) have received federal funding for a three-site clinical trial to test the effects of a collaborative, multidisciplinary intervention (Collaborative Care to Alleviate Symptoms and Adjust to Illness [CASA]). It addresses physical (breathlessness, fatigue, pain) and psychological (depression) symptoms and their relationships to functional status and health-related QOL. The design of the study and the intervention are based on an integration of the TOUS into Wilson and Cleary's (1995) Model of Health-Related Quality of Life.

A majority of investigators who have based their research on the TOUS have addressed the practice implications. A few of the practice applications that would be consistent with the TOUS are listed in the following.

1. Because the symptom experience is highly individualized, nursing care would be patient-centered, not strictly illness-centered.
2. The theory suggests that a very comprehensive assessment of the patient's situation at baseline is warranted. The assessment would include a wide range of possible symptoms, not only those that are most commonly associated with the patient's illness, and would address all four dimensions of the symptoms.
3. The three categories of influencing factors would also be explored as part of the patient history. The TOUS emphasizes going beyond the physical aspects of the patient's background. A guide to such a comprehensive assessment could be incorporated into the intake form in the electronic patient record to guide the interview.
4. A TOUS-based treatment plan would be highly individualized and comprehensive, targeting the important influencing factors that could be changed and providing continuous symptom monitoring in both inpatient settings and following discharge. In most cases, that will require including strategies that help reduce stress and depression in addition to the usual physical care measures.
5. Finally, TOUS-based treatment also includes monitoring changes in performance outcomes that have been identified as markers for the

patient's condition. Although short-term performance changes are typically monitored during hospitalization to determine readiness for discharge or step-down, longer-term performance outcomes that indicate changes in the patient's ability to function need to be identified and included in the treatment plan for follow-up and community-based care. It is the long-term functional outcomes that influence QOL (Dong et al., 2016).

As expressed in the strategic plan of the NINR, symptom management is one of the most important issues addressed in nursing practice. More specific models at lower levels of abstraction, such as the middle range Theory of Acute Pain Management (Good, 1998), the related middle range Theory of Pain: A Balance Between Analgesia and Side Effects (Good, 2013), or the Conceptual Model of Chemotherapy-Related Changes in Cognitive Function (Myers, 2009) can and should be applied in managing individual symptoms. Likewise more illness-specific theories and models that address multiple symptoms, such as the Model of the Symptom Experience of Acute Rejection After Lung Transplantation by Dabbs et al. (2004), and more inclusive middle range theories make contributions to practice and may provide the advantage of a slightly different perspective than those that are highly specific. The Theory of Symptom Management (Humphreys et al., 2014) and the Dynamic Symptoms Model (Brant, Dudley, Beck, & Miaskowski, 2016) are more explicit than the TOUS in addressing symptom management strategies.

Although the TOUS does not explicitly include an intervention component, it does help highlight certain aspects of the symptom experience and potential strategies for symptom management that are not addressed by more symptom-specific models (Lenz, Gift, Pugh, & Milligan, 2013; Lenz et al., 2017). For example, the TOUS suggests that multiple management strategies may need to be applied simultaneously, given the multivariate nature of the symptoms and the factors influencing them. It also underscores the importance of addressing the possibility of several symptom experiences occurring concurrently, because co-occurrence can affect the individual's perception of any one of the symptoms as well as the patient's functioning (Jurgens et al., 2009). Admittedly, the TOUS does not address explicitly the many intervention-related concepts that Brant et al. (2009) recommend be included in theories that will help advance symptom management science, such as self-care, self-efficacy, decision-making processes, and change theory–related considerations.

According to Cooley (2000), the TOUS is valuable, because it "proposes a way to integrate information about the complexity and interactive nature of the symptom experience" (p. 146). Matthie and McMillan (2014) also note that the TOUS is an excellent guide for comprehensive symptom assessment. Hutchinson and Wilson (1998) and Jurgens et al. (2009) stressed the theory's encouragement of nurses to design interventions in a way that takes into account the multiple dimensions and the interactive nature of symptoms, influencing factors, and consequences, thereby making them client-specific. In its most recent version, the TOUS, with its emphasis on the interplay among the model's components, encourages creative thinking about new and different approaches to symptom management. Many clinicians have described it as having intuitive appeal because it is relatively straightforward, easy to understand and apply, and focused on relevant concerns.

## ■ CONCLUSIONS: AREAS FOR CONTINUING DEVELOPMENT

The TOUS, which was grounded in clinical research and practice, is a middle range theory that is valuable as a basis for additional research and as a guide to nursing practice. Although it is one of the few middle range theories that has undergone revision based on empirical findings, the TOUS remains a work in progress. The updated version addressed several of the weaknesses of the original; however, we acknowledge that some aspects of the theory remain underdeveloped and more updating is needed. The authors are committed to continued development and publication of updates.

A recent review of the TOUS was carried out by S. E. Lee et al. (2016) using Fawcett and DeSanto-Madeya's (2013) framework for theory analysis and evaluation. They concluded that improvement is needed in the theory's semantic clarity, semantic and structural consistency, and parsimony. More specifically they found problematic the use of more than one term for some of the concepts (e.g., symptom and symptom experience). Additionally, they suggested that the inclusion of both directional and reciprocal relationships between influencing factors and symptoms was a contradiction, and recommended inclusion of the bidirectional relationship only. (The TOUS authors believe that the reciprocity between influencing factors and symptoms is implicit in the arrow depicting feedback from symptoms to influencing factors.) S. E. Lee et al. (2016) also noted that while the TOUS diagram shows that symptoms can mediate the relationship between influencing factors and performance, it does not depict a moderating relationship. Despite these criticisms, they concluded that the TOUS is sound, and has acceptable significance, testability, and empirical and pragmatic adequacy. It highlights concepts and relationships that are important for guiding practice, particularly the reality of multiple, simultaneously occurring symptoms.

The changes that were made to the theory in the 1997 revision added to the complexity of the model but also made it more consistent with the reality that constitutes the symptom experience. The modifications have been validated in several ill and well samples. Thus far, the symptoms that have been described in these studies have included pain, dyspnea, nausea, vomiting, insomnia and other sleep problems, hair loss, not looking like myself, loss of appetite, hot flashes, weakness, and fatigue. More research is needed in additional clinical populations and with more symptoms.

The current research suggests that the symptom dimensions identified in the TOUS are both relevant and measurable; however, additional elaboration is warranted with regard to conceptualization and measurement, particularly the dimensions of quality and time. For example, it may be prudent to add abruptness of symptom onset. The theory needs to address explicitly the dynamics of the symptom experience, including the notions of possible recurrence (Brant et al., 2009; Henley et al., 2003). Addition of a meaning dimension has been suggested; thus, a clearer explanation of how it is incorporated in the existing distress dimension is needed.

The inclusion of multiple symptoms in the model introduces a number of areas of complexity that have not yet been addressed in detail. The sequence in which symptoms appear and the extent to which a given symptom tends to influence the appearance and characteristics of others are examples. The notion of primary and secondary symptoms should be included explicitly. For example, on the basis of their study of persons with multiple sclerosis, Motl et al. (2010) noted that findings about the relative importance of individual symptoms within clusters in predicting outcomes have important practice implications. They suggested that targeting one symptom rather than several co-occurring symptoms may be the most effective and efficient approach to improving outcomes. They recommend extending the TOUS "by examining pathways among multiple, co-occurring symptoms with performance outcomes" (p. 409).

Additional conceptual/theoretical work is needed to address several of the issues that have been pointed out by investigators who have used the theory. For example, a question exists as to whether the theory is relevant for both signs and symptoms. Likewise, its potential applicability to subjects or patients who have perceptual deficits or are unable to describe the symptom experience (e.g., infants, unconscious patients, or some of the older adults) has been assumed by some investigators, but has not yet been explored fully. Another criticism of the theory is that some of the key components—specifically the antecedent influencing factors and the outcomes—need to be better defined and variables within the categories specified (Brant et al., 2009; S. E. Lee et al., 2016). The complex relationships among the three categories of influencing factors and the symptom experience need fuller elaboration and clarification.

Although the potential relevance of all three types of influencing factors has been quite well supported, there are some inconsistencies that need to be examined. The most robust influencing factors need to be identified and the nature of their complex relationships to the symptom experience explicated. Psychological factors have been found repeatedly to play a key role in exacerbating or mitigating symptoms; however, there is potential for conceptual and empirical overlap between psychological factor variables (anxiety and depression in particular) and the affective or distress component of the symptom experience. Overlap between measures of psychological factors (e.g., depression) and symptoms (e.g., fatigue) also needs to be addressed, but cannot be eliminated when many of the legacy instruments are used. There is also inconsistency as to whether mood states (anxiety, depression) are to be treated as symptoms themselves or as psychological influencing factors. The interplay between these two model components needs to be examined.

The performance component of the model needs additional development. Several investigations have revealed it to be more complex than originally thought. The notions of primary and secondary outcomes and temporally proximal and distal outcomes will be important to incorporate in the TOUS. Although the functional, pragmatic focus of the performance outcome was chosen purposefully, it does de-emphasize other, more inclusive outcomes that may be important consequences of symptoms. QOL, particularly the affective aspects thereof, is a prime example. Functioning is generally included as a component of QOL, but the latter is more inclusive. The possible place of QOL within the TOUS is a topic that needs to be explored conceptually and empirically.

Finally, more attention needs to be paid to symptom assessment and management. As noted earlier, the TOUS has many practice implications and recent findings suggest potentially useful interventions; however, these remain to be detailed and possible patterns discerned. The place of interventions as an explicit component of the model should be determined. Brant et al. (2009) set forth a considerable challenge in their recommendation that "future models and theories should depict the global concepts that define not only the symptom intervention but the healthcare interactions and the patient's physiological, psychological and sociocultural responses to the intervention" (p. 238).

The process of developing the TOUS has been and continues to be the product of exciting group interaction. Multiple practice-grounded observations, a growing body of literature documenting its application, and lively discussions with colleagues and students, have led to its continued development. Its richness can only increase as the developers continue to address the input of others who have used the theory in research and practice.

# ■ REFERENCES

Abbott, A. A., Baranson, S., & Zimmerman, L. (2010). Symptom burden clusters and their impact on psychosocial functioning following coronary artery bypass surgery. *Journal of Cardiovascular Nursing*, 4, 301–310. doi:10.109/JCN .ob013e3181cfbb46

Ameringer, S. E., Erickson, J. M., Macpherson, C. F., Stegenga, K., & Linder, L. A. (2015). Symptoms and symptom clusters identified by adolescents and young adults with cancer using a symptom heuristics app. *Research in Nursing & Health*, 38, 436–448. doi:10.1002/NUR.21697

Armstrong, T. S. (2003). Symptoms experience: A concept analysis. *Oncology Nursing Forum*, 30, 601–606. doi:10.1188/03.ONF.601.606

Armstrong, T. S., Cohen, M. Z., Eriksen, L. R., & Hickey, J. V. (2004). Symptom clusters in oncology patients and implications for symptom research in people with primary brain tumors. *Journal of Nursing Scholarship*, *36*(3), 197–206. doi:10.111/j.1547.5069.2004.04038.x

Atay, S., Conk, Z., & Hahar, Z. (2012). Identifying symptom clusters in paediatric cancer patients using the Memorial Symptom Assessment Scale. *European Journal of Cancer Care*, *21*, 460–468. doi:10.1111/j.13652354.2012.01324.x

Badke, M. B., & Boissonnault, W. G. (2006). Changes in disability following physical therapy intervention for patients with low back pain: Dependence on symptom duration. *Archives of Physical Medicine & Rehabilitation*, *87*, 749–756. doi:10.1016/j.apmr.2006.02.033

Baggott, C., Cooper, B. A., Matthay, M., & Miaskowski, C. (2012). Symptom cluster analysis based on symptom occurrence and severity ratings among pediatric oncology patients during myelosuppressive chemotherapy. *Cancer Nursing*, *35*(1), 19–28. doi:10.1097/NCC.ob.013e.31822909fd

Barsevick, A. M. (2007). The elusive concept of the symptom cluster. *Oncology Nursing Forum*, *34*, 971–980. doi:10.1188/07.ONF.971-980

Barsevick, A. M., Dudley, W. N., & Beck, S. L. (2006). Cancer-related fatigue, depressive symptoms, and functional status: A mediation model. *Nursing Research*, *55*(5), 366–372.

Barsevick, A. M., Whitmore, K., Nail, L. M., Beck, S. L., & Dudley, W. N. (2006). Symptom cluster research: Conceptual, design, measurement and analysis issues. *Journal of Pain and Symptom Management*, *31*(1), 85–95. doi:10.1016/j.jpainsymman.2005.05.015

Beck, S. L., Dudley, W. N., & Barsevick, A. M. (2005). Pain, sleep disturbance, and fatigue in patients with cancer: Using a mediation model to test a symptom cluster. *Oncology Nursing Forum*, *32*(3), E48–E55. doi:10.1188/04.ONF.E48-E55

Bekelman, D. B., Allen, L. A., Peterson, J., Hattler, B., Havranek, E. P., Fairclough, D. L., . . . Meek, P. M. (2016). Rationale and study design of a patient-centered intervention to improve health status in chronic heart failure: The Collaborative Care to Alleviate Symptoms and Adjust to Illness (CASA), randomized trial. *Contemporary Clinical Trials*, *51*, 1–7. doi:10.1016/j.cct.2016.09.002

Brant, J. M., Beck, S., & Miaskowski, C. (2009). Building dynamic models and theories to advance the science of symptom management research. *Journal of Advanced Nursing*, *66*(1), 228–240. doi:10.1111/j.1365-2648.2009.05179.x

Brant, J. M., Dudley, W. N., Beck, S., & Miaskowski, C. (2016). Evolution of the dynamic symptoms model. *Oncology Nursing Forum*, *43*, 651–654. doi:10.1188/16.ONF.651-654

Carpenter, J. S., Elam, J. L., Ridner, S. H., Carney, P. H., Cherry, G. J., & Cucullu, H. L. (2004). Sleep, fatigue, and depressive symptoms in breast cancer survivors and matched health women experiencing hot flashes. *Oncology Nursing Forum*, *31*(3), 591–598. doi:10.1188/04.ONF.591-598

Cashion, A. K., & Grady, P. A. (2015). The National Institutes of Health/National Institutes of Nursing Research Intramural Research Program and the development of the National Institutes of Health Symptom Science Model. *Nursing Outlook*, *63*, 484–487. doi:10.1016/j.OUTLOOK.2015.03.001

Chan, C. W. H., Richardson, A., & Richardson, J. (2011). Managing symptoms in patients with advanced lung cancer during radiotherapy: Results of a psychoeducational randomized clinical trial. *Journal of Pain and Symptom Management, 41*, 347–357. doi:10.1016/j.jpainsymman.2010.04.024

Chen, E., Nguyen, J., Cramarossa, G., Kahn, L. O., Leung, A., Lutz, S., & Chow, E. (2011). Symptom clusters in persons with lung cancer: A literature review. *Expert Review of Pharmacoeconomics & Outcomes Research, 11*, 433–439. doi:10.1586/erp.11.56

Chen, L.-H., Li, C.-Y., Shieh, S.-M., Yin, W.-H., & Chiou, A.-F. (2010). Predictors of fatigue in patients with heart failure. *Journal of Clinical Nursing, 19*, 1588–1596. doi:10.1111/j.1365-2702.2010.03218.x

Chen, M. L., & Huang, P. H. (2007). Symptom patterns of patients with nasopharyngeal cancer receiving radiation therapy. *Oncology Nursing Forum, 34*, 185.

Cheng, K. K. F., & Lee, D. T. F. (2011). Effects of pain, fatigue, insomnia, and mood disturbance on functional status and quality of life of elderly patients with cancer. *Critical Reviews in Oncology Hematology, 78*, 127–137. doi:10.1016/j.critrevonc.2010.03.002

Cherwin, C. H. (2012). Gastrointestinal symptom representation in cancer symptom clusters: A synthesis of the literature. *Oncology Nursing Forum, 39*, 157–165. doi:10.1188/12ONF.157-165

Chow, E., & Merrick, J. (2010). A critical discussion of symptom clusters in metastatic cancer. In E. Chow & J. Merrick (Eds.), *Advanced cancer: Pain and quality of life* (pp. 129–143). New York, NY: Nova Science.

Clayton, M. F., Mishel, M. M., & Belyea, M. (2006). Testing a model of symptoms, communication, uncertainty and well-being in older breast cancer survivors. *Research in Nursing & Health, 29*, 18–39. doi:10.1002/NUR.20108

Cleeland, C. S., Zhao, F., Chang, V. T., Sloan, J. A., O'Mara, A. M., Gilman, P. B., . . . Fisch, M. J. (2013). The symptom burden of cancer: Evidence for a core set of cancer-related and treatment-related symptoms from the Eastern Cooperative Oncology Group Symptom Outcomes and Practice Patterns study. *Cancer, 119*, 4333–4340. doi:10.1002/cncr.28376

Coolbrandt, A., Wildiers, H., Aertgeerts, B., Van der Elst, E., Laenen, A., de Casterlé, . . . Koen, M. (2014). Characteristics and effectiveness of complex nursing interventions aimed at reducing symptom burden in adult patients treated with chemotherapy: A systematic review of randomized controlled trials. *International Journal of Nursing Studies, 51*, 495–510. doi:10.1016/j.ijnurstu.2013.08.008

Cooley, M. (2000). Symptoms in adults with lung cancer: A systematic research review. *Journal of Pain and Symptom Management, 19*, 137–153. doi:10.1016/S0885-3924(99)00150-5

Corwin, E. J., Brownstead, J., Barton, N., Heckar, S., & Morin, K. (2005). The impact of fatigue on the development of postpartum depression. *Journal of Obstetric, Gynecologic, & Neonatal Nursing, 34*(5), 577–586. doi:10.1177/0884217505279997

Crane, P. B. (2005). Fatigue and physical activity in older women after myocardial infarction. *Heart & Lung, 34*, 30–38. doi:10.1016/jhrting.2004.08.007

Crosta, Q. R., Ward, T. M., Walker, A. J., & Peters, L. M. (2014). A review of pain measures for hospitalized children with cognitive impairment. *Journal for Specialists in Pediatric Nursing, 12*(2), 109–118. doi:10.1111/jspn.12069

Dabbs, A. D., Dew, M. A., Stilley, C. S., Manzetti, J., Zullo, T., McCurry, K. R., & Iacono, A. (2003). Psychosocial vulnerability, physical symptoms and physical impairment after lung and heart-lung transplantation. *Journal of Heart and Lung Transplantation, 22*(11), 1268–1275. doi:10.1016/51053.2498(02)01227-5

Dabbs, A. D., Hoffman, L. A., Swigart, V., Happ, M. B., Iacono, A. T., & Dauber, J. H. (2004). Using conceptual triangulation to develop an integrated model of the symptom experience of acute rejection after lung transplantation. *Advances in Nursing Science, 27*, 136–149.

Dodd, M. J., Miaskowski, C., & Lee, K. A. (2004). Occurrence of symptom clusters. *Journal of the National Cancer Institute, 32*, 76–78. doi:10.1093/jncimonographs/lgh008

Dong, S. T., Costa, D. S. J., Butow, P. H., Lovell, M. R., Agar, M., Velikova, G., . . . Fayers, P. M. (2016). Symptom clusters in advanced cancer patients: An empirical comparison of statistical methods and the impact on quality of life. *Journal of Pain and Symptom Management, 51*, 88–98. doi:10.1016/j.jpainsymman.2015.07.013

Duncan, J. G., Bott, M. J., Thompson, S. A., & Gajewski, B. J. (2009). Symptom occurrence and associated clinical factors in nursing home residents with cancer. *Research in Nursing and Health, 32*, 453–464. doi:10.1002/nur.20331

Eckhardt, A., DeVon, H., Piano, M., Ryan C., & Zerwic, J. (2014). Fatigue in the presence of coronory heart disease. *Nursing Research, 63*(2), 83–93. doi:10.1097/NNR.0000000000000019

Ely, E. W., Gautam, S., Margolin, R., Francis, J., May, L., Speroff, T., . . . Inouye, S. K. (2001). The impact of delirium in the intensive care unit on hospital length of stay. *Intensive Care Medicine, 27*(12), 1892–1900. doi:10.1007/s00134-001-1132-2

Ely, E. W., Shintani, A., Truman, B., Speroff, T., Gordon, S. M., Harrell, F. E., . . . Dittus, R. S. (2004). Delirium as a predictor of mortality in mechanically ventilated patients in the intensive care unit. *Journal of the American Medical Association, 291*(14), 1753–1762. doi:10.1001/jama.291.14.1753

Ensari, I., Adamson, B. C., & Motl, R. W. (2015). Longitudinal association between depressive symptoms and walking impairment in people with relapsing-remitting multiple sclerosis. *Journal of Health Psychology, 21*, 2732–2741. doi:0.1177/1359105315584837

Farrell, D., & Savage, E. (2010). Symptom burden in inflammatory bowel disease: Rethinking conceptual and theoretical underpinnings. *International Journal of Nursing Practice, 16*, 437–442. doi:10.1111/j.1440-172X.2010.01867.x

Fawcett, J., & DeSanto-Madeya, S. (2013). *Contemporary nursing knowledge: Analysis and evaluation of nursing models and theories* (3rd ed.). Philadelphia, PA: F. A. Davis.

Fox, S. W., & Lyon, D. E. (2006). Symptom clusters and quality of life in survivors of lung cancer. *Oncology Nursing Forum, 33*(5), 931–936.

Franck, L. S., Kools, S., Kennedy, C., Kong, S. K. F., Chen, J.-L., & Wong, T. K. S. (2004). The symptom experience of hospitalized Chinese children and adolescents and relationship to pre-hospital factors and behavior problems. *International Journal of Nursing Studies, 41,* 661–669. doi:10.1016/j.ijnurstu.2004.02.001

Francoeur, R. B. (2005). The relationship of cancer symptom clusters to depressive affect in the initial phase of palliative radiation. *Journal of Pain and Symptom Management, 29*(2), 130–155. doi:10.1016/j.jpainsymman.2004.04.014

Gift, A. G. (1990). Dyspnea. *Nursing Clinics of North America, 25,* 955–965.

Gift, A. G., & Cahill, C. (1990). Psychophysiologic aspects of dyspnea in chronic obstructive pulmonary disease: A pilot study. *Heart & Lung, 19,* 252–257.

Gift, A. G., Jablonski, A., Stommel, M., & Given, C. W. (2004). Symptom clusters in elderly patients with lung cancer. *Oncology Nursing Forum, 31*(2), 203–210. doi:10.1188/04.ONF.203-212

Gift, A. G., & Pugh, L. C. (1993). Dyspnea and fatigue. *Nursing Clinics of North America, 28,* 373–384.

Good, M. (1998). A middle-range theory of acute pain management: Use in research. *Nursing Outlook, 436,* 120–124. doi:10.1016/S0029-6554(98)90038-0

Good, M. (2013). Pain: A balance between analgesia and side effects. In S. J. Peterson & T. S. Bredow (Eds.), *Middle range theories: Application to nursing research* (3rd ed., pp. 51–67). Philadelphia, PA: Wolters Kluwer/Lippincott Williams & Wilkins.

Henley, S. M., Kallas, K. D., Klatt, C. M., & Swenson, K. K. (2003). The notion of time in symptom experiences. *Nursing Research, 52*(6), 410–417.

Herr, J. K., Salyer, J., Flattery, M., Goodloe, L., Lyon, D. E., Kabban, C. S., & Clement, D. G. (2014). Heart failure symptom clusters and functional status: A cross-sectional study. *Journal of Advanced Nursing, 71*(6), 1274–1287.

Hoffman, A. J. (2013). Enhancing self-efficacy for optimized patient outcomes through the theory of symptom self-management. *Cancer Nursing, 36,* E16–E26. doi:10.1097/NCC.0b013e31824a730a

Hsiao, C.-P., Moore, E. M., Insel, K. C., & Merkle, C. J. (2014). Symptom self-management strategies in patients with non-metastatic prostate cancer. *Journal of Clinical Nursing, 23,* 440–449. doi:10.1111/jocn.12178

Hsu, M.-C., & Tu, C.-H. (2014). Improving quality-of-life outcomes for patients with cancer through mediating effects of depressive symptoms and functional status: A three-path mediation model. *Journal of Clinical Nursing, 23*(17–18), 2461–2472. doi:10.1111/jocn.12399

Huang, J., Gu, L. Y., Zhang, L. J., Lu, X. Y., Zhuang, W., & Yang, Y. (2016). Symptom clusters in ovarian cancer patients with chemotherapy after surgery: A longitudinal survey. *Cancer Nursing, 39*(2), 106–116. doi:10.1097/NCC .0000000000000252

Huang, T.-Y., Moser, D. K., Hsieh, Y.-S., Gau, B.-S., Chiang, F.-T., & Hwang, S.-L. (2013). Moderating effect of psychosocial factors for dyspnea in Taiwanese and American heart failure patients. *Journal of Nursing Research, (21),* 49–58. doi:10.1097/jnr.0b013e3182828d77

Humphreys, J., Janson, S., Donesky, K., Dracup, K., Lee, K. A., Puntillo, K . . . The UCSF Symptom Management Faculty Group. (2014). In M. J. Smith & P. Liehr

(Eds.). *Middle range theory for nursing* (3rd ed., pp. 141–164). New York, NY: Springer Publishing.

Hutchinson, S. A., & Wilson, H. S. (1998). The theory of unpleasant symptoms and Alzheimer's disease. *Scholarly Inquiry for Nursing Practice*, 22, 143–158.

Jablonsky, A. (2007). The multidimensional characteristics of symptoms reported by patients on hemodialysis. *Nephrology Nursing Journal*, 34, 29–37.

Jaremka, L. M., Andridge, R. R., Fagundes, C. P., Alfano, C. M., Povoski, S. P., Lipari, A. M . . . Kiecolt-Glaser, J. K. (2014). Pain, depression, and fatigue: Loneliness as a longitudinal risk factor. *Health Psychology*, 33, 948–957. doi:10.1037/a0034012

Johnson, D., & Robertson, A. (2014). The evaluation of the effectiveness of relaxation training and sleep hygiene education for insomnia of depressed patients. *Clinical Scholars Review*, 6, 39–46. doi:10.1891/1939-2095.6.1.39

Jurgens, C. Y. (2006). Somatic awareness, uncertainty and delay in care-seeking in acute heart failure. *Research in Nursing and Health*, 29, 74–76. doi:10.1002/nur.20118

Jurgens, C. Y., Lee, C. S., Reitano, J. M., & Riegel, B. (2013). Heart failure symptom monitoring and response training. *Heart & Lung*, 42, 273–280. doi:10.1016/j.hrtlng.2013.03.005

Jurgens, C. Y., Moser, D. K., Armola, R., Carlson, B., Sethares, K., Riegel, B., & The Heart Failure Quality of Life Trialist Collaborators. (2009). Symptom clusters of heart failure. *Research in Nursing & Health*, 32, 551–560. doi:10.1002/nur.20343

Kapella, M. C., Larson, J. L., Patel, M. K., Covey, M. K., & Berry, J. K. (2006). Subjective fatigue, influencing variables and consequences in chronic obstructive pulmonary disease. *Nursing Research*, 55(1), 10–17. doi:10.1097/00006199 -200601000-00002

Keller, V. E. C. (2004). Symptom assessment for preverbal and early verbal children: assessment for pain and nausea in children 1 through 5 years of age. *Dissertation Abstracts International*, DAI-B 65/07.

Keller, V. E., & Keck, J. F. (2006). An instrument for observational assessment of nausea in young children. *Pediatric Nursing*, 32, 420–426.

Kim, H.-J. [Hee-Ju], Barsevick, A. M., & Tulman, L. (2009). Predictors of the intensity of symptoms in a cluster in patients with breast cancer. *Journal of Nursing Scholarship*, 41, 158–165. doi:10.1111/j.1547-5069.2009.01267.x

Kim, H.-J. [Hee-Ju], Malone, P. S., & Barsevick, A. M. (2014). Subgroups of cancer patients with unique pain and fatigue experiences during chemotherapy. *Journal of Pain and Symptom Management*, 48, 558–568. doi:10.1016/j.jpainsymman.2013.10.025

Kim, H.-J. [Hee-Ju], McDermott, P. A., & Barsevick, A. M. (2014). Comparison of groups with different patterns of symptom cluster intensity across the breast cancer treatment trajectory. *Cancer Nursing*, 37, 88–96. doi:10.1097/NCC.0b013e31828293e0

Kim, H.-J. [Hee-Ju], McGuire, D. B., Tulman, L., & Barsevick, A. M. (2005). Symptom clusters: Concept analysis and clinical implications for cancer nursing. *Cancer Nursing*, 28(4), 270–282.

Kim, H.-J. [Hyo-Jin], Kim, S., Lee, H., & Oh, S. E. (2014). Factors affecting symptom experience of breast cancer patients: based on the Theory of Unpleasant Symptoms. *Asian Oncology Nursing, 14*, 7–14. doi:10.5388/aon.2014.14.1.7

Kim, H.-S., Oh, E.-G., Lee, H., Kim, S.-H., & Kim, H.-K. (2015). Predictors of symptom experience in Korean patients with cancer undergoing chemotherapy. *European Journal of Oncology Nursing, 19*, 644–653. doi:10.1016/j.ejon.2015.04.003

Kim, S.-H., Oh, E.-G., & Lee, W.-H. (2006). Symptom experience, psychological distress, and quality of life in Korean patients with liver cirrhosis: A cross-sectional survey. *International Journal of Nursing Studies, 43*, 1047–1056. doi:10.1016/j.ijnurstu.2005.11.012

Kim, S.-H., Oh, E.-G., Lee, W.-H., Kim, O.-S., & Han, K.-H. (2006). Symptom experience in Korean patients with liver cirrhosis. *Journal of Pain and Symptom Management, 31*(4), 325–334. doi:10.1016/j.jpainsymman.2005.08.015

Kiser, D. W., Greer, T. B., Wilmoth, M. C., Dmochowski, J., & Naumann, R. W. (2010). Peripheral neuropathy in patients with gynecologic cancer receiving chemotherapy: Patient reports and provider assessments. *Oncology Nursing Forum, 37*, 758–764. doi:10.1188/10.onf.758.764

Kugler, C., Geyer, S., Gottlieb, J., Simon, A., Haverich, A., & Dracup, K. (2009). Symptom experience after solid organ transplantation. *Journal of Psychosomatic Research, 66*, 101–110. doi:10.1016/j.jpsychores.2008.07.017

Laird, B. J. A., Scott, A. C., Colvin, L. A., McKeon, A., Murray, G. D., Fearon, K. C., & Fallon, M. T. (2011). Pain, depression, and fatigue as a symptom cluster in advanced cancer. *Journal of Pain and Symptom Management, 42*, 1–11. doi:10.1016/j.jpainsymman.2010.10.261

Lang, C. A., Conrad, S., Garrett, L., Battistutta, D., Cooksley, W. G. E., Dunne, M., & Macdonald, G. A. (2006). Symptom prevalence and clustering of symptoms in people living with chronic hepatitis C infection. *Journal of Pain and Symptom Management, 31*(4), 335–344. doi:10.1016/j.jpainsymman.2005.08.016

Lee, E.-H., Chung, B. Y., Park, H. B., & Chun, K. H. (2004). Relationships of mood disturbance and social support to symptom experience in Korean women with breast cancer. *Journal of Pain and Symptom Management, 27*(5), 425–433. doi:10.1016/j.jpainsymman.2003.10.007

Lee, K., Song, E. K., Lennie, T. A., Frazier, S. K., Chung, M. L., Heo, S., . . . Moser, D. K. (2010). Symptom clusters in men and women with heart failure and their impact on cardiac event-free survival. *Journal of Cardiovascular Nursing, 25*, 263–272. doi:10.1097/JCN.0b013e3181cfbb88

Lee, S. E., Vincent, C., & Finnegan, L. (2016). An analysis and evaluation of the theory of unpleasant symptoms. *Advances in Nursing Science, 40*(1), E16–E39. doi:10.1097/ANS.0000000000000141

Lenz, E. R., Gift, A. G., Pugh, L. C., & Milligan, R. A. (2013). Unpleasant symptoms. In S. J. Peterson & T. S. Bredow (Eds.), *Middle range theories: Application to nursing research* (3rd ed., pp. 68–81). Philadelphia, PA: Wolters Kluwer/Lippincott Williams & Wilkins.

Lenz, E. R., Pugh, L. C., Milligan, R., & Gift, A. (2017). Unpleasant symptoms. In S. J. Peterson & T. S. Bredow (Eds.). *Middle range theories: Application to nursing research and practice* (4th ed, pp. 67–77). Philadelphia, PA: Wolters Kluwer.

Lenz, E. R., Pugh, L. C., Milligan, R., Gift, A., & Suppe, F. (1997). The middle-range theory of unpleasant symptoms: An update. *Advances in Nursing Science, 19*(3), 14–27.

Lenz, E. R., Suppe, F., Gift, A. G., Pugh, L. C., & Milligan, R. A. (1995). Collaborative development of middle-range nursing theories: Toward a theory of unpleasant symptoms. *Advances in Nursing Science, 17*(3), 1–13.

Lester, J., & Bernhard, L. (2009). Urogenital atrophy in breast cancer survivors. *Oncology Nursing Forum, 36,* 993–698. doi:10.1188/09.onf.693-698

Lester, J., Bernhard, L., & Ryan-Wenger, N. (2012). A self-report instrument that describes urogenital atrophy symptoms in breast cancer survivors. *Western Journal of Nursing Research, 34,* 72–96. doi:10.1177/0193945910391483

Liu, H. E. (2006). Fatigue and associated factors in hemodialysis patients in Taiwan. *Research in Nursing and Health, 29,* 40–50. doi:10.1002/nur.20109

Loutzenhizer, L., McAuslan, P., & Sharpe, D. P. (2015). The trajectory of maternal and paternal fatigue and factors associated with fatigue across the transition to parenthood. *Clinical Psychology, 19,* 15–27. doi:10.1111/cp.12048

Matthie, N., & McMillan, S. C. (2014). Pain: A descriptive study in patients with cancer. *Clinical Journal of Oncology Nursing, 18,* 205–210. doi:10.1188/14.cjon.205-210

McCann, K., & Boore, J. R. P. (2000). Fatigue in persons with renal failure who require maintenance haemodialysis. *Journal of Advanced Nursing, 32,* 1132–1142.

Miaskowski, C., Dodd, M., & Lee, K. (2004). Symptom clusters: The new frontier in symptom management research. *Journal of the National Cancer Institute Monographs, 2004*(32), 17–21. doi:10.1093/jncimonographs/lgh023

Michael, K. M., Allen, J. K., & Macko, R. F. (2006). Fatigue after stroke: Relationship to mobility, fitness, ambulatory activity, social support and falls efficacy. *Rehabilitation Nursing, 31*(5), 210–217.

Milligan, R. A. (1989). Maternal fatigue during the first three months of the postpartum period. *Dissertation Abstracts International, 50,* 7B.

Milligan, R. A., Flenniken, P., & Pugh, L. C. (1996). Positioning intervention to minimize fatigue in breastfeeding women. *Applied Nursing Research, 9,* 67–70.

Milligan, R. A., Lenz, E. R., Parks, P. L., Pugh, L. C., & Kitzman, H. (1996). Postpartum fatigue: Clarifying a concept. *Scholarly Inquiry for Nursing Practice, 10*(3), 279–291.

Motl, R. W., & McAuley, E. (2009). Symptom cluster as a predictor of physical activity in multiple sclerosis: Preliminary evidence. *Journal of Pain and Symptom Management, 38,* 270–280. doi:10.1016/j.jpainsymman.2008.08.004

Motl, R. W., McAuley, E., & Sandoff, B. M. (2013). Longitudinal change in physical activity and its correlates in relapsing remitting multiple sclerosis. *Physical Therapy, 93,* 1037–1048. doi:10.2522/ptj.20120479

Motl, R. W., McAuley, E., Wynn, D., Suh, S., Weikert, M., & Dlugonsky, D. (2010). Symptoms and physical activity among adults with relapsing-remitting multiple sclerosis. *Journal of Nervous and Mental Disease, 198,* 213–219. doi:10.1097/NMD.0b013e3181d14131

Motl, R. W., Suh, Y., & Weikert, M. (2010). Symptom cluster and quality of life in multiple sclerosis. *Journal of Pain and Symptom Management, 39,* 1025–1032. doi:10.1016/j.jpainsymman.2009.11.312

Motl, R. W., Weikert, M., Suh, Y., & Dlugonski, D. (2010). Symptom cluster and physical activity in relapsing-remitting multiple sclerosis. *Research in Nursing and Health, 33,* 398–412. doi:10.1002/nur.20396

Myers, J. S. (2009). A comparison of the theory of unpleasant symptoms and the conceptual model of chemotherapy-related changes in cognitive function. *Oncology Nursing Forum, 36,* E1–E10. doi:10.1188/09.onf.e1-e10

National Institute of Nursing Research. (2016). *The NINR Strategic Plan: Advancing science, improving lives.* Retrieved from https://www.ninr.nih.gov/sites/www .ninr.nih.gov/files/NINR_StratPlan2016_reduced.pdf

Oh, E.-G., Kim, C.-J., Lee, W.-H., & Kim, S.-S. (2004). Correlates of fatigue in Koreans with chronic lung disease. *Heart & Lung, 33*(1), 13–20. doi:10.1016/ j.hrtlng.2003.09.001

Park, S. K., Stotts, N. A., Douglas, M. K., Donesky-Cuenco, D., & Carrieri-Kohlman, V. (2012). Symptoms and functional performance in Korean immigrants with asthma or chronic obstructive pulmonary disease. *Heart & Lung, 41*(3), 226–237. doi:10.1016/j.hrtlng.2011.09.014

Phligbua, W., Pongthavornkamol, K., Knobf, T. M., Junda, T., Viwatwongkasem, C., & Srimuninnimit, V. (2013). Symptom clusters and quality of wife in women with breast cancer receiving aedjuvant chemotherapy. *Pacific Rim International Journal of Nursing Research, 17,* 249–267.

Pugh, L. C. (1990). Psychophysiologic correlates of fatigue during childbearing. *Dissertation Abstracts International, 51,* 1B.

Pugh, L. C., & Milligan, R. A. (1993). A framework for the study of childbearing fatigue. *Advances in Nursing Science, 15*(4), 60–70. doi:10.1097/00012272-199306000 -00007

Pugh, L. C., & Milligan, R. A. (1995). Patterns of fatigue during pregnancy. *Applied Nursing Research, 8,* 140–143. doi:10.1016/S0897-1897(95)80593-1

Pugh, L. C., & Milligan, R. A. (1998). Nursing intervention to increase the duration of breastfeeding. *Applied Nursing Research, 11,* 190–194. doi:10.1016/ S0897-1897(98)80318-2

Pugh, L. C., Milligan, R. A., & Brown, L. P. (2001). The breastfeeding support team for low-income predominantly minority women: A pilot intervention study. *Health Care for Women International, 22,* 501–515. doi:10.1080/073993301317094317

Pugh, L. C., Milligan, R. A., Frick, K. D., Spatz, I. D., & Bronner, Y. (2002). Breastfeeding duration and cost effectiveness of a support program for low-income breastfeeding women. *Birth, 29*(2), 95–100. doi:10.1046/j.1523-536X .2002.00169.x

Pugh, L. C., Milligan, R. A., & Lenz, E. R. (2000). Response to "insomnia, fatigue, anxiety, depression, and quality of life of cancer patients undergoing chemotherapy." *Scholarly Inquiry for Nursing Practice, 14,* 291–294.

Pugh, L. C., Serwint, J. R., Frick, K. D., Nanda, J. P., Sharps, P. W., Spatz, D. L., & Milligan, R. A. (2010). A randomized controlled community-based trail to improve breastfeeding rates among urban low-income mothers. *Academic Pediatrics, 10,* 14–20. doi:10.1016/j.acap.2009.07.005

Redeker, N. S., Anderson, R., Bakken, S., Corwin, E., Docherty, S., Dorsey, S. G., . . . Grady, P. (2015). Advancing symptom science through use of common data elements. *Journal of Nursing Scholarship, 47*, 379–388. doi:10.1111/jnu.12155

Redeker, N. S., Lev, E. L., & Ruggiero, J. (2000). Insomnia, fatigue, anxiety, depression and quality of life of cancer patients undergoing chemotherapy. *Scholarly Inquiry for Nursing Practice: An International Journal, 14*, 275–290.

Rhodes, V., & Watson, P. (1987). Symptom distress–the concept past and present. *Seminars in Oncology Nursing, 3*(4), 242–247. doi:10.1016/s0749-2081(87)80014-1

Rodgers, C. C., Hooke, M. C., & Hockenberry, M. J. (2013). Symptom clusters in children. *Current Opinion in Supportive & Palliative Care, 7*, 67–72. doi:10.1097/SPC.0b013e32835ad551

Roland, R. A., & Hendrich, S. M. (2011). Symptom clusters and quality of life in older adult breast cancer survivors. *Oncology Nursing Forum, 38*, 672–680. doi:10.1188/11.onf.672-680

Runquist, J. J., Morin, K., & Stetzer, F. C. (2009). Severe fatigue and depressive symptoms in lower-income urban postpartum women. *Western Journal of Nursing Research, 31*, 599–612. doi:10.1177/0193945909333890

Scordo, K. A. (2005). Mitral valve prolapsed syndrome health concerns, symptoms and treatments. *Western Journal of Nursing Research, 27*, 390, 405. doi:10.1177/0193945904273617

Shahrbanian, S., Duquette, P., Kuspinar, A., & Mayo, N. E. (2015). Contributions of symptom clusters to multiple sclerosis consequences. *Quality of Life Research, 24*, 617–629. doi:10.1007/s11136-014-0804-7

Skerman, H. M., Yates, P. M., & Battistutta, D. (2012). Cancer-related symptom clusters for symptom management in outpatients after commencing adjuvant chemotherapy, at 6 months, and 12 months. *Supportive Care in Cancer, 20*, 95–105. doi:10.1007/s00520-010-1070-z

So, W. K. W., Leung, D. Y. P., Ho, S. S. M., Lai, E. T. L., Sit, J. W. H., & Chang, C. W. H. (2013). Associations between social support, prevalent symptoms and health-related quality of life in Chinese women undergoing treatment for breast cancer: A cross-sectional study using structural equation modeling. *European Journal of Oncology Nursing, 17*, 442–448. doi:10.1016/j.ejon.2012.11.001

Song, J.-E., Chang, S.-B., Park, S.-M., Kim, S., & Nam, C.-M. (2010). Empirical test of an explanatory theory of postpartum fatigue in Korea. *Journal of Advanced Nursing, 66*, 2627–2639. doi:10.1111/j.1365-2648.2010.05380.x

Spector, R. E. (2017). *Cultural diversity in health and illness* (9th ed.). New York, NY: Pearson.

Sudradhar, R., Atzema, C., Seow, H., Earle, C., Porter, J., Howell, D., . . . Barbera, L. (2014). Is performance associated with symptom scores? A population-based longitudinal study among cancer outpatients. *Journal of Palliative Care, 30*(2), 99–107.

Tankumpuan, T., Utriyaprasit, K., Chayaput, P., & Itthimathin, P. (2015). Predictors of physical functioning in postoperative brain tumor patients. *Journal of Neuroscience Nursing, 47*, E11–E21. doi:10.1097/jnn.0000000000000113

Thompson, P. (2007). The relationship of fatigue and meaning in life in breast cancer survivors. *Oncology Nursing Forum, 34*, 653–660. doi:10.1188/07.onf.653-660

Tyler, R., & Pugh, L. C. (2009). Application of the theory of unpleasant symptoms in bariatric surgery. *Bariatric Nursing and Surgical Care, 4*, 271–276. doi:10.1089/bar.2009.9953

Tzeng, Y., Teng, Y., Chou, F., & Tu, H. (2009). Identifying trajectories of birth-related fatigue of expectant fathers. *Journal of Clinical Nursing, 18*, 1674–1683. doi:10.1111/j.1365-2702.2008.02751.x

Waltz, C. F., Strickland, O. L., & Lenz, E. R. (2017). *Measurement in nursing and health research* (5th ed). New York, NY: Springer Publishing.

Wang, F., & Fu, J. (2014). Symptom clusters and quality of life in China patients with lung cancer undergoing chemotherapy. *African Health Sciences, 14*, 49–55 doi:10.4314/ahs.v14i.8

Wilmoth, M. C., Coleman, E. A., Smith, S. C., & Davis, C. (2004). Fatigue, weight gain, and altered sexuality in patients with breast cancer: Exploration of a symptom cluster. *Oncology Nursing Forum, 31*(6), 1069–1075. doi:10.1188/04.onf.1069-1075

Wilmoth, M. C., Coleman, E. A., & Wahab, H. T. (2009). Initial validation of the symptom cluster of fatigue, weight gain, psychologic distress and altered sexuality. *Southern Online Journal of Nursing Research, 9*(3).

Wilmoth, M. C., Hatmaker-Flanigan, E., LaLoggia, V., & Nixon, T. (2011). Ovarian cancer survivors: Qualitative analysis of the symptom of sexuality. *Oncology Nursing Forum, 38*, 699–708. doi:10.1188/11.onf.699.708

Wilson, I. B., & Cleary, P. D. (1995). Linking clinical variables with health-related quality of life: A conceptual model of patient outcomes. *Journal of the American Medical Association, 273*(1), 59–65. doi:10.1001/jama.273.1-59

Wu, X. D., Qin, H. Y., Zhang, H. E., Zheng, J. E., Xin, M. A., Liu, L., . . . Zhang, M. F. (2015). The prevalence and correlates of symptom distress and quality of life in Chinese oesophageal cancer patients undergoing chemotherapy after radical oesophagectomy. *European Journal of Oncology Nursing, 19*, 502–508. doi:10.1016/j.ejon.2015.02.010

Xiao, C. H., Polomano, R., & Bruner, D. W. (2013). Comparison between patient-reported and clinician-observed symptoms in oncology. *Cancer Nursing, 36*, E1–E16. doi:10.1097/ncc.06013e318269040f

Yang, C.-Y., Tsai, J.-C., Huang, Y.-C., & Lin, C.-C. (2011). Effects of a home-based walking program on perceived symptom and mood status in postoperative breast cancer women receiving adjuvant chemotherapy. *Journal of Advanced Nursing, 67*, 158–168. doi:10.1111/j.1365-2648.2010.05492.x

# CHAPTER 10

## Theory of Self-Efficacy

**Barbara Resnick**

Self-efficacy is defined as an individual's judgment of his or her capabilities to organize and execute courses of action. The core of Self-Efficacy Theory means that people can exercise influence over what they do. Through reflective thought, generative use of knowledge and skills to perform a specific behavior, and other tools of self-influence, a person will decide how to behave (Bandura, 1997). To determine self-efficacy, an individual must have the opportunity for self-evaluation or the ability to compare individual output to some sort of evaluative criterion. This comparative evaluation process enables an individual to judge performance capability and establish self-efficacy expectation.

## ■ PURPOSE OF THE THEORY AND HOW IT WAS DEVELOPED

The Theory of Self-Efficacy is based on the Social Cognitive Theory and conceptualizes person–behavior–environment interaction as triadic reciprocality, the foundation for reciprocal determinism (Bandura, 1977, 1986). Triadic reciprocality is the interrelationship among person, behavior, and environment; reciprocal determinism is the belief that behavior, cognitive, and other personal factors as well as environmental influences operate interactively as determinants of each other. Reciprocality does not mean that the influence of behavioral and personal factors as well as environment is equal. Depending on the situation, the influence of one factor may be stronger than the other, and these influences may vary over time.

Cognitive thought—which is a critical dimension of the person–behavior–environment interaction—does not arise in a vacuum. Bandura (1977, 1986) suggested that individuals' thoughts about themselves are developed and verified through four different processes: (a) direct experience of the effects produced by their actions, (b) vicarious experience, (c) judgments voiced by others, and (d) derivation of further knowledge of what they already know by using rules of inference. Human functioning is viewed as a dynamic interplay of personal, behavioral, and environmental influences.

## Initial Theory Development and Research

In 1963, Bandura and Walters wrote *Social Learning and Personality Development*, which expanded on the Social Learning Theory to incorporate observational learning and vicarious reinforcement. In the 1970s, Bandura incorporated what he considered to be the missing component to that theory, self-efficacy beliefs, and published *Self-Efficacy: Toward a Unifying Theory of Behavior Change* (Bandura, 1977). The work supporting self-efficacy belief was based on research testing the assumption that exposure to treatment conditions could result in behavioral change by altering an individual's level and strength of self-efficacy. In the initial study (Bandura, Adams, & Beyer, 1977; Bandura, Reese, & Adams, 1982), 33 subjects with snake phobias were randomly assigned to three different treatment conditions: (a) enactive attainment, which included actually touching the snakes; (b) role modeling or seeing others touch the snakes; and (c) the control group. The results suggested that self-efficacy was predictive of subsequent behavior, and enactive attainment resulted in stronger and more generalized (to other snakes) self-efficacy expectations.

Expansion of the early research included three additional studies (Bandura et al., 1982): (a) 10 subjects with snake phobias, (b) 14 subjects with spider phobias, and (c) 12 subjects with spider phobias. Similar to the initial self-efficacy study, enactive attainment and role modeling were effective interventions for strengthening self-efficacy expectations and impacting behavior. The study of 12 subjects with spider phobias also considered the physiological arousal component of self-efficacy. Pulse and blood pressure were measured as indicators of fear arousal when interacting with spiders. After interventions to strengthen self-efficacy expectations (enactive attainment and role modeling), heart rate decreased and blood pressure stabilized.

This early self-efficacy research used an ideal controlled setting in that the individuals with snake phobias were unlikely to seek opportunities to interact with snakes when away from the laboratory setting. Therefore, there was controlled input of efficacy information. Although this ideal situation is not possible in the clinical setting, the Theory of Self-Efficacy has been used to study and predict health behavior change and management in a variety of settings.

The literature explores factors that influenced the willingness of older adults to participate in functional activities and exercises. There was a recurring theme that suggested self-efficacy and outcome expectations mattered to an individual's willingness. Therefore, the theory helps to understand behavior and guide the development of interventions to change behavior.

## ▪ CONCEPTS OF THE THEORY

Bandura, a social scientist, differentiated two components of Self-Efficacy Theory: self-efficacy expectations and outcome expectations. These two components are the major ideas of the theory. Self-efficacy expectations are judgments about personal ability to accomplish a given task, whereas outcome expectations are judgments about what will happen if a given task is successfully accomplished. Both were differentiated because individuals can believe that a certain behavior will result in a specific outcome; however, they may not believe that they are capable of performing the behavior required for the outcome to occur. For example, Mrs. White may believe that rehabilitation will enable her to go home independently; however, she may not believe that she is capable of ambulating across the room. Therefore, Mrs. White may not participate in the rehabilitation program or be willing to practice ambulation.

Bandura (1977, 1986, 1995, 1997) suggests that outcome expectations are based largely on the individual's self-efficacy expectations. People anticipate that the types of outcomes generally depend on their judgments of how well they will be able to perform the behavior. Those individuals who consider themselves highly efficacious in accomplishing a given behavior will expect favorable outcomes for that behavior. Expected outcomes are dependent on self-efficacy judgments. Therefore, Bandura postulated that expected outcomes may not add much on the prediction of behavior.

Bandura (1986) postulates that there are instances when outcome expectations can be dissociated from self-efficacy expectations. This occurs either when no action will result in a specific outcome or when the outcome is loosely linked to the level or quality of the performance. For example, if Mrs. White knows that *even if she* regains functional independence by participating in rehabilitation, she will still be discharged to a skilled nursing facility rather than back home, her behavior is likely to be influenced by her outcome expectations (discharge to the skilled nursing facility). In this situation, no matter what Mrs. White's performance, the outcome is the same; thus, outcome expectancy may influence her behavior independent of her self-efficacy beliefs.

Expected outcomes are also partially separable from self-efficacy judgments when extrinsic outcomes are fixed. For example, when a nurse provides care to six patients during an 8-hour shift or to 10 patients in the same shift, she receives the same salary. This could negatively impact the performance. It is also possible for an individual to believe that he or she is capable of performing a specific behavior rather than the outcome of performing that behavior is worthwhile. For example, older adults in rehabilitation may believe that they are capable of performing the exercises and activities involved in the rehabilitation process, but they may not believe that performing the exercises will result in improved functional ability. Some older adults believe that resting rather than exercising will lead to recovery. In this situation, outcome expectations may have a direct impact on performance.

Both self-efficacy and outcome expectations influence the performance of functional activities (Galik, Pretzer-Aboff, & Resnick, 2011; Pretzer-Aboff, Galik, & Resnick, 2011; Quicke, Foster, Ogollah, Croft, & Holden, 2016; Resnick,

2011; Resnick & D'Adamo, 2011; Scarapicchia et al., 2015), adoption and maintenance of exercise behavior (Chase, 2011; Grim, Hortz, & Petosa, 2011; Hays, Pressler, Damush, Rawl, & Clark, 2010; Nahm et al., 2010; Qi, Resnick, Smeltzer, & Bausell, 2011), dietary intake (Resnick, Hammersla, et al., 2014), smoking cessation (Kamish & Öz, 2011), sex education for children (Akers, Holland, & Bost, 2011), and hip fracture prevention behaviors (Nahm et al., 2010). Outcome expectations are particularly relevant to older adults. These individuals may have high self-efficacy expectations for exercise, but if they do not believe in the outcomes associated with exercise (e.g., improved health, strength, or function), then it is unlikely that there will be adherence to a regular exercise program (Chase, 2011).

Generally, it is anticipated that self-efficacy will have a positive impact on behavior. However, it must be recognized that there are times when self-efficacy will have no or a negative effect on performance. Some research found that there is a negative effect of self-reported personal goals on performance such that higher personal goals can cause low performance (Vancouver & Kendell, 2006; Vancouver, Thompson, & Williams, 2001). Consistent with a multiple goal process conceptualization, self-efficacy was also found to relate positively to directing resources toward a goal but negatively to the magnitude of resources allocated for accepted goals (Vancouver, More, & Yoder, 2008). High self-efficacy expectations can actually be counterproductive. High self-efficacy may lead people to have a false sense of confidence and not put in as much effort as needed to perform optimally (Jones, Harris, Waller, & Coggins, 2005). This may be particularly true of behaviors such as exercise in which adequate resources to perform are needed (i.e., adequate physical strength), and the individual may have limited experience on which to draw and appropriately evaluate his or her self-efficacy expectations.

## Sources of Self-Efficacy Judgment

Bandura (1986) suggested that judgment about one's self-efficacy is based on four informational sources: (a) enactive attainment, which is the actual performance of a behavior; (b) vicarious experience or visualizing other similar people perform a behavior; (c) verbal persuasion or exhortation; and (d) physiological state or physiological feedback during a behavior, such as pain or fatigue. The cognitive appraisal of these factors results in a perception of a level of confidence in the individual's ability to perform certain behavior. The positive performance of this behavior reinforces self-efficacy expectations (Bandura, 1995).

### ENACTIVE ATTAINMENT

Enactive attainment, the actual performance of behavior, has been described as the most influential source of self-efficacy information (Bandura, 1977,

1986), and it is the most common intervention that is used to strengthen effi-cacy expectations in older adults. There has been repeated empirical verifi-cation that actually performing an activity strengthens self-efficacy beliefs. Specifically, the impact of enactive attainment has been demonstrated with regard to snake phobias, smoking cessation, exercise behaviors, performance of functional activities, and weight loss. Enactive attainment generally results in greater strengthening of self-efficacy expectations compared to informational sources. However, performance alone does not establish self-efficacy beliefs. Other factors such as preconceptions of ability, the perceived difficulty of the task, the amount of effort expended, the external aid received, the situational circumstance, and past successes and failures impact the individual's cognitive appraisal of self-efficacy (Bandura, 1995). An older adult who strongly believes that he or she is able to bathe and dress independently because he or she has been doing so for 90 years will not likely alter self-efficacy expectations if he or she wakes up with severe arthritic changes one morning and is consequently unable to put on a shirt. However, repeated failures to perform the activity will impact self-efficacy expectations. The relative stability of strong self-efficacy expectations is important; otherwise an occasional failure or setback could severely impact both self-efficacy expectations and behavior.

## VICARIOUS EXPERIENCE

Self-efficacy expectations are also influenced by vicarious experiences or see-ing other similar people successfully performing the same activity (Bandura, 1977; Chase, 2011; Martin et al., 2011). However, there are some conditions that impact the influence of vicarious experience. If the individual has not been exposed to the behavior of interest or has had little experience with it, vicari-ous experience is likely to have a greater impact. Additionally, when clear guidelines for performance are not explicated, self-efficacy will be more likely to be impacted by the performance of others. Among older adults with cogni-tive impairment, vicarious experiences are particularly effective in increasing activity (Galik, Resnick, Lerner, Sabol, & Gruber-Baldini, 2015; Resnick, Galik, Nahm, Shaughnessy, & Michael, 2009).

## VERBAL PERSUASION

Verbal persuasion involves telling an individual that he or she has the capabili-ties to master the given behavior. Empirical support for the influence of verbal persuasion has been documented since Bandura's early research of phobias (Bandura et al., 1977). Verbal persuasion has proven effective in supporting recovery from chronic illness and in health promotion research. Persuasive health influences lead people with a high sense of self-efficacy to intensify efforts at self-directed change of risky health behavior. Verbal encouragement from a trusted, credible source in the form of counseling and education has been used alone and with performance behavior to strengthen efficacy expectations (Bennett et al., 2011; Chase, 2011; Clark et al., 2015; Gau, Chang, Tian, & Lin, 2011; Irvine et al., 2011; Kamish & Öz, 2011; Martin et al., 2011; Oberg, Bradley, Allen, & McCrory, 2011; Resnick, Wells, et al., 2016; Reifegerste & Rossmann, 2017; Rosal et al., 2011; Skinner et al., 2011; van Stralen, de Vress, Mudde, Bolman, & Lechner, 2011; Williams, 2011). For example, verbal encouragement through telephone calls and email support was successful in increasing adherence to relevant self-care behaviors among adults with congestive heart failure (Clark et al., 2015) and encouragement through the computer was effective in strengthening self-efficacy associated with behaviors to prevent unintended pregnancy and infections (Swartz et al., 2011) and in improving coping self-efficacy associated with HIV (Brown, Vanable, Carey, & Elin, 2011).

### PHYSIOLOGICAL FEEDBACK

Individuals rely in part on information from their physiological state to judge their abilities. Physiological indicators are especially important in relation to coping with stressors, physical accomplishments, and health functioning. Individuals evaluate their physiological state or arousal, and if aversive, they may avoid performing the behavior. For example, if the older adult has a fear of falling or getting hurt when walking, a high arousal state associated with the fear can limit the performance and decrease the individual's confidence in ability to perform the activity. Similarly, if the rehabilitation activities result in fatigue, pain, or shortness of breath, these symptoms may be interpreted as physical inefficacy and the older adult may not feel capable of performing the activity.

Interventions can be used to alter the interpretation of physiological feedback and help individuals to cope with physical sensations, enhancing self-efficacy and resulting in improved performance. Interventions include (a) visualized mastery, which eliminates the emotional reactions to a given situation (Bandura et al., 1977); (b) enhancement of physical status (Bandura, 1995); and (c) altering the interpretation of bodily states (Resnick, Galik, Gruber-Baldini, & Zimmerman, 2011; Resnick, Gruber-Baldini, Galik, et al., 2009; Resnick, Gruber-Baldini, Zimmerman, et al., 2009; Resnick, Wells, et al., 2016; Schnoll et al., 2011; Van der Maas et al., 2015). Interventions that decrease the pain associated with the use of pain medication or ice treatments and interventions focused on decreasing fear of falling have been shown to increase participation in rehabilitation and exercise among older adults (Resnick et al., 2011; Resnick, Gruber-Baldini, Galik, et al., 2009; Resnick, Gruber-Baldini, Zimmerman, et al., 2009; Schnoll et al., 2011; Van der Maas et al., 2015).

### ■ RELATIONSHIPS AMONG THE CONCEPTS: THE MODEL

The Theory of Self-Efficacy was derived from the Social Cognitive Theory and must be considered within the context of reciprocal determinism. The four sources of experience (direct experience, vicarious experience, judgments by others, and derivation of knowledge by inference) that can potentially influence self-efficacy and outcome expectations interact with characteristics of the individual and the environment. Ideally, self-efficacy and outcome expectations are strengthened by these experiences and subsequently moderate behavior. Since self-efficacy and outcome expectations are influenced by performance of a behavior, it is likely that there is a reciprocal relationship between performance and efficacy expectations (see Figure 10.1).

## Measurement of Self-Efficacy and Outcome Expectations

Operationalization of self-efficacy constructs is based on Bandura's (1977) early work with snake phobias. Self-efficacy measures were developed as paper and pencil measures that list activities—from least to most difficult—in a specific behavioral domain. In Bandura's (1977, 1986) early work, participants were asked to indicate whether they could perform the activity (magnitude of self-efficacy expectations) and then evaluated the level of confidence they had in performing the given activity (strength of self-efficacy).

Traditionally in the development of self-efficacy measures, items are derived based on the combined quantitative and qualitative research exploring factors that influenced adherence to a specific behavior, such as exercise (Bandura, 1986; Resnick & Jenkins, 2000). For example, the self-efficacy for exercise scale includes nine items, with each item reflecting a commonly recognized challenge associated with exercise for older individuals (Resnick & Jenkins, 2000). Participants then responded by indicating that they have no confidence (0) or are very confident (10).

Development of outcome expectation measures has been less well-defined, although the process of establishing appropriate items is the same as it is for self-efficacy expectations. However, there is increasing evidence of measurement of

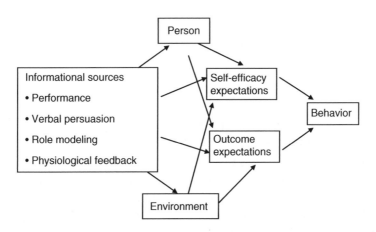

**FIGURE 10.1**  Self-Efficacy.

outcome expectations across a few behaviors, such as physical activity, specifically exercise (M. Choi, Ahn, Jung, 2015; Hall, Wójcicki, Phillips, & McAuley, 2012; Millen & Bray, 2009; Resnick, 2005; Sriramatr, Berry, & Rodgers, 2013; Wilcox, Castro, & King, 2006), function (Harnirattisai & Johnson, 2002), medication adherence (Qi et al., 2011), and breast cancer treatment (Rogers et al., 2005).

## ■ USE OF THE THEORY IN NURSING RESEARCH

The Theory of Self-Efficacy has been used in nursing research focusing on clinical aspects of care, education, nursing competency, and professionalism. The number of studies exploring the relationship between self-efficacy and exercise or testing the impact of exercise interventions on exercise behavior over the past 5 years was approximately 5,774. Of these, 4,637 were published in nursing journals. Increasingly these studies incorporate outcome expectations as well as self-efficacy expectations and address both nursing behavior and patient behavior across the entire life span.

Self-efficacy expectations are used in cross-sectional work to describe the sample and consider the relationship between demographic factors and self-efficacy, psychosocial factors, performance of behaviors, and/or outcome expectations. Alternatively, self-efficacy expectations are used to predict behavior in longitudinal research and to guide interventions and change behavior in intervention studies. These studies cover behaviors associated with exercise, physical activity, function, parenting, nursing skills, health promotion behaviors, and management of chronic illness, among others. The majority of these studies have been done within the United States, although there is an increasing literature supporting the use of this theory among Asians as well as other cultural groups. The most important with regard to the use of the Theory of Self-Efficacy in nursing research is that the researcher maintains the behavioral specificity by developing a specific fit between the behavior that is being considered and efficacy and outcome expectations. If the behavior of interest is walking for 20 minutes every day, the self-efficacy measure should focus on the challenges related to this specific behavior (time, fatigue, pain, or fear of falling).

### Self-Efficacy Studies Related to Managing Chronic Illness

Self-efficacy is commonly used to explain and improve the management of chronic illnesses (Horowitz, Eckhardt, Talavera, Goytia, & Lorig, 2011; Quicke et al., 2016). Gortner and colleagues were some of the first nurses to initiate self-efficacy intervention research in chronic illness management with the focus of the work being on cardiovascular disease (Gortner & Jenkins, 1990; Gortner, Rankin, & Wolfe, 1988). Jenkins's work built off that of Gortner et al., and she tested a self-efficacy intervention on recovery of 156 patients following cardiac surgery (Gortner & Jenkins, 1990). The use of Self-Efficacy Theory to help individuals manage chronic illness continues to be prevalent in patients with congestive heart failure (Granger, Moser, Germino, Harrell, & Ekman, 2006; Han, Lee, Park, Park, & Cheol, 2005; Johansson, Dahlström, & Bromström, 2006), after an acute coronary event (Blanchard, Arthur, & Gunn, 2015; Flora, Anderson, & Brawley, 2015), with hypertension (Grant, 2014; Martin et al., 2011); those with diabetes (Lorig et al., 2010; Muzaffar, Castelli, Scherer, & Chapman-Novakofski, 2014; Oberg et al., 2011; Rosal et al., 2011), rheumatoid arthritis (Niedermann et al., 2011), stroke (Shaughnessy & Resnick, 2009), cancer (McCorkle et al., 2011), renal disease (Patterson, Meyer, Beaujean, & Bowden, 2014), multiple sclerosis (Suh, Joshi, Olsen, & Motl, 2014), osteoporosis (Qi et al., 2011), and mental illness (Druss et al., 2010; Kramer, Helmes, Sellig, Fuchs, & Bengel, 2014), among others. In addition, the self-efficacy work in chronic illness has focused on self-management of the symptoms associated with chronic problems such as pain (Bennett et al., 2011; Gustavsson, Denison, & von Koch, 2011; Quicke et al., 2016).

Consistently, self-efficacy expectations have been associated with outcome behavior (e.g., management of pain, medication use; Davis et al., 2017; Johnson et al., 2016; Qi et al., 2011) and more recent work focuses on interventions geared to strengthening self-efficacy and associated outcome behavior relevant for the chronic medical problem. Innovative approaches such as using text messages to remind adolescents with asthma to use their inhalers have been tested and shown to lead to improvements in self-efficacy related to medication and increase adherence to inhaler usage (Johnson et al., 2016). Text messaging was also used to improve adherence to oral cancer medications among a group of adults (Spoelstra et al., 2015). Combined pharmacological and behavioral interventions used to strengthen self-efficacy and symptom management with regard to pain and depression have been shown to be effective (Damusch et al., 2016; Tahmassian & Jalali Moghadam, 2011). For example, a 12-month study with primary care patients exposed to therapy sessions to manage these two symptoms led to improvements in self-efficacy and improvements in both pain and depression (Damusch et al., 2016).

## Self-Efficacy for Health-Promoting Activities Such as Exercise and Weight Loss

Self-efficacy approaches are most commonly used to influence exercise and diet behaviors. Self-efficacy expectations have generally been positively associated with exercise (Chase, 2011; Der Ananian, Churan, & Adams, 2015; Flora et al., 2015; Grim et al., 2011; Nahm et al., 2010; Quicke et al., 2016; Scarapicchia et al., 2015; van Stralen et al., 2011). Specifically, findings noted that self-efficacy was significantly associated with the adoption and maintenance of exercise behavior across the life span including adolescents (Elkins, Nabors, King, & Vidourek, 2015), adults (Irvine et al., 2011; Pretzer-Aboff et al., 2011; Qi et al.,

2011), and those with chronic illness (Blanchard et al., 2015; Der Ananian et al., 2015; Flora et al., 2015; Quicke et al., 2016; Simons et al., 2015; Suh, Joshi, Olsen, & Motl, 2014). Expected outcomes in the form of perceived benefits from exercise were likewise associated with exercise behavior among older adults (Blanchard et al., 2015; J. Y. Choi, Chang, & Choi, 2015; Elkins et al., 2015; Muzaffar et al., 2014; Quicke et al., 2016; Resnick, Nahm, et al., 2014; Scarapicchia et al., 2015; Short, Vandelanotte, Rebar, & Duncan, 2014).

Using the Theory of Self-Efficacy, interventions have been developed and tested to increase exercise behavior in healthy community-dwelling adults (Resnick, Hammersla, et al., 2014; Scarapicchia et al., 2015; Short et al., 2014; Stephens, Resinicow, Latimer-Sport, & Walker, 2015) as well as those who have sustained a hip fracture or orthopedic event or have osteoporosis (Hays et al., 2010; Orwig et al., 2011; Resnick, Nahm, et al., 2014), or among those who have cardiac disease (Blanchard et al., 2015; Duncan, Pozehl, Norman, & Hertzog, 2011; Flora et al., 2015; Grant, 2014; Yaping et al., 2013), in cancer survivors (Bennett et al., 2011; Cox et al., 2015; Henriksson, Arving, Johansson, Igelstrom, & Nordin, 2016; Lee, Von Ah, Szuck, & Yiu-Keung, 2016; McCorkle et al., 2011), in patients with chronic obstructive pulmonary disease (Donesky et al., 2011; Hospes, Bossenbroek, Ten Hacken, van Hengel, & de Greef, 2009), in patients with diabetes (Collins et al., 2011; Muzaffar et al., 2014), and to help manage pain and anxiety associated with childbirth (Byrne, Hauck, Fisher, Bayes, & Schutze, 2014; Gau et al., 2011), to help young adults cope with life events (Simons et al., 2015), to manage childhood obesity (Bagherniya, Sharma, Mostafavi, Firoozeh, & Seyed, 2015; Webber, 2014), to manage multiple sclerosis (Suh, Joshi, Olsen, & Motl, 2014), to manage depression (Kramer et al., 2014), and for those undergoing dialysis (Patterson, Meyer, Beaujean, & Bowden, 2014).

Innovative examples of how to strengthen self-efficacy for exercise include such things as using social media; for instance, a social marketing campaign as was done in the MoveU study (Scarapicchia et al., 2015). Likewise, the Healthy Outcome for Teens Project (HOT) also used an online educational intervention for middle school children to prevent diabetes and obesity by balancing food intake with physical activity (Muzaffar et al., 2014). For older adults, face-to-face interventions continue to be those most successfully implemented. An example of such a program was a 24-month intervention that included exercise classes and motivational techniques (verbal encouragement, self and role modeling, and elimination of unpleasant sensations associated with exercise; Resnick, Hammersla, et al., 2014). These interventions led to some improvement in time spent in physical activity.

Dietary interventions have also been developed and tested to improve the quality of dietary intake and maintain or facilitate weight loss (Bagherniya et al., 2015; Huang, Yeh, & Tsai, 2011; Oberg et al., 2011; Rejeski, Mihalko, Ambrosius, Bearon, & McClelland, 2011; Rosal et al., 2011; Stephens et al., 2015). For example, a group-mediated intervention for weight loss among older, obese adults was tested to determine if it resulted in changes in self-regulatory self-efficacy for eating behavior and weight loss (Rejeski et al., 2011). A significant treatment effect was observed for self-efficacy for weight loss as well as weight among those who were exposed to both the diet intervention and physical activity. Similarly, a dietary intervention that was not focused on weight loss but rather on improving dietary intake for individuals with diabetes was noted to be effective. This intervention resulted in strengthening self-efficacy around healthy eating and improved hemoglobin A1c levels among those exposed to the intervention (Oberg et al., 2011).

## Self-Efficacy Interventions for Symptom and Disease Management

In addition to using self-efficacy–based interventions to increase adherence to healthy behaviors, such as exercise and healthy diets, self-efficacy interventions have been developed and tested to manage symptoms across a variety of areas. Most commonly these focus on symptoms, such as pain management (Bennett et al., 2011; Damusch et al., 2016), fear of falling (Yoo, Jun, & Hawkins, 2010; Zijlstra et al., 2011), and memory changes (McDougall, Becker, Acee, Vaughan, & Delville, 2011; Williams, 2011). For example, a multicomponent cognitive behavioral group intervention was tested with a sample of 540 community-dwelling adults aged 70 years or older who reported a fear of falling and avoided physical activity (Zijlstra et al., 2011). Testing showed that the multicomponent cognitive behavioral intervention improved control beliefs, self-efficacy, outcome expectations, and social interactions. Moreover, these variables mediated the association between the intervention and concerns about falling or daily activity in community-dwelling older adults.

Another example of symptom-focused interventions recently reported was focused on memory in cancer survivors 65 years of age and older who experience treatment-induced memory impairments. This study compared a memory versus health training intervention in a convenience sample of older adults (McDougall et al., 2011). The memory training was designed to increase cognitive performance, reduce anxiety, decrease negative attributions, promote health, and increase memory self-efficacy. Moderate-to-large effects were revealed in everyday and verbal memory performance scores, memory self-efficacy, strategy use, and memory complaints. There were also moderate effects for group-by-time interactions on the visual memory performance, memory self-efficacy, depression, trait anxiety, and complaints. The memory intervention group tended to improve more than the health training group, although this was not always consistent.

Management of symptoms associated with atopic dermatitis (Mitchella, Fraser, Ramsbotham, Morawska, & Yates, 2015) have also been addressed using self-efficacy approaches to help parents of children with the disease. Likewise, apathy associated with depression has been addressed with self-efficacy–based interventions (Kramer et al., 2014). Self-efficacy approaches are also used to help improve adherence to medication and treatments for diseases.

For example, self-efficacy approaches have been used to increase adherence to osteoporosis-related medications (Nahm et al., 2015) and adherence to use of glaucoma medication (Sleath et al., 2014).

## Self-Efficacy Interventions for Education of Healthcare Providers

In addition to a clinical focus, self-efficacy–based research has also guided the exploration of education techniques for nurses and other healthcare providers. Studies of undergraduates have focused on self-efficacy expectations related to academic performance (McVicar, Andrew, & Kemble, 2015; Phillips, Phillips, Lalonde, & Tormohlen, 2015) and clinical skills (Adelman et al., 2014; Darkwah, Ross, Williams, & Madill, 2011; Jeffries et al., 2011; Sherriff, Burston, & Wallis, 2011; Sung, Huey-Hwa, Ru-Rong, & Chao, 2016). For example, one study focused on undergraduate education (Sherriff et al., 2011) and evaluated the effect of an online, medication calculation education and testing program. The outcome measures used with the nursing students included medication calculation proficiency and self-efficacy expectations associated with medication calculation. Participants were registered nurses and nursing students. Outcome measures included number of test attempts, self-efficacy, medication calculation error rates, and satisfaction with the program. Medication calculation scores at the first test attempt showed improvement following 1 year of access to the program. Two of the self-efficacy subscales improved over time and nurses reported satisfaction with the online program.

One example of the type of self-efficacy–based interventions used with advanced practice nurses includes a simulation-based cardiovascular assessment curriculum (Jeffries et al., 2011). The educational interventions included faculty-led, simulation-based case presentations using the Harvey® cardiopulmonary patient simulator (CPS), and independent learning sessions using the CPS and a multimedia, computer-based CD-ROM program. Outcome measures included a cognitive written exam, a skills checklist, learner self-efficacy, and a satisfaction survey. The 36 students who received the simulation-based training showed statistically significant pre- to posttest improvement in cognitive knowledge and cardiovascular assessment skills.

Self-efficacy–based interventions have been used with other healthcare professionals as well (Salerno, Delaney, Swartwout, & Tsui-Sui, 2015). For example, a self-efficacy–based approach was used to strengthen self-efficacy and outcome expectations related to being involved in research for social workers. This was an intervention that focused on adolescent-focused motivational interviewing training to improve health professionals' knowledge, skills, and confidence in risk reduction counseling with adolescents. Following the intervention there was a significant improvement in knowledge, skills, and confidence associated with implementing motivational interviewing.

## Self-Efficacy Expectations, Outcome Expectations, and Behavior

Bandura postulates that self-efficacy and outcome expectations increase following self-efficacy–based interventions, particularly performance of the behavior of interest (Bandura, 1995). However, the theory is not always supported. There have been multiple studies in which older adults have been exposed to self-efficacy–based interventions for exercise and there was no change in efficacy expectations, even though there were improvements in behavior (Flora et al., 2015; Muzaffar et al., 2014; Orwig et al., 2011; Resnick, Gruber-Baldini, Zimmerman, et al., 2009). These findings may, in part, be due to measurement issues in that the individuals who volunteered for these intervention studies generally had strong self-efficacy and outcome expectations at baseline and thus there was a ceiling effect. In addition, the measures used may not have been specific enough for the behavior of interest. For example, in many of these studies self-efficacy and outcome expectations were measured in light of the challenges that can influence engaging in an exercise activity rather than simply asking about confidence in, for example, walking 10 feet, 20 feet, and so on. It is also possible that the intervention was not strong enough to result in a change in self-efficacy and outcome expectations.

Alternative explanations for a lack of significant increase in self-efficacy or outcome expectations following an intervention have been proposed by McAuley (McAuley et al., 2006). Specifically, he suggested that a decline in self-efficacy following exposure to an exercise intervention can also occur when there is a decrease in exposure to exercise classes, when exposed to a new exercise that is challenging, when there is a change in clinical condition or ability so that the exercise program is perceived to be more difficult, or when the exercise program is progressively more challenging. Therefore, it is critical to consider these aspects when implementing exercise intervention studies.

## ■ USE OF THE THEORY IN NURSING PRACTICE

Translation of research findings into practice is not often done in a timely fashion. This is particularly true of research findings that focus on behavior change. However, there is evidence to demonstrate that the Theory of Self-Efficacy can help direct nursing care. The theory has been particularly helpful with regard to motivating individuals to participate in health-promoting activities, such as regular exercise, smoking cessation, weight loss, and going for recommended cancer screenings. For example, Resnick and her research teams (Nahm et al., 2010; Orwig et al., 2011; Qi et al., 2011; Resnick, Gruber-Baldini, Zimmerman, et al., 2009; Resnick, Galik, Vigne, & Payne, 2016; Shaughnessy & Resnick, 2009) have used the Self-Efficacy Theory as a foundation for programs that encourage exercise and physical activity in older adults. Among these interventions, the function-focused care (FFC) approach has been tested the most extensively and is described as an exemplar.

## Function-Focused Care

Function-focused care (FFC), also referred to as restorative care, is a philosophy of care that focuses on evaluating the older adult's underlying capability with regard to function and physical activity and helping him or her to optimize and maintain abilities and continually increase time spent in physical activity. Implementation of FFC is guided overall by a social ecological model. This model provides an overarching framework for understanding the interrelations among diverse personal and environmental factors that can influence behavior change and specifically addresses intrapersonal, interpersonal, environmental, and policy factors. At the interpersonal level, self-efficacy–based interventions are used to facilitate an FFC approach and change behavior among caregivers as well as older individuals. The ultimate goal is to optimize function and physical activity among older adults.

FFC is implemented using the following four components: (a) environment and policy/procedure assessments; (b) education; (c) developing function-focused goals; and (d) mentoring and motivating. Component a involves completing assessments of the environment and policies/procedures relevant to function and physical activity within the settings. The findings from these assessments guide environmental and policy/procedure change, such as making pleasant walking areas on units or in facilities, establishing transportation policies that allow patients/residents to ambulate to tests or procedures, or allowing residents to walk in outside areas when living in long-term care settings.

Component b involves teaching nursing staff, other members of the interdisciplinary team (e.g., social work, physical therapy), patients, and families about the philosophy of FFC. Teaching is done both formally and informally in small groups or one on one and incorporates self-efficacy techniques including verbal encouragement, use of role models, and actual performance of skills and activities (e.g., use of demonstrations by caregivers for how to interact with older individuals using an FFC approach).

Component c involves establishing individualized goals for older individuals geared toward increasing their function and time spent in physical activity. Goals are established after evaluating the older adult's underlying function and ability (e.g., ability to follow a one-, two-, or three-step command, ability to get up from a chair). Individualized goals provide important encouragement as they indicate to the older individual that the goal established is something that the healthcare team or family in the home setting believes he or she is capable of achieving.

Component d is implemented using all four sources of self-efficacy–based information for both the caregivers being exposed to FFC and the patient/resident. Building off the initial education done with caregivers (this includes nurses, nursing assistants, home healthcare workers, and family caregivers, and other members of the interdisciplinary team including physicians, social workers, physical therapists, etc.), an identified champion in a facility or home setting will provide the ongoing verbal encouragement, support, recognition, and positive reinforcement around performing FFC with the older individual. For example, this might be a simple "it was terrific that you worked with Mrs. Jones to have her walk to the dining room today"; or "that was great this morning when you led the residents in a few minutes of dance prior to eating breakfast." The champion also can provide one-on-one mentoring and role modeling as needed. This might include intervening in a situation in which FFC is not occurring. For example, a nursing assistant or a family might be pushing Mrs. Jones to the dining room in a wheelchair because she wanted to get a ride. The champion might interrupt and role-model FFC interactions by indicating to Mrs. Jones that she did a great job walking to the dining room this morning and encourage her to "show Jane [the caregiver] how well you can walk!" Other formalized activities the champion might do include: (a) observing performance of caregivers within a setting and providing one-on-one mentoring of ways in which to incorporate FFC into routine care, (b) providing caregivers with positive reinforcement for doing FFC interactions, (c) meeting in groups or informally with caregivers to address their beliefs about physical activity and feelings and experiences associated with providing FFC, (d) reinforcing the benefits associated with FFC for both caregivers and older adults as a way to strengthen outcome expectations, (e) highlighting role models (other caregivers who successfully implemented the program), and (f) identifying change aides and positive opinion leaders to help with dissemination and implementation of FFC and eliminate the influence of negative opinion leaders.

In addition, caregivers are taught to implement self-efficacy–based approaches to motivate older adults to engage in function and physical activity. As with all types of behaviors, actual performance is the best way to strengthen self-efficacy and outcome expectations. Therefore, caregivers are taught to engage the resident in an activity he or she is capable of performing well and without uncomfortable sensations such as fear or pain. Once performance occurs, the caregivers are encouraged to provide critically important positive reinforcement to older individuals for engaging in the activity. This might be a hug, a smile, or a round of applause! Goals are set with the older individual. The individual, particularly those with cognitive impairment may need help to establish realistic and beneficial goals. The best way to establish these goals is to talk with the individual and identify what is important to them in terms of quality of life and what they want to be able to do functionally and physically. This might be working toward going out on a trip or going to a granddaughter's wedding. Activities and goals are individualized and should reflect what the person has done and enjoyed throughout his or her lifetime. Walking, shopping, delivering televisions, or working on a nursing unit can all be used to motivate the older individual to engage in those well-known activities yet again.

Role modeling is very useful as is self-modeling as a way to motivate older individuals. The role model may be the caregiver, a relative, or a peer and may be as simple as showing the older individual what to do at any given moment. For example, with older adults with significant cognitive impairment sitting next to them and getting up from a chair will cue (i.e., model for) them to do likewise. Likewise, reminding the older individual that he or she was able to walk to the bathroom successfully yesterday and thus can do so today is a form of self-modeling that is often effective.

For older adults, the experience of engaging in functional and physical activity must occur free of uncomfortable physiological feedback. Due to multi-morbidities, there is a high prevalence of symptoms associated with physical activity such as pain, fatigue, and fear of exacerbating underlying disease or falling. These symptoms need to be anticipated, acknowledged, and addressed. It is extremely challenging to eliminate these sensations and yet maintain function and physical activity; thus, acknowledging the sensations, talking about them, and assuring the individual that we "won't let them fall" or "won't have them do anything that will cause them more pain" are important. Pain medications and use of ice or heat to a joint are other ways to manage the pain before ambulation or a given activity.

In addition to addressing the uncomfortable sensations associated with an activity, the positive and pleasant outcomes and sensations can be highlighted. Making function and physical activity fun is important—music, dance, and the use of humor through what may be slower and more tedious personal care activities are useful interventions. Associating exercise activities with improvements in blood pressure readings, blood sugars, and weight loss is another way to demonstrate the benefits of activity.

# ■ CONCLUSION

The studies that nurse researchers have done using the Theory of Self-Efficacy provide support for the importance of self-efficacy and outcome expectations with regard to behavior change. The studies also provide support for the effectiveness of specific interventions that have been tested to strengthen both self-efficacy and outcome expectations and thereby improve behavior. However, it is important to note that studies have also demonstrated that self-efficacy and outcome expectations may not be the only predictors of behavior. Other variables, such as genetic predispositions, tension/anxiety, barriers to behavior, and other psychosocial experiences, impact behavior. Bandura (1986) recognized that expectations alone would not result in behavior change if there were no incentives to perform or if there were inadequate resources or external constraints. Certainly, an individual may believe that he or she can participate in a rehabilitation program but may not have the resources (i.e., transportation or money) to do so. In addition, when considered over time, it is possible that self-efficacy and outcome expectations will not get stronger. Rather, the individual may recognize that it is not as easy to perform a given behavior, and self-efficacy and outcome expectations may actually weaken.

Self-Efficacy Theory is situation-specific. Therefore, it is difficult to generalize an individual's self-efficacy from one type of behavior to the other. If an individual has high self-efficacy with regard to diet management, this may or may not generalize to persistence in an exercise program. Future nursing research needs to focus on the degree to which specific self-efficacy behaviors can be generalized. To what degree is self-efficacy, a dimension of individual humanness, distinct for each person but consistent across a range of related behaviors for one person? Future consideration should also be given to the relationship between self-efficacy and resilience, particularly with regard to specific areas. Resilience refers to the capacity to spring back from a physical, emotional, financial, or social challenge. Self-efficacy is an important component of resilience. Future research should also begin to consider the genetic variability in individuals and how this may impact self-efficacy. Resilient individuals will tend to have stronger self-efficacy and thus are more likely to engage in an activity on a regular basis.

Measurement of self-efficacy and outcome expectations requires the development of situation-specific scales with a series of activities listed of increasing difficulty or by a contextual arrangement in nonpsychomotor skills such as dietary modification (Bandura, 1997). It is important to carefully construct these scales and establish evidence of reliability and validity. Behavior-specific scales can be used as the foundation for assessing an individual's self-care abilities in a particular area. Interventions can then be developed that are relevant for that individual.

Increasingly, outcome expectations are being included along with self-efficacy beliefs. This is critically important as there is evidence that some interventions may strengthen outcome expectations (e.g., education) but have no impact on self-efficacy beliefs (Flora et al., 2015). There may also be differences in response to an intervention in terms of impact on self-efficacy versus outcome expectations based on gender. In a study of sex differences in physical activity among Korean college students (J. Y. Choi et al., 2015), for example, it was noted that only self-efficacy was associated with physical activity for males while only outcome expectations were associated with physical activity for females. The influence of self-efficacy expectations and outcome expectations as they relate to initiation versus long-term adherence to behaviors is currently not well understood and ongoing research in this area is needed. Social Cognitive Theory and the Theory of Self-Efficacy have helped guide nursing research related to behavior change. Ongoing studies are needed to continue to build and utilize this work to improve the health of individuals in this country and globally.

## ■ REFERENCES

Adelman, E. E., Meurer, W. J., Nance, D. K., Kocan, M. J., Maddox, K. E., Morgenstern, L. B., & Skolarus, L. E. (2014). Stroke awareness among inpatient nursing staff at an academic medical center. *Stroke, 45*(1), 271–273.

Akers, A. Y., Holland, C. L., & Bost, J. (2011). Interventions to improve parental communication about sex: A systematic review. *Pediatrics, 127*(3), 494–510.

Bagheriya, M., Sharma, M., Mostafavi, F., & Keshavarz, S. A. M. (2015). Application of social cognitive theory in predicting childhood obesity prevention behaviors in overweight and obese Iranian adolescents. *International quarterly of Community Health Education, 35*(2), 133–147.

Bandura, A. (1977). Self-efficacy: Toward a unifying theory of behavioral change. *Psychological Review, 84*, 191–215.

Bandura, A. (1986). *Social foundations of thought and action.* Upper Saddle River, NJ: Prentice Hall.

Bandura, A. (1995). *Self-efficacy in changing societies.* New York, NY: Cambridge University Press.

Bandura, A. (1997). *Self-efficacy: The exercise of control.* New York, NY: W. H. Freeman.

Bandura, A., Adams, N., & Beyer, J. (1977). Cognitive processes mediating behavioral change. *Journal of Personality and Social Psychology, 35*(3), 125–149.

Bandura, A., Reese, L., & Adams, N. (1982). Microanalysis of action and fear arousal as a function of differential levels of perceived self-efficacy. *Journal of Personality and Social Psychology, 43*, 5–21.

Bennett, M., Bagnall, A. M., Raine, G., Closs, S. J., Blenkinsopp, A., Dickman, A., & Ellershaw, J. (2011). Educational interventions by pharmacists to patients with chronic pain: Systematic review and meta-analysis. *Clinical Journal of Pain, 27*(7), 623–630.

Blanchard, C., Arthur, H. M., & Gunn, E. (2015). Self-efficacy and outcome expectations in cardiac rehabilitation: Associations with women's physical activity. *Rehabilitation Psychology, 60*(1), 59–66.

Brown, J., Vanable, P. A., Carey, M. P., & Elin, L. (2011). Computerized stress management training for HIV+ women: A pilot intervention study. *AIDS Care, 23*(12), 1525–1532.

Byrne, J., Hauck, Y., Fisher, C., Bayes, S., & Schutze, R. (2014). Effectiveness of a mindfulness-based childbirth education pilot study on maternal self-efficacy and fear of childbirth. *Journal of Midwifery & Women's Health, 59*(2), 192–197.

Chase, J. (2011). Systematic review of physical activity intervention studies after cardiac rehabilitation. *Journal of Cardiovascular Nursing, 26*(5), 351–358.

Choi, J. Y., Chang, A. K., & Choi, E.-J. (2015). Sex differences in social cognitive factors and physical activity in Korean college students. *Journal of Physical Therapy Science, 27*(6), 1659–1664.

Choi, M., Ahn, S., & Jung, D. (2015). Psychometric evaluation of the Korean Version of the Self-Efficacy for Exercise Scale for older adults. *Geriatric Nursing, 36*(4), 301–305.

Clark, A. P., McDougall, G., Riegel, B., Joiner-Rogers, G., Innerarity, S., Meraviglia, M., . . . Davila, A. (2015). Health status and self-care outcomes after an education-support intervention for people with chronic heart failure. *Journal of Cardiovascular Nursing, 30*(4 Suppl.), S3–S13.

Collins, T., Lunos, S., Carlson, T., Henderson, K., Lightbourne, M., Nelson, B., & Hodges, J. S. (2011). Effects of a home-based walking intervention on mobility and quality of life in people with diabetes and peripheral arterial disease: A randomized controlled trial. *Diabetes Care, 34*(10), 2174–2179.

Cox, M., Carmack, C., Hughes, D., Baum, G., Brown, J. Jhingran, A., . . . Basen-Engquist, K. (2015, October). Antecedents and mediators of physical activity in endometrial cancer survivors: Increasing physical activity through steps to health. *Health Psychology, 34*(10), 1022–1032. doi:10.1037/hea0000188

Damusch, T. M., Kroenke, K., Bair, M. J., Wu, J., Tu, W., Krebs, E. E., & Poleshuck, E. (2016). Pain self-management training increases self-efficacy, self-management behaviours and pain and depression outcomes. *European Journal of Pain, 20*(7), 1070–1078.

Darkwah, V., Ross, C., Williams, B., & Madill, H. (2011). Undergraduate nursing student self-efficacy in patient education in a context-based learning program. *Journal of Nursing Education, 50*(10), 579–582.

Davis, S. A., Carpenter, D., Cummings, D. M., Lee, C., Blalock, S. J., Scott, J. E., . . . Sleath, B. (2017). Patient adoption of an internet based diabetes medication tool to improve adherence: A pilot study. *Patient Education & Counseling, 100*(1), 174–178.

Der Ananian, C. A., Churan, C., & Adams, M. A. (2015). Correlates of physical activity among blacks and whites with arthritis. *American Journal of Health Behavior, 39*(4), 562–572.

Donesky, D., Janson, S. L., Nguyen, H. Q., Neuhaus, J., Neilands, T. B., & Carrieri-Kohlman, V. (2011). Determinants of frequency, duration, and continuity of home walking in patients with COPD. *Geriatric Nursing, 32*(3), 178–187.

Druss, B., Zhao, L., von Esenwein, S. A., Bona, J. R., Fricks, L., Jenkins-Tucker, S., . . . Lorig, K. (2010). The Health and Recovery Peer (HARP) program: A peer-led intervention to improve medical self-management for persons with serious mental illness. *Schizophrenia Research, 118*(1–3), 264–270.

Duncan, K., Pozehl, B., Norman, J. F., & Hertzog, M. (2011). A self-directed adherence management program for patients with heart failure completing combined aerobic and resistance exercise training. *Applied Nursing Research, 24*(4), 207–214.

Elkins, R. L., Nabors, L., King, K., & Vidourek, R. (2015). Factors influencing expectations of physical activity for adolescents residing in Appalachia. *American Journal of Health Education, 46*(1), 7–12.

Flora, P. K., Anderson, T. J., & Brawley L. R. (2015). Illness perceptions and adherence to exercise therapy in cardiac rehabilitation participants. *Rehabilitation Psychology, 60*(2), 179–186.

Galik, E., Pretzer-Aboff, I., & Resnick, B. (2011). Nurses perspective of function focused care in acute care. *International Journal of Older Adults, 15*(1), 48–55.

Galik, E., Resnick, B., Lerner, N., Sabol, M., & Gruber-Baldini, A. L. (2015). Function focused care for assisted living residents with dementia. *Gerontologist, 55*(Suppl. 1), S13–S26.

Gau, M., Chang, C.-Y., Tian, S.-H., & Lin, K.-C. (2011). Effects of birth ball exercise on pain and self-efficacy during childbirth: A randomised controlled trial in Taiwan. *Midwifery, 27*(6), e293–e300.

Gortner, S., & Jenkins, L. (1990). Self-efficacy and activity level following cardiac surgery. *Journal of Advanced Nursing, 15,* 1132–1138.

Gortner, S., Rankin, S., & Wolfe, M. (1988). Elders' recovery from cardiac surgery. *Progress in Cardiovascular Nursing, 3*(2), 54–61.

Granger, B., Moser, D., Germino, B., Harrell, J., & Ekman, I. (2006). Caring for patients with chronic heart failure: The trajectory model. *European Journal of Cardiovascular Nursing, 5*(3), 222–227.

Grant, S. (2014). *Self-monitoring blood pressure in patients with hypertension: Who self-monitors and why?* (Doctoral dissertation research). University of Birmingham, United Kingdom. AN: 109763284.

Grim, M., Hortz, B., & Petosa, R. (2011). Impact evaluation of a pilot web-based intervention to increase physical activity. *American Journal of Health Promotion, 25*(4), 227–230.

Gustavsson, C., Denison, E., & von Koch, L. (2011). Self-management of persistent neck pain: Two-year follow-up of a randomized controlled trial of a multicomponent group intervention in primary health care. *Spine, 36*(25), 2105–2115.

Hall, K. S., Wójcicki, T. R., Phillips, S. M., & McAuley, E. (2012). Validity of the multidimensional outcome expectations for exercise scale in continuing-care retirement communities. *Journal of Aging & Physical Activity, 20*(4), 456–468.

Han, K., Lee, S. J., Park, E. S., Park, Y., & Cheol, K. H. (2005). Structural model for quality of life in patients with chronic cardiovascular disease in Korea. *Nursing Research, 54,* 85–96.

Harnirattisai, T., & Johnson, R. (2002). *Reliability of self-efficacy and outcome expectations scales for exercise and functional activity in Thai elder.* Paper presented at the Health Science Research Day, University of Missouri-Columbia.

Hays, L., Pressler, S., Damush, T., Rawl, S., & Clark, D. (2010). Exercise adoption among older, low-income women at risk for cardiovascular disease. *Public Health Nursing, 27*(1), 79–88.

Henriksson, A., Arving, C., Johansson, B., Igelstrom, H., & Nordin, K. (2016). Perceived barriers to and facilitators of being physically active during adjuvant cancer treatment. *Patient Education Counseling, 99*(7), 1220–1226.

Horowitz, C., Eckhardt, S., Talavera, S., Goytia, C., & Lorig, K. (2011). Effectively translating diabetes prevention: A successful model in a historically under-served community. *Translational Behavioral Medicine, 1*(3), 443–452.

Hospes, G., Bossenbroek, L., Ten Hacken, N. H., van Hengel, P., & de Greef, M. H. (2009). Enhancement of daily physical activity increases physical fitness of outclinic COPD patients: Results of an exercise counseling program. *Patient Education & Counseling, 75*(2), 274–278.

Huang, T., Yeh, C.-Y., & Tsai, Y.-C. (2011). A diet and physical activity intervention for preventing weight retention among Taiwanese childbearing women: A randomised controlled trial. *Midwifery, 27*(2), 257–264.

Irvine, A., Philips, L., Seeley, J., Wyant, S., Duncan, S., & Moore, R. W. (2011). Get moving: A web site that increases physical activity of sedentary employees (includes abstract). *American Journal of Health Promotion, 25*(3), 199–206.

Jeffries, P. R., Beach, M., Decker, S. I., Dlugasch, L., Groom, J., Settles, J., & O'Donnell, J. M. (2011). Multi-center development and testing of a simulation-based cardiovascular assessment curriculum for advanced practice nurses. *Nursing Education Perspectives, 32*(5), 316–322.

Johansson, P., Dahlström, U., & Bromström, A. (2006). Consequences and predictors of depression in patients with chronic heart failure: Implications for nursing care and future research. *Progress in Cardiovascular Nursing, 21*(4), 202–211.

Johnson, K. B., Patterson, B. L., Ho, Y., Chen, Q., Nian, H., Davison, C., . . . Mulvaney, S. A. (2016). The feasibility of text reminders to improve medication adherence in adolescents with asthma. *Journal of the American Medical Informatics Association, 23*(3), 449–455.

Jones, F., Harris, P., Waller, H., & Coggins, A. (2005). Adherence to an exercise prescription scheme: The role of expectations, self-efficacy stage of change and psychological well-being. *British Journal of Health Psychology, 10*, 359–378.

Kamish, S., & Öz, F. (2011). Evaluation of a smoking cessation psychoeducational program for nurses. *Journal of Addictions Nursing, 22*(3), 117–123.

Kramer, L. V., Helmes, A. W., Seelig, H., Fuches, R., & Bengel, J. (2014). Correlates of reduced exercise behavior in depression: The role of motivational and volitional deficits. *Psychology & Health, 29*(10), 1206–1225.

Lee, E. E., Von Ah, B. S., Szuck, B., & Yi-Keung, J. L. (2016). Determinants of physical activity maintenance in breast cancer survivors after a community–based intervention. *Oncology Nursing forum, 43*(1), 93–102.

Lorig, K., Ritter, P. L., Laurent, D. D., Plant, K., Green, M., Jernigan, V. B., & Case, S. (2010). Online diabetes self-management program: A randomized study. *Diabetes Care, 33*(6), 1275–1281.

Martin, M. Y., Kim, Y. I., Kratt, P., Litaker, M. S., Kohler, C. L., Schoenberger, Y. M., . . . Williams, O. D. (2011). Medication adherence among rural, low-income hypertensive adults: A randomized trial of a multimedia community-based intervention. *American Journal of Health Promotion, 25*(6), 372–378.

McAuley, E., Konopack, J. F., Motl, R. W., Morris, K. S., Doerksen, S. E., & Rosengren, K. R. (2006). Physical activity and quality of life in older adults: Influence of health status and self-efficacy. *Annals of Behavioral Medicine, 31*(1), 99–103.

McCorkle, R., Ercolano, E., Lazenby, M., Schulman-Green, D., Schilling, L. S., Lorig, K., & Wagner, E. H. (2011). Self-management: Enabling and empowering patients living with cancer as a chronic illness. *A Cancer Journal for Clinicians, 61*(1), 50–62.

McDougall, G., Becker, H., Acee, T. W., Vaughan, P. W., & Delville, C. L. (2011). Symptom management of affective and cognitive disturbance with a group of cancer survivors. *Archives of Psychiatric Nursing*, 25(1), 24–35.

McVicar, A., Andrew, S., & Kemble, R. (2015). The 'bioscience problem' for nursing students: An integrative review of published evaluations of Year 1 bioscience, and proposed directions for curriculum development. *Nurse Education Today*, 35(3), 500–509.

Millen, J., & Bray, S. R. (2009). Promoting self-efficacy and outcome expectations to enable adherence to resistance training after cardiac rehabilitation. *Journal of Cardiovascular Nursing*, 24(4), 316–327.

Mitchella, A. E., Fraser, J. A., Ramsbotham, J., Morawska, A., & Yates, P. (2015). Childhood atopic dermatitis: A cross-sectional study of relationships between child and parent factors, atopic dermatitis management and disease severity. *International Journal of Nursing Studies*, 52(1), 216–228.

Muzaffar, H., Castelli, D. M., Scherer, J., & Chapman-Novakofski, K. (2014). The impact of Web-Based HOT (Health Outcomes for Teens) Project on risk for type 2 diabetes: A randomized controlled trial. *Diabetes Technology & Therapeutics*, 16(12), 846–852.

Nahm, E. S., Barker, B., Resnick, B., Covington, B., Magaziner, J., & Brennan, P. (2010). Effects of a social cognitive theory-based hip fracture prevention web site for older adults. *Computers, Informatics, Nursing*, 28(6), 371–377.

Nahm, E. S., Resnick, B., Bellantoni, M., Zhu, S., Brown, C., Brennan, P. F., . . . Plummer, L. (2015). Dissemination of theory-based online bone health programs: Two intervention approaches. *Health Informatics Journal*, 21, 120–136.

Niedermann, K., de Bie, R. A., Kubli, R., Ciurea, A., Steurer-Stey, C., Villiger, P. M., & Büchi, S. (2011). Effectiveness of individual resource-oriented joint protection education in people with rheumatoid arthritis: A randomized controlled trial. *Patient Education & Counseling*, 82(1), 42–48.

Oberg, E. B., Bradley, R., Allen, J., & McCrory, M. A. (2011). CAM: Naturopathic dietary interventions for patients with type 2 diabetes. *Complementary Therapies in Clinical Practice*, 17(3), 157–161.

Orwig, D., Hochberg, M., Yu-Yahiro, J., Resnick, B., Hawkes, W. G., Shardell, M., . . . Magaziner, J. (2011). Delivery and outcomes of a yearlong home exercise program after hip fracture: A randomized controlled trial. *Journal of Archives of Internal Medicine*, 171(4), 323–331.

Patterson, M. S., Meyer, M. R. U., Beaujean, A. A., & Bowden, R. G. (2014). Using the social cognitive theory to understand physical activity among dialysis patients. *Rehabilitation Psychology*, 59(3), 278–288.

Phillips, K. T., Phillips, M. M., Lalonde, T. L., & Tormohlen, K. N. (2015). Marijuana use, craving and academic motivation and performance among college students: An in-the-moment study. *Addictive Behaviors*, 47, 42–47.

Pretzer-Aboff, I., Galik, E., & Resnick, B. (2011). Feasibility and impact of a function focused care intervention for Parkinson's disease in the community. *Nursing Research*, 60(4), 276–283.

Qi, B., Resnick, B., Smeltzer, S. C., & Bausell, B. (2011). Self-efficacy enhanced education program in preventing osteoporosis among Chinese immigrants: A randomized controlled trial. *Nursing Research, 60*(6), 393–404.

Quicke, J. G., Foster, N. E., Ogolah, R. O., Croft, P. R., & Holden, M. A. (2016). The relationship between attitudes, beliefs and physical activity in older adults with knee pain: Secondary analysis of a randomized controlled trial. *Arthritis Care & Research, 68*(1), 215–219.

Reifegerste, D., & Rossmann, C. (2017). Promoting physical activity with group pictures. Affiliation-based visual communication for high-risk populations. *Health Communication, 32*(2), 161–168.

Rejeski, W. J., Mihalko, S. L., Ambrosius, W. T., Bearon, L. B., & McClelland, J. W. (2011). Weight loss and self-regulatory eating efficacy in older adults: The cooperative lifestyle intervention program. *Journals of Gerontology Series B: Psychological Sciences & Social Sciences, 66B*(3), 279–286.

Resnick, B. (2005). Reliability and validity of the outcome expectations for exercise scale-2. *Journal of Aging and Physical Activity, 13*(4), 382–394.

Resnick, B. (2011). *Implementing restorative care nursing in all setting.* New York, NY: Springer Publishing.

Resnick, B., & D'Adamo, C. (2011). Wellness center use and factors associated with physical activity among older adults in a retirement community. *Rehabilitation Nursing, 36*(2), 47–53.

Resnick, B., Galik, E., Vigne, E., & Payne, A. (2016). Dissemination and implementation of function focused care-assisted living. *Health Education & Behavior, 43*(3), 296–304.

Resnick, B., Galik, E., Gruber-Baldini, A., & Zimmerman, S. (2011). Testing the impact of function focused care in assisted living. *Journal of the American Geriatrics Society, 59*(12), 2233–2240.

Resnick, B., Galik, E., Nahm, E., Shaughnessy, M., & Michael, K. (2009). Optimizing adherence in older adults with cognitive impairment. In S. Shumaker, J. Ockene, & K. Riekert (Eds.), *The handbook of health behavior change* (3rd ed., pp. 519–544). New York, NY: Springer Publishing.

Resnick, B., Gruber-Baldini, A., Galik, E., Pretzer-Aboff, I., Russ, K., Hebel, J., & Zimmerman, S. (2009). Changing the philosophy of care in long-term care: Testing of the restorative care intervention. *The Gerontologist, 49*(2), 175–184.

Resnick, B., Gruber-Baldini, A., Zimmerman, S., Galik, E., Pretzer-Aboff, I., Russ, K., & Hebel, J. R. (2009). Nursing home resident outcomes from the Res-Care intervention. *Journal of the American Geriatrics Society, 57*(7), 1156–1165.

Resnick, B., Hammersla, M., Michael, K., Galik, E., Klinedinst, J., & Demehin, M. (2014). Changing behavior in senior housing residents: Testing of Phase I of the PRAISEDD-2 Intervention. *Applied Nursing Research, 27*(3), 162–169.

Resnick, B., & Jenkins, L. (2000). Reliability and validity testing of the self-efficacy for exercise scale. *Nursing Research, 49*, 154–159.

Resnick, B., Nahm, E. S., Zhu, S., Brown, C., An, M., Park, B., & Brown, J. (2014). The impact of osteoporosis, falls, fear of falling and efficacy expectations on exercise among community-dwelling older adults. *Orthopaedic Nursing, 33*(5), 277–288.

Resnick, B., Wells, C., Galik, E., Holtzman, L., Zhu, S., Gamertsfelder, E., . . . Boltz, M. (2016). Feasibility and efficacy of function focused care for orthopedic trauma patients. *Journal of Trauma Nursing, 23*(3), 144–155.

Rogers, L., Shah, P., Dunnington, G., Greive, A., Shanmugham, A., Dawson, B., & Courneya, K. S. (2005). Social cognitive theory and physical activity during breast cancer treatment. *Oncology Nursing Forum, 32*(4), 807–815.

Rosal, M. C., Ockene, I. S., Restrepo, A., White, M. J., Borg, A., Olendzki, B., . . . Reed, G. (2011). Randomized trial of a literacy-sensitive, culturally tailored diabetes self-management intervention for low-income Latinos: Latinos en control. *Diabetes Care, 34*(4), 838–844.

Salerno, J., Delaney, K. R., Swartwout, K. D., & Tsui-Sui, A. K. (2015). Improving interdisciplinary professionals' capacity to motivate adolescent behavior change. *Journal for Nurse Practitioners, 11*(6), 626–632.

Scarapicchia, T. M., Sabiston, C. M., Brownrigg, M., Blackburn-Evans, A., Cressy, J., Robb, J., & Faulkner, G. E. (2015). MoveU? Assessing a social marketing campaign to promote physical activity. *Journal of American College Health, 63*(5), 299–306.

Schnoll, R., Martinez, E., Tatum, K. L., Glass, M., Bernath, A., Ferris, D., & Reynolds, P. (2011). Increased self-efficacy to quit and perceived control over withdrawal symptoms predict smoking cessation following nicotine dependence treatment. *Addictive Behaviors, 36*(1–2), 144–147.

Shaughnessy, M., & Resnick, B. (2009). Using theory to develop an exercise intervention for patients post stroke. *Topics in Stroke Rehabilitation, 16*(2), 140–146.

Sherriff, K., Burston, S., & Wallis, M. (2011). Effectiveness of a computer based medication calculation education and testing programme for nurses. *Nurse Education Today, 32*(1), 46–51.

Short, C. E., Vandelanotte, C., Rebar, A., & Duncan, M. J. (2014). A comparison of correlates associated with adult physical activity behavior in major cities and regional settings. *Health Psychology, 33*(11), 1319–1327.

Simons, D., Rosenberg, M., Salmon, J., Knuiman, M., Granich, J., Deforche, B., & Timperio, A. (2015). Psychosocial moderators of associations between life events and changes in physical activity after leaving high school. *Preventive Medicine, 72*, 30–33.

Skinner, C., Buchanan, A., Champion, V., Monahan, P., Rawl, S., Springston, J., . . . Bourff, S. (2011). Process outcomes from a randomized controlled trial comparing tailored mammography interventions delivered via telephone vs. DVD. *Patient Education & Counseling, 85*(2), 308–312.

Sleath, B. L., Blalock, S. J., Muir, K. W., Carpenter, D. M., Lawrence, S. D., Giangiacomo, A. L., . . . Robin, A. L. (2014). Determinants of self-reported barriers to glaucoma medicine administration and adherence: A multisite study. *Annals of Pharmacotherapy, 48*(7), 856–862.

Spoelstra, S. L., Given C. W., Sikorskii, A., Coursaris, C. K., Majumder, A., Dekoekkoer, T., . . . Given, B. A. (2015). A randomized controlled trial of the feasibility and preliminary efficacy of a texting intervention on medication adherence in adults prescribed oral anticancer agents: Study protocol. *Journal of Advanced Nursing, 71*(12), 2965–2976.

Sriramatr, S., Berry, T. R., & Rodgers, W. M. (2013). Validity and reliability of Thai versions of questionnaires measuring leisure-time physical activity, exercise-related self-efficacy, outcome expectations and self-regulation. *Pacific Rim International Journal of Nursing Research*, *17*(3), 203–216.

Stephens, T. T., Resinicow, K., Latimer-Sport, M., & Walker, L. (2015). Social cognitive predictors of dietary behavior among African Americans. *American Journal of Health Education*, *46*(3), 174–181.

Suh, Y. U., Joshi, I., Olsen, C., & Motl, R. (2014). Social cognitive predictors of physical activity in relapsing-remitting multiple sclerosis. *International Journal of Behavioral Medicine*, *21*(6), 891–898.

Sung, S.-C., Jiang, H.-H., Chen, R.-R., & Chao, J.-K. (2016). Bridging the gap in sexual healthcare in nursing practice: Implementing a sexual healthcare training programme to improve outcomes. *Journal of Clinical Nursing*, *25*(19/20), 2989–3000.

Swartz, L., Sherman, C. A., Harvey, S. M., Blanchard, J., Vawter, F., & Gau, J. (2011). Midlife women online: Evaluation of an internet-based program to prevent unintended pregnancy & STIs. *Journal of Women & Aging*, *23*(4), 342–359.

Tahmassian, D., & Jalali Moghadam, N. (2011). Relationship between self-efficacy and symptoms of anxiety, depression, worry and social avoidance in a normal sample of students. *Iranian Journal of Psychiatry and Behavioral Science*, *5*(2), 91–98.

Van der Maas, L. C. C., Köke, A., Pont, M., Bosscher, R. J., Twisk, J. W. R., Janssen, T. W. J., & Peters, M. L. (2015). Improving the multidisciplinary treatment of chronic pain by stimulating body awareness: A cluster-randomized trial. *Clinical Journal of Pain*, *31*(7), 660–669.

van Stralen, M. M., de Vress, H., Mudde, A. N., Bolman, C., & Lechner, L. (2011). The long-term efficacy of two computer-tailored physical activity interventions for older adults: Main effects and mediators. *Health Psychology*, *30*(4), 442–452.

Vancouver, J. B., & Kendell, L. (2006). When self-efficacy negatively relates to motivation and performance in a learning context. *Journal of Applied Psychology*, *91*(5), 1146–1153.

Vancouver, J. B., More, K., & Yoder, R. J. (2008). Self-efficacy and resource allocation: Support for a nonmonotonic, discontinuous model. *Journal of Applied Psychology*, *93*(1), 35–47.

Vancouver, J. B., Thompson, C., & Williams, A. A. (2001). The changing signs in the relationships among self-efficacy, personal goals and performance. *Journal of Applied Psychology*, *86*(4), 605–620.

Webber, K. (2014). *The relationship of personal and environmental factors and physical activity in parents of young African American children* (Doctoral Dissertation page 187). University of Arizona, AZ. (AN: 109786493)

Wilcox, S., Castro, C., & King, A. (2006). Outcome expectations and physical activity participation in two samples of older women. *Journal of Health Psychology*, *11*(1), 65–77.

Williams, K. N. (2011). Targeting memory improvement in assisted living: A pilot study. *Rehabilitation Nursing*, *36*(6), 225–232.

Yaping, D., Brehm, W., Strobl, H., Tittlbach, S., Zhijian, H., & Gangyan, S. (2013). Steps to and correlates of health enhancing physical activity in adulthood: An intercultural study between German and Chinese individuals. *Journal of Exercise Science & Fitness*, 11(2), 63–77.

Yoo, E. J., Jun, T. W., & Hawkins, S. A. (2010). The effects of a walking exercise program on fall-related fitness, bone metabolism, and fall-related psychological factors in elderly women. *Research in Sports Medicine*, 18(4), 236–250.

Zijlstra, G., van Haastregt, J. C., van Eijk, J. T., de Witte, L. P., Ambergen, T., & Kempen, G. I. (2011). Mediating effects of psychosocial factors on concerns about falling and daily activity in a multicomponent cognitive behavioral group intervention. *Aging & Mental Health*, 15(1), 68–77.

# CHAPTER 11

## Story Theory

**Patricia R. Liehr and Mary Jane Smith**

Our belief in the healing potential of story and recognition of the importance of building theory at the intersection of practice and research has been essential to the development of Story Theory. The theory was first published in 1999 (Smith & Liehr, 1999) with the name Attentively Embracing Story. Since that time, we simplified the name to focus on story. The central otology and epistemology of the theory remains as Reed (1999) described it over a decade ago. The ontology affirms that "story is an inner human resource for making meaning," and the epistemology is based in the understanding that "middle range theory bonds research and practice in a method of knowledge development" (p. 205).

### ■ PURPOSE OF THE THEORY AND HOW IT WAS DEVELOPED

Stories are a fundamental dimension of the human experience, connecting past, present, and future for individuals, families, and communities. Stories express who people are, where they have been, and where they are going. They shape connections with those who share the journey. The purpose of Story Theory is to describe and explain story as a foundation for a nurse–person health-promoting process in practice and for systematic data gathering and analysis in research. The core concept of the theory is intentional dialogue occurring in a nurse–person relationship. In this relationship, the nurse gathers a story about a health challenge that matters to the person who is sharing the story.

The foundation and ongoing development of the theory rests in the long-standing relationship of its authors. Their relationship started in an educational program that cultivated discussion of common values about nursing practice and research. Smith began studying rest in 1975 with her dissertation research (Smith, 1975). Later, she conceptualized rest as "easing with the flow of rhythmic change in the environment" (Smith, 1986, p. 23). Liehr's (1992) dissertation examined the blood pressure (BP) effects of talking about the usual day and listening to a story. These early works were harbingers of what was to come in collaboration.

Years passed and we both pursued our own work. Smith was working with pregnant teens and Liehr was working with people attending cardiac rehabilitation. A serendipitous meeting at a nursing conference led to discussion of the importance of story for promoting health and human development. In talking about our individual work, we were struck by the commonalities that surfaced when we gathered stories. It became clear that we both recognized and tapped into story-sharing as a powerful resource for health and healing. This clarity and our common ground experience with story-gathering offered an opportunity to articulate a theory as a basis for further work. We believed it was important that the theory be at the middle range level of abstraction to ensure applicability in both nursing research and practice. The theory was constructed with attention to critical story elements, including complicating, developmental, and resolving phases of narrative creation (Franklin, 1994).

We began trying to name the theory to reflect our experience with patients and research participants. We had an image of the way story-sharing mattered to people when we listened with full attention. It took time to engage in the creative process of naming the theory. After several months and many names, we had the name that we believed accurately captured what we were describing. Once the theory was named, each of us began to view practice and research situations through the lens of attentively embracing story. As we used this lens to consider practice and research and discussed the theory with colleagues and students, we recognized that all people do not attentively embrace their story even when given the opportunity for story-sharing with someone who truly cares to listen. Readiness for embracing story and experiencing ease varies from individual to individual; it even varies from time to time for a single individual.

We changed the theory name between 2003 and 2006. Although the process of attentive embracing is incorporated into the theory's meaning, the words were removed from the theory name. The current name, Story Theory, is more precise, parsimonious, and at the middle range level of discourse while still reflecting the essential idea that we wished to describe. The name change is consistent with the original intent of theory applicability to any situation where a nurse engages a person to intentionally dialogue about what matters most regarding a health challenge that complicates everyday living. We describe story as a narrative happening of connecting with self-in-relation through intentional dialogue to create ease. Ease emerges in the midst of accepting the whole story as one's own . . . a process of attentive embracing.

## Foundation Literature and Assumptions

Story Theory is at the middle range level of abstraction, holding assumptions congruent with unitary and neomodernist perspectives (Parse, 1981; Reed, 1995; M. E. Rogers, 1994). In these nonreductionistic views, human beings are transforming and transcending in mutual process with their environment. The mutual, ever-changing motion of creating meaning is essential to the unitary perspective expressed by the narrative happening of story in and through time. Developing personal history and human potential for health and healing is essential to the neomodernist perspective. In this view, the healing power of story is a manifestation all through life.

The human story is a health story in the broadest sense. It is a recounting of one's current life situation to clarify present meaning in relation to the past with an eye toward the future. The idea of story is not new to nursing. Nursing's story roots date back to Nightingale (1946), who called for a rejection of mindless chattering and a devotion to listening to the patient: "He feels what a convenience it would be, if there were any single person to whom he could speak simply and openly . . . to whom he could express his wishes and directions" (p. 96). Nurses have long known the importance of listening and have known how to listen so that they could understand what matters most. Several extant nursing theories relate listening to story in their theory structure (Boykin & Schoenhofer, 2001; Newman, 1999; Parse, 1981; Peplau, 1991; Watson, 1997). In addition, nurse scholars have affirmed its importance over decades (Banks, 2014; Benner, 1984; Burkhardt & Nagai-Jacobson, 2002; Chinn & Kramer, 1999; Ford & Turner, 2001).

In the field of medicine, Charon (2006) pioneered the use of "narrative medicine" distinguishing narrative from story. She identified narrative as a "repository" from which story emerges. Ultimately, story and narrative are intricately intertwined with narrative providing strings of facts. Story weaves context, spirit, and meaning through the facts to create a complex tapestry.

For the purpose of this work, we refer to stories within the context of narrative . . . story is a narrative happening of connecting with self-in-relation through intentional dialogue to create ease. Story expresses the narration of events as remembered while infusing unique personal perspectives. These perspectives offer a glimpse into thoughts and feelings, shape meaning, and guide choices in the moment. The assumptions of the theory create a value-laden niche that supports essential theory ideas.

The assumptions of the theory are that persons (a) change as they interrelate with their world in a vast array of flowing connected dimensions, (b) live an expanded present where past and future events are transformed in the here and now, and (c) experience meaning as a resonating awareness in the creative unfolding of human potential. The first assumption grounds sensitivity to the complexity of entangled health story dimensions to highlight persons moving with, through, and beyond their unfolding story. The second assumption invites a focus on the story-sharer's present health experience with the listener's understanding that the story-sharer's unique perspective incorporates the past and future in the here and now. The third assumption supports the human propensity to create meaning through awareness of thoughts, feelings, behavior, bodily experience, and other human expressions, all in the rhythm of the unfolding health story.

# ■ CONCEPTS OF THE THEORY

Story Theory is composed of three interrelated concepts: (a) intentional dialogue, (b) connecting with self-in-relation, and (c) creating ease. According to the theory, story is a narrative happening of connecting with self-in-relation through intentional dialogue to create ease. Ease emerges in the midst of accepting the whole story as one's own.

## Intentional Dialogue

Intentional dialogue is purposeful engagement with another to summon the story of a health challenge that complicates everyday living. There is intention to engage in dialogue about the unique life experience of one's pain, confusion, joy, broken relationships, satisfaction, or suffering as a catalyst to seek understanding and begin a process of change. Sharing one's story happens in a trusting relationship, where the nurse walks with another along a path, journeying a little further along to uncover what is happening, and paying attention to the unfolding movement of a story to ascertain current positions and future direction. Intentional dialogue energizes the experience of being alive by touching that which matters most to the person sharing a story about a health challenge.

There are two dimensions of intentional dialogue: true presence and querying emergence. True presence is the nurse's nonjudgmental rhythmical focusing/refocusing of energy on the other, which is open to what was, is, and can be. It is "bringing one's humanness to the moment while simultaneously giving self over to the other who is exploring the meaning of the situation" (Liehr, 1989, p. 7). True presence is the substance of the nurse's activity during story-sharing. In giving full attention to the other, the nurse "conveys to the speaker that his contribution is worth listening to, that as a person he is respected enough to receive the undivided attention of another" (C. R. Rogers, 1951, p. 34).

Attending to the emergence of the unfolding health story assumes true presence and focuses on seeking clarification of the patterns that connect the beginning, middle, and end of a story. The nurse lives true presence by staying in while staying out. There is an all-at-once staying close to the story rhythm from the perspective of the person sharing the story while simultaneously distancing to discern patterns of connectedness. If the story is told over many encounters, it helps the nurse to make notes about story progress, possible patterns, and hunches about meaning. These notes may be a source of guidance when follow-up encounters occur, especially when issues resurface over multiple encounters.

Querying the emergence of the health story is clarification of vague story directions. Both the nurse and the story-sharer attend to the story of the health challenge. The nurse concentrates and tries to understand the story from the other's perspective. Nothing can be assumed about the story; only the person who is sharing knows the details. The story is never finished. There is always more to the story, including parts that the individual may not want to tell. The nurse in true presence stays with the longing to tell and the desire to tell only so much at a time.

## Connecting With Self-in-Relation

Connecting with self-in-relation is the active process of recognizing self as related with others in an unfolding story. In Story Theory, connecting with self-in-relation is composed of personal history and reflective awareness. Personal history is the unique narrative uncovered when individuals reflect on where they have come from, where they are now, and where they are going in life. The nurse encourages reckoning with a personal history by traveling to the past to arrive at the story beginning, moving through the middle, and into the future all in the present, thus going into the depths of the story to find unique meanings that often lie hidden in the ambiguity of puzzling dilemmas. Self is affirmed in recognition and acceptance of nuances, faults, and strengths, as well as understanding of how one has lived, is currently living, and how one envisions future hopes and dreams.

Reflective awareness, the second dimension of the concept, is the opposite of taking life for granted. It is being in touch with bodily experience, thoughts, and feelings. Reflective awareness enables thoughtful observation of self so that bodily experience, thoughts, and feelings are recognized for what they are as separate and distinct entities rather than personal defining qualities. For instance, when people in pain recognize that their pain is separate and distinct from who they are, they simultaneously recognize that they are more than their pain; that the pain is not a personal life-defining entity; and that they can be with the pain rather than being defined by it. With this mindful way of being in the moment, there is "a profound shift in one's relationship to thoughts and emotions, the result being greater clarity, perspective, objectivity and ultimately, equanimity" (Shapiro, Carlson, Astin, & Freedman, 2006, p. 379).

As the nurse guides reflective awareness on bodily experiences, thoughts, and feelings in a given moment of story, the story-sharer becomes present to what is known and unknown, allowing unrecognized meaning to surface. Meaning changes when the unknown comes to light as known in an expanded present moment. In sharing the story, the person is telling the story to the nurse who is fully present and at the same time telling the story to self. Reflective awareness on personal history enlivens one's connection with self-in-relation to others and the world. It establishes an environment for creating ease.

## Creating Ease

Creating ease is an energizing release experienced as story moments/events/ perspectives come together. It happens in the context of a person's innate human drive to be at ease and the nurse's intention to enable ease. The two dimensions of creating ease are remembering disjointed story moments and flow in the midst of anchoring. Remembering disjointed story moments is connecting events in time through the realization, acceptance, and understanding that comes as health story fragments sort, converge, and come together. Polanyi (1958) discusses understanding as "a grasping of disjointed parts into a comprehensive whole" (p. 28). In the nurse–person dialogue, there is a remembering of disconnected moments as the nurse moves with the person through the story. Patterns surface as individuals shed a momentary light on the meaning of important experiences. Often, the nurse does not divert attention to the highlighted experiences when they are first introduced but tucks them into the background while staying with the foreground story. With focused presence over time, the nurse enables the other to illuminate issues, values, ideas, and context, uncovering coherent patterns of meaning in the tapestry of life experience.

Flow is an experience of dynamic harmony, and anchoring is an experience of settling on meaning in the moment. As patterns are discerned, named, and made explicit, anchoring and flowing occur all at the same time. Meaning surfaces while anchoring in a moment of pattern clarity, allowing a sense of flow and calmness. Csikszentmihalyi describes the harmony that ensues when one anchors to meanings, which captures purposeful unity and focus on life direction. He provides descriptions of individuals who used changing health situations to achieve clarity of purpose, noting that "a person who knows how to find flow from life is able to enjoy even situations that seem only to allow despair" (Csikszentmihalyi, 1990, p. 193). The defining feature of flow is "intense experiential involvement in moment-to-moment activity" (Csikszentmihalyi, Abuhamdeh, & Nakamura, 2005, p. 600).

As a whole story surfaces, it often encompasses disparate moments, like gladness and melancholy, restriction and freedom, fear and security, and discrepancy and coherence, to name only a few of the juxtaposed realities that characterize any and every whole story. No story is one-sided. The person experiencing loss is also experiencing gain and the one who is lonely often has uplifting interactions with others. When story-sharing becomes a vehicle for healing, "embracing story" happens. Embracing story energizes release from the confines of a disjointed story where story moments are scattered making it difficult to discern direction. Ease is resonating energy, enabling vision even for only a moment—a powerful moment creating possibilities for human development.

## ▪ RELATIONSHIPS AMONG THE CONCEPTS: THE MODEL

The theory comes to life in practice and research through traditional dimensions of story: complicating, developmental, and resolving processes (Franklin,

1994). When gathering story guided by the theory, the complicating process focuses on a health challenge that is pursued through intentional dialogue; the developmental process is composed of the story plot, a thread that connects the story-sharer to self-in-relation to meaningful others and relevant contexts; and, the resolving process has the potential to create ease when the story-sharer shifts views, enabling progression with new understanding . . . an accomplishment identified as movement toward resolving the health challenge. The relationships among the concepts of the theory are depicted in Figure 11.1. This model is different from the first model of the theory (Smith & Liehr, 1999), which attempted to show the dynamic nature of the theory but failed to capture the all-at-once happening of intentional dialogue, connecting with self-in-relation, and creating ease.

The current model attempts to depict a common flow of energy between nurse and person where story emerges. In this shared flux of energy all the concepts of story come together. The model incorporates story processes (complicating health challenge, developing story plot, movement toward resolving) that provide a base for gathering story in research and practice.

Story is a narrative happening of connecting with self-in-relation through intentional dialogue to create ease. Ease emerges in the midst of accepting the whole story as one's own. Implicit in the description is the suggestion that the story process begins with intentional dialogue to support connecting with oneself in relationship with others and with one's world with the possibility of experiencing ease. There is no doubt that the relationship among the concepts appears on the printed page as linear. However, the intent is that these concepts are in a dynamic interrelationship, a complex quality that is difficult to depict in a two-dimensional space (Liehr & Smith, 2011a). For example, moments of ease surface when the nurse first engages the person in a caring way to identify what really matters. Even a brief encounter with a caring nurse enables a connection before story parts come together as a whole. Needless to say, the complexity of human interaction defies linearity. As nurse scientists

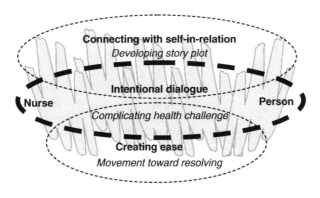

**FIGURE 11.1**  Story.

we are called to fit language to the relationships among the concepts as best we can, recognizing that the simplicity necessary for models conflicts with the complexity recognized in most nursing phenomena.

## Theory-Guided Story-Gathering

The theory proposes common processes for gathering a story, whether the nurse is doing research or practice. To gather a story is to engage in intentional dialogue and invite another to share a story about a health challenge that complicates everyday living. One of the defining elements calling for Story Theory guidance is the nurse's focus on addressing a health challenge. Implicit in any story about a health challenge is connection with others, with one's environment, with oneself—the thread of the story plot rests in this connection. Working through this connection offers potential for movement toward resolving the health challenge—for creating ease. The methodological processes of story are: complicating health challenge, developing story plot, and movement toward resolving.

### COMPLICATING HEALTH CHALLENGE

A complicating health challenge is any circumstance where life change or pattern disruption generates uneasiness in everyday living. The health challenge may be an obvious illness-related phenomenon, such as the diagnosis of a serious illness, or it may be a naturally occurring developmental event like sending the youngest child off to college. It may be discomfort brought on by life circumstances such as bullying experienced by a middle school child or by a novice nurse in a new practice setting. It may be instigated by demands such as required lifestyle change following a cardiac event or the initiation of hemodialysis. Whatever the health challenge, story-gathering begins when the nurse asks about "what matters most" to the person sharing the health challenge story. Attentive presence to "what matters" is a way of "being with," which places the story-sharer at the center of attention. It carries the story-sharer into the moment so that the present moment can be explored as a mystery. For the nurse, movement into the moment calls for connecting with the clear and centered intention to listen and hear the story with the story-sharer leading the way.

### DEVELOPING STORY PLOT

The developing story plot ties moments together in a meaningful way. When the nurse invites reflection on the past, focusing on issues that have importance for the present health challenge, these issues are introduced because they "matter most" in a way that is known only to the person sharing the story; they are essential to the developing story plot and are critical to understanding self-in-relation. At the empirical level, story plot may be documented as high points, low points, and turning points emerging in the description of the health challenge. High points include times when things are going well, low points are times when things are not going so well, and turning points are times identified as deciding moments or perspective-shaping twists that subtly or dramatically alter one's life direction.

Sometimes, the high points, low points, and turning points that create the story plot can be uncovered by taking pen to paper and drawing relationship structures. For instance, a family tree can be used to note important relationships and serve as a base for understanding connecting with self-in-relation. Story path is another example of a relationship structure, in this case linking present, past, and future of an unfolding story plot. When using this approach, the nurse generally begins with a line on a blank piece of paper and labels the line "the story of . . ." to orient the person sharing the story to the dialogue. The story will always be about a health challenge. Most often, the story begins with the present . . . asking the storyteller to identify where he or she is right now, today, on his or her life/health journey in relation to the health challenge he or she is facing. Then, attention turns to the past and finally to the future. The following box provides an example of a story path collected from a young adult, Joe, who was undertaking lifestyle change due to a recent diagnosis of hypertension. Joe's brief story is provided and high points, low points, and turning points noted on the story path are categorized. Although simplistic, this example provides the basic story path structure that has been reported previously in other Story Theory descriptions (Liehr & Smith, 2015) and in the nurse coaching literature (Dossey, 2015).

---

**A Brief Story of Joe**

Joe is a 35-year old White male who works as a computer programmer. He is the third of four children and he has 10-year-old and 3-year-old children with his wife, Debby, who is the primary supporter of his lifestyle change. Joe's mom has hypertension and her father died from a stroke at age 52. She is "pleased" that Joe is taking on a lifestyle change. Joe describes his job as most stressful with never-ending deadlines. At home, he is forever telling the kids "no . . . stop doing this or that." Joe says that he routinely "holds anger and frustration in," a pattern he attributes to learning as a child. His blood pressure was 164/99 at the beginning of the story-gathering session. The health challenge that was complicating Joe's life on the first story-sharing session was his experience of overwhelming stress that contributed to a sense that he was much older than his 35 years.

*(continued)*

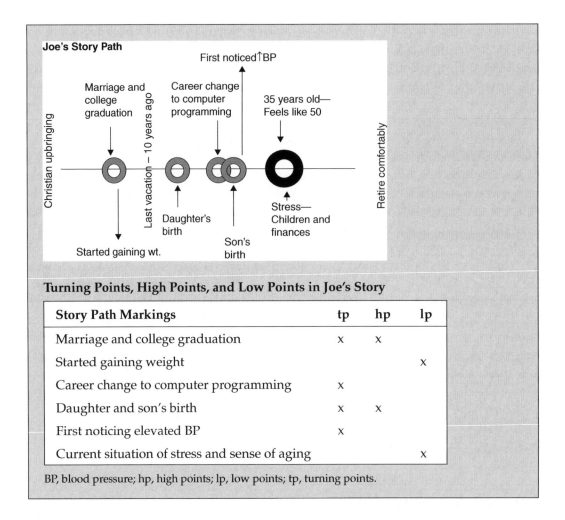

**Turning Points, High Points, and Low Points in Joe's Story**

| Story Path Markings | tp | hp | lp |
|---|---|---|---|
| Marriage and college graduation | x | x | |
| Started gaining weight | | | x |
| Career change to computer programming | x | | |
| Daughter and son's birth | x | x | |
| First noticing elevated BP | x | | |
| Current situation of stress and sense of aging | | | x |

BP, blood pressure; hp, high points; lp, low points; tp, turning points.

When using the story path for research, we have found that the time-oriented dimension of this approach is more important than the actual line on a piece of paper. Sometimes participants engage with the researcher to "populate" the line, marking meaningful life events and sometimes the line is seemingly dismissed by the participant as the present–past–future story unfolds. When this approach for gathering stories was first described (Liehr & Smith, 2000), its utility for collecting practice evidence was emphasized. As a research approach, story path enables collection of stories about a particular health challenge with the consistent structure of present–past–future focus. Researchers have used the story path approach to gather data from participants across a broad age range and across diverse cultural backgrounds (see the section Use of the Theory in Nursing Research). For instance, Charbonneau-Dahlen, Lowe, and Morris (2016) adapted story path for use in research with Native American women who had been removed from their families to live in boarding schools as children. These researchers report development of a Dream Catcher–Medicine Wheel Model as being culturally meaningful for story-gathering. Their adaptation of the story path created relevance for this Native American population enabling past, present, and future story elements to surface from the perspective of the Medicine Wheel while the Dream Catcher overlay provided a familiar filter for "catching bad dreams" and diminishing uneasiness for the story-sharer.

Possible approaches for story-gathering are limited only by the imagination of the nurse scholar. The underlying principles to keep in mind when identifying a story-gathering structure is the meaning of the structure for the persons from whom the story is being gathered; and the potential of the structure to stay true to the intent of story-gathering. For instance, use of a linear story path may be confusing for people from cultures who view time as overlapping/extending in the moment; this was the incentive for development of the Dream Catcher–Medicine Wheel Model (Charbonneau-Dahlen, Lowe, & Morris, 2016). Another circumstance that may demand adjusting occurs when gathering stories from people at the end of life, who have difficulty envisioning and talking about a future. In gathering stories for research, the nurse will adjust the story-gathering approach to allow for cultural and situational circumstances that reflect attention to making the story-gathering relevant for each unique population group.

## MOVEMENT TOWARD RESOLVING

Movement toward resolving happens in keeping the story-sharer immersed in the "now" health experience, while realizing that the pace of story progression is an ever-changing self-directing metric . . . and it is never really finished. For the nurse and for the story-sharer, finding a center of stillness and letting go of busyness and distraction energizes mindful attention to the story and propels potential for movement toward resolving. In a present-centered focus, one is free to take on the health challenge and to view it in a manageable way. Oftentimes this shift to a manageable view energizes a sense of ease as a person attentively embraces the fullness of life emerging in the moment. It is an opportunity to change thinking and feeling and to move on differently.

Over the years, we have learned that movement toward resolving emerges along a spectrum including subtle recognition as well as all-out embracing the now moment. There is no final resolution for any story and resolving does not close when story-sharing ends; it occurs in its own time. On some occasions, subtle recognition is a huge step along the path of human development, opening doors and pointing directions, enabling next steps.

# ■ USE OF THE THEORY IN NURSING RESEARCH

Since Story Theory was first published over a decade ago, we have explored ways to investigate what is learned from practice stories and we have debated the best qualitative approach as well as the value of a quantitative approach for analyzing story data when guided by the theory. We have learned that there is neither a simple destination for the exploration nor an answer to the debate. To some extent, we ourselves, our students, our colleagues, and anyone who uses Story Theory to guide research is pushing the edge of understanding about how nursing practice stories collected through research can best be gathered and analyzed to access their inherent wisdom. Several examples of published research will be presented, highlighting the place Story Theory has had in the research process. In these examples, the reader will find that the theory has been used to guide a story-centered care intervention; and, it has been used to guide story analysis with both quantitative and qualitative methods. Regardless of the place of Story Theory in a study design, health stories gathered for the purpose of scholarly inquiry require an analysis strategy based on a research question. It is the wording of the question that guides the method of analysis.

## Research on a Story-Centered Care Intervention

In an effort to assess the power of story-gathering guided by Story Theory, Liehr et al. (2006) tested the effect of adding story-centered care to exercise and diet for people with stage one hypertension. The research question was: What is the difference in 24-hour ambulatory BP when story-centered care is added to structured exercise and nutrition counseling for people with stage one hypertension? Participants who received story-centered care had lower systolic BP while awake than those who received only the exercise and nutrition intervention ($p < .05$). During story-centered care, advanced practice nurses engaged participants in four sessions using: a family tree to access connection with significant others; a story path to focus on what mattered most in the present within the context of past and future; and BP self-monitoring diaries to foster connection with self. Although the number of participants was small ($N = 24$), significant findings suggested that the Story Theory–guided intervention was promising.

Summers (2016) tested the effect of story-centered care on disclosure for adolescents attending an urgent care clinic. Rather than research questions, she proposed hypotheses. The specific hypothesis relevant to story-centered care outcomes suggested that: Story-centered care would increase adolescent disclosure during the visit compared to standard care. To test this hypothesis, Summers used a quantitative word analysis approach that is more thoroughly described in the next section. However, provider–adolescent word-use ratios indicated that adolescents used twice the number of words relative to the provider when receiving story-centered care as compared to standard care. The quantity of words used by adolescents in the story-centered care group was significantly greater ($p < .01$), averaging 876 words compared to 217 words for adolescents in the standard care group.

## Analyzing Story Data: Quantitative

When word use in a story about a health challenge is quantified, quantification is not intended to represent a measure of the story but rather a numeric chronicle of story word qualities (e.g., negative emotion words; positive emotion words; cognitive process words; linguistic elements) over time or an opportunity for understanding story–health outcome connections. When quantifying story data, researchers have used Linguistic Inquiry and Word Count (LIWC), a software program developed by Pennebaker, Chung, Ireland, Gonzales, and Booth (2007). LIWC is a computerized text analysis software that discerns linguistic elements (e.g., word count and sentence punctuation); affective, cognitive, sensory, and social words; and words that reflect relativity and personal concerns. The structure has had psychometric testing, and reliability and validity estimates are reported by Pennebaker and King (1999).

Hain (2008) studied people undergoing hemodialysis focusing on the question: "What is the relationship between word use (LIWC) in stories of lifestyle change and cognitive function (modified minimental) for older adults undergoing hemodialysis?" She found statistically significant relationships between global cognitive function and the linguistic elements of words per sentence ($r = .41$; $p < .01$) and use of big words ($r = .37$, $p < .01$). She suggests that these linguistic elements could be readily detected by nurses who work with hemodialysis patients, allowing timely referral for cognitive assessments, which could contribute to better quality of care and quality living (Hain, 2008).

As part of a manuscript describing varying approaches to mixed methods design (Chiang-Hanisko, Newman, Dyess, Piyakong, & Liehr, 2016), Liehr provides an exemplar that raises two research questions: (a) What are the turning points described by veterans in stories about surviving the bombings of Pearl Harbor? (qualitative); and (b) What percentage of personal pronouns, positive/negative emotion words, and cognitive process words were used by the veterans in their stories of survival? (quantitative).

The second question guided a quantitative analysis using LIWC. Descriptive statistics quantified word-use components. "I" words (X = 7.1%) predominated over "we" words (X = 2.1%). Also, while negative (X = 1.4%) and positive emotion word use (X = 1.0%) was comparable, cognitive process word use (X = 6.5%) outranked the emotion word use. In response to the second research question, the conclusion was: seventy years after their experience, survivors were reflecting rather than emoting and their perspectives were self-owned (I) rather than shared (we). These findings generated questions about the power of reflecting on and owning one's story of trauma, particularly related to the strong evidence for human connection as a resource, a finding that emerged from the qualitative component of the study.

## Analyzing Story Data: Qualitative

Stories are the substance of qualitative research, and traditional approaches can be used when analyzing stories gathered with the guidance of Story Theory. For instance, phenomenological analysis is an example of an established way to analyze story data when the research question addresses the human experience (Giorgi, 1985; Smith & Liehr, 1999; Van Manen, 1990). Content analysis (Hsieh & Shannon, 2005) is another approach that can be combined with Story Theory to address relevant concepts (health challenge, movement to resolve health challenge).

Ramsey (2012) addressed the question: What is the structure of meaning for women living with migraine headache? The study was guided by Story Theory and phenomenology (van Manen, 1990). Data were gathered using story path and analyzed using a phenomenological approach. Interrelated themes in the structure of meaning included: (a) recalling the significant experience that reshaped life; (b) experiencing self as vulnerable; (c) being overcome by unrelenting torturous pain; (d) pushing through to hold self together to do what needs to be done; (e) surrendering to the compelling call to focus on self; (f) making the most of pain-free time; and (g) being on guard against an unpredictable attack and yet hopeful that it is possible to outsmart the next attack. Ramsey's findings provide guidance for nurses who work with women who experience unrelenting migraine headaches.

Maiocco and Smith (2016) also used the combination of Story Theory and phenomenology (van Manen, 1990) to study woman veterans coming back from war. Data were gathered using story path and analyzed using a phenomenological approach. Themes included: (a) arriving home with mixed sentiments; (b) evolving to changed view of self, family, others; (c) permeating aggravation from conversations and actions of others; (d) confounding broken relationships, frequent deployments, and leaving the military; (e) remembering war experiences that never end; and (f) seeking opportunity for what is possible. The authors concluded that it was important to ascertain military experience when working with women and to be sensitive to mental health issues that arise for female veterans, who generally do not tell their stories of deployment but may benefit from the experience of sharing stories of deployment and postdeployment challenges.

Walter and Smith (2016) combined Story Theory for data collection with phenomenology (van Manen, 1990) for analysis to address a research question about the challenge of mothering a child with autism. Four themes emerged from the data: acknowledging that the child's development was not normal; coming face to face with the reality of autism; taking on challenges of living every day; and living with an uneasiness about the future of the child. The authors indicate that the mothering experience is an emergent challenge that warrants research attention over the course of time.

Songwathana and Liehr (2015) reported a preliminary study that used story-guided content analysis to address the question of approaches followed by a Muslim woman to move beyond abrupt widowhood. Data collected over time indicated four approaches: accepting support from close friends and family; connecting with Muslim faith; holding on to concern for children's well-being; and reaching out to other widows. The strong thread of "connection" in the study findings is noted by the authors as a potential direction for intervention for women who have suffered abrupt widowhood.

Rateau studied the stories of persons who encountered catastrophic loss from flood using story theory as the theoretical foundation (Rateau, 2017). Stories were gathered using a story path from eight persons who experienced substantial loss of material possessions and property due to a flood. Three turning points were uncovered across all stories. The turning points are: facing the devastation, embracing the rebuilding, and developing inner strength (p. 562). These findings suggest a transformational movement beyond that is critical for recovery and healing.

## Story Inquiry Method

Story inquiry method is a systematic approach that uses Story Theory to guide data collection and analysis (Liehr & Smith, 2011b). The five processes of the inquiry method are: (a) gather stories about a complicating health challenge using a meaningful consistent structure to encourage story-sharing; (b) begin deciphering the dimensions of the complicating health challenge; (c) describe the developing story plot (high points, low points, turning points); (d) identify movement toward resolving; and (e) synthesize findings to address the research question. In any single study, a researcher may address all of the story analysis processes (health challenge; story plot; approaches for resolving challenges) or only select one through articulation of the research question/s.

Since story inquiry was first introduced, five studies have reported findings guided by the method (Carpenter, 2014; Hains, Wands, & Liehr, 2011; Kelley & Lowe, 2012; Liehr, Nishimura, Ito, Wands, & Takahashi, 2011; Walter, 2017). Each study is briefly described culminating with the lessons learned about using the story inquiry method.

Hain et al. (2011) posed the questions: (a) What are the health challenges of making lifestyle change for older adults undergoing hemodialysis and (b) How do they resolve the challenges? Data were analyzed to address the first research question, beginning with the words of the participants, isolating the excerpts related to health challenges, grouping like statements together, eliminating redundancy, and naming each of the groups. The health challenge themes described by participants were: living a restriction-driven existence; balancing independence/dependence; and struggling with those providing care. Similar analysis was conducted to address the second research question. Approaches used by participants to resolve the health challenges were: unhappy passive acceptance; taking lifestyle change in stride; active attitudinal effort to accept reality; and assertive behavior to get what you want.

Lessons learned from the use of story inquiry method in this study primarily focused on the most appropriate way to articulate the research question related to the health challenge. Rather than querying the health challenge as a whole, the research question will query the dimensions of the health challenge. So when the researcher identifies a focus for study, such as making lifestyle change, being obese, or being admitted to a nursing home, the health challenge is named. The dimensions of the challenge will enable the researcher to arrive at the nuances and complexities of the health challenge.

In a study of survivors from Pearl Harbor and Hiroshima, Liehr et al. (2011) posed the research question: What turning points marked movement over time in stories of health for survivors? Turning points for Hiroshima survivors were: (a) facing the disorienting aftermath; (b) becoming Hibakusha (A-bomb survivor); and (c) reaching out to create meaning/purpose. For the Pearl Harbor survivors, the turning points were: (a) coming to grips with the reality of a Japanese attack; (b) honoring the memory of their war experience; and (c) embracing connection as a source of comfort. Each of these turning points was imbued with themes that enriched the meaning and contributed to understanding (Liehr et al., 2011).

The major lesson learned about story inquiry method while conducting this study was related to the importance of defining "turning points" for use by all analysts. This is especially important when more than one researcher is engaged in analyzing but it is even important when one researcher is conducting the analysis over time. Liehr et al. (2011) defined turning points as "twists in the stories, where there was a shift in living through and with wartime trauma." (p. 219). Staying true to the definition at the start of each analysis session was critical to the integrity of the data analysis.

Kelley and Lowe (2012) used story inquiry method to analyze stories of stress for Cherokee-Keetoowah adolescents. The research questions posed were: (a) What is the health challenge of stress experienced by Cherokee-Keetoowah adolescents? and (b) How do these adolescents resolve stress? Dimensions of the health challenge of stress became the focus for the first research question. Cherokee-Keetoowah adolescents identified the burden of expectations, relationship disruption, and imposing feelings and actions of others as dimensions of the health challenge of stress. They described connecting with valued others, engaging in meaningful activities, and choosing a positive attitude about change as the approaches they used to manage stress.

One implicit lesson in this work with Cherokee adolescents relates to the potential of story methods to assure cultural sensitivity. Issues of cultural sensitivity in research are addressed if people are approached with humility and intention to understand. Story-gathering guided by the theory is a vehicle for humble understanding. A second lesson from the Kelley and Lowe (2012) study relates to the method for story exchange. Stories were written rather than collected in a face-to-face format in this study. Adolescents were given instructions to write for 15 minutes about their stress and how they managed it without regard for punctuation, spelling, or sentence structure. The potential for story-centered writing sessions that cultivate personal reflection warrants further exploration in future research using the story inquiry method.

Carpenter (2014) used the story inquiry method to address the challenge of living with diabetes, exploring dimensions of the health challenge and approaches for resolving the challenge. The dimensions of the challenge were: caught up in knowing, yet not knowing life circumstances; engaged in daily struggle with everyday life choices; and paralyzed in the present. Approaches for resolving the challenge were: making effort to take control of self with hope; striving to do what is right with an eye to the future; and accepting supportive efforts from family and healthcare providers.

Carpenter's study called attention to the practical wisdom of guidance from people living with chronic illness that occurs when movement toward resolving a health challenge is queried. Although the dimensions of the health challenge provide an understanding of the experience, how people manage the experience has potent application for nursing practice.

Walter (2017) used story inquiry to guide research on the experience of living with headache for adolescents. The research questions were related to three areas: (a) dimensions of the complicating health challenge; (b) high points, low points, and turning points; and (c) approaches used to address living with headache. The challenge of living with headache was described as enduring distress inclusive of pain, uncertainty, distancing from significant others, and a sense of not knowing how to resolve the headache. High points were: contentment with school achievement, supportive relationships, and times of comfort. Low points were difficulty pursuing sports and exercise, and conflicting family relationships. Turning points were developing hope, insight, and the possibility of moving toward resolution. Approaches to address the headache were medication, sleep, and moving beyond the pain (e.g., piano playing, music). Unlike the other researchers, Walter queried all aspects of the theory using the story inquiry method. In her conclusion, she suggests that including the adolescent's story as an integral dimension of practice contributes to the development of an effective plan of care.

## ■ USE OF THE THEORY IN NURSING PRACTICE

The question leading the story when the foremost intention is caring–healing is "what matters" to the client about the complicating health challenge. In eliciting the story, the nurse leads the client along, clarifying meaningful connections about what is happening in everyday living in the context of the client's complicating health challenge. Sharing the health challenge story brings developing story plot and movement toward resolving to the surface. The resulting story about "what matters" to the client provides distinct information about how one person lived the health challenge.

Stories are so integral to nursing practice that they are often gathered by nurses and used to guide healthcare decision making without a second thought about their potential for knowledge development. One approach for analyzing practice stories guided by Story Theory (Smith & Liehr, 2005) that has been embraced by the nurse coaching movement (Dossey, 2015) has been modified to create a five-phase process that merges scholarly attention with the empirical evidence of practice stories to contribute to knowledge development. The phases of this modified process are: (a) gather a story about a health challenge in your practice setting and write the story immediately after collecting it; (b) identify the story's high points, low points, and turning points; (c) identify approaches for moving to resolve the health challenge; (d) connect the existing literature to each component of the process (health challenge; high, low, turning points; movement to resolve the health challenge); and (e) collect additional stories about the health challenge to confirm developing knowledge.

Health stories collected through application of Story Theory during nursing practice include those about patients with dementia who expressed disagreement through behavioral messages (Ito, Takahashi, & Liehr, 2007) and coming to know the voice of vulnerable adolescents in an urban practice setting (Jolly, Weiss, & Liehr, 2007). Summers (2002) used the theory as a foundation for mutual timing, a concept she believes is critical for effective healthcare encounters.

Rateau (2010) described her personal story of a catastrophic loss from a house fire and explosion. Through recounting her story, she experienced an increased understanding of the event leading to a transformation of meaning and a deepened level of well-being. She offers implications for using Story Theory–guided practice for persons experiencing traumatic catastrophic loss to find meaning and move beyond the loss.

Two scholars used Story Theory to provide culturally sensitive care. Millender (2011) described application of Story Theory for a hospitalized Guatemalan Mayan patient to develop a culturally relevant plan of care. She found that the medical history did not offer evidence of the patient's cultural beliefs and values and concluded that engaging in intentional dialogue guided by Story Theory provided the nurse with useful cultural information. In reference to the Appalachian culture, Gobble (2009) described application of Story Theory to uncover religious and cultural perspectives that guided culturally sensitive advanced practice nursing for a woman living in a rural community.

Performance Excellence and Accountability in Kidney Care (PEAK) is a voluntary movement to reduce mortality among first-year dialysis patients at a national level. On their website (www.kidneycarequality.com/CampLearnCenter.htm) under Best Practice 2, practitioners are referred to Story Theory as a means to achieve this best practice. Theory-based website guidance for health professionals engaging with dialysis patients includes the following dialogue-leading questions and statements:

1. Tell me about the challenges you are facing as you begin dialysis.
2. What is most important to you right now?
3. Can you think of a past challenge or "difficult time" that you "got through?" Tell me about that time and what helped you get through it.
4. Tell me about your future hopes and dreams.

## ■ USE OF THE THEORY IN NURSING EDUCATION

Story Theory has begun to establish a literature base supporting use in nursing research: practice applicability that extends to guidance for nurse coaching (Dossey, 2015) and best practice guidance for nurses working with people starting hemodialysis (www.kidneycarequality.com/CampLearnCenter.htm). However, judging by publications, less attention has been given to the theory in nursing education. The few publications indicating use of theory are briefly described here.

Liu, Wu, Yang, and Chen (2016), a team of scholars from China, have described the theory for Chinese scholars, noting its application to nursing practice and research. Graduate students working with this team have begun to use the theory to guide research.

Carpenter (2010) described applying Story Theory to structure an undergraduate clinical course for a student in the honors program. The result was an innovative teaching strategy that increased the quality for all students in the practicum experience. This was accomplished by guiding students to develop skill in intentional dialogue and the use of story path. It was concluded that taking the course beyond the biomedical/technical aspects of care to show the importance of nursing presence through gathering the patient's story enriched the practice experience.

These beliefs about the importance of story for health and human caring are confirmed by the Carnegie Foundation report (Benner, Sutphen, Leonard, & Day, 2010), calling for a radical transformation in nursing education. In their guidelines for improving nursing education, the authors say:

Because injuries and illness occur in the context of a person's life, the nurse must formulate a narrative of the patient's immediate clinical history, his concerns, and even an account of his life and lifeworld. Reasoning across time involves the ability to construct a sensible story of immediate events, their sequence, and their consequences in terms of illness trajectory and life concerns. (p. 225)

As nursing moves toward educating greater and greater numbers of nurses with practice doctorates, it is important to honor the wisdom found in practice stories; to consider the potential of practice stories for advancing nursing practice scholarship; and to identify systematic approaches for using practice stories for nursing knowledge development.

## ■ CONCLUSION

Collaborative work on Story Theory began in 1996, and the theory was first published in 1999. In the years since we first began thinking through the meaning of story for health, we have stayed with the theory and continued to reflect on next directions. In this process, we have grown stronger and stronger in our belief about the power of story wisdom for contributing to nursing practice and knowledge development. Each time we share our understanding of Story Theory with the nursing community, we learn more about the theory and formulate next directions. Middle range theory development is scholarship in progress weaving practice and research threads into intricate patterns for practical use. As these thoughts are shared, new questions are realized, and so the story goes.

## ■ REFERENCES

Banks, J. (2014). "And that's going to help Black women how?": Storytelling and striving to stay true to the task of liberation in the academy. In P. N. Kagan, M. C. Smith & P. L. Chinn. *Philosophies and practices of emancipatory nursing: Social justice as Praxis* (pp. 188–204). New York, NY: Routledge.

Benner, P. (1984). *From novice to expert.* Menlo Park, CA: Addison-Wesley.

Benner, P., Sutphen, M., Leonard, V., & Day, L. (2010). *Educating nurses: A call for radical transformation.* San Francisco, CA: Jossey-Bass.

Boykin, A., & Schoenhofer, S. (2001). The role of nursing leadership in creating caring environments in health care delivery systems. *Nursing Administration Quarterly, 25*(3), 1–7.

Burkhardt, M. A., & Nagai-Jacobson, M. G. (2002). *Spirituality: Living our connectedness.* Albany, NY: Delmar.

Carpenter, R. D. (2010). Using Story Theory to create an innovative honors level nursing course. *Nursing Education Perspectives, 31*(1), 28–32.

Carpenter, R. D. (2014). Challenges and movement to resolution for persons living with diabetes. *Archives in Psychiatric Nursing, 28*, 352–353.

Chiang-Hanisko, L., Newman, D., Dyess, S., Piyakong, D., & Liehr, P. (2016). Guidance for using mixed methods design in nursing practice research. *Applied Nursing Research, 31*, 1–5.

Charbonneau-Dahlen, B., Lowe, J., & Morris, S. L. (2016). Giving voice to historical trauma through storytelling: The impact of boarding school experience on American Indians. *Journal of Aggression, Maltreatment & Trauma.* doi:10.1080/10926771.2016.1157843

Charon, R. (2006). *Narrative medicine: Honoring the stories of illness.* New York, NY: Oxford University Press.

Chinn, P. L., & Kramer, M. K. (1999). *Theory and nursing integrated knowledge development.* New York, NY: Mosby.

Csikszentmihalyi, M. (1990). *Flow: The psychology of optimal experience.* New York, NY: Harper & Row.

Csikszentmihalyi, M., Abuhamdeh, S., & Nakamura, J. (2005). Flow. In A. J. Elliot & C. S. Dweck (Eds.), *Handbook of competence and motivation* (pp. 598–608). New York, NY: Guilford.

Dossey, B. M. (2015). Stories, strengths, and the nurse coach 5-step process. In B. M. Dossey, S. Luck, B. G. Schaub. *Nurse coaching: Integrative approaches for health and wellbeing* (pp. 85–108). North Miami, FL: International Nurse Coach Association.

Ford, K., & Turner, D. (2001). Stories seldom told: Pediatric nurses' experiences of caring for hospitalized children with special needs and their families. *Journal of Advanced Nursing, 33*, 288–295.

Franklin, J. (1994). *Writing for story.* Middlesex, England: Penguin.

Giorgi, A. (1985). *Phenomenology and psychological research.* Pittsburgh, PA: Duquesne University Press.

Gobble, C. D. (2009). The value of story theory in providing culturally sensitive advanced practice nursing in rural Appalachia. *Online Journal of Rural Nursing and Health Care, 9*(1), 94–105. Retrieved from http://rnojournal.binghamton.edu/index.php/RNO/article/view/108

Hain, D. J. (2008). Cognitive function and adherence of older adults undergoing hemodialysis. *Nephrology Nursing Journal, 35*(1), 23–30.

Hain, D. J., Wands, L. M., & Liehr, P. (2011). Approaches to resolve health challenges in a population of older adults undergoing hemodialysis. *Research in Gerontological Nursing, 4*(1), 53–62.

Hsieh, H. F., & Shannon, S. E. (2005). Three approaches to qualitative content analysis. *Qualitative Health Research, 15*(9), 1277–1288.

Ito, M., Takahashi, R., & Liehr, P. (2007). Heeding the behavioral message of elders with dementia in day care. *Holistic Nursing Practice, 21*(1), 12–18.

Jolly, K., Weiss, J. A., & Liehr, P. (2007). Understanding adolescent voice as a guide for nursing practice and research. *Issues in Comprehensive Pediatric Practice, 30*(3), 3–13.

Kelley, M., & Lowe, J. (2012). The health challenge of stress experienced by Native American adolescents. *Archives in Psychiatric Nursing, 26*(1), 71–73.

Liehr, P. (1989). A loving center: The core of true presence. *Nursing Science Quarterly*, 2, 7–8.

Liehr, P. (1992). Uncovering a hidden language: The effects of listening and talking on blood pressure and heart rate. *Archives of Psychiatric Nursing*, 6, 306–311.

Liehr, P., Meininger, J. C., Vogler, R., Chan, W., Frazier, L., Smalling, S., & Fuentes, F. (2006). Adding story-centered care to standard lifestyle intervention for people with stage 1 hypertension. *Applied Nursing Research*, 19, 16–21.

Liehr, P., Nishimura, C., Ito, M., Wands, L. M., & Takahashi, R. (2011). A lifelong journey of moving beyond wartime trauma for survivors from Hiroshima and Pearl Harbor. *Advances in Nursing Science*, 34(3), 215–228.

Liehr, P., & Smith, M. J. (2000). Using story theory to guide nursing practice. *International Journal of Human Caring*, 4, 13–18.

Liehr, P., & Smith, M. J. (2011a). Modeling the complexity of story theory for nursing practice. In A. W. Davidson, M. A. Ray, & M. C. Turkel (Eds.), *Nursing, caring, and complexity science* (pp. 241–248). New York, NY: Springer Publishing.

Liehr, P., & Smith, M. J. (2011b). Refining story inquiry as a method for research. *Archives of Psychiatric Nursing*, 25(1), 74–75.

Liehr, P., & Smith, M. J. (2015). Patricia Liehr and Mary Jane Smith's story theory. In M. C. Smith & M. E. Parker (Eds.), *Nursing theories and nursing practice* (4th ed., pp. 421–434). Philadelphia, PA: F. A. Davis.

Liu, H., Wu, X., Yang, Q., & Chen, Y. (2016). Story theory and its application to nursing science. *Chinese Nursing Research*, 30, 776–778.

Maiocco, G., & Smith, M. J. (2016). The experience of women veterans coming back from war. *Archives in Psychiatric Nursing*, 30, 393–399.

Millender, E. (2011). Using stories to bridge cultural disparities, one culture at a time. *Journal of Continuing Education in Nursing*, 42(1), 37–42.

Newman, M. A. (1999). The rhythm of relating in a paradigm of wholeness. *Image: Journal of Nursing Scholarship*, 31, 227–230.

Nightingale, F. (1946). *Notes on nursing: What it is and what it is not*. Philadelphia, PA: J. B. Lippincott.

Parse, R. R. (1981). *Man-living-health: A theory of nursing*. New York, NY: Wiley.

PEAK: Performance Excellence and Accountability in Kidney Care. *Patient "Tools of Engagement." Best practice 2*. Retrieved from http://www.kidneycarequality.com/CampLearnCenter.htm

Pennebaker, J. W., Chung, C. K., Ireland, M., Gonzales, A., & Booth, R. J. (2007). *The development and psychometric properties of LWIC2007*. Austin, TX: LIWC.net. Retrieved from https://pdfs.semanticscholar.org/5842/736189064114be6cbe04e6e8c239a9312c4e.pdf

Pennebaker, J. W., & King, L. A. (1999). Linguistic styles: Language use as an individual difference. *Journal of Personality and Social Psychology*, 77, 1296–1312.

Peplau, H. (1991). *Interpersonal relations in nursing*. New York, NY: Springer Publishing.

Polanyi, M. (1958). *The study of man*. Chicago, IL: University of Chicago Press.

Ramsey, A. R. (2012). Living with migraine headache: A phenomenological study of women's experiences. *Holistic Nursing Practice*, 26(6), 297–307.

Rateau, M. R. (2010). A story of transformation following catastrophic loss. *Archives in Psychiatric Nursing, 24*(4), 260–265.

Rateau, M. R. (2017). An analysis of stories from those who have encountered catastrophic loss from flood. *Archives of Psychiatric Nursing, 31,* 561–565. doi:10.1016/j.apnu.2017.07.009

Reed, P. A. (1995). Treatise on nursing knowledge development for the 21st century: Beyond postmodernism. *Advances in Nursing Science, 17,* 70–84.

Reed, P. A. (1999). Response to "Attentively embracing story: A middle-range theory with practice and research implications." *Scholarly Inquiry for Nursing Practice: An International Journal, 13,* 205–209.

Rogers, C. R. (1951). *Client-centered therapy.* Boston, MA: Houghton Mifflin.

Rogers, M. E. (1994). The science of unitary human beings: Current perspectives. *Nursing Science Quarterly, 7,* 33–35.

Shapiro, S. L., Carlson, L. E., Astin, J. A., & Freedman, B. (2006). Mechanisms of mindfulness. *Journal of Clinical Psychology, 62*(3), 373–386.

Smith, M. J. (1975). Changes in judgment of duration with different patterns of auditory information for individuals confined to bed. *Nursing Research, 24,* 93–98.

Smith, M. J. (1986). Human-environment process: A test of Rogers' principle of integrality. *Advances in Nursing Sciences, 9,* 21–28.

Smith, M. J., & Liehr, P. (1999). Attentively embracing story: A middle-range theory with practice and research implications. *Scholarly Inquiry for Nursing Practice: An International Journal, 13,* 187–204.

Smith, M. J., & Liehr, P. (2005). Story theory: Advancing nursing practice scholarship. *Holistic Nursing Practice, 19*(6), 272–276.

Songwathana, P., & Liehr, P. (2015). Approaches for moving beyond abrupt widowhood: A case study analysis with one Muslim Thai woman. *Archives in Psychiatric Nursing, 29,* 361–362.

Summers, L. (2002). Mutual timing: An essential component of provider/patient communication. *Journal of the Academy of Nurse Practitioners, 14,* 19–25.

Summers, L. (2016). Adolescent disclosure. *The International Journal of Health, Wellness and Society, 6*(2), 39–56.

van Manen, M. (1990). *Researching lived experience.* Albany: State University of New York Press.

Walter, S. M. (2017). The experience of adolescents living with headache. *Holistic Nursing Practice, 31*(6), 280–289.

Walter, S. M., & Smith, M. J. (2016). Mothering a child with autism. *Archives in Psychiatric Nursing, 30*(5), 600–601.

Watson, J. (1997). The theory of human caring: Retrospective and prospective. *Nursing Science Quarterly, 10,* 49–52.

# CHAPTER 12

## Theory of Transitions

Eun-Ok Im

Nursing phenomena occur around various life transitions such as during pregnancy and at midlife. There are transitions from a critical care unit to a long-term care facility, from hospital to community, from one country to a different country, and within a hospital due to changes in administrators. People sometimes go through transitions smoothly and successfully, but frequently they have issues, concerns, and/or problems in transitions due to the disequilibrium caused by changes (Meleis, 2010). Nurses have played a central role in providing care for people in transitions, especially for individuals, families, and communities experiencing changes that trigger new roles, losses of networks, and support systems (Meleis, 2010, p. xv). Nurses could facilitate successful transitions by providing information, support, and/or direct care, which subsequently help prevent diseases, reduce health risks, enhance health/well-being, and facilitate rehabilitation of those in transitions. Meleis (2010) asserted that transitions are central to the mission of nursing.

Transitions Theory started from the point of view that nursing phenomena could be explained as a health/illness experience during life changes. The theory has frequently been used to explain nursing phenomena across diverse circumstances related to change in health/ illness, life situations, developmental stages, and organizations (Im, 2009; Meleis, 2010). Furthermore, Transitions Theory has provided a structure for nursing curriculum, a framework for research questions/hypotheses, and directions for nursing care (Im, 2009). In this chapter, the purpose and development process of Transitions Theory are described. Then, the major concepts of Transitions Theory and the relationships among the concepts are described. Finally, the current use of Transitions Theory in nursing research and practice is presented.

## ■ PURPOSE OF THE THEORY AND HOW IT WAS DEVELOPED

The purpose of this middle range theory is to describe, explain, and predict human beings' experiences in various types of transitions including health/ illness transitions, situational transitions, developmental transitions, and organizational transitions. Because nursing phenomena frequently involve transition, Transitions Theory has been used in nursing research and practice (Im, 2011). Furthermore, due to its comprehensiveness, Transitions Theory has been widely accepted in nursing research and practice (Im, 2011). An entire issue of *Advances in Nursing Science* (Chinn, 2012) was recently dedicated to transitions, and in her editorial, Chinn recognizes Meleis's contribution, noting the central importance of transitions for the discipline: "I believe that the concept of transitions, along with the central concept of caring, forms a core around which the practice of nursing is constructed" (p. 191). In 2015, Meleis was designated as a living legend, the highest honor given by the American Academy of Nursing, to honor her lifelong contributions to the nursing discipline, including her tremendous contributions to nursing theory. Transitions Theory was formulated with the goal of integrating what is known about transition experience across different types of life change to provide direction for nursing therapeutics. This theory also provides a framework guiding direction about integrating the results of previous research related to transitions and manipulating transition-related concepts for further study.

The development of Transitions Theory can be characterized by the following descriptors (Im, 2011): a borrowed view; research program and collaborative works; and mentoring.

## From a Borrowed View

The theory has been developed over the past 50 years. Meleis (2007) initiated her conceptualization of Transitions Theory in her master's and PhD dissertation research. Then, through her early theoretical works on Role Supplementation Theory and her research on immigrant health, she began to inquire about the nature of transitions and the human experience of transitions. Thus, we can say that development of Transitions Theory started with the Role Insufficiency Theory (Meleis, 1975, 2007; Meleis & Swendsen, 1978; Meleis, Swendsen, & Jones, 1980), which has its theoretical roots in symbolic interactionism and role theories in sociology. In her first theoretical work, Meleis claimed role insufficiency was a result of unhealthy transitions. Role insufficiency was defined as any difficulty in the cognizance and/or performance of a role or in the attainment of its goals, as well as difficulty in the sentiments associated with the role behavior, as perceived by the self or by significant others (Meleis, 1975; Meleis & Swendsen, 1978; Meleis et al., 1980). In the early work, the goal of healthy transitions was the mastery of behaviors, sentiments, cues, and symbols associated with new roles and identities and nonproblematic processes (Meleis, 1975). Meleis (2007) later mentioned her difficulties in conceptualizing the nature of transitions and the nature of responses to different transitions, but also thought that the goal of nursing knowledge development should be on developing nursing therapeutics (Jones, Zhang, & Meleis, 1978; Meleis, 1975; Meleis & Swendsen, 1978). Her work in the 1970s shows her efforts to develop the idea of role supplementation with a focus on defining the components, processes, and strategies that may be related to role supplementation.

## From a Research Program and Collaborative Works

Meleis's well-known research interests were on immigrant populations and their health (Im & Meleis, 2000; Im, Meleis, & Lee, 1999; Jones et al., 1978; Lipson & Meleis, 1983, 1985; Lipson, Reizian, & Meleis, 1987; Meleis, 1981; Meleis, Lipson, & Dallafar, 1998; Meleis & Rogers, 1987; Meleis & Sorrell, 1981). Most of her publications in the 1980s and 1990s focused on the health/illness experience of Arab immigrants in the United States. Through her research, immigration was conceptualized as a situational transition (Budman, Lipson, & Meleis, 1992; Im et al., 1999; Laffrey, Meleis, Lipson, Solomon, & Omidian, 1989; Lipson & Meleis, 1983, 1985; Lipson et al., 1987; Meleis, 1981; Meleis & La Fever, 1984; Meleis & Rogers, 1987; Meleis & Sorrell, 1981; Meleis et al., 1998).

This is also the period when Chick and Meleis (1986) conceptualized transition as a concept central to nursing. While working as a faculty member at the University of California, San Francisco (UCSF), Meleis met Chick—who was a visiting scholar at UCSF at that time—and they worked together to develop transitions as a concept (Chick & Meleis, 1986). This was the first theoretical work on Transitions Theory. In addition, Meleis's collaborative works with international colleagues helped conceptualize transitions as central to nursing (Lane & Meleis, 1991; May & Meleis, 1987; Meleis, Arruda, Lane, & Bernal, 1994; Meleis, Douglas, Eribes, Shih, & Messias, 1996; Meleis, Kulig, Arruda, & Beckman, 1990; Meleis, Mahidal, Lin, Minami, & Neves, 1987; Shih et al., 1998; Stevens, Hall, & Meleis, 1992).

## From Mentoring

The development of Transitions Theory also results from the mentoring process. Meleis's first major paper on Transitions Theory in 1997 (Schumacher & Meleis, 1994) resulted from working with and mentoring a student. Based on the work of Chick and Meleis, Schumacher, who was a doctoral student at UCSF at that time, worked with Meleis to conduct an extensive literature review on transitions in nursing and developed the transition framework based on 310 articles (Schumacher & Meleis, 1994). This integrated literature review led to a definition of transitions and creation of a conceptual framework in nursing. This framework was well received by nursing researchers, and a few researchers began to use it in their studies.

Transitions Theory was later developed based on the research studies by Meleis's former students who investigated diverse populations in various types of transitions. Former students of Meleis conducted an analysis of their research findings related to transition experiences and responses, and integrated similarities and differences to further develop transitions as a middle range theory (Meleis, Sawyer, Im, Hilfinger Messias, & Schumacher, 2000). As a group, the researchers compared, contrasted, and integrated the findings, and developed Transitions Theory through extensive reading, reviewing, and dialoguing with constant analysis and comparison of the findings related to the major concepts of the theory.

With the emergence of situation-specific theories as a new type of nursing theory (Meleis, 1997), several situation-specific theories were developed based on Transitions Theory by Meleis's former students (Im, 2006; Im & Meleis, 1999a, 1999b; Schumacher, Jones, & Meleis, 1999). These situation-specific theories include the Situation-Specific Theory of Low-Income Korean Immigrant Women's Menopausal Transition (Im & Meleis, 1999a), the Situation-Specific Theory of Elderly Transition (Schumacher, Dodd, & Paul, 1993; Schumacher et al., 1999), and the Situation-Specific Theory of Caucasian Cancer Patients' Pain Experience (STOP; Im, 2006). As a whole, Meleis (2010) published all the theoretical works related to Transitions Theory in a book in 2010. Im (2011) also published a literature review on Transitions Theory to identify a trajectory of theoretical development in nursing and provide direction for future theoretical development. Recently, Meleis (2015) published a book chapter that presents her new theoretical ideas and developments in Transitions Theory. This book chapter is based on the most widely and frequently used middle range theory of Transitions that was published in *Advances in Nursing Science* (Meleis et al., 2000).

## ■ CONCEPTS OF THE THEORY

The major concepts of Transitions Theory suggested by Meleis et al. (2000) include the following: types and patterns of transitions, properties of transition experiences, transition conditions (facilitators and inhibitors), patterns of response/process and outcome indicators, and nursing therapeutics. The definitions of each of these concepts were described in two manuscripts (Meleis et al., 2000; Schumacher & Meleis, 1994) more than a decade ago. The definitions are summarized here.

### Types and Patterns of Transitions

#### TYPES OF TRANSITIONS

The concept of types of transitions includes four different types: developmental transitions, health and illness transitions, situational transitions, and organizational transitions. Developmental transitions are those due to developmental events including birth, adolescence, menopause, aging (or senescence), and death. Health and illness transitions are events such as a recovery process, hospital discharge, and diagnosis of chronic illness (Meleis & Trangenstein, 1994). Situational transitions are those due to changes in life circumstances such as entering an educational program, immigrating from one country to another, and moving from home to a nursing home (Chick & Meleis, 1986). Organizational transitions are those related to changing environmental conditions that affect the lives of clients and workers (Schumacher & Meleis, 1994).

## PATTERNS OF TRANSITIONS

In the Transitions Theory (Meleis et al., 2000), patterns of transitions include multiplicity and complexity. Multiple transitions frequently occur simultaneously; people experience several different types of transitions at the same time rather than experiencing a single transition. Meleis et al. (2000) suggested that multiple transitions could happen sequentially or simultaneously, and the degree of overlap among multiple transitions and the associations between separate events that initiate different transitions should be considered because of the complexities involved.

# Properties of Transition Experience

In the Transitions Theory (Meleis et al., 2000), the properties of transition experiences include awareness, engagement, change and difference, time span, and critical points and events. These properties of transition experience are interrelated as a complex process.

## AWARENESS

Awareness is perception, knowledge, and recognition of a transition experience (Meleis et al., 2000, p. 18). The level of awareness could be reflected in the degree of congruency between what is known about processes and responses and what constitutes an expected set of responses and perceptions of individuals undergoing similar transitions (Meleis et al., 2000, p. 18). According to Chick and Meleis (1986), a person's awareness of change may not necessarily mean that the person has begun his or her transition. Meleis et al. (2000) proposed later that a lack of the awareness also does not always mean that the transition has not begun.

## ENGAGEMENT

Properties of transitions also include engagement (Meleis et al., 2000). Engagement is the degree to which a person demonstrates involvement in the process of transition (Meleis et al., 2000, p. 19). According to Meleis et al. (2000), the level of awareness influences the level of engagement, and there will be no engagement without awareness.

## CHANGES AND DIFFERENCES

The properties of transition also include changes and differences (Meleis et al., 2000). Changes in a person's identities, roles, relationships, abilities, and behaviors result in a sense of movement or direction in internal and external processes (Schumacher & Meleis, 1994). All transitions are considered to be associated with change although not all change indicates a transition. In the theory, Meleis et al. (2000) proposed that disclosing and explaining the meaning, influence, and scope of change (e.g., nature, temporality, perceived importance or severity, personal, familial, and societal norms and expectations) are essential in understanding transition. Differences are conceptualized as a property of transitions. Unsatisfied or atypical expectations, feeling dissimilar, being realized as dissimilar, or viewing the world and others in dissimilar ways could mean challenging differences. Transitions Theory suggests that nurses need to consider a client's level of comfort and mastery in dealing with changes and differences to provide adequate and appropriate care for people in transitions.

## TIME SPAN

Another property of transitions is time span (Meleis et al., 2000). Transitions Theory indicates that all transitions could be characterized as flowing and moving over time (Meleis et al., 2000). Actually, transition refers to a span of time with an identifiable starting point, extending from the first signs of anticipation, perception, or demonstration of change; moving through a period of instability, confusion, and distress; and to an eventual ending with a new beginning or period of stability (Meleis et al., 2000). However, Meleis et al. (2000) also warned that framing the time span of some transition experiences can be problematic or even impossible.

## CRITICAL POINTS AND EVENTS

Critical points and events are markers such as birth, death, the cessation of menstruation, or the diagnosis of an illness (Meleis et al., 2000). In Transitions Theory, it was acknowledged that some transitions may not have specific marker events although most transitions have critical marker points and times. The critical points and times are frequently associated with an awareness of changes or challenging engagement in transition processes. Final critical points are identified by a sense of comfort in new schedules, competence, lifestyles, and self-care behaviors.

## Transition Conditions

Transition conditions are those circumstances that influence the way a person moves through a transition that facilitate or hinder progress toward achieving a healthy transition (Schumacher & Meleis, 1994). Transition conditions are the personal, community, or societal factors that may facilitate or inhibit the transition processes and outcomes.

### PERSONAL CONDITIONS

Personal conditions refer to meanings, cultural beliefs and attitudes, socioeconomic status, preparation, and knowledge (Meleis et al., 2000). The meaning attached to a transition and the transition process facilitates or inhibits successful transitions. Personal conditions also include cultural beliefs and attitudes (e.g., stigma associated with cancer), socioeconomic status, anticipatory preparation, or lack of preparation.

### COMMUNITY AND SOCIETAL CONDITIONS

Community conditions and societal conditions could facilitate or inhibit successful transitions. An example of community conditions is community resources and an example of societal conditions is marginalized immigrants' status in the host country (Meleis et al., 2000).

## Patterns of Response—Process and Outcome Indicators

In the framework by Schumacher and Meleis (1994), indicators of healthy transitions were included as a major concept. In Transitions Theory, indicators of healthy transitions were replaced with patterns of response that include process indicators and outcome indicators (Meleis et al., 2000). Process indicators lead clients toward health or vulnerability and risk. Thus, process indicators help nurses assess and intervene to facilitate healthy transitions. Outcome indicators can be used to assess if a transition is healthy or not. However, outcome indicators can sometimes be linked to events in people's lives if they are assessed early in a transition process. The process indicators include feeling connected, interacting, being situated, and developing confidence and coping. The need to feel and stay connected is included as a process indicator of a healthy transition because immigrants are usually in a healthy transition when they add new contacts to their old contacts with their family members and friends. The meaning of the transition and the resulting behaviors can be discovered, analyzed, and understood, and this interactive process may result in a healthy transition. In most transitions, place, time, space, and relationships indicate whether the person is in the process of a healthy transition. The extent of increased confidence that people in transition have indicates whether the person is in the process of a healthy transition. As an outcome indicator, mastery and fluid integrative identities are included in the theory. A healthy transition can be indicated by the extent of mastery of skills and behaviors that people in transition use to manage changes in their situations. Integrative identities through which identities are reformulated can also indicate a healthy transition.

## Nursing Therapeutics

In the framework by Schumacher and Meleis (1994), nursing therapeutics are described as three measures that are widely applicable to therapeutic intervention during transitions. The three measures include assessment of readiness, preparation of transition, and role supplementation (Schumacher & Meleis, 1994). Assessment of readiness requires multidisciplinary efforts and should be based on a comprehensive understanding of the client. This requires the evaluation of each transition condition to produce a comprehensive sketch of people's readiness during transitions and helps determine various patterns of different transition experiences. The preparation for transition refers to education to produce the best condition/situation for enabling transition. Role supplementation as the last nursing therapeutic was originally suggested by Meleis (1975) and used by several researchers (Brackley, 1992; Dracup et al., 1985; Gaffney, 1992; Meleis & Swendsen, 1978). In the recent book chapter by Meleis (2015), she presented her current ideas on nursing therapeutics with major focus areas for interventions. The areas included: (a) clarifying roles, meanings, competencies, expertise, goals, and role training; (b) identifying milestones and using critical points; (c) providing supportive resources, rehearsals, reference groups, and role models; and (d) debriefing (communicating with others regarding transition experience at critical points of transition).

## ■ RELATIONSHIPS AMONG THE CONCEPTS: THE MODEL

The relationships among the major concepts can be illustrated as in Figure 12.1 (Meleis et al., 2000). This relationship is based on the transition framework by Schumacher and Meleis (1994) and the middle range theory of Transitions by Meleis et al. (2000). The following statements regarding the relationships have been explicated by Im (2011, p. 423):

- Transitions are complex and multidimensional. Transitions have patterns of multiplicity and complexity.
- All transitions are characterized by flow and movement over time.
- Transitions cause changes in identities, roles, relationships, abilities, and patterns of behavior.
- Transitions involve a process of movement and change in fundamental life patterns, which are manifested in all individuals.
- Change and difference are neither interchangeable nor synonymous with transition. Transitions result in change and are the result of change.
- The daily lives of clients, environments, and interactions are shaped by the nature, conditions, meanings, and processes of transition experiences.

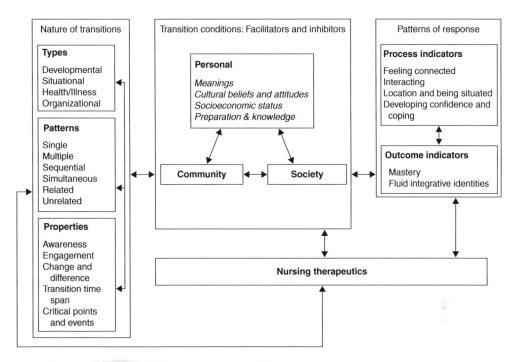

**FIGURE 12.1**   The middle range Transitions Theory.

*Source:* Reprinted with permission from Meleis, A. I., Sawyer, L. M., Im, E. O., Messias, D. K. H., & Schumacher, K. (2000). Experiencing transitions: An emerging middle range theory. *Advances in Nursing Science*, *23*(1), 12–28.

- Vulnerability is related to transition experiences, interactions, and environmental conditions that expose individuals to potential damage, problematic or extended recovery, or delayed or unhealthy coping.
- Nurses are the primary caregivers of clients and their families who are undergoing transitions.

Transitions Theory also has the following theoretical assertions (Im, 2011, p. 424; Meleis et al., 2000; Schumacher & Meleis, 1994):

- Developmental, situational, health and illness, and organizational transitions are central to nursing practice.
- Patterns of transition include whether the client is experiencing a single transition or multiple transitions; whether multiple transitions are sequential or simultaneous; the extent of overlap among transitions; and the nature of the relationship between the different events that are triggering transitions for a client.
- Properties of transition experience are interrelated parts of a complex process.
- The level of awareness influences the level of engagement, in which engagement may not happen without awareness.

- Human perceptions of and meanings attached to health and illness situations are influenced by and in turn influence the conditions under which a transition occurs.
- Healthy transition is characterized by both process and outcome indicators.
- Negotiating successful transitions depends on the development of an effective relationship between the nurse and the client (nursing therapeutic). This relationship is a highly reciprocal process that affects both the client and the nurse.

## Derivatives of Transitions Theory

In this section, three situation-specific theories that were derived from Transitions Theory are presented: STOP, Situation-Specific Theory of Pain Experience for Asian American Cancer Patients (SPEAC), and Situation-Specific Theory of Asian Immigrant Women's Menopausal Symptom Experience in the United States (AIMS).

### THE SITUATION-SPECIFIC THEORY OF CAUCASIAN CANCER PATIENTS' PAIN EXPERIENCE

The STOP (Im, 2006) is a derivative of Transitions Theory. The reason for developing the STOP was to provide a better theoretical basis for the explanation of ethnic-specific cancer pain experience by narrowing the scope of the theory specifically to the pain experience of Caucasian cancer patients. STOP was developed to be a comprehensive theory that could be easily applied to nursing research and practice for management of Caucasian cancer patients' pain. To derive and develop STOP, an integrative approach was used. First, several assumptions were made, which include the following: The theory development process considered the diversity and complexity of the phenomenon from a nursing perspective; it was based on philosophical, theoretical, and methodological plurality; Caucasian cancer patients' pain experience occurred in a specific sociopolitical context; and it was based on a feminist nursing perspective. Multiple theorizing sources were used, which included a systematic literature review and research findings from a multiethnic study on cancer pain experience and Transitions Theory.

**Deduction From Transitions Theory.** Transitions Theory provided the theoretical basis for development of STOP. Caucasian cancer patients' pain experience can be easily linked to the health/illness transition. The major concepts of Transitions Theory are related to the pain experience of Caucasian cancer patients. For instance, the concept of transition conditions includes personal, community, and societal conditions (Meleis et al., 2000): Socioeconomic status can influence selection of pain management strategies; community resources can influence support for pain management; and societal conditions can make women's pain experience different from that of men.

**Induction Through a Literature Review and a Research Study.** To develop STOP, a systematic integrated literature review was conducted and used as a source for theorizing. PubMed was searched for the years of 1995 to 2000 using key words of Caucasian, White, cancer, pain, and/or experience. A total of 114 articles were included in the literature review (78 retrieved articles and 36 from the reference lists of the retrieved articles). All the articles were sorted by the major concepts of STOP. The literature review findings were analyzed and incorporated into the theorizing process.

In addition to the literature review, findings of a study on cancer pain that developed a decision support computer program for cancer pain management (DSCP study; Im, Guevara, & Chee, 2007; Im, Liu, Clark, & Chee, 2008; Im, Liu, Kim, & Chee, 2008; Im, Chee, et al., 2007; Im et al., 2009) were used as a source for theorizing. The overall purpose of the study was to explore gender and ethnic differences in cancer pain experience among 480 cancer patients from four major ethnic groups in the United States. The study included a quantitative Internet survey and four qualitative ethnic-specific online forums. Multiple measurement scales, including questions on sociodemographic characteristics and health/illness status, three unidimensional cancer pain scales, two multi-dimensional cancer pain scales, the Memorial Symptom Assessment Scale, and the Functional Assessment of Cancer Therapy Scale—General, were used for the quantitative Internet survey. Nine online forum topics were used for the qualitative online forums. The quantitative data were analyzed using descriptive and inferential statistics including analysis of variance (ANOVA) and hierarchical multiple regression analyses, and the qualitative data were analyzed using a thematic analysis.

The relationships among the five major concepts of STOP (Im, 2006) are the nature of transition, transition conditions, patterns of response, Caucasian cancer patients' pain experience, and nursing therapeutics. These five concepts are basically those of the Transitions Theory except the concept of Caucasian cancer patients' pain experience, the focus of STOP. Through the literature review and the findings of the DSCP study, all major concepts are confirmed to impact Caucasian cancer patients' pain experience. For instance, the nature (terminal or chronic) of transitions influences Caucasian cancer patients' pain experience. Cancer patients' religion can influence the patients' attitudes toward pain, which subsequently influences their pain experience.

**Uniqueness of STOP.** Compared with the middle range Transitions Theory, STOP has unique subconcepts (under the major concepts), which are frequently ethnic-specific. For example, although cancer experience could be a health/illness transition that all ethnic groups go through in a common way, most Caucasian cancer patients tend to perceive the health/illness transition as a highly individualistic transition. In other words, depending on individual situations, they perceive health/illness transitions differently. Some experience horrible pain during the transition, while others rarely notice pain. Similarly, under the concept of patterns of response, the STOP has several ethnic-specific sub-concepts such as control and transcendence. In the DSCP study, many patients thought they did not have control of their pain and/or disease and needed to bear the experience. On the contrary, others tried to control their pain and/or disease by selecting a specific healthcare provider whom they wanted to work with. In the DSCP study, the participants tried to transcend their cancer and cancer pain experience by "living life to the fullest" or by "not sweating the small things" (Im, 2006, p. 242). Because of these ethnic-specific subconcepts, STOP can be directly applied in nursing research and practice for Caucasian cancer patients' pain experience.

## THE SITUATION-SPECIFIC THEORY OF PAIN EXPERIENCE FOR ASIAN AMERICAN CANCER PATIENTS

The SPEAC (Im, 2008) was also derived from Transitions Theory. An integrative approach was used to develop the SPEAC. The theoretical development started from the following multiple assumptions: There is diversity and complexity in cancer pain experience; theory development is cyclic and evolutionary; the pain experience of Asian American cancer patients occurs in specific sociopolitical contexts; and a feminist nursing perspective is different from other perspectives. The SPEAC was developed using the following multiple sources: Transitions Theory, an integrative literature review, and research findings from a research study focused on cancer pain.

**Deduction From Transitions Theory.** Transitions Theory was used for the development of the SPEAC primarily because Asian American cancer patients' pain experience can be easily linked to the health/illness transition. Also, the major concepts of Transitions Theory are appropriate for a theory about the pain experience of Asian American cancer patients. For example, Asian American cancer patients' pain experience could be linked to their health/illness transition. Transitions Theory has a major concept of properties of transitions that includes awareness, engagement, change and difference, time span, and critical points and events (Meleis et al., 2000). All these properties can be easily linked to Asian American cancer patients' pain experience (Im, 2008). For example, Asian American cancer patients have an awareness of their health/illness transition, are engaged in the diagnosis and treatment process during the transition, experience changes in their physical, psychological, and social selves due to the health/illness transition, and have specific critical points in their transition process (e.g., diagnosis as a start point of the transition, death or ultimate survival as an ending point of the transition; Im, 2008).

**Induction Through a Literature Review and a Research Study.** A systematic integrated literature review was conducted to provide the basis for theorizing. First, the literature was searched through PubMed from 1998 to 2008 with the key words of Asian American, cancer pain, and experience; Asian American, cancer, and pain; and Asian American and cancer. There were 24 retrieved articles and 15 additional articles from the reference lists of the retrieved articles. All the articles were sorted by the major concepts that were the focus of the SPEAC, and major findings were analyzed and incorporated into the theory development process.

The findings of the DSCP study were also used as the basis for the theorizing process of the SPEAC. As mentioned earlier, the overall goal of the DSCP study was to explore differences in cancer pain experience by gender and ethnicity. The study was conducted among 480 cancer patients from four major ethnic groups in the United States using multiple measurement scales and nine online forum topics. Then data were analyzed using descriptive and inferential statistics and a thematic analysis. Only the findings among Asian American cancer patients were the focus of the SPEAC.

The SPEAC includes five major concepts (Im, 2008): (a) the nature of transition, (b) transition conditions, (c) patterns of response, (d) Asian American cancer patients' pain experience, and (e) nursing therapeutics. These major concepts are identical to those of the Transitions Theory except for the concept of Asian American cancer patients' pain experience. All major concepts were found to influence Asian American cancer patients' pain experience in the literature review or in the DSCP study findings. The nature of transitions (terminal or chronic) can influence Asian American cancer patients' pain experience. Transition conditions such as background characteristics can also influence Asian American cancer patients' pain experience; for example, cancer patients' gender can influence the patients' cultural attitudes toward pain, which subsequently influences pain experience in their unique culture.

**Uniqueness of the SPEAC.** The unique aspects of the SPEAC compared to the Transitions Theory are the subconcepts (under the major concepts) that are ethnic-specific. For example, although cancer experience is a universal health/illness transition, most Asian American cancer patients tend to experience the health/illness transition with a situational transition (immigration transition), which is a unique aspect of the SPEAC. Similarly, under the major concept of transition conditions, the SPEAC includes several ethnic-specific subconcepts such as being Asian American, country of birth, and subethnicity. Finally, the major concept of pattern of response includes ethnic-specific subconcepts such as tolerance, natural, normal, and mind control. In the DSCP study, Asian American cancer patients tended to tolerate pain instead of treating it aggressively.

They also tended to consider their pain experience natural, and they tried to normalize or minimize their conditions to overcome cultural stigma attached to cancer. Many of them also tried to manage their pain through mind control by having a strong will, hope, and positive thinking. These ethnic-specific subconcepts give the SPEAC the power to uniquely explain Asian American cancer patients' pain experience, and the SPEAC can be directly applied to nursing research or practice related to Asian Americans' cancer pain experience.

THE SITUATION-SPECIFIC THEORY OF ASIAN IMMIGRANT WOMEN'S MENOPAUSAL SYMPTOM EXPERIENCE IN THE UNITED STATES

The AIMS (Im, 2010; Im, Lee, & Chee, 2010, 2011) was also derived from Transitions Theory. The AIMS was developed using an integrative approach like STOP and SPEAC. The theorizing process began with multiple assumptions of theorizing (Im, 2010, p. 145):

- There are diversities and complexities in Asian immigrant women's menopausal symptom experience.
- The theory development process is cyclical and evolutionary and occurs in specific sociopolitical contexts.
- The inadequate management of menopausal symptoms reported by Asian immigrant women stems from biology and women's continuous interactions with their environments.
- The menopausal symptom experience is influenced by ethnicity and thus significantly interacts with gender, race, and class to structure relationships among individuals.

**Deduction From the Transitions Theory.** The reason for developing the AIMS beginning with Transitions Theory was that Asian immigrant women's menopausal symptom experience could be linked to the health/illness and developmental transitions that they experience in their menopausal transition and to the situation transition due to their immigration from one country to another. The major concepts of Transitions Theory are relevant to a theory about Asian immigrant women's menopausal symptom experience. For example, Transitions Theory has a subconcept of critical points and events under a major concept of properties of transitions (Meleis et al., 2000). This subconcept can be easily linked to the nature of menopausal symptom experience that Asian immigrant women go through. For instance, women's menopausal symptom experience has a specific beginning point with physical and psychological changes and a specific ending point even though it can be vague for some women (Im, 2010).

**Induction Through a Literature Review and a Research Study.** A systematic integrated literature review was also conducted to provide the basis for theorizing. A literature search through PubMed, PsycINFO, and CINAHL for the past 5 years was conducted using various key words including midlife, women, menopause, symptom, Asian, immigrant, Chinese, Korean, Japanese, predictors, and/or factors. The literature review included a total of 75 articles written in English and published in nursing and clinical journals. The articles were sorted by the major foci of AIMS to explain the menopausal symptom experience of Asian immigrant women in the United States. Finally, the major findings of the retrieved articles were analyzed and incorporated into the AIMS theory.

A study on menopausal symptom experience of four major ethnic groups of midlife women in the United States (MOMS) provided another element of foundation for the AIMS (Im et al., 2011; Im, Lee, Chee, Brown, & Dormire, 2010; Im, Lee, Chee, Dormire, & Brown, 2010). The overall goal of the study was to explore ethnic differences in menopausal symptom experience among four major ethnic groups of midlife women in the United States (White, African American, Asian, and Hispanic). The study included a quantitative Internet survey and four qualitative ethnic-specific online forums. For the Internet survey, the questions on background, self-reported ethnic identity, and health and menopausal status and the Midlife Women's Symptom Index were used. For the online forums, seven online forum topics related to the menopausal symptom experience were used. The data analysis process included descriptive and inferential statistics including ANOVA and hierarchical multiple regression analyses for the Internet survey data and thematic analysis for the qualitative online forum data.

The AIMS includes three major concepts illustrated in Figure 12.2 (Im, 2010): (a) transition conditions, (b) patterns of response, and (c) nursing therapeutics. These major concepts came from the middle range theory of Transitions; however, the subconcepts under the major concepts are different for AIMS, the

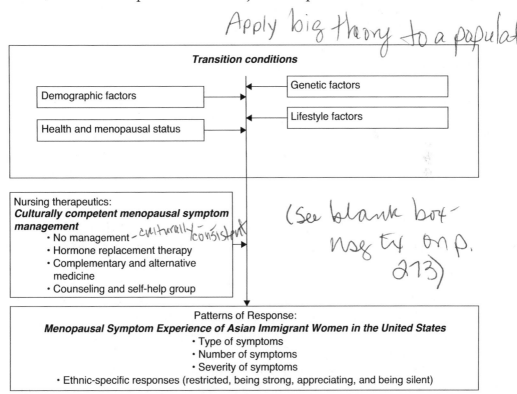

FIGURE 12.2 The Situation-Specific Theory of Asian Immigrant Women's Menopausal Symptom Experience in the United States.

*Source:* Reprinted with permission from Im, E. O. (2010). A situation specific theory of Asian immigrant women's menopausal symptom experience in the U.S. *Advances in Nursing Science, 33*(2), 143–157.

Situation-Specific Theory. Transition conditions include four subconcepts: (a) demographic factors, (b) genetic factors, (c) health and menopausal status, and (d) lifestyle factors.

The subconcepts under the pattern of response for AIMS include the type, number, and severity of symptoms, and ethnic-specific response to menopausal transition. Process and outcome indicators are not separated because they tend to be mingled in the symptom experience. For instance, the types of symptoms (e.g., hot flash) experienced during the menopausal transition could indicate both the process of menopausal transition and the outcome of the menopausal transition. The subconcept of ethnic-specific response includes four major themes from the MOMS study: restricted, being strong, appreciating, and being silent. In the MOMS study, women perceived certain restrictions in their menopausal symptom experience; for example, women perceived some restrictions given that their cultural heritage limits behaviors, emotions, and actions related to menopausal symptom experience. Women thought that the difficulties in their menopausal transition were nothing compared with what they had gone through with their immigration transition and that they became strong and faced their menopausal transition without problems. Women also considered menopause a relief and benefit because they would not need to worry about potential pregnancies or purchase feminine products for their menstrual periods. Finally, women considered silence the best strategy to cope with their menopausal symptoms. The concept of nursing therapeutics includes the following subconcepts: no management, hormone replacement therapy, complementary and alternative therapies, and counseling and self-help groups (Im, 2010). Finally, transition conditions influence menopausal symptom experience and nursing therapeutics to intervene and influence (enhance/worsen) the menopausal symptom experience of Asian immigrant women in the United States.

**Uniqueness of the AIMS.** The AIMS is unique from the middle range theory of Transitions because the specific subconcepts can be applied only to Asian immigrant women in menopausal transition. For example, menopausal transition could be a universal health/illness transition, but Asian immigrant women's menopausal transition is different from other ethnic groups because of their unique cultural attitudes and values related to women's health and menopausal symptoms. Thus, AIMS includes several ethnic-specific subconcepts such as responses like restricted, being strong, appreciating, and being silent. As in the SPEAC, these ethnic-specific subconcepts give AIMS the power to explain the menopausal symptom experience of Asian immigrant women in the United States. Also, the ethnic specificity makes the AIMS directly applicable to nursing research and practice with Asian immigrant women in the United States.

# ▨ USE OF THE THEORY IN NURSING RESEARCH

Transitions Theory has been nationally and internationally used in research studies across a broad spectrum of life transitions (Davies, 2005; Weiss et al., 2007). In addition, the theory was often used as the parent theory for situation-specific theories (Im, 2006; Im & Meleis, 1999a; Schumacher et al., 1999). The theory has been translated for use in Sweden, Taiwan, and many other countries (Im, 2009). After testing Transitions Theory in her investigation of transition experience of relatives related to older people's move to nursing homes, Davies (2005) concluded that the nature of transitions, transition conditions, and patterns of response could be helpful in explaining diverse factors that influence each person's transition and his or her unique experience. Weiss et al. (2007) concluded that their study findings supported Transitions Theory as a useful theoretical basis for conceptualizing and investigating predictors and outcomes of adult medical–surgical patients' perceptions of their readiness for hospital discharge. In addition, Weiss and Lokken (2009) concluded that Transitions Theory was a useful basis to determine predictors and outcomes of postpartum mothers' perceived readiness for hospital discharge. In 2015, there was an international conference dedicated to Transitions Theory in Japan. Based on the thoughts and discussion from the conference, a special issue dedicated to Transitions Theory was published in the *Japanese Journal of Nursing Research* in March–April, 2016.

In a relatively recent review on situation-specific theories (Im, 2014b), Transitions Theory was the most frequently used parent theory of situation-specific theories. In 2007, Meleis (2007) envisioned that many situation-specific theories could be developed based on Transitions Theory, which actually happened during the past decade. During the past decade, nine situation-specific theories were developed based on the middle range Transitions Theory, theorists' own research studies, and/or integrated literature reviews on existing research studies (Im, 2014a). They include the situation-specific theories of: Migration Transition for Migrant Farmworker Women (Clingerman, 2007); Transition to Adult Day Health Services (Bull & McShane, 2008); Guiding Interventions for People with Heart Failure (Davidson, Dracup, Phillips, Padilla, & Daly, 2007); Care Transitions (Geary & Schumacher, 2012); Well-being in Refugee Women Experiencing Cultural Transition (Baird, 2012); Pain Experience for Asian American Cancer Patients (Im, 2008); Caucasian Cancer Patients' Pain Experience (Im, 2006); and Asian Immigrant Women's Menopausal Symptom Experience (Im, 2010; Im et al., 2010, 2011). This capability to readily generate situation-specific theories from the middle range theory of Transitions is a big contrast to other theories; it may reflect higher usability and applicability of the middle range theory of Transitions for nursing practice and research.

# ■ USE OF THE THEORY IN NURSING PRACTICE

Transitions Theory has been widely used in nursing practice for people across unique health-related transitions, including illness, recovery, birth, death, loss, and immigration (Meleis & Trangenstein, 1994). It has been used with geriatric populations, psychiatric populations, maternal populations, family caregivers, menopausal women, Alzheimer's patients, immigrant women, and people with chronic illness (Aroian & Prater, 1988; Brackley, 1992; Im, 1997; Kaas & Rousseau, 1983; Schumacher et al., 1993; Shaul, 1997). The theory has provided a comprehensive perspective on the nature and type of transitions, transition conditions, and process and outcome indicators of patterns of response to transitions. In addition, the theory can be used to develop nursing therapeutics that are congruent with the unique experience of clients and their families, to facilitate healthy successful transitions.

# ■ USE OF THE THEORY IN NURSING EDUCATION

Other than clinical practice, Transitions Theory has been nationally and internationally used in nursing education (Meleis, personal communication, December 29, 2011). It has been incorporated into university nursing curricula (Meleis, personal communication, January 2008), including the University of Connecticut and Clayton State University in Morrow, Georgia. At UCSF, Meleis taught an independent graduate elective course on transitions and health to address student learning needs and requests of graduate students. In 2007, a center called Transitions and Health was established at the University of Pennsylvania (Mary Naylor, Director), which is the first center of its kind based on Transitions Theory. In addition, Transitions Theory has been used in a number of doctoral dissertations.

# ■ CONCLUSION

The middle range theory of Transitions has evolved from a borrowed perspective—through research studies and international and national collaborative works—and from the mentoring process. The theory has been developed based on multiple sources including research studies among diverse groups of people in various types of transitions. An increasing number of situation-specific theories have been derived from the middle range theory of Transitions. Also, Transitions Theory has guided nursing education and practice in current healthcare systems that are characterized by diversities and complexities. However, as Meleis et al. (2000, p. 27) mentioned nearly two decades ago, Transitions Theory needs to be further developed, tested, and refined. Transitions Theory could be further developed through research studies, nursing practice, and nursing education. The recent book chapter by Meleis (2015) could be an example of further development of the middle range Transitions Theory through theoretical deduction. Yet, the theory still needs to be further refined and tested to explain the major concepts and relationships among the major concepts with diverse populations in both common human transitions and unique health transitions. This testing will increase the theory's explanatory and predictive power. Most of all, future studies need to specifically aim to develop and test interventions based on the theory, through which it will gain prescriptive power to direct nursing practice.

## ■ REFERENCES

Aroian, K., & Prater, M. (1988). Transitions entry groups: Easing new patients' adjustment to psychiatric hospitalization. *Hospital and Community Psychiatry*, *39*, 312–313.

Baird, M. B. (2012). Well-being in refugee women experiencing cultural transition. *Advances in Nursing Science*, *35*(3), 249–263. doi:10.1097/ANS.0b013e31826260c0

Brackley, M. H. (1992). A role supplementation group pilot study: A nursing therapy for potential parental caregivers. *Clinical Nurse Specialist*, *6*(1), 14–19.

Budman, C. L., Lipson, J. G., & Meleis, A. I. (1992). The cultural consultant in mental health care: The case of an Arab adolescent. *The American Journal of Orthopsychiatry*, *62*(3), 359–370.

Bull, M. J., & McShane, R. E. (2008). Seeking what's best during the transition to adult day health services. *Qualitative Health Research*, *18*(5), 597–605. doi:10.1177/1049732308315174

Chick, N., & Meleis, A. I. (1986). Transitions: A nursing concern. In P. L. Chin (Ed.), *Nursing research methodology: Issues and implantation* (pp. 237–257). Gainsburg, MD: Aspen.

Chinn, P. (2012). Transitions: A core nursing concept. *Advances in Nursing Science*, *35*(3), 191.

Clingerman, E. (2007). A situation-specific theory of migration transition for migrant farmworker women. *Research and Theory for Nursing Practice*, *21*(4), 220–235.

Davidson, P. M., Dracup, K., Phillips, J., Padilla, G., & Daly, J. (2007). Maintaining hope in transition: a theoretical framework to guide interventions for people with heart failure. *Journal of Cardiovascular Nursing*, *22*(1), 58–64.

Davies, S. (2005). Meleis's theory of nursing transitions and relatives' experiences of nursing home entry. *Journal of Advanced Nursing*, *52*(6), 658–671.

Dracup, K., Meleis, A. I., Clark, S., Clyburn, A., Shields, L., & Staley, M. (1985). Group counseling in cardiac rehabilitation: Effect on patient compliance. *Patient Education and Counseling*, *6*(4), 169–177.

Gaffney, K. F. (1992). Nurse practice-model for maternal role sufficiency. *Advances in Nursing Sciences*, *15*(2), 76–84.

Geary, C. R., & Schumacher, K. L. (2012). Care transitions: integrating transition theory and complexity science concepts. *Advances in Nursing Science, 35*(3), 236–248. doi:10.1097/ANS.0b013e31826260a5

Im, E.-O. (1997). *Negligence and ignorance of menopause within gender multiple transition context: Low income Korean immigrant women* (Unpublished doctoral dissertation). University of California, San Francisco, CA.

Im, E.-O. (2006). A situation-specific theory of Caucasian cancer patients' pain experience. *Advances in Nursing Science, 29*(3), 232–244.

Im, E.-O. (2008). The situation specific theory of pain experience for Asian-American cancer patients. *Advances in Nursing Science, 31*(4), 319–331.

Im, E.-O. (2009). Afaf Ibrahim Meleis: Transition theory. In M. R. Alligood & A. M. Tomey (Eds.), *Nursing theorists and their work* (7th ed., pp. 416–433). St. Louis, MO: Mosby.

Im, E.-O. (2010). A situation specific theory of Asian immigrant women's menopausal symptom experience in the U.S. *Advances in Nursing Science, 33*(2), 143–157.

Im, E.-O. (2011). Transitions theory: A trajectory of theoretical development in nursing. *Nursing Outlook, 59*(5), 278–285.

Im, E.-O. (2014a). Situation-specific theories from the middle-range transitions theory. *Advances in Nursing Science, 37*(1), 19–31. doi:10.1097/ANS.0000000000000014

Im, E.-O. (2014b). The status quo of situation-specific theories. *Research and Theory for Nursing Practice, 28*(4), 278–298.

Im, E.-O., Chee, W., Guevara, E., Liu, Y., Lim, H. J., Tsai, H., . . . Shin, H. (2007). Gender and ethnic differences in cancer pain experience: A multiethnic survey in the U.S. *Nursing Research, 56*(5), 296–306.

Im, E.-O., Guevara, E., & Chee, W. (2007). The pain experience of Hispanic patients with cancer in the United States. *Oncology Nursing Forum, 34*(4), 861–868.

Im, E.-O., Lee, B. I., Chee, W., Brown, A., & Dormire, S. (2010). Menopausal symptoms among four major ethnic groups in the United States. *Western Journal of Nursing Research, 32*(4), 540–565.

Im, E.-O., Lee, B. I., Chee, W., Dormire, S., & Brown, A. (2010). A national multiethnic online forum study on menopausal symptom experience. *Nursing Research, 59*(1), 26–33.

Im, E.-O., Lee, S. H., & Chee, W. (2010). Subethnic differences in the menopausal symptom experience of Asian American midlife women. *Journal of Transcultural Nursing, 21*(2), 123–133.

Im, E.-O., Lee, S. H., & Chee, W. (2011). "Being conditioned, yet becoming strong": Asian American women in menopausal transition. *Journal of Transcultural Nursing, 22*(3), 290–299.

Im, E.-O., Lee, S. H., Liu, Y., Lim, H. J., Guevara, H., & Chee, W. (2009). A national online forum on ethnic differences in cancer pain experience. *Nursing Research, 58*(2), 86–94.

Im, E.-O., Liu, H. J., Clark, M., & Chee, W. (2008). African-American cancer patients' pain experience. *Cancer Nursing, 31*(1), 38–46.

Im, E.-O., Liu, Y., Kim, Y. H., & Chee, W. (2008). Asian–American cancer patients' pain experience. *Cancer Nursing, 31*(3), E17–E23.

Im, E.-O., & Meleis, A. I. (1999a). Situation-specific theories: Philosophical roots, properties, and approach. *Advances in Nursing Science, 22*(2), 11–24.

Im, E.-O., & Meleis, A. I. (1999b). A situation-specific theory of Korean immigrant women's menopausal transition. *Journal of Nursing Scholarship, 31*(4), 333–338.

Im, E.-O., & Meleis, A. I. (2000). Meanings of menopause: Low-income Korean immigrant women. *Western Journal of Nursing Research, 22*(1), 84–102.

Im, E.-O., Meleis, A. I., & Lee, K. (1999). Symptom experience of low-income Korean immigrant women during menopausal transition. *Women and Health, 29*(2), 53–67.

Jones, P. S., Zhang, X. E., & Meleis, A. I. (1978). Transforming vulnerability. *Western Journal of Nursing Research, 25*(7), 835–853.

Kaas, M. J., & Rousseau, G. K. (1983). Geriatric sexual conformity: Assessment and intervention. *Clinical Gerontologist, 2*(1), 31–44.

Laffrey, S. C., Meleis, A. I., Lipson, J. G., Solomon, M., & Omidian, P. A. (1989). Assessing Arab-American health care needs. *Social Science and Medicine, 29*(7), 877–883.

Lane, S. D., & Meleis, A. I. (1991). Roles, work, health perceptions, and health resources of women: A study in an Egyptian delta hamlet. *Social Science and Medicine, 33*(10), 1197–1208.

Lipson, J. G., & Meleis, A. I. (1983). Issues in health care of Middle Eastern patients. *Western Journal of Medicine, 139*(6), 854–861.

Lipson, J. G., & Meleis, A. I. (1985). Culturally appropriate care: The case of immigrants. *Topics in Clinical Nursing, 7*(3), 48–56.

Lipson, J. G., Reizian, A. E., & Meleis, A. I. (1987). Arab-American patients: A medical record review. *Social Science and Medicine, 24*(2), 101–107.

May, K. M., & Meleis, A. I. (1987). International nursing: Guidelines for core content. *Nurse Educator, 12*(5), 36–40.

Meleis, A. I. (1975). Role insufficiency and role supplementation: A conceptual framework. *Nursing Research, 24*, 264–271.

Meleis, A. I. (1981). The Arab American in the health care system. *American Journal of Nursing, 81*(6), 1180–1183.

Meleis, A. I. (1997). *Theoretical nursing: Development and progress* (3rd ed.). Philadelphia, PA: Lippincott Williams & Wilkins.

Meleis, A. I. (2007). *Theoretical nursing: Development and progress* (4th ed.). Philadelphia, PA: Lippincott Williams & Wilkins.

Meleis, A. I. (Ed.) (2010). *Transitions theory: Middle range and situation specific theories in nursing research and practice.* New York, NY: Springer Publishing.

Meleis, A. I. (2015). Transitions theory. In M. C. Smith & M. E. Parker (Eds.), *Nursing theories and nursing practice* (4th ed., pp. 361–380). Philadelphia, PA: F. A. Davis.

Meleis, A. I., Arruda, E. N., Lane, S., & Bernal, P. (1994). Veiled, voluminous, and devalued: Narrative stories about low-income women from Brazil, Egypt, and Colombia. *Advances in Nursing Science, 17*(2), 1–15.

Meleis, A. I., Douglas, M. K., Eribes, C., Shih, F., & Messias, D. K. (1996). Employed Mexican women as mothers and partners: Valued, empowered, and overloaded. *Journal of Advanced Nursing, 23*(1), 82–90.

Meleis, A. I., Kulig, J., Arruda, E. N., & Beckman, A. (1990). Maternal role of women in clerical jobs in southern Brazil: Stress and satisfaction. *Health Care for Women International*, *11*(4), 369–382.

Meleis, A. I., & La Fever, C. W. (1984). The Arab American and psychiatric care. *Perspectives in Psychiatric Care*, *22*(2), 72–76.

Meleis, A. I., Lipson, J., & Dallafar, A. (1998). The reluctant immigrant: Immigration experiences among Middle Eastern groups in Northern California. In D. Baxter & R. Krulfeld (Eds.), *Beyond boundaries: Selected papers on refugees and immigrants* (Vol. V, pp. 214–230). Arlington, VA: American Anthropological Association.

Meleis, A. I., Mahidal, V. T., Lin, J. Y., Minami, H., & Neves, E. P. (1987). International collaboration in research: Forces and constraints-by leaders from Thailand, People's Republic of China, Japan, and Brazil. *Western Journal of Nursing Research*, *9*(3), 390–399.

Meleis, A. I., & Rogers, S. (1987). Women in transition: being vs. becoming or being and becoming. *Health Care for Women International*, *8*, 199–217.

Meleis, A. I., Sawyer, L., Im, E., Schumacher, K., Messias, D., & Schumacher, K. (2000). Experiencing transitions: An emerging middle range theory. *Advances in Nursing Science*, *23*(1), 12–28.

Meleis, A. I., & Sorrell, L. (1981). Bridging cultures. Arab American women and their birth experiences. *American Journal of Maternal and Child Nursing*, *6*(3), 171–176.

Meleis, A. I., & Swendsen, L. (1978). Role supplementation: An empirical test of a nursing intervention. *Nursing Research*, *27*, 11–18.

Meleis, A. I., Swendsen, L., & Jones, D. (1980). Preventive role supplementation: A grounded conceptual framework. In M. H. Miller & B. Flynn (Eds.), *Current perspectives in nursing: Social issues and trends* (Vol. 2, pp. 3–14). St. Louis, MO: Mosby.

Meleis, A. I., & Trangenstein, P. A. (1994). Facilitating transitions: Re-definition of the nursing mission. *Nursing Outlook*, *42*, 255–259.

Schumacher, K. L., Dodd, M. J., & Paul, S. M. (1993). The stress process in family caregivers of persons receiving chemotherapy. *Research in Nursing & Health*, *16*, 395–404.

Schumacher, K. L., Jones, P. S., & Meleis, A. I. (1999). Helping elderly persons in transition: A framework for research and practice. In L. Swanson & T. Tripp-Reimer (Eds.), *Advances in gerontological nursing: Life transitions in the older adult* (Vol. 3, pp. 1–26). New York, NY: Springer Publishing.

Schumacher, K. L., & Meleis, A. I. (1994). Transitions: A central concept in nursing. *Image: Journal of Nursing Scholarship*, *26*(2), 119–127.

Shaul, M. P. (1997). Transition in chronic illness: Rheumatoid arthritis in women. *Rehabilitation Nursing*, *22*, 199–205.

Shih, F. J., Meleis, A. I., Yu, P. J., Hu, W. Y., Lou, M. F., & Huang, G. S. (1998). Taiwanese patients' concerns and coping strategies: Transitions to cardiac surgery. *Heart and Lung*, *27*(2), 82–98.

Stevens, P. E., Hall, J. M., & Meleis, A. I. (1992). Examining vulnerability of women clerical workers from five ethnic/racial groups. *Western Journal of Nursing Research*, *14*(6), 754–774.

Weiss, M. E., & Lokken, L. (2009). Predictors and outcomes of postpartum mothers' perceptions of readiness for discharge after birth. *Journal of Gynecological and Neonatal Nursing, 38*(4), 406–417.

Weiss, M. E., Piacentine, L. B., Lokken, L., Ancona, J., Archer, J., Gresser, S., . . . Vega-Stromberg, T. (2007). Perceived readiness for hospital discharge in adult medical-surgical patients. *Clinical Nurse Specialist, 21*(1), 31–42.

# CHAPTER 13

## Theory of Self-Reliance

**John Lowe**

Growing up Cherokee has everything to do with my understanding of self-reliance. Being one of 22 doctoral prepared Native American nurses in the United States provides another perspective of who I am. The historical context of my people has shaped me and my scholarly work.

Cherokee historians, scholars, and tribal leaders have noted that the historical background and distinct culture of the Cherokee should be known in order to understand and respect the Cherokee today (Henson, 2001; Mooney, 1975; Perdue, 1989). Historically, the Cherokee were the mountaineers of the South. They considered themselves inheritors of a dignity beyond their simple means and referred to themselves as the "principle people" (Ehle, 1988). The way of life and roles for them began to change under the new federal government of George Washington. Most of the land owned by the Cherokee was taken away through government treaties and force of arms. The federal government also established the Indian Boarding Schools where the language and practice of traditions were prohibited. This restriction was done in an attempt to strip the Native American of his or her identity.

It is important to me that Cherokee identity shines through in this chapter on the middle range theory of Self-Reliance. The theory arose from Cherokee values and the work is being shared because I think these core values have meaning for the broader population of Native American people as well as indigenous people throughout the world. In fact, the values that I learned as a Cherokee have the potential to affect health for populations beyond Native American and indigenous people.

### ■ PURPOSE OF THE THEORY AND HOW IT WAS DEVELOPED

Self-reliance has been noted by Native American leaders to be the mainstay and way of life that influence the health among Native American people (Tyler, 1973). Additionally, self-reliance has been recognized as a key variable for keeping Cherokees in balance (Stuart, 1993). The history of the Cherokee has continued to affect the physical, emotional, psychosocial, economic, and spiritual well-being of the people. Formal and informal leaders and tribal members of Cherokee communities have expressed concern about the lack of self-reliance among their members. Historical events are viewed as undermining self-reliance, which in turn decreases well-being. The purpose of the middle range theory of Self-Reliance is to articulate a process for promoting well-being with attention to appreciation for one's culture.

Growing up Cherokee, I observed that Native American people who became disconnected from the culture were plagued with health problems. These observations were the foundation of my commitment to make a difference for my people. My father, who stayed connected and grounded in Cherokee values, often said: "The Cherokee way is best." I later came to understand that self-reliance characterized the Cherokee way. Then, in my PhD program, I conducted an ethnographic study to understand the meaning of self-reliance for Cherokee people and how it was exhibited in daily life (Lowe, 2002b). A follow-up ethnographic study was conducted to explore how self-reliance was characterized and achieved during adolescence particularly among Cherokee males (Lowe, 2003). The three concepts of the Self-Reliance Theory, being responsible, disciplined, and confident, were the themes that emerged from these studies. The self-reliance instrument was developed based on these concepts (Lowe, 2006).

## Foundational Literature

The knowledge of the historical background and distinct culture of Native Americans has been noted as important to increase the understanding of this group today (Henson, 2001). Historically, the Cherokee inhabited the southeast region of the United States that now includes the states of Virginia, West Virginia, Tennessee, Kentucky, North Carolina, South Carolina, Georgia, and Alabama (Mooney, 1982). The way of life and roles of the Cherokee and most Native Americans changed dramatically as a result of the dispossession of land and culture through government treaties and force of arms. The establishment of the Indian Boarding Schools was among the events that undermined self-reliance of Native Americans. The traditional dress and speaking the tribal language were prohibited in an attempt to strip Native Americans of their identity. The physical, emotional, psychosocial, economic, and spiritual well-being of the Cherokee continues to be impacted today by prohibitions enforced decades ago.

Self-reliance is a concept within the Cherokee holistic worldview where all things are believed to come together to form a whole (Altman & Belt, 2008). Cherokee tribal leaders have noted self-reliance to be the mainstay and way of life that influences the health of the Cherokee people, helping them to find and keep balance (Henson, 2001; Stuart, 1993).

Social change has been widespread in Native American populations, challenging the traditional way of life, values, and relational systems. The Native American family is changing rapidly as family members must now work outside the home, threatening the closeness of the family, in contrast to earlier years when families worked closely together to survive in a hostile environment (Frank, Moore, & Ames, 2000). Many Cherokee elders and tribal leaders report that the interdependence (Cherokee self-reliance) of the family, clan, and the tribe of earlier years has eroded (Lowe, 2002a), leading to stress-related health outcomes. Stress and coping processes have been reported to play an important role in physical and mental health outcomes among Native Americans (Walters & Simoni, 2002). For instance, Native American youth have significantly greater emotional distress than their White peers, and much of their distress is related to social and cultural factors (Bergstrom, Miller, & Peacock, 2003).

## Assumptions

The cultural themes that constitute the assumptions of the theory are "being true to oneself" and "being connected." These assumptions cut across all the three concepts of self-reliance. The first assumption, "being true to oneself," refers to acknowledging one's heritage and living in keeping with the worldview of one's culture. The worldview of the Cherokee that provides the roots for this theory is considered to be circular and holistic where all things are believed to come together to form a whole (Altman & Belt, 2008). The second assumption, "being connected," refers to identifying and utilizing resources within creation. According to this dimension of the worldview, each person is a resource within the creation. The gifts and talents of each person will benefit not only the person but also the family, community, and cultural group. One identifies and utilizes his or her own gifts and talents and those of others.

## ■ CONCEPTS OF THE THEORY

Self-reliance is being true to self and is lived by being responsible, disciplined, and confident while staying connected to one's cultural roots. The three concepts of self-reliance are (a) being responsible, (b) being disciplined, and (c) being confident.

**Being responsible** is being accountable to care for self and to care for others by getting assistance, respecting self, respecting others, and respecting the Creator. Respecting others occurs by being dependable and accountable. Honoring traditions, values, and language is a way to respect the Creator. The Creator in this context is the life force that grounds a sense of self.

**Being disciplined** is setting goals and pursuing goals by taking the initiative to make decisions and taking risks necessary to achieve goals. After decisions are made and goals are set, the pursuit of goals occurs by creating a plan, getting assistance, and redirecting one's effort.

**Being confident** refers to having a sense of identity and self-worth. Self-worth refers to knowing self within one's cultural heritage, being proud of one's heritage, and accepting cultural values and beliefs.

## ■ RELATIONSHIPS AMONG THE CONCEPTS: THE MODEL

The Model of Self-Reliance (Figure 13.1) depicts a pattern of interrelating circles in keeping with a holistic world view. The three interlocking circles in the center of the model describe the interrelatedness through intertwining and interlacing of the concepts.

## ■ USE OF THE THEORY IN NURSING RESEARCH

Lowe began a program of research focused on substance abuse in Native American communities while in graduate school at the master's level. His thesis research explored the social support that contributes to abstinence after substance-use treatment in the Native American young adult. The research identified the overall concept of self-reliance as the mainstay and way of life that influences the health and well-being of Native Americans. During his PhD

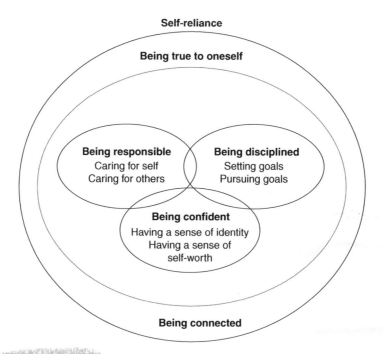

**FIGURE 13.1** Self-Reliance.

*Source:* Reprinted with permission from Lowe, J. (2003). The self-reliance of the Cherokee male adolescent. *Journal of Addictions Nursing*, *14*, 209–214.

studies, he continued to explore how the concept of self-reliance is defined by the Cherokee since self-reliance for the Cherokee had not been defined or researched previously. His PhD dissertation utilized the ethnographic method to identify how (a) self-reliance is conceptualized by the Cherokee; (b) the adult Cherokee perceives, achieves, and demonstrates self-reliance; and (c) nurses and healthcare professionals can incorporate the Cherokee concept of self-reliance in healthcare (Lowe, 2002b).

Lowe investigated the Cherokee adolescent's perception of self-reliance and its relationship to health (Lowe, 2003), finding that self-reliance was a way to keep the Cherokee from abusing drugs or alcohol. Participants in his studies reported a mentoring relationship, described as "being influenced," that is essential to enhance self-reliance (Lowe, 2005). The Cherokee Self-Reliance Model that emerged from the findings of these studies was used to guide the development of a series of intervention studies. A Cherokee self-reliance instrument was developed and tested in the intervention studies. The instrument is a 24-item questionnaire with a 5-point Likert scale. A reliability coefficient alpha of 0.84 was documented for the instrument when it was used with Cherokee adolescents (Lowe, 2006).

Lowe first conducted a pilot study funded by the Association of Nurses in AIDS Care/Biotech. The "Cherokee Teen Talking Circle" was evaluated for its effect on HIV/AIDS knowledge and attitudes as well as protective behaviors. Cherokee self-reliance was also measured as a variable in this pilot study. The participants included 41 high school students who completed a 2-hour Talking Circle intervention. Pretest to posttest scores on HIV/AIDS knowledge and attitudes and protective behaviors were studied with paired $t$ tests. There were significant differences in knowledge (pretest mean: 4.44 + 0.92; posttest mean: 4.83 + 0.38) and attitudes (pretest mean: 9.88 + 0.38; posttest mean: 10.68 + 1.31). Cherokee self-reliance and HIV/AIDS knowledge, attitude, and protective behavior at posttest was significantly ($p < .01$) correlated (knowledge [0.499]; attitude [0.421]; behavior [0.254]; Lowe, 2008). In addition, the Talking Circle was demonstrated to be a feasible cultural approach, resulting in meaningful participation with study participants.

In a postdoctoral study funded by the National Institute on Alcohol Abuse and Alcoholism (NIAAA) Minority Supplement to R01 AA 10246-05 S1 Teen Intervention Project (TIP), Lowe conducted a Talking Circle intervention to help adolescents address alcohol and substance abuse problems. The parent TIP research was built on the standardized Student Assistance Program (SAP). The SAP involved a 10-session motivational, skills-building group intervention, developed for use with eighth through 12th graders (Wagner & Waldron, 2001; Wagner, Drinklage, Cudworth, & Vyse, 1999). This group intervention utilized a traditional group setting, approach, and process. The core ideas of the SAP were merged with Cherokee values through the Talking Circle intervention to create the Teen Intervention Project—Cherokee (TIP-C; Lowe, 2006).

Findings of the pilot TIP-C research revealed that the average Drug Use Screening Inventory—Revised (DUSI-R) score of the TIP-C participants ($N$ = 108) reduced from 24.74 to 20.94 ($t = -13.82, p < .001$). The participants' average stress score also decreased from 43.60 at the baseline to 41.44 postintervention ($t = -6.41, p < .001$). By contrast, the participants' average Cherokee self-reliance score increased from 90.51 at baseline to 110.92 postintervention ($t = 26.97, p < .001$; Lowe, 2006). During each follow-up assessment, TIP-C participants were encouraged to write about the impact of the intervention. One participant, who completed his 1-year follow-up assessment, had been diagnosed and was receiving treatment for cancer at the time of his written feedback. He said: "I am so thankful that I went through the TIP-C groups . . . even though I have been very sick, this has been one of the best years of my life . . . I have been clean and sober and I now know what it means to live the Cherokee way."

Lowe conducted another 3-year study "Community Partnership to Affect Keetoowah–Cherokee Adolescent Substance Abuse" funded by the National Institute on Drug Abuse (NIDA; 1 R01 DA021714). A community-based participatory research (CBPR) approach was used to develop and test the culturally competent school-based intervention—Cherokee Talking Circle (CTC)—a revision of the TIP-C intervention. The difference in substance abuse, Cherokee self-reliance, and stress between Keetoowah–Cherokee adolescents who received the CTC prevention and those who received standard substance abuse education (SE) was evaluated. Findings revealed that higher self-reliance and less focus on self were related with the ability to express feelings, which was higher for those who scored higher on self-reliance. Substance abuse scores between the CTC and SE groups were significantly different (F = 13.14.10, $p < .001$) with the CTC group having lower substance abuse scores. There was also a significant interaction effect between time and group (F = 27.95, $p < .001$) with the greatest differences between the groups noted immediately after the intervention ($t = -3.89, p < .001$) and at the 3-month follow-up ($t = -4.69, p = .001$). At each time point, self-reliance was higher for the CTC group than the SE group and the difference between the groups increased over time (Lowe, Liang, Riggs, & Henson, 2012).

Lowe conducted a 2-year NIDA (R34DA029724) funded study to examine the feasibility of using the CTC for Native American sixth graders as they transition to middle school. In this study, results revealed a trend toward statistical significance. At 6 months postintervention, the CTC group had significantly lower substance involvement/interest scores than the SE control group. CTC substance abuse/use scores decreased from 2.3 to 1.3 ($t$ (33) = 1.8, $p = .007$). Cherokee self-reliance scores increased from 90.5 at baseline to 110.9 postintervention ($t = 26.97, p < .001$; Lowe, Liang, & Henson, 2016).

A 5-year NIDA (R01DA029779) funded study was recently conducted by Lowe and colleagues that was guided by the Self-Reliance Theory. This study tested a school-based, brief motivational intervention for substance abuse among Native American high school students. At the time when this study was conducted, there was no evidence from research concerning the use and effect of motivational interviewing among Native American youth guided by a cultural-specific theory such as the Self-Reliance Theory.

Lowe is currently conducting a NIDA/NIAAA funded (R01DA035143) project that proposes to evaluate an after-school substance abuse prevention intervention; the Intertribal Talking Circle (ITC), targeting sixth grade Native American youth in three tribal communities: Ojibwe/Chippewa in Minnesota, Choctaw in Oklahoma, and Lumbee in North Carolina. A CBPR approach is being used to culturally and technologically adapt the ITC as an innovative virtual Talking Circle intervention. A two-condition controlled study is being used to evaluate the efficacy of the ITC to increase Native American youth self-reliance while decreasing Native American youth substance-use involvement. An adult training program second-level intervention study is also being conducted to train tribal personnel from the three regional tribes on how to implement the ITC intervention as a tribal program beyond the study period. Effectiveness is being determined by a small partial crossover randomized trial comparing ITC intervention to a Wait-List Control (WLC) condition. Process evaluations are focusing on the future adoption and implementation of the ITC, and recommendations for sustainable adaptations. The project is also building Native American capacity to address health disparities, as experienced native investigators are mentoring three junior native investigators.

Lowe has collaborated with researchers nationally and internationally, sharing the self-reliance work and the community-based participatory approach that he uses for his research. For instance, he collaborated with Native American colleagues to expand the Cherokee Self-Reliance Model so that it is appropriate for other tribes, renaming the model "Native Self-Reliance." The Native Self-Reliance Model has been used to guide a study where the Talking Circle intervention was implemented with Plains tribal youth (Patchell, Lowe, Robbins, & Hoke, 2015). From an international perspective, Lowe has begun work with indigenous people in Australia (Aboriginal and Torres Straight Islanders), Canada (First Nation), New Zealand (Maori), and Panama (Kuna) who are interested in a community-based approach to research, the Self-Reliance Theory, and the process of using the Talking Circle. Australian, Canadian, New Zealand, and Panamanian colleagues recognize Lowe as a scholar who advocates for culturally competent healthcare of Native Americans and indigenous people globally. When in international settings, Lowe meets with indigenous nurses as well as community elders who seek his counsel.

## ■ USE OF THE THEORY IN NURSING PRACTICE

The Talking Circle is a meaningful approach to nursing practice. It is described here as it is lived in the Native American tradition. Nurses in practice are invited to consider how the Talking Circle may be used in other cultural traditions.

In the Native American tradition, a Talking Circle is a coming together and a place where stories are shared in a respectful manner and in a context of complete acceptance by participants. Native Americans have long used the circle to celebrate the sacred interrelationship that is shared with one another and with their world (Simpson, 2000). The idea of the Talking Circle permeates the traditions of Native Americans to this day. It symbolizes an entire approach to life and to the universe in which each being participates in the circle and each one serves an important and necessary function that is valued no more or no less than that of any other being.

By honoring the circle, human beings honor the process of life and the process of growth that is an ever-flowing stream in the movement of life energy (Garrett & Carroll, 2000). Cherokees consider the whole greater than the sum of its parts and have always believed that healing and transformation should take place in the presence of the group since they are all related to one another in very basic ways (Reed, 1993). Through use of the Talking Circle, Native Americans can use the support and insight of their brothers and sisters to move away from something, such as substance abuse, and toward something else. In this way, the Talking Circle has served a very sacred function of healing or cleansing, while also serving as a way of bringing people together.

The traditional sense of belonging and comfort provides healing for all and the circle reminds the Cherokee of life and their place in it (Ywahoo, 1987). Each person comes to the circle as a human being with his or her own concerns, and together participants seek harmony and balance by sharing stories, praying, singing, talking, and sometimes even just sitting together in silence.

## ■ USE OF THE THEORY IN NURSING EDUCATION

Lowe has long used the Talking Circle approach in his work with nursing students. Every semester he takes a group of students to tribal communities in Oklahoma to participate in a service learning cultural immersion experience where the Native American culture and community become the classroom. Self-reliance is threaded throughout this learning experience. The Talking Circle became a powerful teaching approach that emerged from the Self-Reliance Theory, offering opportunities for personal growth that extend beyond the community nursing content that is the focus for the course. Lowe and a former doctoral student conducted a study using the Talking Circle approach to gain a deeper understanding of what was learned and meaningful about the cultural immersion experience (Lowe & Cirilo, 2016). A Native American elder, leader, and cultural expert facilitated the Talking Circle sessions. The students who participated in the Native American cultural immersion experience and study were from various cultural backgrounds such as Caucasian, African American, Haitian, Hispanic/Latino, Middle Eastern, Asian, Caribbean, Russian, Irish, and South African. The Talking Circle approach for the study provided a setting that facilitated the nursing students to share openly and with ease concerning the cultural immersion experience. The nursing students shared how they were required to leave their work/job situations, school duties, families, and children behind during the cultural immersion experience in Oklahoma. This encouraged and allowed them to let go of their usual responsibilities and make themselves completely available for the experience. As a result, the nursing students described the experience as an opportunity to learn about others, teach them, grow with them, be with them, and to learn about themselves in a self-reliant way they have never experienced.

## ■ CONCLUSION

The Theory of Self-Reliance has roots in Native American culture and values. It has grown over time as a foundation guiding the Talking Circle intervention used in nursing research, practice, and education. The theory is strengthened by the existence of a psychometrically sound instrument that enables evaluation of self-reliance through self-report. The middle range theory of Self-Reliance in this chapter is an expression of invitation to nurses who may choose to use the theory for practice, research, and education. Use of the theory will honor the Native American people who cultivated self-reliance in the midst of unimaginable historical trauma. The theory is shared in a spirit of gratitude for the wisdom of ancestors and in a spirit of generosity, wishing to extend their wisdom to others who may benefit from the middle range theory of Self-Reliance.

## ■ REFERENCES

Altman, H. M., & Belt, T. N. (2008). Reading history: Cherokee history through a Cherokee lens. *Native South*, 1(1), 90–98.

Bergstrom, A., Miller, L., & Peacock, T. (2003). The seventh generation: Native students speak about finding the good path. Retrieved from https://eric.ed.gov/?id=ED472385

Ehle, J. (1988). *Trail of tears: The rise and fall of Cherokee Nation*. New York, NY: Doubleday.

Frank, J., Moore, R., & Ames, G. (2000). Historical and cultural roots of drinking problems among American Indians. *American Journal of Public Health*, 90(3), 344–350.

Garrett, M., & Carroll, J. (2000). Mending the broken circle: Treatment of substance dependence among Native Americans. *Journal of Counseling and Development*, 78(4), 379–388.

Henson, J. (2001). *Letter of research support*. Tahlequah, OK: United Keetoowah Band.

Lowe, J. (2002a). Balance and harmony through connectedness: The intentionality of Native American nurses. *Holistic Nursing Practice, 16*(4), 4–11.

Lowe, J. (2002b). Cherokee self-reliance. *Journal of Transcultural Nursing, 13*(4), 287–295.

Lowe, J. (2003). The self-reliance of the Cherokee adolescent male. *Journal of Addictions Nursing, 14*, 209–214.

Lowe, J. (2005). Being influenced: A Cherokee way of mentoring. *Journal of Cultural Diversity, 12*(2), 37–49.

Lowe, J. (2006). Teen intervention project–Cherokee (TIP-C). *Pediatric Nursing, 32*(5), 495–500.

Lowe, J. (2008). A cultural approach to conducting HIV/AIDS and HCV education among Native American adolescents. *Journal of School Nursing, 24*(4), 229–238.

Lowe, J., & Cirilo, R. (2016). The use of talking circles to describe a Native American transcultural caring immersion experience. *Journal of Holistic Nursing, 34*(3), 280–290.

Lowe, J., Liang, H., & Henson, J. (2016). Preventing substance use among Native American early adolescents. *Journal of Community Psychology, 44*(8), 997–1010.

Lowe, J., Liang, H., Riggs, C., & Henson, J. (2012). Community partnership to affect substance abuse among Native American adolescents. *The American Journal of Drug and Alcohol Abuse, 38*(5), 250–255.

Mooney, J. (1975). *Historical sketch of the Cherokee.* Chicago, IL: Aldine Publishing.

Mooney, J. (1982). *Myths of the Cherokee and sacred formulas of the Cherokee.* Nashville, TN: Charles and Randy Elder Publishers.

Patchell, B., Lowe, J., Robbins, L., & Hoke, M. K. (2015). The effect of a culturally tailored substance abuse prevention intervention with Plains Indian adolescents. *Journal of Cultural Diversity: An Interdisciplinary Journal, 22*(1), 3–8.

Perdue, T. (1989). *The Cherokee.* New York, NY: Chelsea House Publishers.

Reed, M. (1993). *Seven clans of the Cherokee society.* Cherokee, NC: Cherokee Publications.

Simpson, L. (2000). Stories, dreams, and ceremonies: Anishinaabe ways of learning. *Tribal College Journal of American Indian Higher Education, 11*(4), 26–29.

Stuart, D. (1993). *Letter of research support.* Tahlequah, OK: Cherokee Nation.

Tyler, S. L. (1973). *A history of Indian policy.* Washington, DC: U.S. Government Printing Office.

Wagner, E. F., Drinklage, S., Cudworth, C., & Vyse, J. (1999). A preliminary evaluation of the effectiveness of a standardized Student Assistance Program. *Substance Use and Misuse, 34*(11), 1571–1584.

Wagner, E. F., & Waldron, H. (Eds.). (2001). *Innovations in adolescent substance abuse intervention.* Oxford, UK: Pergamon.

Walters, K. L., & Simoni, J. M. (2002). Reconceptualizing Native women's health: An "indigenist" stress coping model. *American Journal of Public Health, 92*(4), 520–524.

Ywahoo, D. (1987). *Voices of our ancestors: Cherokee teachings from the wisdom fire.* Boston, MA: Shambala.

# CHAPTER 14

## Theory of Cultural Marginality

**Heeseung Choi**

As transportation and communication technology advance, there is a complementary increase in contacts between culturally distinct populations. The number of immigrants has continued to grow; as of 2015, about 13.5% (43.3 million) of the U.S. population was foreign-born (Migration Policy Institute, 2017). Approximately 16% of these immigrants reported entry since 2010 (Migration Policy Institute, 2017). Although society is becoming more and more ethnically and culturally diverse, the lack of mutual understanding between healthcare providers and clients from different cultural backgrounds remains a barrier to progress in healthcare services for immigrants. The Theory of Cultural Marginality was developed to increase understanding of the unique experiences of individuals who are straddling distinct cultures and to offer direction for providing culturally relevant care.

## ■ PURPOSE OF THE THEORY AND HOW IT WAS DEVELOPED

While working with immigrant adolescents and living in the United States as an immigrant, I noticed unique circumstances that immigrant adolescents encountered as a result of the immigration process and the impact of the process on their mental health. A review of related theories and research on immigrant adolescents' mental health issues provided the foundation for developing a program of research that began with Korean American adolescents. In a community-based study, I discovered that Korean American adolescents demonstrated significantly lower levels of self-esteem, coping skills, and mastery in addition to higher levels of depression and somatic symptoms than American adolescents (Choi, Stafford, Meininger, Roberts, & Smith, 2002). The response pattern was more prominent among foreign-born Koreans than U.S.-born Koreans. In a subsequent school-based study, compared with Whites, Asian and Hispanic American adolescents experienced higher levels of social stress and somatic symptoms and depression (Choi, Meininger, & Roberts, 2006). Among White, African, Hispanic, and Asian Americans, Asian American adolescents reported the lowest scores on self-esteem, coping, and family cohesiveness, and the highest score in family conflicts (Choi et al., 2006).

These findings led to an exploration of the reasons for the adolescents' vulnerability and to examining the stress of the immigration process as a significant risk factor for mental distress. The next step in building my program of research required an extensive literature review searching for theories that contributed to understanding how distress was associated with immigration for Asian American adolescents.

Theories contributing to the development of the Theory of Cultural Marginality were acculturation, acculturative stress, and marginality. Acculturation was first defined by the Social Science Research Council (SSRC) as "phenomena which result when groups of individuals having different cultures come into continuous first-hand contact, with subsequent changes in the original cultural patterns of either or both groups" (Redfield, Linton, & Herskovits, 1936, p. 149). Theories addressing acculturation have undergone many changes over time, expressed originally through unidimensional models to current expression as multidimensional and orthogonal models (Berry, Poortinga, Segall, & Dasen, 1992; Keefe & Padilla, 1987; Oetting & Beauvais, 1990–1991; Vega, Gil, & Wagner, 1998). The Unidimensional Bipolar Model suggested that individuals inevitably lost their culture of origin as they became acculturated into a new culture (Redfield et al., 1936). Individuals were believed to have only two options: either they acculturated or they remained in their old culture. On the other hand, the Multidimensional Model focuses on the complex nature of acculturation and selective, or uneven, acculturation across domains of social life (Berry et al., 1992; Keefe & Padilla, 1987; Vega et al., 1998). The Orthogonal Model proposes biculturality and assumes that acculturating individuals could maintain two different cultural identities simultaneously (Oetting & Beauvais, 1990–1991). An individual may identify himself or herself as a member of both cultural groups, not necessarily choosing either cultural group. These two models opened a new era for theories of acculturation.

One of the popular approaches to acculturation is the Fourfold Theory of Acculturation (Berry, 1995; Berry & Kim, 1988; Berry et al., 1992). The Fourfold Theory explains strategies that acculturating individuals use. Depending on the chosen culture of reference, strategies are categorized as assimilation, separation, integration, and marginalization.

In assimilation, individuals give up their cultural identity and are absorbed into the dominant, or new, culture. Separation, by contrast, is withdrawal from the dominant culture to reside within the old culture. Integration is regarded as the ideal response and involves "making the best of both worlds" (Berry et al., 1992, p. 279). In marginalization, individuals lose their cultural and psychological contacts with both cultures. Theories of acculturation are broad-ranging and complex, incorporating social, economic, and political components, as well as values, attitudes, self-identity, and behavior change components (Berry & Kim, 1988; Berry et al., 1992).

Acculturative stress—a second theory that contributed to cultural marginality—was developed to highlight the link between acculturation and mental health outcomes. Acculturative stress was defined by Vega et al. (1998) as "a by-product of acculturation that is specific to personal exposure to social situations and environments that challenge individuals to make adjustments in their social behavior or the way they think about themselves" (p. 125). Individuals experience acculturative stress during the acculturating process or as a result of discrimination or being different (Chavez, Moran, Reid, & Lopez, 1997). Acculturative stress has been associated with declining mental health status in acculturating immigrants (Gil, Wagner, & Vega, 2000; Hovey & Magana, 2002; Noh & Kaspar, 2003). The intensity of the relationship between acculturative stress and mental health outcomes is determined by a number of moderating factors including the nature of the dominant culture and the characteristics of the acculturating individuals and groups (Berry & Kim, 1988; Berry et al., 1992).

The third theory to contribute to the development of the Theory of Cultural Marginality was the Theory of Marginality. The Theory of Marginality was first proposed by Park in 1928. Park introduced the "marginal man" concept with special attention to social context (Park, 1928, p. 893). He described the marginal man as experiencing conflicts of the divided self, the old and new self, a lack of integrity, spiritual instability, restlessness, malaise, and moral turmoil between at least two cultural lives. Stonequist (1935) further explored the nature, variations, social situations, and life cycle of the marginal man. By Stonequist's (1935) definition, life cycles consist of an introductory period of preparation, a crisis period, and an adjustment period that may provide opportunities and impetus for social and psychological growth. The Theory of Marginality has been applied to a wide range of situations, such as middle managers' experiences in the social hierarchy of the workplace (Ziller, 1973), student nurses' experiences (Andersson, 1995), and menopause experiences (Im & Lipson, 1997).

In nursing, Hall, Stevens, and Meleis (1994) defined marginality as the condition of being peripheralized from mainstream society or the center of the society based on identity, status, and experience. Marginalization and marginality were viewed from a sociopolitical perspective in relation to racial, gender, political, or economic oppression and were scrutinized along with inequities in economic, political, and social power and resources (Hall, 1999; Hall et al., 1994).

The broad perspective that characterizes the theories of acculturation, acculturative stress, and marginality has led to criticisms that cite vagueness and a lack of empirical support (Del Pilar & Udasco, 2004; Rudmin, 2003) as major weaknesses. Del Pilar and Udasco (2004) claimed that marginality contains so many different layers of experiences that it is impossible to explain it in a unified way. Keeping in mind the strengths as well as the limitations and criticisms of the previous theories, I began by defining cultural marginality. The first definition of cultural marginality was "situations and feelings of passive betweenness when people exist between two different cultures and do not yet perceive themselves as centrally belonging to either one" (Choi, 2001, p. 198). With continued contemplation of this definition, thoughtful ongoing review of the literature, and research with immigrant adolescents, the Theory of Cultural Marginality developed. Schwartz-Barcott and Kim (2000) emphasized the importance of an empirical component in the process of theory development. To validate the Theory of Cultural Marginality with empirical data, I conducted a qualitative study exploring Korean American adolescents' and their parents' perceptions of being in between two different cultures. Twenty Korean American adolescents between the ages of 11 and 14 years and 21 parents were interviewed.

The qualitative study revealed that the main sources of stress for Korean American adolescents were managing a balanced peer relationship, discrimination, pressure to excel academically and to be successful, and lack of in-depth parent–child (P–C) relationships. Parents experienced feeling uneasy and insecure about parenting children in the American culture, lacked a sense of belonging, felt ambivalent toward their children's ethnic identity, and found they were unable to advocate for children. Parents also reported struggling with a lack of depth in P–C relationships (Choi & Dancy, 2009). As a result of these experiences, parents often felt inadequate, guilty, and regretful. The findings were integrated into the conceptual structure of the theory. This process provides a strong empirical foundation for the Theory of Cultural Marginality. I introduce relevant quotes as I discuss the main concepts of the theory.

## ■ CONCEPTS OF THE THEORY

The major concepts of the Theory of Cultural Marginality are across-culture conflict recognition, marginal living, and easing cultural tension. As an individual recognizes conflicts between cultures, he or she engages in marginal living and initiates adjustment responses to ease cultural tension. Therefore, cultural marginality is marginal living while recognizing across-culture conflicts and striving to ease cultural tension. An important dimension of cultural marginality, in addition to the major concepts, is contextual/personal influences that create the foundation for a person's experience of cultural marginality. Each of the major concepts of the theory as well as contextual/personal influences is discussed. In describing the major concepts of the theory, quotes shared by parents and adolescents in my qualitative study are shared.

## Marginal Living

Marginal living—a major concept of the theory—is defined as passive betweenness in the pushing/pulling tension between two cultures while forging new relationships in the midst of old and living with simultaneous conflict/promise. In the Theory of Cultural Marginality, marginal living is viewed as a process of being in between two cultures with emphasis on being in transition rather than being on the periphery of one culture.

Passive betweenness is the essential quality of marginal living. Park (1928) described the marginal experience as a situation that "condemned him to live in two worlds, in neither of which he ever quite belonged" (p. 893). Nobody chooses to be on the edge of two different cultures or to be in between. It is especially true for children who usually have no option when moving from one country to another (Guarnaccia & Lopez, 1998). They simply follow their parents' choice of new country for a better life. Even adults who decide to live in a new country really do not want to be in an "in between" position. Some people who have experienced marginality recalled the time as "a period when they stand with both feet in different boots" (Andersson, 1995, p. 131). The experience has been described as "trapped," "being betwixt and between," and "being located within a structure of double ambivalence" (Bennett, 1993, p. 113; Weisberger, 1992, p. 429). The following quotes capture the quality of passive betweenness. A mother said:

> I, myself, have to live a life of the crippled in this country . . . I feel like I am floating in the air. I don't know if I will be able to stand on my feet before I die. I worry whether my children will grow up well . . . I know for sure that I came here for my children, but I was in agony because I thought I made a wrong decision . . . I am so worried about how to live my life as a mother.

An adolescent said:

> I go crazy over . . . Korean pride and World Cup. But my friends are like, "Outside, you are Korean, but inside, you are White." So I feel like I'm part of them. Sometimes I'm like that and sometimes I'm not.

When people move to a new country or a different culture, they inevitably must become engaged in new relationships (Rogler, 1994). New relationships do not form in a single day, and building them is not as simple as taking off old clothes and changing into new ones. One of the qualities of marginal living is forging new relationships in the midst of old relationships. This quality is often more prominent among adolescents since forming new allegiances with peers and confirming their identities and values within the peer group are critical developmental tasks. Adolescents, who are eager to forge new relationships in the midst of old relationships, often encounter contradiction and conflicts. While moving forward to engage in new relationships, adolescents are concerned about losing connection with their old relationships. As adolescents actively forge new relationships while parents dwell in the past, the P–C relationship gets untied. The following quote describes the experience of an adolescent who began to engage in new relationships in a new world:

> We [mom and herself] will grow apart since we will be living in two different cultures, using different languages. I think she's already having a hard time . . . I wish you had a program to help her overcome such barriers so we may stay close.

Adolescents who are living "in between" face tension between two cultures. Parents encourage their children to mingle with new friends, to pursue further opportunities, so that they will be successful in the new society. This phenomenon is prominent especially among families who emigrated for better education and opportunities. However, parents feel threatened and become anxious about losing control over their children as their children blend into the new culture. The following quote illustrates the pushing/pulling quality of tension from the perspective of the father of a 12-year-old boy:

> Many of their parents have double standards for them. They want their children to be successful in America as American citizens, yet they want them to remain Koreans at the same time. And that gives children an ambiguous message, which confuses them. . . . If you keep giving such contradicting messages to children, especially at a sensitive stage when they start questioning their parents' authority, they will surely get confused and it might lead to creating other problems. I think that is the real problem.

Complicating matters, the new society or dominant culture has similarly contradictory attitudes toward immigrants: It welcomes immigrants warmly and promises to provide them abundant opportunities and resources; however, in reality, what immigrants often face is overt and covert discrimination, as reported by both Korean American adolescents and their parents during the interviews. Korean American adolescents encountered teachers' insensitive attitudes toward different cultures, experienced limited opportunities, and got unfair grades and punishments. Korean American adolescents also reported that they had been teased or bullied because of their accent and physical appearance.

There is a demand for immigrants to make choices among contradicting norms, expectations, roles, and values. They often find themselves struggling in simultaneous conflict and promise. Conflict couched in promise is a quality of marginal living causing identity confusion, anxiety, ambivalence, feelings of alienation, loss, helplessness, worthlessness, a feeling of uncertainty, and apprehension about the future (Andersson, 1995; Berry et al., 1992; Fuertes & Westbrook, 1996; Scribner, 1995; Weisberger, 1992). However, conflict does not always create negative outcomes. Depending on how the individual perceives and manages conflict, it may offer possibility for change. In a previous article on the concept of cultural marginality (Choi, 2001), conflict and promise were categorized as two distinct attributes; however, subsequent research has indicated that promise is integral to conflict. Thus, for the Theory of Cultural Marginality, conflict/promise is conceptualized as a single quality of marginal living. Hall and colleagues (Hall, 1999, p. 100; Hall et al., 1994) identified resilience and a "hope-positive view of the future" as well as vulnerabilities when marginalized people struggled to acquire their own survival strategies to protect themselves and enhance their sense of well-being. Marginal living presents both a conflict and a promise as well as a crisis and a turning point, thus providing an impetus for growth.

During the interviews, Korean American parents expressed hopes for their children's future even in the midst of feelings of alienation, powerlessness, worthlessness, and uncertainty. They expected their children to blend into mainstream society and move up the social ladder by obtaining high educational status, leading children to feel pressured to excel academically and to be successful. Integral to this experience of marginal living is the recognition of across-culture conflict, a second concept of the Theory of Cultural Marginality.

## Across-Culture Conflict Recognition

Across-culture conflict recognition is a beginning understanding of differences between two contradicting cultural values, customs, behaviors, and norms. Just as people feel and react to perceived temperature, not measured temperature, people feel and react to their recognition of differences while in between cultures. Conflict emerges as individuals face distinct value systems with accompanying expectations and are forced to make difficult choices. Korean American adolescents reported encountering two distinct cultural values and expectations between peers and their parents and between Korean and American friends.

Identifying across-culture conflict recognition as a concept of the Theory of Cultural Marginality has significant implications for research and practice because it allows for individual differences in perception, responses, and mental health outcomes associated with cultural marginality. This is consistent with the theorizing of Lazarus (1997), who identified cognitive appraisal of cultural environment as one of the significant determinants of mental health outcomes. An adolescent said:

> You know how parents raise their kids based on how they were raised. . . . Well, if I compare my style with regular White friends, it's completely different. They are always out and my parents think you play too much or you do this too much but if you compare me with them, that's not really true. Well, I know it's best for me what they say but sometimes it's like that's how we live here in America.

## Easing Cultural Tension

Easing cultural tension resolves across-culture conflict. Adjustment responses proposed in the Theory of Cultural Marginality are adapted from Weisberger's work on marginality among German Jews (Weisberger, 1992). Four responses, assimilation, reconstructed return, poise, and integration, are processes for easing cultural tension. The responses are not mutually exclusive; rather, they are mixed empirically (Weisberger, 1992) and will be referred to as response patterns to connote their contextual, situational, dynamic nature.

The first response pattern is assimilation. It is a process whereby individuals are absorbed into the dominant or new culture (Berry, 1995; Berry & Kim, 1988; Berry et al., 1992). This is usually the first response pattern exhibited by new immigrants, particularly when the dominant or new culture is unfavorable to the newcomers. Immigrants strive hard to acquire new language and customs and to mingle with people of the new society. It is a useful strategy for survival in the new culture; however, it may create self-denial, self-hatred, and feelings of guilt (Weisberger, 1992).

After encountering the new culture, individuals may return to their own culture, exhibiting the pattern of reconstructed return. They may choose to return as a result of resistance, obstacles, and conflicts with a new culture or as a result of reminiscence and longing for one's own culture. When they return, they do so with a new perspective toward their own culture as well as to the new culture since they cannot be free from the influences of the new culture (Anderson & Levy, 2003; Weisberger, 1992). Thus, every return is a reconstructed return. A typical characteristic of people who return to or remain in their culture is an overidentification with their own culture. Weisberger (1992, p. 442) describes the characteristics among the returning German Jews as "more Jewish than Jewish." The following quote is from a mother of a 14-year-old daughter who was referred by her teacher to a school counselor for her misbehavior at school:

> Even if she was born here [United States] and has never been to Korea, she always hangs out with Korean friends, particularly Korean kids who recently moved from Korea. She likes to have Korean clothes, accessories, phone, and stuff . . . I think it is because [of] her longing for Korea and Korean culture.

Poise is a response pattern characterized by a tentative fit on the margin regardless of emotional conflict and struggle. Individuals who respond with poise may become free from obligation or attachment to a certain culture, but they have to be "homeless in a cultural sense" (Weisberger, 1992, p. 440). Even when responding with a pattern of poise, individuals will continue to experience emotional conflicts and a period of personal crisis continues. Accumulated effects of crisis may include stress and poor mental health outcomes such as personality changes, substance abuse, depression, and even suicidal ideation (Hovey & Magana, 2002; Park, 1928; Vega et al., 1998; Williams & Berry, 1991).

Integration is an adjustment response pattern where an individual creates a third culture by merging and integrating the old and new cultures. Through integration, individuals surpass cultural boundaries, contexts, and identities and acquire superior social functioning, gaining access to multiple cultural worlds (Guarnaccia & Lopez, 1998; Park, 1928; Weisberger, 1992) and easing cultural tension. They will experience a sense of cultural home, a sense of belonging, integration of identity, and psychological and cognitive growth (Bennett, 1993; Vivero & Jenkins, 1999). For them, the possibility of returning to the cultural tension of marginal living is minimized. When faced with another circumstance of cultural tension, it is likely that they will respond successfully. The level of ease experienced during the process will influence the mental health and well-being of the individual. A 14-year-old boy who used to struggle to fit in with peers due to language and cultural barriers now becomes comfortable with both American and Korean cultures and feels confident:

> I feel very special in a positive way. There are my friends who think I'm cool. They rather look UP to me . . . I explain to my friends what Korean culture is. Like New Year's Day, they called me to go with them and watch fireworks. I was like, "I can't" and I explained to them what "Duk-gook" [Korean traditional food] is and "Sae-bae." Like I have to bow down and I get money. And they are like, "Can we come to your house and do 'Sae-bae' so we get money too?" I explained to them and they want to know more about it. One of my friends can actually count from 1 to like 25. They actually go to Web sites so they can learn, so they can talk to me. And I actually gave them Korean music, and he's like, can you type the lyrics in English? So they are more into Koreanness. They are more interested.

One adjustment response pattern may have more constructive impact on an individual's mental health than the others; however, there is no ideal or most useful pattern that works for everyone, nor is there one pattern that works for one person all of the time. For instance, integration may be a feasible adjustment response pattern for immigrant adolescents but not for immigrant older adults. For older adults, remaining in contact with the old culture and returning to old-culture ways may make them more comfortable; the pattern of reconstructed return may be most useful for them. For healthcare providers working with immigrant populations, it is important to assess unique experiences and perceptions rather than to categorize individuals based on their adjustment response pattern. However, knowledge about the response patterns individuals use to ease cultural tension may enable understanding of the complex processes that are central to the struggle that many immigrants face.

## Contextual/Personal Influences

Scholars of Acculturation Theory recognize nature or types of the dominant society and characteristics of acculturating individuals as significant factors in the acculturation process (Berry & Kim, 1988; Williams & Berry, 1991). In this Theory of Cultural Marginality, the factors influencing the process of across-culture conflict recognition, marginal living, and easing cultural tensions are described as contextual/personal influences.

Contextual influences identified in literature reviews and shared in interviews with Korean Americans are the nature of the dominant society, such as openness or tolerance to diversity, available social and healthcare resources for immigrants, racial and/or ethnic composition of school and neighborhood, and support from teachers and peers. Particularly, healthcare providers' beliefs and attitudes toward an individual from a different cultural background play a significant role in this model since their beliefs and attitudes could result in undesirable ethical consequences of patient care as well as inappropriate care (Johnstone, 2016).

The personal influences include the knowledge about the dominant society, age at immigration, length of stay in the dominant society, educational backgrounds, socioeconomic status, language proficiency, ethnic identity, preimmigration experiences, reasons for immigration, loyalty to own culture, resilience, or ability to endure the hardship, openness, P–C relationships, coping strategies, and significant others' attitude toward the dominant culture (Berry, 1995; Berry & Kim, 1988; Berry et al., 1992; Trueba, 2002).

These influences govern not only the individuals who are in the midst of cultural marginality but also the dominant culture that is a source of interaction for immigrant people. Existing theories describing acculturation have been criticized for ignoring the influences of the acculturating individuals or groups to the dominant culture (Rudmin, 2003). The theories viewed acculturating individuals only as passive recipients. When two cultures clash, the interaction is reciprocal although the strength of the influence may not be comparable. Contextual/personal influences make the interaction between two cultures and the effect of one culture on another a mutual process.

## ■ RELATIONSHIPS AMONG THE CONCEPTS: THE MODEL

Figure 14.1 depicts the relationships among the major concepts of the theory.

Marginal living begins with the recognition of across-culture conflict. As individuals encounter marginal living, they strive to ease cultural tension through adjustment response patterns. The four response patterns are assimilation, reconstructed return, poise, and integration. Although not an explicit concept in the theory, the importance of contextual/personal influences is recognized by inclusion as a foundation for the Theory of Cultural Marginality.

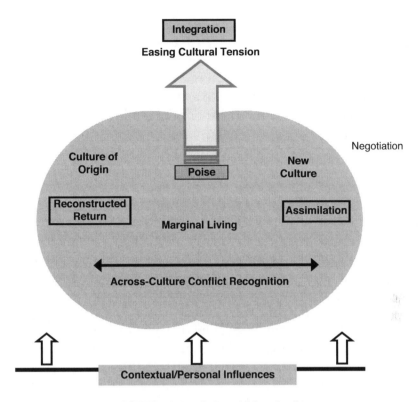

**FIGURE 14.1**  Cultural Marginality.

# ■ USE OF THE THEORY IN NURSING RESEARCH AND EDUCATION

The concept of cultural marginality (Choi, 2001) and the Theory of Cultural Marginality (Choi, 2008) have been cited in various areas of nursing research and practice (Alexander, Kinman, Miller, & Patrick, 2003; Buscemi, 2011; Horback & Rothery-Jackson, 2007; Loue & Sajatovic, 2012). The concept was used to understand experiences of Mexican American families caring for children with serious chronic conditions (Rehm, 2003), analyze the concept of acculturation in Mexican immigrants (Page, 2006), study the stress experienced by Pakistani Ismaili Muslim girls (Khuwaja, Selwyn, Kapadia, McCurdy, & Khuwaja, 2007), and explore the cultural identity of Afro-Caribbean Americans (Archibald, 2011).

Since the theory was introduced, it has been used to guide research and practice for people experiencing marginal living. First, based on the Social Cognitive Theory and Cultural Marginality Theory, I developed an individually administered, computer-based mental health promotion program, **P**romoting **I**ntergenerational **D**ialogue on **E**motions (PRIDE). (Note: The program name was changed from "Be Connected" to PRIDE; Choi, 2012.) Using a two-group, repeated-measures, and controlled randomized study design, I tested the feasibility of PRIDE and compared the efficacy of PRIDE with an attention control (AC) group on parental knowledge, parental stress, parental self-efficacy, filial self-efficacy, P–C communication, P–C conflict, and P–C satisfaction. A total of 58 parents (28 fathers and 30 mothers) and 30 Korean American adolescents aged 11 to 14 years participated in the study (16 families in PRIDE and 14 families in the AC group). PRIDE had good feasibility for Korean American families and was favored by both parents and adolescents. Efficacy results of the study were also promising at 1 month postintervention. Particularly, fathers' parental knowledge ($d = 0.82$), mothers' parental knowledge ($d = 1.95$), fathers' report on P–C communication ($d = 0.61$), and Korean American adolescents' report on conflicts with the father ($d = 0.44$) showed medium-to-large effects of PRIDE compared with an AC condition. As PRIDE is taken to a larger trial, this computer-based program may then be disseminated to multicity community settings. The development and pilot testing of PRIDE is reported in detail elsewhere (Choi, 2012).

A second area of research for the Theory of Cultural Marginality is instrument development. Researchers have developed scales to measure levels of acculturation and acculturative stress and to explain the relationships between these concepts and mental health outcomes (Hovey & King, 1997; Padilla, Alvarez, & Lindholm, 1986; Phinney, 1992; Sam & Berry, 1995; Williams & Berry, 1991). In addition, cultural competence has been studied and I have collaborated with a team of researchers to develop a Korean version of the Cultural Awareness Scale (K-CAS; Choi, Suh, Park, Park, & Hernandez, 2015) with good reliability (alpha = .83) and construct validity. However, there is no scale specifically designed to measure cultural marginality.

The phenomenon of globalization is not limited to the United States. As of 2015, about 1.90 million foreigners (3.9% of total population) reside in Korea and about 8% of them (151,608) immigrated to Korea for marriage (Korean Immigration Service, 2015). Currently, about 278,036 interracial families live in Korea and 207,693 children are growing up in interracial families (Ministry of Gender Equality and Family, 2016). To assess marginal living experiences of immigrant children living in South Korea, including biracial children, I developed the cultural marginality scale.

The items on this 13-item scale were derived from the qualitative descriptive study of Korean American adolescents and their parents and the existing acculturative stress scale, the Societal, Attitudinal, Familial, and Environmental Acculturative Stress Scale for Children (SAFE-C; Chavez et al., 1997). Responses range from 0 = *hardly ever or never* to 3 = *almost always.* As a next step in developing a reliable and valid instrument, I conducted cognitive interviews with nine children, aged 10 to 13. The main purpose of the cognitive interview was to explore the cognitive processes that respondents use to answer the questions (i.e., how respondents understand, mentally process, and respond to the questions; Knafl et al., 2007; Willis, 2005). The cognitive interview helps the researcher clarify intention of questions and identify problems with wording, readability, item or section sequence, and length of the instrument. The cognitive interview is generally conducted with a small number of respondents (5–25 people) before field-testing a newly developed instrument.

All participants were born in interracial families; self-identify themselves as having multiple cultural identities or heritages; and currently reside in Korea. Seven out of nine children reported that one of their parents was from China. One child reported having an Indonesian mother and another child reported having a Japanese mother.

During the cognitive interviews, any difficult or confusing words were identified and rephrased to increase clarity and reduce possible errors in responses. The 13-item cultural marginality scale assessing children's experiences of marginal living was finalized based on the findings of the interviews. These 13 items generally address topics like ethnic identity, peer relationship problems, and perceived discrimination. Example items with this specific sample include: I don't feel like I am Korean or Chinese; My parents want me to understand and remember their respective cultures; I think that kids don't want to play with me because of my mixed background; and I think that being raised in interracial families could be my unique strength. Psychometric testing will occur for the Korean version of this instrument before proceeding with translation and testing in an English-speaking population.

The cultural marginality scale with items aligned according to the concepts of the theory will allow assessment of the structure of the associated concepts and of the extent to which cultural marginality influences health. Assessing the relationship between cultural marginality and mental health outcomes has significant implications for the healthcare of immigrants. It has particular relevance for preventive care, where nurses caring for immigrants develop approaches for recognizing those who are at risk for mental health problems.

An education research project guided by the Theory of Cultural Marginality was the study titled *Cultural Competency Among Nursing.* This was the study that enabled testing of the K-CAS (Choi et al., 2015). One of the most critical contextual influences affecting an individual's experience of cultural marginality is the nurse's openness to diversity and competency in caring for patients from diverse sociocultural backgrounds. The specific aims of this mixed-method study were to (a) assess perceived levels of openness to diversity and cultural competence among Korean nursing students; (b) explore Korean nursing students' nursing care experiences with patients from diverse cultural backgrounds; and (c) explore Korean nursing students' needs for cultural competence education integrated into the nursing curriculum. The ultimate goal of the study was to develop a nursing curriculum that would prepare students for a culturally diverse patient population in Korea. A total of 515 nursing students (364 undergraduate and 151 graduate students) from four nursing schools in Korea completed the questionnaire. Additionally, 18 undergraduate and 20 graduate students ($n = 38$) participated in one of six focus groups.

The study indicated a lack of understanding of the concept of cultural competence among Korean nursing students (Choi et al., 2015). In addition, the findings from the qualitative data demonstrated that participants encountered their personal boundaries regarding openness to other cultures and they experienced prejudice when caring for ethnically diverse patients. The findings confirmed that the interaction between two cultures is reciprocal and that healthcare providers and patients were mutually influenced by each other.

The findings were incorporated into a nursing course called "Sociocultural diversity and health." The objective of this course was to help students understand the influence of various cultures (e.g., racial, ethnic, socioeconomic, educational, and geographic) on healthcare services and research.

The study conducted by Cardona (2016) is the most recent work guided by the Theory of Cultural Marginality. Cardona used the theory to develop a culturally relevant eating disorder assessment tool for Hispanic women and identify healthcare providers' behaviors that could promote culturally relevant interactions with these women. Even though it was a pilot study, conducted with five Hispanic women who were diagnosed with eating disorders, it demonstrated that the women had experienced feelings of alienation while dealing with symptoms of their eating disorders (e.g., dietary restrictions, weight fluctuations) influenced by both American and Hispanic cultures.

## ■ USE OF THE THEORY IN NURSING PRACTICE

Previously, the concept of cultural marginality has been used to discuss adherence issues of Mexican clients (Barron, Hunter, Mayo, & Willoughby, 2004) and to address the gap in healthcare provider–client relationships and its impact on health disparities. The theory can also be applied to school nurse practice to foster awareness of culturally distinct adolescent needs (Labun, 2003).

Another example of use of the theory in nursing practice is the application of it to the case of a 23-year-old, English-speaking African refugee to the United States (Burke, 2011). At the age of 13, she experienced the most severe type of female genital mutilation (FGM) by an elder in Djibouti, Africa, and suffers from candidiasis and hematocolpos. In her article, Burke analyzed experiences of the patient using the concepts of the theory and discussed how the Theory of Cultural Marginality can be used as a framework to guide culturally sensitive, evidence-based nursing care for women with FGM. Particularly, she emphasized the need for nurses to constantly assess contextual and personal influence factors, to serve as a significant contextual influence, to provide culturally relevant care, and to support patients' integration of cultures while assisting with health decisions.

Use of the theory in practice is limited; however, the aforementioned examples of research and practice demonstrate possible applications for the Theory of Cultural Marginality. Possible areas include education or health promotion programs assessing and modifying an individual's personal influences, culturally relevant therapeutic nurse–patient interactions, and development of cultural competence training for healthcare providers.

In this chapter, the Theory of Cultural Marginality was described mainly in the context of immigrant adolescents' experiences; however, the theory is applicable to any immigrant who is encountering marginal living. The Theory of Cultural Marginality can be used as a framework to explore unique experiences of diverse groups of immigrants and people caught between two distinct cultures and to provide care for them. Particularly, recognizing the influence of the contextual/personal factors has significant implications for healthcare providers. For instance, adjustment response patterns and healthcare needs among immigrants who came to a new country for freedom cannot be the same as those for people who immigrated for educational opportunities. By recognizing these influences and modifying them when appropriate, healthcare providers may ease the adjustment process, promote healthy development, and elicit desirable health outcomes.

## ■ CONCLUSION

What is it like to be caught between cultures? How does that experience impact one's health? How can healthcare providers ease the experience? These questions have inspired the development of the Theory of Cultural Marginality. The goal of the theory is to highlight the complexity of living between two cultures by emphasizing the challenge to the health of people encountering marginal living, and thereby, enlighten healthcare providers to provide appropriate care for them. The theory elucidates essences of marginal living, across-culture conflict recognition, and striving to ease cultural tension while recognizing the fundamental importance of contextual/personal influences. Understanding of the theory and the relationships among the concepts promises a framework for culturally relevant healthcare for immigrant people. Nowadays, health issues related to immigration affect many different countries. To better meet the needs of the increasingly diverse groups of people (e.g., children from interracial families, third-culture individuals), the theory needs to continuously evolve and be refined through further research and practice within and outside the United States.

## ■ REFERENCES

Alexander, G. L., Kinman, E. L., Miller, L. C., & Patrick, T. B. (2003). Marginalization and health geomatics. *Journal of Biomedical Informatics, 36,* 400–407.

Anderson, T. L., & Levy, J. A. (2003). Marginality among older injectors in today's illicit drug culture: Assessing the impact of ageing. *Addiction, 98,* 761–770.

Andersson, E. P. (1995). Marginality: Concept or reality in nursing education? *Journal of Advanced Nursing, 21,* 131–136.

Archibald, C. (2011). Cultural tailoring for an Afro-Caribbean community: A naturalistic approach. *Journal of Cultural Diversity, 18*(4), 114–119.

Barron, F., Hunter, A., Mayo, R., & Willoughby, B. (2004). Acculturation and adherence: Issues for health care providers working with clients of Mexican origin. *Journal of Transcultural Nursing, 15,* 331–337.

Bennett, J. M. (1993). Cultural marginality: Identity issues in intercultural training. In R. M. Paise (Ed.), *Education for intercultural experience* (pp. 109–135). Yarmouth, ME: Intercultural Press.

Berry, J. W. (1995). Psychology of acculturation. In N. R. Goldberger & J. B. Veroff (Eds.), *The culture and psychology reader* (pp. 457–488). New York: New York University.

Berry, J. W., & Kim, U. (1988). Acculturation and mental health. In P. R. Dasen, J. W. Berry, & N. Sartorius (Eds.), *Health and cross-cultural psychology: Toward applications* (pp. 207–236). Newbury Park, CA: Sage.

Berry, J. W., Poortinga, Y. H., Segall, M. H., & Dasen, P. R. (1992). *Cross-cultural psychology: Research and applications.* New York, NY: Cambridge University.

Burke, E. (2011). Female genital mutilation: Applications of nursing theory for clinical care. *The Nurse Practitioner, 36,* 45–50.

Buscemi, C. P. (2011). Acculturation: State of the science in nursing. *Journal of Cultural Diversity, 18*(2), 39–42.

Cardona, G. R. (2016). *Initial testing of the risk assessment of eating disorders (RAED) tool for use in primary care of Hispanic women* (Unpublished doctoral dissertation). University of Arizona, Tuscon, Arizona.

Chavez, D. V., Moran, V. R., Reid, S. L., & Lopez, M. (1997). Acculturative stress in children: A modification of the SAFE Scale. *Hispanic Journal of Behavioral Sciences, 19,* 34–44.

Choi, H. (2001). Cultural marginality: A concept analysis with implications for immigrant adolescents. *Issues in Comprehensive Pediatric Nursing, 24,* 193–206.

Choi, H. (2008). Theory of cultural marginality. In M. J. Smith & P. R. Liehr (Eds.), *Middle range theory for nursing* (2nd ed., pp. 243–260). New York, NY: Springer Publishing.

Choi, H. (2012). The development of a culturally relevant preventive intervention. *Open Journal of Nursing, 2,* 123–129.

Choi, H., & Dancy, B. L. (2009). Korean American adolescents' and their parents' perceptions of acculturative stress. *Journal of Child and Adolescent Psychiatric Nursing, 22,* 203–210.

Choi, H., Meininger, J. C., & Roberts, R. E. (2006). Ethnic differences in adolescents' mental distress, social stress, and resources. *Adolescence, 41*(162), 263–283.

Choi, H., Suh, E. E., Park, C., Park. J., & Fernandez, E. (2015). Reliability and validity of a Korean version of the Cultural Awareness Scale (K-CAS). *Korean Journal of Adult Nursing*, 27(4), 472–479.

Choi, H., Stafford, L., Meininger, J. C., Roberts, R. E., & Smith, D. P. (2002). Psychometric properties of the DSM Scale for Depression (DSD) with Korean American youths. *Issues in Mental Health Nursing*, 23, 735–756.

Del Pilar, J. A., & Udasco, J. O. (2004). Marginality theory: The lack of construct validity. *Hispanic Journal of Behavioral Sciences*, 26, 3–15.

Fuertes, J. N., & Westbrook, F. D. (1996). Using the Social, Attitudinal, Familial, and Environmental (SAFE) Acculturation stress scale to assess the adjustment needs of Hispanic college students. *Measurement and Evaluation in Counseling and Development*, 29, 67–76.

Gil, A. G., Wagner, E. F., & Vega, W. A. (2000). Acculturation, familism, and alcohol use among Latino adolescent males: Longitudinal relations. *Journal of Community Psychology*, 28, 443–458.

Guarnaccia, P. J., & Lopez, S. (1998). The mental health and adjustment of immigrant and refugee children. *The Child Psychiatrist in the Community*, 7, 537–553.

Hall, J. M. (1999). Marginalization revisited: Critical, postmodern, and liberation perspectives. *Advances in Nursing Science*, 22(2), 88–102.

Hall, J. M., Stevens, P. E., & Meleis, A. I. (1994). Marginalization: A guiding concept for valuing diversity in nursing knowledge development. *Advances in Nursing Science*, 16(4), 23–41.

Horback, S., & Rothery-Jackson, C. (2007). Cultural marginality: Exploration of self-esteem and cross cultural adaptation of the marginalized individual: An investigation of the second generation Hare Krishnas. *Journal of Intercultural Communication*, 14. Retrieved from https://www.immi.se/intercultural/nr14/horback.htm

Hovey, J. D., & King, C. A. (1997). Suicidality among acculturating Mexican Americans: Current knowledge and directions for research. *Suicide and Life-Threatening Behavior*, 27, 92–103.

Hovey, J. D., & Magana, C. G. (2002). Exploring the mental health Mexican migrant farm workers in the midwest: Psychosocial predictors of psychological distress and suggestions for prevention and treatment. *Journal of Psychology*, 136, 493–513.

Im, E.-O., & Lipson, J. G. (1997). Menopausal transition of Korean immigrant women: A literature review. *Health Care for Women International*, 18, 507–520.

Johnstone, M.-J. (2016). *Bioethics: A nursing perspective* (6th ed.). Chatswood, Australia: Elsevier.

Keefe, S. E., & Padilla, A. M. (1987). *Chicano ethnicity*. Albuquerque: University of New Mexico Press.

Khuwaja, S. A., Selwyn, B. J., Kapadia, A., McCurdy, S., & Khuwaja, A. (2007). Pakistani Ismaili Muslim adolescent females living in the United States of America: Stresses associated with the process of adaptation to U.S. culture. *Journal of Immigrant Health*, 9, 35–42.

Knafl, K., Deatrick, J., Gallo, A., Holcombe, G., Bakitas, M., Dixon, J., & Grey, M. (2007). The analysis and interpretation of cognitive interviews for Instrument development. *Research in Nursing and Health, 30,* 224–234.

Korean Immigration Service. (2015). Korean immigrant service statistics. Retrieved from https://www.immigration.go.kr/HP/COM/bbs_003/ListShowData.do?str NbodCd=noti0096&strWrtNo=129&strAnsNo=A&strOrgGbnCd=104000&strRtn URL=IMM_6050&strAllOrgYn=N&strThisPage=1&strFilePath=imm

Labun, E. (2003). Working with a Vietnamese adolescent. *Journal of School Nursing, 19,* 319–325.

Lazarus, R. S. (1997). Acculturation isn't everything. *Applied Psychology, 46,* 39–43.

Loue, S., & Sajatovic, M. (Eds.). (2012). *Encyclopedia of immigrant health.* New York, NY: Springer Publishing.

Migration Policy Institute. (2017). State immigration data profiles. Retrieved from http://www.migrationpolicy.org/data/state-profiles/state/demographics/US

Ministry of Gender Equality and Family. (2016). *2015 National Multicultural Family Survey (Report 2016-03).* Seoul, South Korea: Hanhak Munhwa.

Noh, S., & Kaspar, V. (2003). Perceived discrimination and depression: Moderating effects of coping, acculturation, and ethnic support. *American Journal of Public Health, 93,* 232–238.

Oetting, E. R., & Beauvais, F. (1990–1991). Orthogonal cultural identification theory: The cultural identification of minority adolescents. *The International Journal of the Addictions, 25,* 655–685.

Padilla, A. M., Alvarez, M., & Lindholm, K. J. (1986). Generational status and personality factors as predictors of stress in students. *Hispanic Journal of Behavioral Sciences, 8,* 275–288.

Page, R. L. (2006). Acculturation in Mexican immigrants: A concept analysis. *Journal of Holistic Nursing, 24*(4), 270–278.

Park, R. E. (1928). Human migration and the marginal man. *The American Journal of Sociology, 33,* 881–893.

Phinney, J. S. (1992). The multigroup ethnic identity measure: A new scale for use with adolescents and youth adults from diverse groups. *Journal of Adolescent Research, 7,* 156–176.

Redfield, R., Linton, R., & Herskovits, M. J. (1936). Memorandum on the study of acculturation. *American Anthropologist, 38,* 149–152.

Rehm, R. S. (2003). Legal, financial, and ethical ambiguities for Mexican American families: Caring for children with chronic conditions. *Qualitative Health Research, 13,* 689–702.

Rogler, L. H. (1994). International migrations: A framework for directing research. *American Psychologist, 49,* 701–708.

Rudmin, F. W. (2003). Critical history of the acculturation psychology of assimilation, separation, integration, and marginalization. *Review of General Psychology, 7,* 3–37.

Sam, D. L., & Berry, J. W. (1995). Acculturative stress among young immigrants in Norway. *Scandinavian Journal of Psychology, 36,* 10–24.

Schwartz-Barcott, D., & Kim, H. S. (2000). An expansion and elaboration of the hybrid model of concept development. In B. L. Rodgers & K. A. Knafl (Eds.), *Concept development in nursing* (2nd ed., pp. 129–159). Philadelphia, PA: Saunders.

Scribner, A. P. (1995). Advocating for Hispanic high school students: Research-based educational practices. *The High School Journal, 78*, 206–214.

Stonequist, E. V. (1935). The problem of the marginal man. *The American Journal of Sociology, 41*, 1–12.

Trueba, H. T. (2002). Multiple ethnic, racial, and cultural identities in action: From marginality to a new cultural capital in modern society. *Journal of Latinos and Education, 1*, 7–28.

Vega, W. A., Gil, A. G., & Wagner, E. (1998). Cultural adjustment and Hispanic adolescent drug use. In W. A. Vega & A. G. Gil (Eds.), *Drug use and ethnicity in early adolescence* (pp. 125–148). New York, NY: Plenum.

Vivero, V. N., & Jenkins, S. R. (1999). Existential hazards of the multicultural individual: Defining and understanding "cultural homelessness." *Cultural Diversity and Ethnic Minority Psychology, 5*, 6–26.

Weisberger, A. (1992). Marginality and its directions. *Sociological Forum, 7*, 425–446.

Williams, C. L., & Berry, J. W. (1991). Primary prevention of acculturative stress among refugees: Application of psychological theory and practice. *American Psychologist, 46*, 632–641.

Willis, G. B. (2005). *Cognitive interviewing.* Thousand Oaks, CA: Sage.

Ziller, R. C. (1973). *The social self.* New York, NY: Pergamon.

# CHAPTER 15

## Theory of Moral Reckoning

**Alvita K. Nathaniel**

Today's healthcare environment—with its spiraling technology, longer life spans, power imbalance, and budget restraints—engenders an atmosphere with moral problems of ever-increasing complexity—problems for which the most basic moral beliefs about life, death, right, and wrong are challenged. An increasing number of researchers have examined nurses' responses to these types of stressors and their impact on patient care, often determining that nurses experience moral distress in many such situations. The Theory of Moral Reckoning began with an interest in this compelling concept.

### ■ PURPOSE OF THE THEORY AND HOW IT WAS DEVELOPED

Andrew Jameton, a philosopher and ethicist, first described moral distress in nursing. When Jameton asked nurses to talk about moral dilemmas, he noticed that their stories failed to meet the definition of dilemma (Jameton, 1984). A moral dilemma forces one to choose between two undesirable, mutually exclusive alternatives—the correct choice is unclear, since all alternatives have nearly equal moral weight and none are more right or wrong than others. The nurses' stories did not fit the definition of moral dilemma. Relating their personal stories, nurses consistently talked to Jameton about situations in which they believed they knew the morally right actions to take, yet they felt constrained from following their convictions (Jameton, 1993). Jameton concluded that nurses were compelled to tell these stories because of their profound suffering and their belief about the importance of the situations. Mentioning this concept only briefly, Jameton proposed that "moral distress arises when one knows the right thing to do, but institutional constraints make it nearly impossible to pursue the right course of action" (Jameton, 1984, p. 6). Jameton also stipulated that nurses who participate in an action that they have judged to be morally wrong experience moral distress (Jameton, 1993). Building upon Jameton's definition, Wilkinson defined moral distress as "the psychological disequilibrium and negative feeling state experienced when a person makes a moral decision but does not follow through by performing the moral behavior indicated by that decision" (Wilkinson, 1987, p. 16). In the intervening years, there has been increasing interest in moral distress. Most subsequent nursing sources rely on Jameton's definition of moral distress (McCarthy & Gastmans, 2015).

For many years, I taught a nursing ethics course and later coauthored an ethics textbook (Burkhardt & Nathaniel, 1998, 2013). The concept of moral distress caught my imagination. I wondered, for example, if we in the profession claim that nurses are autonomous professionals, why do so many nurses violate their own moral codes when faced with constraints to action? How can institutional pressure override an individual's moral values that were formed over a lifetime? Why do highly educated professionals view themselves as powerless in morally troubling situations? How does moral distress affect nurses, patients, and the healthcare system as a whole?

Even though the early literature offered emotionally charged descriptions of nurses' moral distress, the knowledge was limited in four essential ways. First, there were few studies, with few informants, so even though many nurses had written about moral distress, we really knew very little about it. Second, only a handful of published studies identified moral distress in their purpose statements. In addition, most published studies were rudimentary and exploratory in nature. Third, theoretical foundations did not adequately explain moral distress. Fourth, there were gaps in the literature in terms of the impact of moral distress on nursing care and patients' health outcomes.

Awareness of these limitations compelled me to try to learn more about the process. I began conducting interviews with nurses who reported that they had experienced morally troubling patient care situations. My purpose was to address gaps in knowledge by seeking answers to one basic research question: What transpires in morally laden situations in which nurses experience distress? Using the inductive approach of classic Grounded Theory (Glaser, 1965, 1978, 1998; Glaser & Strauss, 1967), I soon recognized that more was going on in these situations than could be explained adequately by the concept of moral distress. Distinct patterns and processes emerged from the data, making it clear that nurses' experiences followed a relatively predictable pattern as each nurse made important choices before, during, and after becoming entangled in a morally significant situational bind.

As required by the classic Grounded Theory method, I laid aside preconceived notions, logical elaborations, and ideas gleaned from the extant literature. New concepts, processes, and tentative hypotheses began to emerge from the empirical data through careful investigation, inductive reasoning, and analysis. Early in the data-gathering phase, I noticed that nurses vividly recalled important junctures in their professional lives that included morally troubling patient care situations, yet seemed to be part of a much bigger process. Extant research focusing on moral distress remained pertinent and was subsequently interwoven into the larger, more explanatory and predictive process of moral reckoning, adding depth and complexity to the resultant theory.

The Theory of Moral Reckoning emerged through the inductive process of the classic Grounded Theory method. I recorded the interviews as field notes immediately after each interview. Analysis began with the first episode of data gathering and was simultaneous with other steps of the process. Using constant comparison as suggested by Glaser (1965), data were analyzed sentence by sentence as they were coded. Data were organized into concepts and further into categories. I composed conceptual-level memos as concepts became evident. As the research continued, social psychological processes began to surface. Nurses' main concern was the situational bind that ensnared them. Moral reckoning emerged as the process by which the nurses continually solved the main concern. Moral reckoning was also the concept to which all other concepts related. These two criteria led me to recognize that moral reckoning was the core category of the theory. Identification of the core category opened the door for subsequent selective theoretical sampling, coding, and memoing. Theoretical sampling began when concepts seemed to require more refinement or areas needed more depth. Memos consisted of the emerging concepts and categories (highly abstract concepts). Saturation occurred when all new data revealed interchangeability of indices. At that point, I began sorting and organizing the memos.

The larger process of moral reckoning overlaps moral distress as described in the extant literature. Both moral reckoning and moral distress include a situational bind (unnamed in moral distress literature) and short- and long-term consequences for nurses. Because it explicates choices and actions and includes precursor conditions and long-term consequences, the substantive and more comprehensive and explanatory Theory of Moral Reckoning effectively synthesizes, organizes, and transcends what was previously known about moral distress.

Moral reckoning captures the culmination of the process as nurses critically and emotionally reflect on motivations, choices, actions, and consequences entangled in a particularly troubling patient care situation. They are alone with their experiences, wrestling with something they have difficulty communicating. According to Strauss (1959), critical events occur in which there is a temporary gap between events and the person's understanding of them. The person is aware of this gap. Under certain social conditions, such as with moral reckoning, a person will undergo so many or such critical experiences for which conventional explanations seem inadequate that the person begins to question large segments of what was previously learned. Subsequently, there is an internal rhetorical battle. The person cannot question what was learned in the past without questioning internal purposes. If the person rejects the explanations once believed, then there will be a type of alienation—a perception of a world lost. The person may feel spiritually dispossessed as he or she embraces a set of counterexplanations to recreate a worldview (Strauss, 1959).

The term *reckon* is especially suitable to describe the name of the theory. To reckon is to enumerate serially or separately; to name or mention one after another in due order; to go over or through (a series) in this manner; to recount, relate, narrate, and tell; to mention; to allege; to calculate, work out, decide the nature or value of; to consider, judge, or estimate by, or as the result of calculation; to consider, think, suppose, be of opinion; to speak or discourse of something; to render or give an account (of one's conduct, etc.); and to regard in a certain light (Simpson & Weiner, 1989, pp. 335–336). Reckoning is "the action of rendering to another an account of one's self or one's conduct; an account, statement of something" (Simpson & Weiner, 1989, p. 336).

## ■ CONCEPTS OF THE THEORY

Concepts in the middle range theory of Moral Reckoning include ease, situational binds, resolution, and reflection. The named concepts of the theory are processes that comprise the stages of moral reckoning that occur over time. The second concept, situational bind, is an event that interrupts the stage of ease.

### Ease

Ease is a state of naturalness, a sense of comfort. Ease assumes a certain measure of freedom from constraint, worry, hardship, and agitation. Ease also denotes readiness and skillfulness. Nurses who experience ease are comfortable. They have technical skills and feel rewarded to practice within the boundaries of self, profession, and institution. They know their patients and witness their suffering, making the implicit promise that they have the skill and knowledge to relieve suffering. These nurses are competent and confident. They know what others expect of them and experience a sense of flow and at-homeness. When at ease, nurses have high standards and are proud of their technical abilities and skill at communicating with patients and others. As long as the work of nursing fulfills the nurse and the nurse experiences a sense of comfort with the integration of core beliefs and professional and institutional norms, then ease continues.

### Situational Binds

Situational binds are serious and complex conflicts within individuals and tacit or overt conflicts between nurses and others—all having moral overtones. The concept *situational bind* was discussed by Strauss (1959), who theorized that when situational binds occur the person questions his or her central purpose, asking to what, for what, or to whom he or she is committed. The person experiences turmoil and inner dialogue that leads to a decision.

Situational binds lead to life turning points. These incidents transform identity and force a person to recognize that "I am not the same as I was, as I used to be" (Strauss, 1959, p. 93). Critical incidents lead to anxiety, tension, and self-questioning—and also the need to explore and validate the new and exciting or frightening ideas (Strauss, 1959, p. 93). Situational binds lead to decisions that ultimately change people's lives.

## Resolution

Resolution is a move to set things right, to resolve the turmoil, and to relieve the tension. Resolution occurs when a person terminates the intolerable condition by finding a solution to the problem, deciding on a course of action, and bringing a situation to a conclusion. The person might make a declaration or carry out a plan. Resolution tends to disentangle one from a situational bind.

## Reflection

Reflection is contemplating, pondering, and thinking about past events. Having made and acted upon a decision, a person reflects as he or she reckons past behavior and actions. The person carefully considers the events and generates opinions. Reflection raises questions about previous judgments, particular acts, and the essential self. Reflection may extend over a lifetime.

## ■ RELATIONSHIPS AMONG THE CONCEPTS: THE MODEL

Moral reckoning consists of a three-stage process and critical juncture as nurses reflect on motivations, choices, actions, and consequences of a morally troubling patient care situation (Nathaniel, 2004, 2006). The relationship among the stages is depicted in Figure 15.1. In the middle range theory of Moral Reckoning, the stage of ease is disrupted by a situational bind and then followed by the processes of resolution and reflection.

## The Stage of Ease

After the initial novice phase, nurses experience a stage of ease in which they enjoy a sense of satisfaction and at-homeness in the workplace. They feel comfortable with their knowledge and skills. Properties central to the stage of ease include becoming, professionalizing, institutionalizing, and working. There is a fragile balance among the properties during the stage of ease such that each property is related to the other, creating a feeling of comfort.

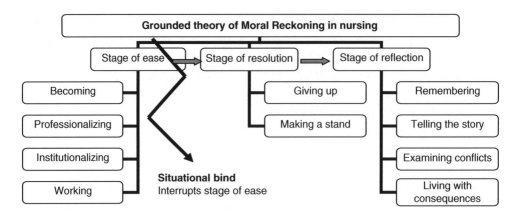

**FIGURE 15.1**  Moral Reckoning.

*Source:* Reprinted from Nathaniel, A. K. (2006). Moral reckoning in nursing. *Western Journal of Nursing Research*, 28(4), 419–438.

## BECOMING

As Strauss once wrote, "The human experience of time is one of process: the present is always a becoming" (Strauss, 1959, p. 31). Through the process of becoming every person evolves a set of core beliefs and values, which are a product of lifelong learning about what is important and how to behave in society. Core beliefs evolve through experience, from the testimony of authority, and from the modeling of parents, teachers, ministers, peers, and others. Integration and consistency of core values produce moral integrity (Beauchamp & Childress, 2013). Through the lifelong process of becoming, nurses develop core beliefs and values.

## PROFESSIONALIZING

The process of becoming a nurse includes inculcation of certain cultural norms learned in nursing school and early practice. Professional norms are conceptual ideals that contribute to the nurse's idea of what a good nurse should be or do. Explicitly, nurses learn that they have unique relationships with patients and are responsible to keep promises, which are sometimes implicit in the relationship. Penticuff identified moral goals that are part of nursing's common perspective, such as "the protection and enhancement of human dignity, the alleviation of vulnerability, the promotion of growth and health, and the enhancement of coping and comfort in the face of hardship" (Penticuff, 1997, p. 51). Likewise, nurses honor the common professional norms of knowing patients as persons, listening to their needs and preferences, supporting their everyday choices through advocacy, and maintaining their dignity (Doutrich, Wros, & Izumi, 2001).

Professionalizing is supported by the theoretical work of Strauss (1959) and Glaser (1998). Strauss suggested that to become a member of a group, a person must invest in the goals of the group. Investment in a group occurs through the transmission of ideas and signifies shared meanings. Insofar as the person thinks of himself or herself as an integral part of the group, he or she embraces its goals. The person, then, has dual commitment to the group and to self. Strauss also suggested that a person may be so heavily identified with the group that "he is no longer quite himself" (Strauss, 1959, p. 37). Validation by the group is so important that the person reinterprets activity and meaning. Thus, as can be seen in moral reckoning, the person's core values may be either supported or challenged by the values of the group as the person becomes professionalized. Similarly, Glaser (1998) proposed that personal identities may merge with the properties of a profession so that members find it difficult to break through the boundaries (Glaser, 1998). In this situation, the unit identity becomes the person's self-image. Professional norms sometimes lead nurses to act according to role-set behavior, governed by blind adherence to professional norms and by their perception of the expectations of others.

### INSTITUTIONALIZING

The third property rests on the premise that the nurse works in an institutional setting with both implicit and explicit institutional norms. This is corroborated by the studies of Liaschenko (1995) and Ehrenreich and Ehrenreich (1990), who propose that institutionalized medicine is a complex interconnected tangle of practice patterns, cultural beliefs, and values. Institutional healthcare delivery norms constitute basic social structural processes within which the practice of nursing takes place. Explicit institutional norms include completing a job according to institutional standards and respecting lines of authority. Implicit institutional norms include such concepts as ensuring that the business makes a profit, following orders, and handling crises without making waves.

### WORKING

The work of nursing is varied, challenging, and rewarding. Nurses attend to the most personal and private needs and learn much about patients' hopes, fears, and desires (Penticuff, 1997). They get to know patients who stay on their unit for extended periods or return many times. Doing the work of nursing includes knowing patients intimately, witnessing their suffering, accepting the responsibility to care, desiring to do the work well, and knowing what to do.

## Situational Binds

Sometimes troubling events occur that challenge the integration of core beliefs, professional norms, and institutional norms. When this happens, nurses find themselves in *situational binds* that force them into a critical juncture in their professional lives (Nathaniel, 2004, 2006).

A situational bind terminates the stage of ease and throws the nurse into turmoil when core beliefs and other claims conflict. Three types of situational binds include conflicts between core values and professional or institutional norms, moral disagreement among decision makers in the face of power imbalance, and workplace deficiencies that cause real or potential harm to patients (Nathaniel, 2004, 2006). These binds produce dramatic consequences for nurses when they must choose one value or belief over another—forcing a turning point in their professional lives.

Situational binds in nursing involve an intricate interweaving of many factors including professional relationships, divergent values, workplace demands, and other implications with moral overtones. Situational binds vary in their complexity, context, and particulars but are similar in terms of their immediate and long-term effects. When situational binds occur, nurses must make critical decisions—choosing one value or belief over another. Specific types of binds include conflict between the nurse's core beliefs and professional or institutional norms, power imbalance complicated by differences in beliefs and values, conflicting loyalty, and serious workplace deficiencies (Nathaniel, 2004, 2006). Types of cases most frequently mentioned in the extant literature included causing needless suffering by prolonging the life of dying patients or performing unnecessary tests and treatments, especially on terminal patients; lying to patients; incompetent or inadequate treatment by a physician; and coercing consent from poorly informed patients (Cavaliere, Daly, Dowling, & Montgomery, 2010; Corley, 1995; Cummings, 2011; Deady & McCarthy, 2010; Dewitte, Piers, Steeman, & Nele, 2010; Dunwoody, 2011; Gaeta & Price, 2010; Hall, Brinchmann, & Aagaard, 2012; Halpern, 2011; Huffman & Rittenmeyer, 2012; McArthur, 2010; Mueller, Ottenberg, Hayes, & Koenig, 2011; Piers et al., 2011, 2012; Rodney, 1988; Whitehead, Herbertson, Hamric, Epstein, & Fisher, 2015; Wilkinson, 1987).

The disruption of ease that nurses experience during situational binds results from a number of dynamic internal and external tensions (Nathaniel, 2004, 2006). For example, the ability to act on moral decisions may be constrained by socialization to follow orders, self-doubt, lack of courage, and conflicting loyalty. Penticuff (1997) also found that nurses struggle with conflicting loyalties to patients, nursing peers, physicians, and institutions. Asymmetrical power relationships and powerlessness often lead to situational binds. Nurses may have insight into the problem at hand yet believe they cannot participate in the decision-making process. They sense a moral responsibility, want the best outcome for patients, know what is needed, and yet believe they are powerless to get it done. In some instances, nurses experience distress when they know the professional and institutional norms, and yet are unable to uphold them because of workplace deficiencies. Workplace deficiencies include such factors as chronic staff shortage, unreasonable institutional expectations, and equipment inadequacy (Nathaniel, 2004, 2006). Situational binds force nurses to make difficult decisions in the midst of crises characterized by intolerable internal conflict. Something must be done to rectify the situation: One must make a choice.

In the midst of the situational bind or soon after, nurses experience consequences such as profound emotions, reactive behaviors, and physical manifestations. Nurses may experience feelings of guilt, anger, powerlessness, conflict, depression, outrage, betrayal, and devastation. Physical manifestations such as lightheadedness, crying, sleeplessness, and vomiting may also occur.

During the time of or after situational binds, nursing care is affected— sometimes negatively and sometimes positively. Some nurses are unable to care for the patient or to even return to the unit after a troubling incident. Some nurses make up for what they consider to be wrongdoing by giving more compassionate care—even to the point of sacrificing personal time. For others, care improves in the long term because of lessons learned in the process.

## The Stage of Resolution

Situational binds constitute crises of intolerable internal conflict. The nurse seeks to resolve the problem and set things right. This signifies the beginning of the stage of resolution. This stage often alters one's professional trajectory. There are two properties of the stage of resolution: making a stand and giving up. These properties are not mutually exclusive. In fact, a nurse might give up, reconsider, and make a stand.

### MAKING A STAND

In the midst of a situational bind, some nurses choose to make a stand. Making a stand takes a variety of forms—all of which include professional risk. Nurses may even make a stand by stepping beyond the proscribed boundaries of the profession to do what, to them, seems to be the morally correct action. Nurses may make a stand by refusing to follow physicians' orders, initiating negotiations, breaking rules, whistle-blowing, and so forth. Making a stand is rarely successful in the short term. Not a single informant in Liaschenko's (1995) study reported an instance where treatment was stopped on his or her testimony. Nevertheless, making a stand may occasionally improve the overall situation in the long term.

### GIVING UP

Sometimes nurses resolve a morally troubling situation by giving up. Giving up may overlap with making a stand in some instances. Nurses often give up because they recognize the futility of making an overt stand. They are simply not willing to sacrifice for no purpose. They may give up to protect themselves or to seek a way or find a place where they can better integrate core beliefs, professional norms, and institutional norms. Giving up includes participating (with regret) in an activity they consider to be morally wrong, such as leaving the unit, the institution, or the profession altogether. Sometimes nurses seem to give up in the short term but move toward more advanced autonomous roles or toward leadership positions—all of which prepare them to make a stand in the future.

## The Stage of Reflection

During the stage of reflection, the nurse thoughtfully examines beliefs, values, and actions. Properties of the stage of reflection include remembering, telling the story, examining conflicts, and living with the consequences. During this stage, which may last a lifetime, nurses reflect on the moral problem and their response. Nurses recall vivid mental pictures and evoked emotions such as feelings of guilt and self-blame, lingering sadness, anger, and anxiety. Moral reckoning continues over time as nurses remember, tell the story, examine conflicts, and live with the consequences.

### REMEMBERING

One of the more intriguing properties of moral reckoning is the manner in which nurses remember critical events. After particularly troubling situations, nurses retain vivid mental pictures, which tend to evoke emotions many years later. Nurses remember sensual particulars of the incident—the sights, sounds, and smells. Even after many years, the images are seared into their minds. Remembering evokes emotions including feelings of guilt and self-blame, lingering sadness, anger, and anxiety. Lingering emotional effects may be profound for many.

Strauss (1959) proposed that a remembered act is never finished. As a person recalls the act, he or she selectively reconstructs it, remembering certain aspects and dropping others. The person reassesses acts many times, seeking new perspectives or new facts. Thus, learning leads to revision of concepts that, in turn, leads to reorganization of behavior. Strauss further proposed that the process of continual learning and revision results in a new identity. This reflection raises challenges and the discovery of new values through which transformation takes place.

### TELLING THE STORY

Nurses want to tell the story to sympathetic others. They may tell a friend or family member immediately after an incident occurs or meet with other nurses to discuss the event. Nurses rely upon others to hear the story and to understand it from their perspective. A listening, nonjudgmental person allows the nurse to tell the story as he or she attempts to seek meaning and to reckon belief and action. Nurses continue the process over time—telling and retelling the story as they try to make sense of it. Smith and Liehr (2014) address story-gathering in the chapter describing Story Theory. They contend that engaging in dialogue about unique human experience catalyzes the beginning of a process of personal change. Through following the story path as recollected, one begins a process of discovery, self-revelation, and reckoning. As the story unfolds, the person attempts to understand the meaning of experiences and gain new perspectives and wisdom. The person goes into the depths of the story to find unique meanings and reconstruct a story that has a beginning, middle, and end. Consistent with the Theory of Moral Reckoning, Smith and Liehr propose that as the person tells the story, he or she gains a full-dimensional, reflective awareness of bodily experiences, thoughts, feelings, emotions, and values. Patterns are discerned, made explicit, and named. Telling the story relieves pain and creates possibilities for human development.

## EXAMINING CONFLICTS

As nurses tell their stories, they begin to examine conflicts in the troubling situation. They examine their values and ask questions about what actually happened, who was to blame, and how they can avoid similar situations in the future. As they thoughtfully examine the conflicts, some intellectualize their participation, some set limits, and some gain strength to make a stand and accept the consequences in future situations.

Nurses continue to struggle with conflicts between personal values and professional ideals. They want to be able to identify themselves as good nurses. Similarly, Kelly (1998) reported that some nurses have a painful awareness of the discrepancy between who they aspired to be and what they have become. These nurses suffer the loss of their own professional self-concept, their vision of the kind of nurses they wanted to be, and their image of nursing as they believed it was.

As nurses think about their roles in what they consider past moral wrongdoing, some set limits or make pronouncements about their future actions. Some identify a point beyond which they will not again be willing to go. Others vow to step outside their boundaries to help a patient in the future, fully aware and willing to accept the consequences of their future actions. Thus, the nurse's ethical practice evolves through the iterative process of experience and reflection.

## LIVING WITH THE CONSEQUENCES

Nurses live with the consequences of morally troubling situations for a prolonged period of time. Consequences other than those already mentioned include fractured professional relationships and a change in one's life trajectory.

Following a situational bind in which the nurse believes another person committed moral wrongdoing, he or she may be unable to work collaboratively with that person or others who were unsupportive. They lose faith in the person's integrity and respect for them as practitioners. Since they are no longer comfortable in the original workplace and have fractured professional relationships, many nurses change their work setting following a situational bind. They may change employers or specialties and are likely to seek further education intending to correct the type of moral wrongs they experienced in the past.

## ■ USE OF THE THEORY IN NURSING RESEARCH

The Theory of Moral Reckoning has been used to expand the knowledge base of nursing and other disciplines. Newly published studies in nursing and medicine use the specific definitions, concepts, findings, or the entire theory to further explore and more fully develop what is known about moral distress and moral reckoning. The Theory of Moral Reckoning served as a theoretical model for several research studies. For example, Pratt, Martin, Mohide, and Black (2013) used the theory to structure research focusing on how moral distress impacts the nurse educator's decisions regarding whether to pass or fail unsatisfactory students, and Allen and Butler (2016) used the theory to show how interventions to alleviate moral distress lead to improvements. Recent research and other scholarship that focuses on moral reckoning has originated from many countries including the United States, Iran, Korea, Brazil, Switzerland, Italy, Sweden, the Netherlands, Ireland, Turkey, Spain, Canada, Uganda, New Zealand, Chile, China, Poland, South Africa, and the United Kingdom (Abbaszadeh, Nozar, & Mostafa, 2013; Barlem & Ramos, 2015; Brisbois, 2016; Bruce, Weinzimmer, & Zimmerman, 2014; Callister, Luthy, Thompson, & Memmott, 2009; Cho, An, & So, 2016; da Costa Cordoza et al., 2012; den Uil-Westerlaken & Cusveller, 2013; DeTienne, Agle, Phillips, & Ingersol, 2012; Edmonson, 2010, 2015; Garros, 2016; Harrowing & Mill, 2010; Hinz, 2016; Laabs, 2011; Langley, Kisorio, & Schmollgruber, 2015; Lazzarin, Biondi, & Di Mauro, 2012; McCarthy & Gastmans, 2015; McClendon & Buckner, 2007; Mumbrue, 2010; Rushton, 2013; Shoorideh, Ashktorab, Yaghmaei, & Alavi Majd, 2015; Sporrong, Hoglund, & Arnetz, 2006; Stanley & Matchett, 2014; Wiegand & Funk, 2012; Winland-Brown & Dobrin, 2009; Wojtowicz & Hagen, 2014; Woods, Rodgers, Towers, & La Grow, 2015; Zuzelo, 2007).

The Theory of Moral Reckoning has been used in many nursing students' scholarly work. Graduate and undergraduate students regularly request information about the theory as they prepare various assignments. Recognizing that moral distress is an integral element of moral reckoning, national and international doctoral dissertations such as those by Deady (2014), Healee (2013), Baxter (2012), and Porter (2010) cited moral reckoning as a reference point or used the theory as a foundation of their research. Relying on substantial elements of the theory, for example, Porter focused on nurse managers' perceptions of the external constraints on moral agency, which lead to moral distress. Master's students have also used the Theory of Moral Reckoning to examine ethical issues in nursing practice. For example, Michael Fulks (2015) related the stages of moral reckoning to the everyday practice of nurses in intensive care areas. Mumbrue (2010) focused heavily on moral reckoning in her master's thesis as she conducted a phenomenological study of nurses who experience the unexpected death of a patient. Moral reckoning has gained an audience among students and experienced scholars, yet more work needs to be done.

Vigorous theoretical sampling is needed to (a) allow a more thorough and useful understanding of the concepts of ease, situational bind, resolution, and reflection; (b) provide a better understanding of core values as they intersect with professional and institutional norms; and (c) modify the theory to include different levels of nursing practice.

In addition, nursing ethics research is needed to shed light on what nurses understand about nursing ethics, the depth of this understanding, how the understanding factors into everyday decision making, and what kind of learning leads to empowered, patient-centered, ethical decision making. Further qualitative and quantitative research is needed to determine the characteristics of nurses who experience moral distress and moral reckoning versus those who do not, including the quality of patient care provided by each group. Correlational research is needed to identify nurses who leave the bedside and those who stay, particularly in relation to whether or not they have experienced situational binds. In the face of the nursing shortage, this has implications for nurse recruiting and retention. If caring and sensitive nurses leave the bedside, it is important to identify strategies to retain them.

Research on moral reckoning should not be limited to the profession of nursing. Investigators have an opportunity to use the theory with a wide variety of populations. For instance, professionals who are forced to face moral problems encountered in crisis situations affecting humanity, such as natural disasters or terrorist events, may experience moral reckoning. Significant losses, such as the death of a child or the loss of a family-sustaining job, create a context for moral reckoning. In addition, the obvious use of the theory with other disciplines deserves consideration, particularly as related to nursing practice and patient outcomes.

## ■ USE OF THE THEORY IN NURSING PRACTICE

Interest in the Theory of Moral Reckoning and moral distress has become intense within the nursing profession in the past several years. The literature reveals that these phenomena are problems for other professions and other cultures as well. The Theory of Moral Reckoning has been cited in innumerable publications worldwide. Literature focusing on nurses, nursing students, bioethicists, physicians, podiatrists, educators, pharmacists, and police has cited the Theory of Moral Reckoning. Moral distress has even been documented among veterinarians.

## Implications for Nursing Ethics Development

Moral reckoning points to a chasm between the ethical practice of nurses and Formal Ethics Theory. This may indicate what MacIntyre (1988) terms an "epistemological crisis" in nursing: a crisis that occurs when events bring into question ideals and convictions of a tradition and when previous methods of inquiry, conceptualization, and principles fall into question. MacIntyre suggests that an epistemological crisis can be resolved successfully through innovations that meet three requirements: (a) new concepts and new theory must furnish a systematic and rational solution to a previously unmanageable problem; (b) innovations must explain what it was that made the tradition ineffective; and (c) the new tradition must carry out tasks in a way that exhibits some fundamental continuity of new conceptual and theoretical structures with shared beliefs (MacIntyre, 1988). Such ethics will allow for consideration of the uniqueness and particularity of patient situations, while acknowledging diverse moral perspectives. As MacIntyre (1988) suggests, nurses should come to understand rival perspectives as different, yet comprising complementary understandings of reality.

## Implications for Nursing Educators

The Theory of Moral Reckoning in nursing caught the attention of many nursing educators. Reference to the theory is seen in educational materials from West Virginia University, University of Manitoba, Breyer State University, Morehead State University, Johns Hopkins University, Ryerson University, University of Minnesota, Haifa University, University of Kentucky, and others. It is also found online on a variety of electronic platforms. There are presentations on moral reckoning and its constituent element of situational binds on YouTube (Boyd, 2013a, 2013b), on educational flashcards that present moral reckoning as one of five types of moral problems (Sijeffer, 2011), and in an animated presentation that describes the theory (Hanson, 2013). It has also been cited in educational materials on the Canadian Nurses Association and American Nurses Association websites (Edmonson, 2010, 2015; Edwards, 2009). Through the educational experiences listed previously, students are guided to find ways to recognize, avoid, or resolve situational binds through values clarification, autonomous decision making, and authentic communication.

The theory has been applied to several research studies. An excellent example is a study by Pratt et al. (2013), who used the theory to guide a descriptive analysis of six studies focusing on moral dilemmas and the impact of moral distress in the educational setting. The Theory of Moral Reckoning served as the theoretical model to help the investigators understand how nurse educators work through moral dilemmas, make decisions, and provide justification. Using the Theory of Moral Reckoning as a theoretical model, Pratt et al. (2013) analyzed findings of six previous studies. Findings of the six studies were determined to fit within the theory, particularly in relation to the situational binds and the stages of resolution and reflection. For example, the investigators were able to identify the property of "giving up" among those nurse educators who assigned passing grades, even when they doubted a student's clinical competency. Perceived pressures, which constituted the situational bind, included educators' thoughts about jeopardizing the students' future career choices, fear of damaging their own reputation with colleagues, and fear of endangering their reappointment or tenure if student evaluations were poor. Pratt et al. (2013) found the Theory of Moral Reckoning to be parsimonious and useful for gaining a deeper understanding of educators' decision making when faced with unsatisfactory students. One of the hallmarks of Grounded Theory research is the idea that theories are always modifiable when new data emerge. The work of these investigators and others adds new dimensions to the theory and adds credence to use of the theory in diverse settings. Even though the Theory of Moral Reckoning has gained the attention of many nurse educators, more work is still to be done.

The Theory of Moral Reckoning brings forth several implications for nursing education. Nurse educators should continue to strengthen nursing ethics education, teaching strategies to improve nurses' empowerment, and helping students learn effective ways to establish intra- and interprofessional relationships. Nurse educators should teach students to be ethically self-aware and provide opportunities for them to learn about normative ethics. Educators can closely examine implicit messages transmitted to students, particularly traditions of the discipline that inhibit meaningful dialogue and sustain conflict and power imbalance. In this manner, they help students learn strategies and language that prepare them to enter into ethical dialogue with other professionals and to prepare students for the realities of practice.

Specifically, the middle range theory of Moral Reckoning uncovers a basic social process that educators should discuss with students in great detail. Nurse educators help to prepare novice nurses through curricula that include recognition of the conditions of the stage of ease—becoming, professionalizing, and institutionalizing. To help prepare students for the real world, educators can facilitate dialogue that uncovers sources of conflict between core beliefs, professional traditions, and institutional expectations. They can acknowledge the unique relationship between nurses and patients, recognizing special elements of the relationship such as knowing intimately and witnessing suffering.

Nurse educators can also prepare students for situational binds related to asymmetrical power relationships, loyalty conflicts, and workplace deficiencies. When students practice dealing with these problems in simulated educational circumstances, they may find better ways to deal with situational binds before encountering them in the workplace. Educators might also prepare students for the stage of resolution and the properties of giving up and making a stand in order to be better prepared to follow integrity-preserving courses of action.

Nurse educators must return to a clear focus on nursing codes of ethics. When nurses internalize professional ethics, they may be less likely to waver when faced with situational binds. Ongoing research of moral reckoning is being conducted utilizing a sample of professionals from other disciplines. Preliminary findings seem to indicate that professionals from disciplines in which educators clearly focus on a code of professional ethics are less likely to experience moral reckoning.

In addition to its use in nursing ethics education and research, the Theory of Moral Reckoning has also been used to teach advanced research techniques. A number of nursing research textbooks have presented the theory as an exemplar for Grounded Theory research (De Chesnay, 2014; Polit & Beck, 2008, 2010; Streubert & Carpenter, 2011).

## Implications for Practicing Nurses

Because it is a middle range theory, Moral Reckoning is easily applicable to nursing practice. In addition to the practice implications that are made explicit in the theory, subsequent research continues to identify implications and recommendations for nurses in practice.

Practicing nurses should internalize their code of professional ethics and claim their professional autonomy. Preliminary findings of the research, mentioned earlier, also seem to indicate that professionals who acknowledge their own autonomy are less likely to experience moral reckoning. When situational binds occur, they may be more likely to act according to their own values, rather than feel compelled to violate them.

Avoiding situational binds and searching for integrity-saving compromise may help practicing nurses engaged in morally troubling situations. A structured discussion of the process of moral reckoning may lead to an increase of satisfaction with nursing care. In these discussion groups, nurses can purposely examine core values and their relationship to professional and institutional norms.

## ■ CONCLUSION

This middle range theory of Moral Reckoning encompasses moral distress yet reaches further—identifying a life event experienced through disruption of ease as one confronts a situational bind demanding resolution and reflection. The concepts of the theory—ease, situational bind, resolution, and reflection—name the stages of the basic social process of moral reckoning. The theory has been developed in the context of the discipline of nursing, but its use in other contexts promises meaningful guidance and ongoing development.

## ■ REFERENCES

Abbaszadeh, A., Nozar, N., & Mostafa, R. (2013). The relationship between moral distress and retention in nurses of Birjand teaching hospital. *Journal of Medical Ethics and History of Medicine*, 6(2), 57–66.

Allen, R., & Butler, E. (2016). Addressing moral distress in critical care nurses: A pilot study. *International Journal of Critical Care and Emergency Medicine*, 2(2). Retrieved from http://clinmedjournals.org/articles/ijccem/international-journal-of -critical-care-and-emergency-medicine-ijccem-2-015.pdf

Barlem, E. L., & Ramos, F. R. (2015). Constructing a theoretical model of moral distress. *Nursing Ethics*, 22(5), 608–615.

Baxter, M. L. (2012). *Being certain: Moral distress in critical care nurses* (PhD Dissertation). Virginia Commonwealth University, Richmond, VA.

Beauchamp, T. L., & Childress, J. F. (2013). *Principles of biomedical ethics* (7th ed.). New York, NY: Oxford University Press.

Boyd, S. (Producer). (2013a). Moral reckoning. Retrieved from https://www .youtube.com/watch?v=SPFZ8M4yzdQ

Boyd, S. (Producer). (2013b). Situational bind scene. Retrieved from https://www .youtube.com/watch?v=ZAOCuv6hUr0

Brisbois, M. D. (2016). The use of critical reflective inquiry among American baccalaureate nursing students in a global service learning experience in Haiti: A qualitative study. *Journal of Nursing Education and Practice*, 6, 84–92.

Bruce, C. R., Weinzimmer, S., & Zimmerman, J. L. (2014). Moral distress in the ICU. In J. L. Vincent (Ed.), *Annual update in Intensive Care and Emergency Medicine 2014*. Swizerland: Springer International.

Burkhardt, M. A., & Nathaniel, A. K. (1998). *Ethics & issues in contemporary nursing*. New York, NY: Cengage.

Burkhardt, M. A., & Nathaniel, A. K. (2013). *Ethics & issues in contemporary nursing* (4th ed., Vol. 4). New York, NY: Cengage.

Callister, L. C., Luthy, K. E., Thompson, P., & Memmott, R. J. (2009). Ethical reasoning in baccalaureate nursing students. *Nursing Ethics*, 16(4), 499–510.

Cavaliere, T. A., Daly, B., Dowling, D., & Montgomery, K. (2010). Moral distress in neonatal intensive care unit RNs. *Advances in Neonatal Care*, 10(3), 145–156.

Cho, H. N., An, J., & So, H. S. (2016). Differences of turnover intention by moral distress of nurses. *Journal of the Korea Contents Association*, 15(5), 403–413.

Corley, M. C. (1995). Moral distress of critical care nurses. *American Journal of Critical Care*, 4(4), 280–285.

Cummings, C. L. (2011). What factors affect nursing retention in the acute care setting? *Journal of Research in Nursing, 16*(6), 489–500. doi:10.1177/1744987111407594

da Costa Cordoza, C. R., Barlem, E. L. D., Lunardi, V. L., Barlem, J. G. T., Vidal, D. A. S., & Botelho, L. R. (2012). Ethical conflicts that have influence in nursing work in obstetrics units. *Journal of Nursing: UFPE On Line, 6*(7), 1523–1529. Retrieved from http://www.academia.edu/9476359/ETHICAL_CONFLICTS_THAT_HAVE_AN_INFLUENCE_IN_NURSING_WORK_IN_OBSTETRICS_UNITS_2012

Deady, R. (2014). *Moral shielding: A grounded theory of integrity maintenance in multidisciplinary teams* (PhD Thesis). University College Cork, Cork, Ireland.

Deady, R., & McCarthy, J. (2010). A study of the situations, features, and coping mechanisms experienced by Irish psychiatric nurses experiencing moral distress. *Perspectives in Psychiatric Care, 46*(3), 209–220.

De Chesnay, M. (2014). *Nursing research using grounded theory: Qualitative designs and methods in nursing.* New York: NY: Springer Publishing.

den Uil-Westerlaken, J., & Cusveller, B. (2013). Competencies in nursing students for organized forms of clinical moral deliberation and decision-making. *Journal of Nursing Education and Practice, 3*(11), 1–8.

DeTienne, K. B., Agle, B. R., Phillips, J. C., & Ingersol, M. C. (2012). The impact of moral stress compared to other stressors on employee fatigue, job satisfaction, and turnover: An empirical investigation. *Journal of Business Ethics, 110,* 337–391.

Dewitte, M., Piers, R., Steeman, E., & Nele. (2010). Moral distress and burn-out in nurses on acute geriatric wards: Fourth European Nursing Congress. *Journal of Clinical Nursing, 19,* 19–20.

Doutrich, D., Wros, P., & Izumi, S. (2001). Relief of suffering and regard for personhood: Nurses' ethical concerns in Japan and the USA. *Nursing Ethics, 8*(5), 448–458.

Dunwoody, D. (2011). Nurses' level of moral distress and perception of futile care in the critical care environment. *Dynamics, 22*(2), 22–24.

Edmonson, C. (2010). Moral courage and the nurse leader. *Online Journal of Issues in Nursing, 15*(3). Retrieved from http://www.nursingworld.org/MainMenu Categories/ANAMarketplace/ANAPeriodicals/OJIN/TableofContents/Vol152010/No3-Sept-2010/Moral-Courage-for-Nurse-Leaders.html

Edmonson, C. (2015). Strengthening moral courage among nurse leaders. *Online Journal of Issues in Nursing, 20*(2), 9. Retrieved from http://www.nursingworld .org/MainMenuCategories/ANAMarketplace/ANAPeriodicals/OJIN/TableofContents/Vol-20-2015/No2-May-2015/Articles-Previous-Topics/Strengthening-Moral-Courage.html

Edwards, M. (2009). *Moral distress in ICU nurses* [PowerPoint Presentation]. Manitoba, Canada: University of Manitoba.

Ehrenreich, B., & Ehrenreich, J. (1990). The system behind the chaos. In N. F. McKenzie (Ed.), *The crisis in health care: Ethical issues* (pp. 50–69). New York, NY: Meridian.

Fulks, M. (2015). *Theoretical and ethical basis of practice: Alarm fatigue.* Mobile: University of South Alabama.

Gaeta, S., & Price, K. J. (2010). End-of-life issues in critically ill cancer patients. *Critical Care Clinics, 26*(1), 219–227.

Garros, D. (2016). Moral distress in the everyday life of an intensivist. *Frontiers in Pediatrics, 4*, 91.

Glaser, B. G. (1965). The constant comparative method of qualitative analysis. *Social problems, 12*, 10.

Glaser, B. G. (1978). *Theoretical sensitivity: Advances in the methodology of grounded theory*. Mill Valley, CA: Sociology Press.

Glaser, B. G. (1998). *Doing grounded theory: Issues and discussion*. Mill Valley, CA: Sociology Press.

Glaser, B. G., & Strauss, A. L. (1967). *The discovery of grounded theory: Strategies for qualitative research*. New Brunswick, NJ: Aldine Transaction.

Hall, E. O. C., Brinchmann, B. S., & Aagaard, H. (2012). The challenge of integrating justice and care in neonatal nursing. *Nursing Ethics, 19*(1), 80–90.

Halpern, S. D. (2011). Perceived inappropriateness of care in the ICU: What to make of the clinician's perspective? *Journal of the American Medical Association, 306*(24), 2725–2726.

Hanson, E. (Producer). (2013). Theory of moral reckoning: A grounded mid-range theory by Alvita Nathaniel. Retrieved from https://prezi.com/sg7cjfk9a1wt/theory-of-moral-reckoning

Harrowing, J. N., & Mill, J. (2010). Moral distress among Ugandan nurses providing HIV care: A critical ethnography. *International Journal of Nursing Studies, 47*, 723–731. doi:10.1016/j.ijnurstu.2009.11.010

Healee, D. (2013). *Restoring: A grounded theory of recovery* (PhD Thesis). University of Aukland, Aukland, New Zealand.

Hinz, C. (2016). Making the most of a moral dilemma. *Daily Nurse*. Retrieved from http://dailynurse.com/making-moral-dilemma

Huffman, D. M., & Rittenmeyer, L. (2012). How professional nurses working in hospital environments experience moral distress: A systematic review. *Critical Care Nursing Clinics of North America, 24*(1), 91–100.

Jameton, A. (1984). *Nursing practice: The ethical issues*. Englewood Cliffs, NJ: Prentice-Hall.

Jameton, A. (1993). Dilemmas of moral distress: Moral responsibility and nursing practice. *Clinical Issues in Perinatal and Women's Health Nursing, 4*(4), 542–551.

Kelly, B. (1998). Preserving moral integrity: A follow-up study with new graduate nurses. *Journal of Advanced Nursing, 28*(5), 1134–1145.

Laabs, C. (2011). Perceptions of moral integrity: Contradictions in need of explanation. *Nursing Ethics, 18*(3), 431–440.

Langley, G. C., Kisorio, L., & Schmollgruber, S. (2015). Moral distress experienced by intensive care nurses. *Southern African Journal of Critical Care, 31*(2), 36–41.

Lazzarin, M., Biondi, A., & Di Mauro, S. (2012). Moral distress in nurses in oncology and haematology units. *Nursing Ethics, 19*(2), 183–195.

Liaschenko, J. (1995). Artificial personhood: Nursing ethics in a medical world. *Nursing Ethics, 2*(3), 185–196.

MacIntyre, A. C. (1988). *Whose justice? Which rationality?* Notre Dame, IN: University of Notre Dame Press.

McArthur, A. (2010). How professional nurses working in hospital environments experience moral distress: A systematic review. *Journal of Advanced Nursing, 66*(5), 962–963.

McCarthy, J., & Gastmans, C. (2015). Moral distress: A review of the argument-based nursing ethics literature. *Nursing Ethics, 22*(1), 131–152.

McClendon, H., & Buckner, E. B. (2007). Distressing situations in the intensive care unit: A descriptive study of nurses' responses. *Dimensions of Critical Care Nursing, 26*(5), 199–206.

Mueller, P. S., Ottenberg, A. L., Hayes, D. L., & Koenig, B. A. (2011). "I felt like the angel of death": Role conflicts and moral distress among allied professionals employed by the US cardiovascular implantable electronic device industry. *Journal of Interventional Cardiac Electrophysiology: An International Journal of Arrhythmias and Pacing, 32*(3), 253–261.

Mumbrue, T. L. (2010). *The lived experience of nurses who encounter the unexpected death of a patient.* MSN, University of Wisconsin, Oshkosh, Oshkosh, WI.

Nathaniel, A. K. (2004). A grounded theory of moral reckoning in nursing. *Grounded Theory Review, 4*(1).

Nathaniel, A. K. (2006). Moral reckoning in nursing. *Western journal of nursing research, 28*(4), 419–438; discussion 439–448.

Penticuff, J. H. (1997). Nursing perspectives in bioethics. In K. Hoshino (Ed.), *Japanese and Western bioethics* (pp. 49–60). The Netherlands: Khower Academic Publishers.

Piers, R. D., Azoulay, E., Ricou, B., Dekeyser Ganz, F., Decruyenaere, J., Max, A., . . . Benoit, D. D. (2011). Perceptions of appropriateness of care among European and Israeli intensive care unit nurses and physicians. *Journal of the American Medical Association, 306*(24), 2694–2703.

Piers, R. D., Magali, Steeman, E., Vlerick, P., Benoit, D. D., & Nele J, N. (2012). End-of-life care of the geriatric patient and nurses' moral distress. *Journal of the American Medical Directors Association, 13*(1), 7–13.

Polit, D. F., & Beck, C. T. (2008). *Nursing research: Generating and assessing evidence for nursing practice* (8th ed.). Philadelphia, PA: Wolters Kluwer Health/Lippincott Williams & Wilkins.

Polit, D. F., & Beck, C. T. (2010). *Essentials of nursing research: Appraising evidence for nursing practice* (7th ed.). Philadelphia, PA: Wolters Kluwer Health/Lippincott Williams & Wilkins.

Porter, R. B. (2010). *Nurse managers' moral distress in the context of the hospital ethical climate* (PhD Dissertation). University of Iowa, Iowa City, Iowa.

Pratt, M., Martin, L., Mohide, A., & Black, M. (2013). A descriptive analysis of the impact of moral distress on the evaluation of unsatisfactory nursing students. *Nursing Forum, 48*(4), 231–239.

Rodney, P. (1988). Moral distress in critical care nursing. *Canadian Critical Care Nursing Journal, 5*(2), 9–11.

Rushton, C. H. (2013). Principled moral outrage: An antidote to moral distress? *AACN Advanced Critical Care, 24*(1), 82–89.

Shoorideh, F. A., Ashktorab, T., Yaghmaei, F., & Alavi Majd, H. (2015). Relationship between ICU nurses' moral distress with burnout and anticipated turnover. *Nursing Ethics, 22*(1), 64–76.

Sijeffer (Producer). (2011). Ethical decision making. *Orbi.* Retrieved from http://www.cram.com/flashcards/ethical-decision-making-3032698

Simpson, J. A., & Weiner, E. S. C. (1989). *The Oxford English dictionary* (2nd ed.). Oxford, UK: Oxford University Press.

Smith, M. J., & Liehr, P. R. (2014). *Middle range theory for nursing* (3rd ed.). New York, NY: Springer Publishing.

Sporrong, S. K., Hoglund, A. T., & Arnetz, B. (2006). Measuring moral distress in pharmacy and clinical practice. *Nursing Ethics, 13*(4), 416–427.

Stanley, M. J. C., & Matchett, N. J. (2014). Understanding how student nurses experience morally distressing situations: Caring for patients with different values and beliefs in the clinical environment. *Journal of Nursing Education and Practice, 4*(10), 133–140.

Strauss, A. L. (1959). *Mirrors and masks: The search for identity.* Glencoe, IL: Free Press.

Streubert, H. S., & Carpenter, D. R. (2011). *Qualitative research in nursing: Advancing the humanistic imperative* (5th ed.). Philadelphia, PA: Wolters Kluwer Health/Lippincott Williams & Wilkins.

Whitehead, P. B., Herbertson, R. K., Hamric, A. B., Epstein, E. G., & Fisher, J. M. (2015). Moral distress among healthcare professionals: Report of an institution-wide survey. *Journal of Nursing Scholarship, 47*(2), 117–125.

Wiegand, D. L., & Funk, M. (2012). Consequences of clinical situations that cause critical care nurses to experience moral distress. *Nursing Ethics, 19*(4), 479–487.

Wilkinson, J. M. (1987). Moral distress in nursing practice: Experience and effect. *Nursing Forum, 23*(1), 16–29.

Winland-Brown, J. E., & Dobrin, A. L. (2009). Medical repatriation: Physicians' and nurses' responses to a dilemma. *Southern Journal of Nursing Research, 9*(4).

Wojtowicz, B., & Hagen, B. (2014). A guest in the house: Nursing instructors' experiences of the moral distress felt by students during inpatient psychiatric clinical rotations. *International Journal of Nursing Education Scholarship, 11*(1), 2013–0086.

Woods, M., Rodgers, V., Towers, A., & La Grow, S. (2015). Researching moral distress among New Zealand nurses: A national survey. *Nursing Ethics, 22*(1), 117–130.

Zuzelo, P. R. (2007). Exploring the moral distress of registered nurses. *Nursing Ethics, 14*(3), 344–359.

# CHAPTER 16

## Theory of Self-Care of Chronic Illness

Barbara Riegel, Tiny Jaarsma, and Anna Stromberg

Populations worldwide are aging (He, Goodkind, & Kowal, 2016). With aging comes a growing prevalence of chronic illness. In the Medicare population of the United States, two thirds have at least two or more chronic conditions or multimorbidity (2011). Similar trends are seen in Europe (Schmidt, Ulrichsen, Pedersen, Botker, & Sorensen, 2016). A recent editorial stated that the epidemic of heart failure, a particularly common chronic illness, has been replaced by a tsunami of comorbidities (Jhund & Tavazzi, 2016). The primary means of caring for these conditions is self-care; it is estimated that 95% of care for chronic illnesses is performed by patients (Funnell & Anderson, 2000).

Over the past 20 years we have been engaged in caring for adults with chronic heart failure and devised the two most widely used measures of self-care of heart failure (Jaarsma, Stromberg, Martensson, & Dracup, 2003; Riegel, Carlson, & Glaser, 2000; Riegel, Lee, Dickson, & Carlson, 2009; Riegel et al., 2004). During the course of those efforts we recognized that few of our patients had only heart failure and many of the required self-care behaviors were similar for different chronic illnesses. We also recognized that those with more than one chronic illness faced unique challenges that were not acknowledged but rather had a "silo" perspective focused on a single condition.

### ■ PURPOSE OF THE THEORY AND HOW IT WAS DEVELOPED

The purpose of the middle range theory of Self-Care of Chronic Illness (Riegel, Jaarsma, & Stromberg, 2012) was to capture a more holistic view of patients—those with varied or multiple chronic conditions. The theory was developed during a period when Professor Riegel was a visiting professor at Linkoping University in Sweden where Professors Jaarsma and Stromberg teach in the Division of Nursing Sciences. Spending time together, talking about self-care, we recognized that the work we had done previously in heart failure was applicable to a wide variety of patient populations. We devoted extended intervals to discussions of our prior work on the Situation-Specific Theory of Heart Failure Self-Care (Riegel & Dickson, 2008; Riegel, Dickson, & Faulkner, 2016), cultural beliefs about self-care in Sweden (Stromberg, Jaarsma, & Riegel,

2012) and other countries (Jaarsma et al., 2013), and the factors influencing self-care. We reviewed other theories of self-care and discussed those at length (Denyes, Orem, Bekel, & SozWiss, 2001). We each drafted content and then met regularly to discuss and refine our ideas as they evolved. Together we wrote assumptions and propositions. The concepts, propositions, and assumptions were reviewed by clinical researchers working with different chronic illness populations and revised based on their recommendations. This process required more than a year.

## ■ ASSUMPTIONS OF THE THEORY

One of the assumptions of this middle range theory is that there are differences between general health-promoting self-care and illness-specific self-care. General self-care is a dynamic, subjective process influenced by age, gender, culture, education, socioeconomic status, and so forth. Self-care that occurs in association with a chronic illness also is influenced by other people (e.g., healthcare providers) and has direct consequences for symptom relief, quality of life, and survival.

A second assumption is that when providers interact with patients, their intention to form a partnership will motivate patients to engage in a level of self-care that can realistically be incorporated into their daily life and lifestyle. It is within this context of a mutually rewarding relationship that the self-care of chronic illness takes place. Engaging in self-care makes the patient an active participant in the management of illness. Self-care behaviors may be recommended by others (e.g., healthcare providers or family members) or may be chosen by the patient to meet his or her own goals.

## ■ MAJOR CONCEPTS OF THE THEORY

### Self-Care

Self-care is the overarching or "umbrella" concept built from the three key concepts of self-care maintenance, self-care monitoring, and self-care management. Self-care is defined as a process of maintaining health through health-promoting practices and managing illness. Self-care is performed in both healthy and ill states. It is important to note that everyone engages in some level of health-promoting self-care daily with toothbrushing, food choices, and so on. However, self-care might have another meaning to patients with a chronic illness, since living optimally with a chronic illness often requires a set of behaviors to control the illness process, decrease the burden of symptoms, and improve survival.

## Self-Care Maintenance

Self-care maintenance is behaviors used by patients with a chronic illness to preserve health, to maintain physical and emotional stability, or to improve well-being. These may be health-promoting behaviors (e.g., smoking cessation, preparing healthy food, coping with stress) or illness-related behaviors (e.g., taking medication as prescribed). Engaging in self-care maintenance benefits from reflection on the usefulness of the behavior, vigilance in performing the behavior, an ongoing evaluation of benefits, and effectiveness of the activities. In addition, adaptation often comes into play to accommodate changing conditions. For example, a person who is prescribed a new medication with food restrictions will need to revise his or her routine to integrate changes into a new lifestyle.

## Self-Care Monitoring

Self-care monitoring is the process of observing oneself for changes in signs and symptoms. Self-care monitoring is a process of routine, vigilant body monitoring, surveillance, or body listening (Dickson, Deatrick, & Riegel, 2008). The goal of self-care monitoring is recognition that a change has occurred. Recognition is facilitated by somatic awareness (Jurgens, Fain, & Riegel, 2006) or somatic perception (Jurgens, Lee, & Riegel, 2015), defined as sensitivity to physical sensations and bodily activity.

Monitoring for changes related to health or well-being is a normal human behavior but in self-care of chronic illness, monitoring needs to be more systematic and part of a daily routine. Activities for monitoring, such as checking blood sugar for patients with diabetes, tracking blood pressure for patients with hypertension, and monitoring anger levels in patients with schizophrenia, help to achieve physical and emotional stability. Three criteria are required for effective self-care monitoring: first, clinically significant changes in the condition must be possible over time; second, a method of reliably detecting these changes must exist; and third, a reasonable action must be possible in response. These three criteria are requisite for effective self-care monitoring.

The monitoring of symptoms is effective when the person or an informal caregiver is able to both recognize and interpret the sign or symptom. In other words, only checking for changes in symptoms or signs without interpreting the meaning or significance of the change is not sufficient. Interpreting symptoms is a challenge for patients with a chronic illness when the illness influences their interoception or the ability to perceive internal sensations such as pain (e.g., sensory neuropathy in persons with diabetes). Cognitive dysfunction is another condition that can make symptom interpretation challenging because of difficulties remembering or interpreting. Individuals with depression may also have distinct problems in monitoring for changes due to impaired motivation.

Self-care monitoring includes both the process of collecting information about a certain aspect of self-care by objective observation (e.g., blood sampling for blood glucose or coagulation time, weighing, peak expiratory flow) or subjective observation such as body listening by noting that something is wrong and interpreting the meaning of the change. In the recently revised and updated Situation-Specific Theory of Heart Failure Self-Care (Riegel et al., 2016), which created the foundation for the middle range theory of Self-Care of Chronic Illness, this self-monitoring process is referred to as symptom perception, which involves both the detection of physical sensations through monitoring and the interpretation of their meaning. Symptom perception processes may be unique to heart failure, so for this middle range theory, the generic behavior of monitoring was used.

## Self-Care Management

Self-care management is the response to occurring signs and symptoms. Self-care management involves an evaluation of changes in physical and emotional signs and symptoms to determine if action is needed. These changes may be due to illness, treatment, or the environment. In this context, situation awareness involves alertness to bodily sensations (somatic awareness or perception) and the ability to reliably determine how these sensations change in response to treatments. Those who are managing self-care comprehend the meaning of changes and are able to mentally simulate options and decide on a course of action (Riegel, Dickson, & Topaz, 2013). If a response is needed, self-care management requires that a treatment be implemented and then evaluated as a method to determine an effective treatment.

Treatments are often specific to the signs and symptoms of a particular chronic illness. For example, shortness of breath due to asthma or chronic obstructive pulmonary disease may require use of a bronchodilator but shortness of breath due to heart failure may require taking an extra diuretic. Another important point about self-care management is that it can be done autonomously or in consultation with a healthcare provider, depending on the messages the patient is given by the provider about independent modifications of therapies. With heart failure patients, some providers encourage patients to titrate their own diuretics but other providers require that the patient call the office for direction. Persons with diabetes who take insulin routinely titrate their medication based on meals and exercise. Self-care management requires attention to the effectiveness of a treatment to evaluate whether or not that approach should be tried again in the future.

## ■ RELATIONSHIPS AMONG THE CONCEPTS: THE MODEL

As illustrated in Figure 16.1, the self-care process begins with self-care maintenance, a process that is generally less complex than the decision making

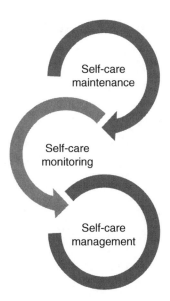

**FIGURE 16.1**   Self-Care of Chronic Illness.

*Source:* Reprinted with permission from Riegel, B., Jaarsma, T., & Stromberg, A. (2012). A middle range theory of self-care of chronic illness. *Advances in Nursing Science, 35,* 194–204.

required of self-care management. Expertise in self-care maintenance often leads to skill in self-care monitoring but mastery of self-care maintenance does not always precede that of self-care monitoring. The relationship between self-care monitoring and management is that monitoring may lead to self-care management or management could stimulate engagement in self-care monitoring.

Self-care is the overarching concept built from the three key concepts of self-care maintenance, self-care monitoring, and self-care management. The three concepts are closely related; therefore the performance of sufficient self-care encompasses all three behaviors. For example, when managing symptoms that worsen, a person has to perform sufficient symptom monitoring. Self-care monitoring is thought to be the link between self-care maintenance and self-care management; however, research is needed to confirm this proposition. These behaviors and activities of self-care maintenance, self-care monitoring, and self-care management do not always take place in the same linear order and certain behaviors might be skipped in some situations. That is, patients are not always consistent in their behaviors. They might choose to perform sufficient self-care related to one illness, but ignore another (Dickson, Buck, & Riegel, 2011). Reasons for this inconsistency have been suggested to be related to confidence or the belief that one illness is more important than another (Buck, Dickson, et al., 2015; Dickson, Buck, & Riegel, 2011, 2013).

## Relationship Between Self-Care Maintenance and Self-Care Monitoring

In previous work that was specific to heart failure patients (Riegel et al., 2010), self-care monitoring was included in the concept of self-care maintenance since daily weighing was seen as treatment adherence. This also can be seen in persons with diabetes self-care where monitoring of blood sugar is seen as treatment adherence. However, self-care maintenance and self-care monitoring are different behaviors and other skills might be needed to perform each one sufficiently. One of the propositions of this middle range theory is that mastery of self-care maintenance precedes that of self-care management because self-care maintenance is less complex than the decision making required for self-care management. Admittedly there are some conditions that require exceedingly complex self-care maintenance (e.g., medication adherence for HIV or organ transplantation), but overall we believe that self-care management is more complex than maintenance because of the decision-making process (Riegel et al., 2013). This does not mean that self-care monitoring cannot be performed without self-care maintenance. In other words, patients could be vigilant in observing their symptoms, but at the same time not be adherent to their medical therapy or their diet. However, in general there is a relationship between self-care maintenance and self-care monitoring. We have found that patients who diligently engage in self-care maintenance tend to be the same people who are observant of their signs and symptoms (Riegel, Vaughan Dickson, Goldberg, & Deatrick, 2007).

## Relationship Between Self-Care Maintenance and Self-Care Management

The relationship between self-care maintenance and self-care management is that if one event occurs the other is also likely to occur (Walker & Avant, 2011). Self-care management is more complex than self-care maintenance, so mastery of self-care maintenance is thought to precede mastery of self-care management, as noted previously. Specifically, if a person engages in self-care maintenance by eating a healthy diet and staying physically active, then it is more likely that this person will engage in self-care management (Riegel et al., 2007). In other words, if someone adheres to therapy they probably also perform (or want to perform) behaviors to manage their symptoms. This relationship is positive in that the behaviors tend to increase together or in sequence. The relationship is asymmetrical because it is rare for someone to master self-care management before self-care maintenance.

## Relationship Between Self-Care Monitoring and Self-Care Management

The type of relationship between self-care monitoring and self-care management is that one set of behaviors leads to the second one. Self-care monitoring is necessary for self-care management in that a decision about a change must first be noticed and evaluated (Riegel et al., 2012). For individuals with a chronic illness, recognition of a sign/symptom begins the process of decision making about what action is needed. When signs and symptoms are detected early and their seriousness is understood, action can be taken before the situation escalates. It is known that some patients dutifully monitor themselves, but do not know what to do with the information they gather. Others know what to do but choose not to do it. Still others monitor and do not detect anything that needs to be managed.

In summary, the three concepts of self-care maintenance, self-care monitoring, and self-care management reflect a sequence in which the behaviors are logically related to each other. Self-care functions well when all the behaviors related to the concepts are performed. However, for a variety of reasons, elements of the process are often skipped, leading to problems in the successful performance of self-care for people with chronic illness.

### ■ USE OF THE THEORY IN NURSING RESEARCH

The middle range theory of Self-Care of Chronic Illness was published in 2012. Since publication, 50 articles from all continents except Africa have cited the theory. Most authors use the definition of self-care and its components to frame their thinking when stating a rationale for a study or when discussing their findings. However, to date no one has empirically tested propositions of the theory. One interesting article by Wärdig et al. (Wärdig, Bachrach-Lindström, Foldemo, Lindström, & Hultsjö, 2013) exploring the prerequisites for a healthy lifestyle as described by individuals diagnosed with psychosis discussed the implications of the theory in individuals with severe mental illness. Although agreeing with our statement that it may be difficult to engage individuals with severe mental illness in self-care, they found that the individuals with psychosis were motivated and wanted to try to perform self-care.

Some researchers have used the theory for developing a new framework, theory, or model. For example, Beacham and Deatrick (Beacham & Deatrick, 2013) used the theory as a framework for self-care in children. They linked self-care maintenance, monitoring, and management to healthcare autonomy and outlined the usefulness of the theory for children and their families. Other researchers have used the theory to guide development of interventions as well as instruments measuring self-care in various conditions, for example, hypertension (Dickson, Lee, Yehle, Abel, & Riegel, 2017).

### ■ USE OF THE THEORY IN NURSING PRACTICE

This middle range theory is intended to be used in a variety of chronic conditions during the process of maintaining health through health-promoting practices, monitoring, and managing illness. At this point a systematic review is needed in order to refine the theory further, judge its clinical relevance, and develop implications for clinical practice. Such a review should assess studies using the theory, case reports, and expert-based evaluations to inform users on how the theory is being applied in different chronic conditions. So far the theory has been used in research with chronic illnesses in general and in a wide variety of specific chronic conditions including Parkinson's disease, psychosis, inflammatory bowel disease, diabetes, sickle cell disease, chronic obstructive pulmonary disease, coronary heart disease, hypertension, and childhood obesity. It has been used in heart failure patients with cardiac resynchronization devices and with left ventricular assist devices. However, clinical reports of implementation in clinical practice are still scarce. A good example of how the theory can be applied in clinical practice (Kato, Jaarsma, & Ben Gal, 2014) uses the theory as a framework for educational initiatives in patients with a left ventricular assist device. Two reports from the Heart Failure Association of the European Society of Cardiology and one from the Canadian Cardiovascular Society Heart Failure Guidelines used the theory to describe the importance of self-care in clinical practice (Cowie et al., 2014; Howlett et al., 2016; Ponikowski et al., 2014).

Caregivers are known to play an important role in supporting self-care in persons suffering from chronic conditions. A systematic review of caregivers (Buck, Harkness, et al., 2015) of patients with heart failure used the middle range theory as a framework to categorize the contribution of caregiver activities into support for self-care maintenance, monitoring, and management. The authors stated that the use of the theory made their analysis more systematic and coherent as well as provided a benchmark against which the contribution of self-care promoting caregiver activities could be determined (Buck, Harkness, et al., 2015). The success of using the theory as an organizing framework provided some evidence for its utility in clinical practice.

Another element with strong implications for clinical practice is reflection, noted in the original publication as a variable influencing the decision-making process (Riegel et al., 2012). In persons with insufficient self-care it is important for healthcare professionals and patients to jointly explore the barriers to self-care and address how to overcome them. Reflection is thought to be key to successful self-care because reflection involves considering the usefulness of a behavior, vigilance in performing it, and an ongoing evaluation of its associated benefits and effectiveness. To reach the goal of reflective and sufficient self-care a person needs to have both the motivation to do it and the knowledge about what to do. In some patients, both are lacking but others lack either knowledge or motivation. Moving from unreflective to reflective sufficient self-care often requires more knowledge and skills (Dickson & Riegel, 2009). When moving from reflective insufficient self-care to reflective sufficient self-care there is a need to increase motivation (Masterson Creber et al., 2016).

The three cornerstones of evidence-based nursing are: use of the best evidence available, clinical judgment, and patient experience/preferences. These are all important areas to use when supporting patients to increase self-care. Adherence to therapies that are evidence-based is associated with the best outcomes (Tan, Chinnappa, Tan, & Hall, 2011). The goal for healthcare providers is to work collaboratively with patients to negotiate the adoption of as many of the advocated behaviors as the patient can tolerate and accept, with an emphasis on those therapies with the best evidence to support them. We currently have evidence for some specific self-care areas such as medication adherence (Golshahi et al., 2015), exercise training in some chronic conditions (Button, Roos, Spasic, Adamson, & van Deursen, 2015), and diet for certain diseases (e.g., diabetes, celiac disease; Austin et al., 2013). In other areas, healthcare professionals have clinical experience that influences their recommendations. Patients often have self-care knowledge based on personal experience about what self-care behaviors are effective. This knowledge must be respected but providers should emphasize mainstream behaviors (e.g., medications known to improve outcomes) rather than behaviors that lack evidence of effects, fail to provide consistent benefit, or may even be harmful (e.g., certain nutritional supplements, herbal products, or restriction in lifestyle or daily life).

## ■ USE OF THE THEORY IN NURSING EDUCATION

The middle range theory of Self-Care of Chronic Illness is used in courses taught at the University of Pennsylvania (Penn) School of Nursing and Linkoping University, Division of Nursing. At Penn, a course on self-care is offered to undergraduate students. Students and faculty discuss the history, definitions, predictors, and outcomes of self-care in various chronically ill populations. Factors (e.g., illness, physiological, treatment regimen, psychological, social, and cultural) that influence how well patients make the transition from health to illness and the performance of self-care behaviors are explored. Students examine what constitutes skilled self-care, the many forces that influence this behavior, and how best to address these forces to prepare them for their role in promoting patient self-care. Fieldwork experiences in the community enable students to gain practical experience in engaging chronically ill individuals in discussions about self-care.

At Linkoping University the theory is presented to all undergraduate and master students when studying chronic illness, representing the theory as a framework useful in understanding and supporting patients in self-care. Students often use the theory in bachelor and master theses. In the doctoral program in nursing science, the theory is presented and analyzed among other self-care theories during a course focused on developing an in-depth understanding of self-care in relation to chronic illness. The course introduces the history, definitions, predictors, measurement, and outcomes of self-care to provide a broadened perspective of the self-care construct, theories and models, and various issues that patients face when dealing with chronic illness. Students write a paper in which they develop or modify a conceptual model/theory of self-care in relation to a chronic illness of their choice. The paper is intended to motivate the use and application of a model/theory in the chosen patient group and reflect on its value, strengths, and weaknesses. Then they describe how they might intervene to modify barriers to self-care (i.e., develop an intervention) and describe how that intervention might be tested in research. This assignment stimulates students to apply a self-care theory/model and think about how it could be used in research.

## ■ CONCLUSION

It is now 5 years since the middle range theory of Self-Care of Chronic Illness was first published. The theory has gained attention and clearly fulfilled the expressed need for a theory of chronic illness that is not disease-specific. The theory has been cited in numerous publications and used to develop instruments measuring self-care of hypertension, diabetes, and coronary heart disease. We have validated a generic instrument measuring self-care maintenance, self-care monitoring, and self-care management in people with any chronic illness. It is still too early to fully judge the clinical relevance of the theory. Although it has already been used in research in a wide variety of chronic conditions, the experiences and conclusions of these studies have not yet been systematically analyzed and summarized. Doing so will illustrate how effectively this theory is guiding evidence-based practice.

## ■ REFERENCES

Austin, S., Guay, F., Senecal, C., Fernet, C., & Nouwen, A. (2013). Longitudinal testing of a dietary self-care motivational model in adolescents with diabetes. *Journal of Psychosomatic Research, 75*(2), 153–159.

Beacham, B. L., & Deatrick, J. A. (2013). Health care autonomy in children with chronic conditions: implications for self-care and family management. *Nursing Clinics of North America, 48*(2), 305–317.

Buck, H. G., Dickson, V. V., Fida, R., Riegel, B., D'Agostino, F., Alvaro, R., &Vellone, E. (2015). Predictors of hospitalization and quality of life in heart failure: A model of comorbidity, self-efficacy and self-care. *International Journal of Nursing Studies, 52*(11), 1714–1722.

Buck, H. G., Harkness, K., Wion, R., Carroll, S. L., Cosman, T., Kaasalainen, S., . . . Arthur, H. M. (2015). Caregivers' contributions to heart failure self-care: A systematic review. *European Journal of Cardiovascular Nursing, 14*(1), 79–89.

Button, K., Roos, P. E., Spasic, I., Adamson, P., & van Deursen, R. W. (2015). The clinical effectiveness of self-care interventions with an exercise component to manage knee conditions: A systematic review. *Knee, 22*(5), 360–371.

Cowie, M. R., Anker, S. D., Cleland, J. G. F., Felker, G. M., Filippatos, G., Jaarsma, T., . . . López-Sendón, J. (2014). Improving care for patients with acute heart failure: before, during and after hospitalization. *ESC Heart Failure, 1*, 110–145.

Denyes, M. J., Orem, D. E., Bekel, G., & SozWiss. (2001). Self-care: A foundational science. *Nursing Science Quarterly, 14*(1), 48–54.

Dickson, V. V., Buck, H., & Riegel, B. (2011). A qualitative meta-analysis of heart failure self-care practices among individuals with multiple comorbid conditions. *Journal of Cardiac Failure, 17*(5), 413–419.

Dickson, V. V., Buck, H., & Riegel, B. (2013). Multiple comorbid conditions challenge heart failure self-care by decreasing self-efficacy. *Nursing Research, 62*(1), 2–9.

Dickson, V. V., Deatrick, J. A., & Riegel, B. (2008). A typology of heart failure self-care management in non-elders. *European Journal of Cardiovascular Nursing, 7*(3), 171–181.

Dickson, V. V., Lee, C. S., Yehle, K., Abel, W. M., & Riegel, B. (2017). Psychometric testing of the self-care of hypertension inventory. *Journal of Cardiovascular Nursing, 32*(5), 431–438

Dickson, V. V., & Riegel, B. (2009). Are we teaching what patients need to know? Building skills in heart failure self-care. *Heart & Lung, 38*(3), 253–261.

Funnell, M. M., & Anderson, R. M. (2000). MSJAMA: The problem with compliance in diabetes. *Journal of the American Medical Association, 284*(13), 1709.

Golshahi, J., Ahmadzadeh, H., Sadeghi, M., Mohammadifard, N., & Pourmoghaddas, A. (2015). Effect of self-care education on lifestyle modification, medication adherence and blood pressure in hypertensive adults: Randomized controlled clinical trial. *Advanced Biomedical Research, 4*, 204.

He, W., Goodkind, D., & Kowal, P. (2016). *An aging world: 2015. International population reports*. Washington, DC: U.S. Government Publishing Office.

Howlett, J. G., Chan, M., Ezekowitz, J. A., Harkness, K., Heckman, G. A., Kouz, S., . . . Zieroth, S. (2016). The Canadian cardiovascular society heart failure companion: Bridging guidelines to your practice. *Canadian Journal of Cardiology, 32*(3), 296–310.

Jaarsma, T., Stromberg, A., Martensson, J., & Dracup, K. (2003). Development and testing of the European heart failure self-care behaviour scale. *European Journal of Heart Failure, 5*(3), 363–370.

Jaarsma, T., Strömberg, A., Ben Gal, T., Cameron, J., Driscoll, A., Duengen, H., & Riegel, B. (2013). Comparison of self-care behaviours of heart failure patients in 15 countries worldwide. *Patient Education and Counseling, 92*(1), 114–120.

Jhund, P. S., & Tavazzi, L. (2016). Has the 'epidemic' of heart failure been replaced by a tsunami of co-morbidities? *European Journal of Heart Failure, 18*(5), 500–502.

Jurgens, C. Y., Fain, J. A., & Riegel, B. (2006). Psychometric testing of the heart failure somatic awareness scale. *Journal of Cardiovascular Nursing, 21*(2), 95–102.

Jurgens, C. Y., Lee, C. S., & Riegel, B. (2015). Psychometric analysis of the heart failure somatic perception scale as a measure of patient symptom perception. *Journal of Cardiovascular Nursing, 32*(2), 140–147.

Kato, N., Jaarsma, T., & Ben Gal, T. (2014). Learning self-care after left ventricular assist device implantation. *Current Heart Failure Reports, 11*(3), 290–298.

Masterson Creber, R., Patey, M., Lee, C. S., Kuan, A., Jurgens, C., & Riegel, B. (2016). Motivational interviewing to improve self-care for patients with chronic heart failure: MITI-HF randomized controlled trial. *Patient Education and Counseling, 99*(2), 256–264.

Ponikowski, P., Anker, S. D., Al Habib, K. F., Cowie, M. R., Force, T. L., Hu, S., . . . Filippatos, G. (2014). Heart failure: preventing disease and death worldwide. *ESC Heart Failure, (1)*1, 4–25.

Riegel, B., Carlson, B., & Glaser, D. (2000). Development and testing of a clinical tool measuring self-management of heart failure. *Heart & Lung, 29*(1), 4–12.

Riegel, B., Carlson, B., Moser, D. K., Sebern, M., Hicks, F. D., & Roland V. (2004). Psychometric testing of the self-care of heart failure index. *Journal of Cardiac Failure, 10*(4), 350–360.

Riegel, B., & Dickson, V. V. (2008). A situation-specific theory of heart failure self-care. *Journal of Cardiovascular Nursing, 23*(3), 190–196.

Riegel, B., Dickson, V. V., Cameron, J., Johnson, J. C., Bunker, S., Page, K., & Worrall-Carter, L. (2010). Symptom recognition in elders with heart failure. *Journal of Nursing Scholarship: An Official Publication of Sigma Theta Tau International Honor Society of Nursing/Sigma Theta Tau, 42*(1), 92–100.

Riegel, B., Dickson, V. V., & Faulkner, K. M. (2016). The situation-specific theory of heart failure self-care: Revised and updated. *Journal of Cardiovascular Nursing, 31*(3), 226–235.

Riegel, B., Dickson, V. V., & Topaz, M. (2013). Qualitative analysis of naturalistic decision making in adults with chronic heart failure. *Nursing Research, 62*(2), 91–98.

Riegel, B., Jaarsma, T., & Stromberg, A. (2012). A middle-range theory of self-care of chronic illness. *Advances in Nursing Science, 35*(3), 194–204.

Riegel, B., Lee, C. S., Dickson, V. V., & Carlson, B. (2009). An update on the self-care of heart failure index. *Journal of Cardiovascular Nursing, 24*(6), 485–497.

Riegel, B., Vaughan Dickson, V., Goldberg, L. R., & Deatrick, J. A. (2007). Factors associated with the development of expertise in heart failure self-care. *Nursing Research, 56*(4), 235–243.

Schmidt, M., Ulrichsen, S. P., Pedersen, L., Botker, H. E., & Sorensen, H. T. (2016). Thirty-year trends in heart failure hospitalization and mortality rates and the prognostic impact of co-morbidity: A Danish nationwide cohort study. *European Journal of Heart Failure, 18*(5), 490–499.

Stromberg, A., Jaarsma, T., & Riegel, B. (2012). Self-care: who cares? *European Journal of Cardiovascular Nursing, 11*(2), 133–134.

Tan, L. B., Chinnappa, S., Tan, D. K., & Hall, A. S. (2011). Principles governing heart failure therapy re-examined relative to standard evidence-based medicine-driven guidelines. *Expert Review of Cardiovascular Therapy, 9*(9), 1137–1146.

Walker, L. O., & Avant, K. C. (2011). *Strategies for theory construction in nursing* (5th ed.). Upper Saddle River, NJ: Pearson/Prentice Hall.

Wärdig, R. E., Bachrach-Lindström, M., Foldemo, A., Lindström, T., & Hultsjö, S. (2013). Prerequisites for a healthy lifestyle-experiences of persons with psychosis. *Issues in Mental Health Nursing*, 34(8), 602–610.

# SECTION THREE

## Concept Building for Research—Through the Lens of Middle Range Theory

*This section includes a beginning chapter that describes a rigorous concept building process that moves the scholar from a practice story to a conceptual foundation that can be used for research. The concept building process described in this chapter includes 10 phases: (1) write a practice story that stirs deep-seated interest; (2) name the phenomenon of interest in the practice story; (3) identify a theoretical lens for viewing the phenomenon, which is now beginning to take shape as an emerging concept; (4) link the emerging concept to existing literature (theoretical; population-based; semantic) and identify a set of preliminary core qualities; (5) gather a story from a person who can experientially describe the emerging concept and the literature-derived core qualities—report this description as a reconstructed story; (6) create a minisaga that captures the spirit of the emerging concept; (7) refine the set of two to four core qualities based on what has been learned from story-gathering— define each core quality; (8) formulate a concept definition that integrates the core qualities; (9) draw a model that depicts relationships between the core qualities of the concept; and (10) create a minisynthesis that integrates the concept definition with a population to suggest a research direction. The concept building process described in the first chapter sets the stage for the next two chapters, where doctoral students who have developed the concepts of nature immersion and sheltering-in-place describe their use of the concept building process. The reader will notice that each doctoral student scholar has embraced the concept building process in a unique way so that the phases of the process are represented in a way that makes sense for the scholar. The concept building processes, as described in these two chapters, are exemplars showing intellectual discipline and a respect for the logical connection essential for creating meaningful conceptual structures to guide research. The last two chapters show how evolution of a concept that was developed using the 10-phase process has blossomed into dissertation research.*

# CHAPTER 17

## Concept Building for Research

**Patricia R. Liehr and Mary Jane Smith**

Over years of working with doctoral students and scholars who were identifying/creating conceptual structures to guide research, this process of concept building has emerged. At its inception, it was an effort to offer a meaningful approach that incorporated both theoretical/scientific and experiential/empirical dimensions of evidence because we believed that both of these dimensions were critical to pursue understanding that had grounding as a guide for research. As we used concept building with scholar colleagues, we have come to see it as a process for articulating one's passion as a thrust for an enduring program of research. With that vision, we continue to shape the process. Although we have retained the 10 phases of the process, we have rearranged and more clearly articulated each phase so that the scholar produces a product with the completion of each phase. Although all phases are necessary for concept building, the product of each phase or a combination of the products may provide a jumping-off point for presentation and publication. For instance, Sopcheck (2015) summarized five of the phases to describe the concept "peaceful letting go," which became the focus for her dissertation research.

Our ongoing work to refine the concept building process affirms three essential beliefs that are relevant to the 10-phase process described in this chapter. First, clearly articulated ideas that stem from practice are critical for the design and implementation of research that has the potential to guide practice and build nursing knowledge. Second, the primary purpose of concept building is to guide research rather than to develop theory. Third, concept building occurs within contexts, both scientific (existing theory and current literature) and experiential (empirical evidence, including stories). Risjord (2009) has referred to concept analysis as either theoretical (inclusive of scientific) or colloquial (inclusive of interview), indicating each as separate but compatible processes. We believe that understanding is enhanced when both the theoretical/scientific and experiential/empirical dimensions of evidence intertwine and therefore, we have included both dimensions in the 10-phase concept building process.

Building concepts for research is a critical thought process central and necessary to becoming a researcher. Critical thought processes include understanding levels of abstraction, abduction/induction/deduction, analysis/synthesis, and appreciation for tacit/explicit knowing. We introduced the ladder of abstraction in Chapter 2, advocating that scholars learn to agilely move up and down the ladder rungs from philosophical to theoretical to empirical perspectives. Discoursing at differing levels of abstraction is a logical endeavor of connecting ideas in a way that makes sense, is coherent, and can be understood by the use of reason. Dimensions of logical reasoning essential for developing concepts for research include abduction, induction, and deduction. These logic dimensions are not separate but move back and forth in an iterative way. Abduction is an interpretative reconstruction drawing on the logic of discovery (Wirth, 2012). Abductive reasoning is inventive; it demands the ability to synthesize. For instance, in concept building, it begins with an incomplete set of observations such as a practice story and moves toward naming a phenomenon of interest. Inductive reasoning takes empirical information, such as observations and comments noted while gathering a story about an emerging concept and moves to a more general synthesis such as a reconstructed story. Deduction moves from a general or theoretical perspective to specifics. An example during concept building occurs when the scholar views a phenomenon through varying theoretical lenses, considering how each lens differentially shapes the core qualities. Learning to respect all levels of abstraction in the logical progression of analysis/synthesis is the rigorous foundation essential for building a concept for research.

Analysis/synthesis shines through the phases of the concept building process. For instance, settling on a final set of two to four concept core qualities demands analysis to distill defining elements from the literature and the empirical story evidence; and synthesis demands a coherent combination of ideas that makes sense to others. Inherent in this synthesis is tacit and explicit knowing. Polanyi (1958, 1966) describes tacit knowing as intuitive and inexpressible . . . beyond what can be made explicit. In contrast, explicit knowing is expressed as full description with details that paint a picture. As scholars become aware of what they tacitly know, for instance through nursing practice experience, they attempt to make what is tacit, explicit. This is an important critical thought process that proceeds with the understanding that some dimension of knowing will always remain tacit.

Each of these critical thought processes is intertwined with the other, challenging the scholar to stay with concept building, revisiting and revising as views that are cloudy become clear, incorporating other dimensions and requiring another cycle of revisiting and revising . . . patient presence with an idea to bring it to a place that enables guidance for practice and research. Smith (1988) has described wallowing while waiting, as a critical skill for scholars who are growing their ideas for research. She describes wallowing as dwelling with the obscure and says:

> In coming through the obscurity, sudden insights illuminate the connections. These insights are moments of coherence, flashes of unity, as though

suddenly the fog lifts and clarity prevails. These moments of coherence push one beyond to deepened levels of understanding. (p. 3)

This chapter offers guidance to graduate students and to faculty teaching courses where students are working to build concepts that will guide research. The chapter may also be helpful to practitioners and junior nursing faculty who are actively engaged in developing their ideas for research. The systematic approach to be described in this chapter includes 10 phases, each with a substantive product (in italics): (1) write a *practice story* that stirs deep-seated interest, (2) name the *phenomenon of interest* in the practice story, (3) identify a *theoretical lens* for viewing the phenomenon, which is now beginning to take shape as an emerging concept, (4) link the emerging concept to existing literature (theoretical; population-based; semantic) and identify a set of *preliminary core qualities*, (5) gather a story from a person who can experientially describe the emerging concept and can address the congruence of the literature-derived core qualities—report this description as a *reconstructed story*, (6) create a *minisaga* that merges what you are learning and captures the spirit of the emerging concept, (7) refine the set of *two to four core qualities* based on what has been learned from story-gathering—*define each core quality*, (8) formulate a *concept definition* that integrates the core qualities, (9) draw a *model* that depicts relationships between the core qualities of the concept, and (10) create a *minisynthesis* that integrates the concept definition with a population to suggest a research direction. This process is not meant to be linear, where the scholar completes one phase and then goes on to the next. Rather, the process begins and then touches back to previous phases, always creating a work in progress taking care to maintain correspondence between the phases and ongoing clarification of the defining core qualities.

It is important to reiterate that the scholar is building a concept rather than building a theory. Sometimes conceptual structures advance through research to become theories (Choi, 2014; Nathaniel, 2014; Williams, 2014) but such development is not the focus of this chapter. In the two chapters that follow, Wallace (Chapter 19) describes the concept building process for sheltering-in-place and Nagata (Chapter 18) describes the process for nature immersion; these are offered as exemplars of the concept building process. This chapter references concept development projects to allow the reader to consider ways that concept building comes to life in the work of doctoral students.

## ■ 1: PRACTICE STORY

The first phase of concept building begins with evidence from a practice story. The practice story addresses a critical incident in nursing practice related to caring in the human health experience that stirs the scholars' interest. The incident might stem from a concern or it might highlight an "ideal" nursing experience. Prior to writing the story, scholars are engaged in a discussion about their research interest . . . what arouses their energy. Then, they write a story that closely ties to both their research interest and their passion to make a difference. Sometimes, scholars are clear about their research interest and discussion about the fit between their interest and their passion can refine their focus. Sometimes, when scholars are unclear about research interests, a detailed practice story that captures their intention to make a difference will help uncover an enduring focus for research.

To generate the practice story, scholars are invited to bring a practice situation into focus, place themselves in a quiet place where they can stay with their focus, and begin writing. They are instructed to begin by describing their first remembrance of the incident writing the story event by event, ending with how the situation came to a close. The practice story has a beginning, middle, and end and is centered on a nurse–person situation. This is not a time for worry about grammar or spelling but it is a time for writing the story as it is remembered with as much detail as possible. Then, the story is set aside. It moves into the background of consciousness for subtle shaping arising in the midst of foreground everyday coming and going. After a few days, scholars can edit their story to enhance sentence structure, eliminate redundancy, and add details that contribute to the essence of the incident being described. Discussion with colleagues often leads to clarification of confusing story elements. These discussions help the scholar craft the final version of the practice story.

There is a range of ways that stories about caring in the human health experience are recounted. Sometimes, the story comes from pressing issues that arise in the nurse's current practice; sometimes, the story source is less direct, coming from roles like clinical instructor or even family member. Sometimes, the story is a composite of more than one patient and or nursing situation. For Wallace, the story of sheltering-in-place surfaced in her practice with women with breast cancer when she noticed their pattern of putting off taking action at the time of diagnosis. For Nagata, the story of nature immersion came to her attention in her holistic nursing practice when she worked to achieve balance for children who were bothered by symptoms such as those associated with allergies or attention deficit disorder. Regardless of the origin, a practice story is created to address observations essential for caring in the human health experience. The practice story is retrospective. It is a recounting of an event that has happened in the past that sticks with the scholar, calling attention to a focus for research. The focus for research is an issue that rouses the scholar's interest to do something to make a difference and the practice story will be a nurse–patient situation that highlights the issue demanding attention. The issue demanding attention is the crux of the story—the phenomenon of interest is often explicit or implicit in the crux of the story.

# ■ 2: PHENOMENON OF INTEREST

The phenomenon of interest is a human health experience. For Wallace (Chapter 19) the phenomenon was "sheltering-in-place." For Nagata (Chapter 18), the phenomenon was "nature immersion" and both are human health experiences that can be applied to many populations across a broad range of age groups. For instance, although "sheltering-in-place" was identified in a group of women diagnosed with breast cancer who had delayed action on their diagnosis, the phenomenon has applicability for older adults with mild cognitive impairment or parents of children on the autism spectrum. Likewise, nature immersion has particular relevance in the increasing technological society, where little time is spent in nature and engagement in cyberspace activities consumes greater proportions of waking hours. The broad range of applicability for these phenomena highlights a place at the middle range level of abstraction, not too high so that they cannot readily translate for use in practice and research and not too low so that they apply to only one population.

The phenomenon begins to emerge as the practice story is analyzed in relation to a scholar's area of research interest. Analysis requires drawing inferences about what is going on in the story that evokes passion. Story analysis is best undertaken with a group of colleagues who raise issues about story dimensions, describe how the storyteller expresses significant dimensions, and articulates where discrepancies arise. Once the phenomenon is identified, it must be named.

Naming the phenomenon requires considerable scrutiny and deliberation. It is an arduous process aimed at addressing a substantive area for study. Usually, several names are considered before settling on a name to move on with concept building. At this point, when a name is selected, it is recognized as a snapshot of a work in progress and therefore may be fine-tuned as the concept building work continues. Maximum flexibility is attained when the phenomenon is named at a middle range level of abstraction. A common mistake made by beginners is that a diagnosis, like congestive heart failure, is named instead of a human health experience. In this situation, scholars are called to focus on the human health experience, such as persistent tiredness, instead of the diagnosis.

# ■ 3: THEORETICAL LENS

The theoretical lens is a perspective for viewing the phenomenon of interest. This perspective can come from a grand theory or from a middle range theory. The perspective shapes the meaning of the phenomenon. For instance, persistent tiredness will be described differently if one is looking through the lens of Human Becoming Theory (Parse, 1992), as compared to the Theory of

Unpleasant Symptoms (Lenz & Pugh, 2014). If viewing persistent tiredness through the lens of Human Becoming grand theory, the meaning of the phenomenon might reflect multidimensional cocreation of the reality of tiredness through recognition of the value placed on feeling energetic. If viewed through the middle range theory of Unpleasant Symptoms, the meaning of the phenomenon could include physiological, psychological, and situational factors influencing persistent tiredness and symptoms that interact and accentuate tiredness.

Paley (1996) argues for the importance of the theoretical niche when clarifying concepts: "The meaning of a term is made specific when it becomes part of a specific theory" (p. 577). He advocates locating concepts within a theoretical niche so that the meaning is specified by the overall structure of the theory. From this perspective, scholars are guided to develop a solid understanding of a theory and its related methodologies, acknowledging the niche for the phenomenon that is shaping as an emerging concept.

When a phenomenon is named at a middle range level of abstraction, a middle range theory can create a contextual niche with a strong logical connection. A stronger logical connection enhances clarity supported through coherence with the theory ontology, epistemology, and methodology. As examples, Wallace selected the middle range theory of Moral Reckoning and Nagata selected the middle range theory of Integrative Nursing Coaching. The reader will recognize the glove-like fit of sheltering-in-place and nature immersion with the selected theoretical niche when they read Chapters 18 and 19. The tightness of this fit contributes significantly to the concept building process.

In the appendix of this book, there is a table of middle range theories published over the past few decades. Theories in this table were identified through a Cumulative Index of Nursing and Health Literature (CINAHL) search using the search terms "middle range theory," "mid-range theory," and "midrange theory." The editors selected these theory citations as ones that: were published in English; focused on theory development and/or presentation; and clearly identified the theory by name. Students can use this table to identify a theoretical lens that fits with their emerging concept. Once the theory is identified, it is important to come to know it so that the nuances of the theory can be fully embraced as a comfortable space for concept building. The phenomenon is now taking shape as an emerging concept.

## ■ 4: LITERATURE-DERIVED PRELIMINARY CORE QUALITIES

The related literature is the existing body of knowledge associated with the emerging concept. The question guiding the literature review is: What core qualities describe the essence of the emerging concept? Three approaches for beginning exploration of related literature are described: theoretical;

population-based; and semantic. While all three are recommended, the order for using the three approaches is not dictated by the concept building process.

One approach for viewing the phenomenon is to explore the foundational literature supporting the theoretical perspective. Oftentimes, if the fit between the theory and the phenomenon is tight, the literature supporting the theory will provide insights that will guide reflective analysis about the emerging concept.

A second approach is population-based. Oftentimes, the population that was the context for the human health experience described in the practice story will provide a literature source. For instance, if the practice story described persistent tiredness in a population with congestive heart failure, the literature related to heart failure symptoms will provide direction about the core qualities of the emerging concept. However, persistent tiredness affects other populations besides those with congestive heart failure. People undergoing chemotherapy may describe persistent tiredness as may pregnant women. In this approach to analyzing related literature, the scholar reviews the literature from multiple population perspectives, seeking to find the recurring descriptors for the emerging concept.

A third approach is to explore the literature associated with the emerging concept name, the semantic approach. For instance, for persistent tiredness, tiredness and fatigue would be search terms that would be explored. If the emerging concept is more abstract, such as cultural belonging, then exploring the literature on social support to identify descriptors of belonging may be helpful. Even literature about gangs might provide insight about the meaning of belonging. There is an element of creative vision in exploring the literature related to the emerging concept. The scholar is challenged to stay with the concept as it is grounded in familiar literature and move beyond familiar literature to access perspectives that may extend understanding. For instance, if a scholar has not encountered the literature from other disciplines while seeking to identify core qualities, it is important to intentionally seek out such literature to consider the emerging concept through cross-disciplinary views.

It is important to remember when undertaking this semantic exploration that context matters . . . so, the meaning of a word like "flow" could refer to blood, to rivers, or to energy and each perspective shapes an alternate meaning. If citing references from an alternate discipline, the scholar is seeking nuances that bring a slightly different but relevant and maybe novel perspective.

Some students have found that a structured approach to analysis/synthesis of the literature enhances the concept building process. One method helpful in reviewing the literature on the emerging concept is a literature matrix set forth on a spreadsheet with rows and columns (Garrard, 2013). Column topics are based on the question guiding the literature search, emphasizing topics that will inform identification of core qualities. Garrard (2013) advocates for the first three columns noting citation information, year of publication, and purpose of the manuscript. We suggest that there also be a column to note whether the source is coming from a theoretical (T), population (P), or semantic (S) perspective; one to specifically identify core qualities suggested by the manuscript; and one to note the core quality definitions indicated by the manuscript author. Other columns may be included to contribute in a way that makes sense to the scholar. For instance, Shapiro (2014) added a column to identify the "nursing substantive foundation." Selection of information to insert in the matrix is a process of analysis that includes both critical reading and thinking to select literature that fits with the column topic and has relevance for the emerging concept. For instance, when exploring the theoretical literature, column headings could be author, title, journal, year, purpose, and theoretical perspective. The columns labeled "purpose" and "theoretical perspective" demand discernment to select appropriate content for the matrix. Matrices reported by Wallace and Nagata provided examples that highlight the usefulness of the matrix for identifying the preliminary set of core qualities.

At the completion of this phase, there will be a preliminary list of core qualities, rooted in the literature. Core qualities are the defining properties of the concept. At this point, before moving to the next phase, the scholar is encouraged to consider the list of core qualities and use an inductive approach to group and name like qualities so that no more than two to four qualities are identified for further exploration during story-gathering.

## ▪ 5: RECONSTRUCTED STORY FROM STORY-GATHERING

We have found that scholars can use guidance regarding systematic story-gathering as an approach for developing the reconstructed story and refining understanding about core qualities of their emerging concept. For the purpose of concept building, we are advocating two phases of story-gathering. In the first phase, the student will query the human health experience designated by the emerging concept and in the second phase, the student will query each of the core qualities identified from the literature.

In the first phase, if the emerging concept is persistent tiredness, the student might ask the person to describe a time when tiredness lasted an unusually long time. Sometimes, it is useful to begin by asking about tiredness now (present); about when it started (past) and how the tiredness was experienced when it first began; then, how it progressed until now (from past to present), noting important markers of change over time; and what hopes (future) are held regarding the experience of tiredness in the days/months/years ahead. This present, past, future perspective has been described as a story path approach (see Chapter 11). The intent of this first phase of story-gathering is to come to know the unbiased thoughts and feelings about the emerging concept.

One of the lessons regarding story-gathering is related to languaging the question for the person sharing the story. For instance, Wallace (Chapter 19) was interested in "sheltering-in-place" for women diagnosed with breast cancer. It would not be appropriate to ask women how they "sheltered-in-place." This question is likely to have little meaning if asked directly. Rather, the scholar might pose a series of statements/questions such as: I would like to know about normal everyday living for you now; how is that different since your diagnosis?; let's talk about what has happened between the time of the diagnosis and now; how do you see the future…what are your hopes and dreams? This approach to engaging will allow the person sharing the story to get to what matters most and it will provide the scholar with critical information that will inform understanding about "sheltering-in-place."

In the second phase of story-gathering the scholar will specifically query the core qualities identified through analysis/synthesis of relevant literature. This phase will be prefaced with an explanation indicating that literature sources have suggested these qualities and the intention of the dialogue is to verify or bring into question each of the qualities noted from the literature. In this case, the person sharing the story is an expert who knows the emerging concept as an embodied experience. This way of knowing contributes powerful evidence to expand the scholar's understanding.

After gathering a story from someone who knows the emerging concept through experience, it may be necessary to return to the literature to seek out a core quality that arose in the dialogue but was not evident in the original literature search. Another reason to go back to the literature is to reexamine a literature-based core quality that was not confirmed in the story-gathering dialogue. When gathering a story to inform concept building, it is important to conduct the story-gathering as the phases direct, so that questions about the core qualities are introduced after an open, unbiased discussion about the human health experience. Sometimes, a core quality will be introduced in the first-phase story-path-guided discussion. When that happens, the scholar should take note and reintroduce the core quality in phase 2 so that further development and enhanced understanding can be pursued.

In writing the reconstructed story, the scholar creates a beginning, middle, and end that highlight the core qualities situated in the human health experience described by the storyteller during story-gathering. The reconstructed story incorporates the personal knowing of the nurse but strives to present a whole story about the emerging concept as shared by the storyteller. This writing asks that the nurse get into the shoes of the other to bring to life the emerging concept. This is not a transcript of the dialogue between the nurse and the story-sharer; it is a succinct synthesis totaling no more than 500 words. In the reconstructed story, the reader comes to know the emerging concept through the experience of one person. Though we understand that a single story is not all-encompassing, this story-gathering process will provide one real-world perspective contributing to shaping the emerging concept. Additional stories could add empirical dimensions to understanding.

## ■ 6: MINISAGA

The minisaga is a short story that synthesizes what has been learned about the emerging concept. According to Pink (2005), "Mini-sagas are *extremely* short stories—just fifty words long . . . no more, no less" (p. 117). Like the reconstructed story, there is a beginning, middle, and end. The minisaga captures the spirit of the emerging concept, so that anyone hearing it has a sense of its importance. The purpose of the minisaga is to crystallize the essence of the emerging concept so that it can be readily shared with others. Writing the minisaga is hard work, requiring dialoguing/critiquing with peers and mentors so that it can be structured to engage attention and authentically represent the scholar's passionate interest. The intent to make a difference for a population often spurs the minisaga about a circumscribed population and/or a pressing societal issue. Two examples of minisagas written by Shapiro (2014) and Greif (2014) are presented here. Shapiro was capturing the spirit of her concept building endeavor focused on "yearning for sleep while enduring distress" and Greif was capturing the spirit of "reconceptualizing normal" for families when one of their children suffered a traumatic brain injury.

> Half of her life, Jenny has endured sleep problems. Night after night she watches the clock, desperately counting hours, waiting for sleep. Anxious and frustrated, the lack of sleep permeates school, work, social life and health. Testing and treatment have brought no relief. Jenny yearns for a good night's sleep. (Shapiro, 2014, p. 375)

Shapiro (2014) is touching on the pressing issue of insomnia in her minisaga about Jenny; this life-disrupting pattern is one that has significant implications for health and well-being.

> Mark's brain injury changed his family in ways his parents and brother could not anticipate. The family is in constant flux, adjusting to ever-changing needs and concerns. His mother manages uncertainty by getting to know Mark all over again, staying open to who he is becoming and always looking forward (Greif, 2014, pp. 392–393).

Greif is addressing the pressing issue of family readjustment to stay whole and normal in the midst of the trauma of brain injury for one of the children. Both Shapiro and Greif stayed with ideas that emerged from concept building when moving on to dissertation research. Their dissertation proposals are shared by these scholars in Chapters 18 and 19.

## ■ 7: REFINED SET OF CORE QUALITIES WITH DEFINITIONS

The core qualities are the defining properties of the emerging concept. The scholar has been formulating the core qualities throughout the phases of this process, beginning with the literature review, which culminated in a set of preliminary core qualities that were taken to the story-gathering. Incorporating the guidance from the story-sharer, the scholar will have reconsidered the preliminary core qualities, perhaps gone back to the literature for affirmation, and finally arrived at a refined set of core qualities. Understandably, at this phase of concept building there is enhanced clarity about the nature of the qualities, enabling an explicit definition of each of two to four core qualities. Each core quality definition will cite the associated literature essential to the definition. The student is asked to stay with the identified core qualities at each phase of the continuing process. At this point, the concept is ready for shaping with a succinct definition.

## ■ 8: CONCEPT DEFINITION

Once the definition is expressed, the concept is established for use. The definition is a sentence that begins with the name of the concept followed by "is" (e.g., Persistent tiredness is . . .). The rest of the sentence arranges the core qualities as related to each other to accurately describe the concept. Although this seems straightforward, it can be difficult to create this defining sentence so that the core qualities are arranged in a meaningful way. Oftentimes, there is much attention to the connecting words, such as *through, to,* or *from*. Repositioning of core qualities and alternate choices of connecting words can create very different definitions. For instance, Wallace (Chapter 19) defined sheltering-in-place: Sheltering-in-place is protecting self in the face of uncertainty in order to preserve normalcy. There are three core qualities: protecting self, uncertainty, and normalcy. Nagata (Chapter 18) defined nature immersion: Nature immersion is personal emergence occurring through connecting with earthy materials. There are two core qualities: personal emergence and connecting with earthy materials. The concept definition is an original contribution of the scholar. It requires that the scholar take a stand and make a unique contribution that sets the stage for ongoing research.

## ■ 9: MODEL

The model is a structural representation of the definition, depicting the relationships between the core qualities of the concept. It is expected that there is congruence between the definition and the model. That is, the core qualities that appear in the definition will appear in the model. It is understood that the model is situated in a theoretical niche, and the student will be able to discuss the link between the theoretical perspective, concept definition, and the model.

## ■ 10: MINISYNTHESIS

The minisynthesis is a three-sentence creation that pulls together the concept building process. The first sentence addresses the significance of the phenomenon in the context of a particular population. The second sentence is the definition of the concept. The third sentence suggests an approach for moving toward a research question.

## ■ CONCLUSION

Although described as a linear process, concept building is iterative and creative with every opportunity to circle back and bring new knowledge to an already accomplished phase. The entire 10-phase process simply brings the scholar to the doorstep of further development through research. Additionally, many components of the concept building process can be the foundation for publication. For instance, the literature review (phase 3) that culminates in a set of preliminary core qualities establishes a state-of-science perspective about the concept that could, with additional development, stand alone as a significant scholarly contribution. Likewise, the systematic story-gathering process and the reconstructed story (phase 5) create the foundation of a case study, which may merit additional story-gathering and/or dissemination to shine a light on the human experience, taking the concept to an empirical level that has the potential to inform nursing practice. The scholar is encouraged to make the concept building process one's own, mining the knowledge gained to establish scholarly focus through dissemination and to shape ongoing work.

## ■ REFERENCES

Choi, H. (2014). Theory of cultural marginality. In M. J. Smith & P. R. Liehr (Eds.), *Middle range theory for nursing* (3rd ed., pp. 289–308). New York, NY: Springer Publishing.

Garrard, J. (2013). *Health sciences literature review made easy* (4th ed.). Sudbury, MA: Jones & Bartlett.

Greif, S. (2014). Reconceptualizing normal. In M. J. Smith & P. R. Liehr (Eds.), *Middle range theory for nursing* (3rd ed., pp. 383–396). New York, NY: Springer Publishing.

Lenz, E. R., & Pugh, L. C. (2014). Theory of unpleasant symptoms. In M. J. Smith & P. R. Liehr (Eds.), *Middle range theory for nursing* (3rd ed., pp. 165–196). New York, NY: Springer Publishing.

Nathaniel, A. (2014). Theory of moral reckoning. In M. J. Smith & P. R. Liehr (Eds.), *Middle range theory for nursing* (3rd ed., pp. 329–346). New York, NY: Springer Publishing.

Paley, J. (1996). How not to clarify concepts in nursing. *Journal of Advanced Nursing, 24*, 572–578.

Parse, R. R. (1992). Human becoming: Parse's theory of nursing. *Nursing Science Quarterly, 5*(1), 35–42.

Pink, D. H. (2005). *A whole new mind: Moving from the information age to the conceptual age.* New York, NY: Penguin Group.

Polanyi, M. (1958). *The study of man.* Chicago, IL: University of Chicago Press.

Polanyi, M. (1966). *The tacit dimension.* London, England: Routledge & Kegan Paul Ltd.

Risjord, M. (2009). Rethinking concept analysis. *Journal of Advanced Nursing, 65*(3), 684–691.

Shapiro, A. L. (2014). Yearning for sleep while enduring distress: A concept for nursing research. In M. J. Smith & P. R. Liehr (Eds.), *Middle range theory for nursing* (3rd ed., pp. 361–382). New York, NY: Springer Publishing.

Smith, M. A. (1988). Theoretical dilemmas: Wallowing while waiting. *Nursing Science Quarterly, 1*(1), 3.

Sopcheck, J. (2015). An emerging concept: Peaceful letting go. *Archives of Psychiatric Nursing, 29*, 71–72.

Williams, L. (2014). Theory of caregiving dynamics. In M. J. Smith & P. R. Liehr (Eds.), *Middle range theory for nursing* (3rd ed., pp. 309–328). New York, NY: Springer Publishing.

Wirth, U. (2012). What is abductive inference. Retrieved from http://user.uni-frankfurt.de/~with/inference.htm

# CHAPTER 18

## Nature Immersion: A Concept for Nursing Research

**Misako Nagata**

This chapter presents a process of concept generation. It requires a critical yet creative logical process that includes induction, deduction, and abduction. Concept building for research described in this chapter is guided by Liehr and Smith's (2014) 10-phase concept building approach: (1) practice story; (2) central phenomenon; (3) theoretical lens; (4) related literature; (5) gather a story; (6) reconstruct story and minisaga; (7) define the core qualities; (8) define the working concept; (9) model; and (10) minisynthesis. The approach guides researchers to identify a phenomenon of interest that flows from practice (Liehr & Smith, 2014, p. 349).

The steps of the concept building approach start with a practice story that sparks interest. In this case, empirical observations during integrative nursing practice were the spark that stimulated the practice story. Writing about a human health experience most interesting to the researcher lays a bridge between empirical and theoretical knowledge (Liehr & Smith, 2014). The nursing practice story consists of a beginning, middle, and end; it is centered on a nurse–patient situation. The concept I developed came from my nursing practice as a private integrative holistic nurse practitioner. Integrative nursing is defined as (Dossey, 2016, p. 4):

A whole-person/whole-system approach that is relationship-centered care where human beings are seen as inseparable from their environments and have an innate capacity for health and well-being. It can be practiced with all patient populations and in all clinical settings and has the potential to strengthen and invigorate the profession. This approach incorporates integrative modalities/complementary and alternative modalities (CAM) as appropriate.

The patient as a person is viewed as having self-harmonizing systems of mind, body, and spirit. The personal capacity for health and healing is integral to the person–environment relationship. Based on a personal interest in the process of healing and well-being, I asked myself the following questions: What are innate capacities for self-harmonizing? How is human–environment self-harmonizing related to the healing process? The phenomenon of interest, nature immersion, unfolded for me in a practice story about a 9-year-old elementary schoolboy with hay fever.

## ■ THE NURSING PRACTICE STORY

Despite a warm spring day, Jiro, a 9-year-old elementary schoolboy, visited me with his mother for his wintry symptomatic condition of a runny nose and red eyes; classical symptoms of hay fever. His life was getting out of balance with his schoolwork and schoolmates, because his symptoms were too severe for him to focus on his studies or play outdoors. His condition was worsening beyond the treatment effectiveness of his prescribed medications. His pediatrician had already doubled the dosage of medication. His mother expressed her woes and wishes to bring back Jiro's true nature of wellness.

Jiro suffered from hay fever every spring since he was 5 years old, with the symptoms increasing and intensifying yearly. In the previous spring, gastrointestinal symptoms of nausea and vomiting with persistent constipation were added to his symptom experience. Once very active and agile, he was now more antsy, anxious, and apprehensive, a condition that snowballed into insomnia. His mother further pointed out skin patches with pinkish, itchy, dry erythema on his right leg that showed up a few days prior to his visit. The story from his mother revealed that the skin problem had repeated each season in the spring since the age of 2.

I made a list of remedies, recipes, and regimens for Jiro: wild wind flowers of Pulsatilla in pellets; Calendula ointment; soybean-based fermented homemade yogurts; plenty of distilled water and green tea; and rest and relaxation through play. We waited to see if his whole nature—body, mind, and spirit—emerged. It was a week later when his mother emailed me that Jiro had a storm of symptoms attacking him so badly, he wasn't able to attend school. Shortly thereafter, his skin patches started to fade away. He soon was able to sleep soundly. The storm waned. His symptoms started to fade away, one by one. He told me his body felt lighter, as did his mind. He felt much better now that the symptoms were more bearable.

## ■ CENTRAL PHENOMENON

Jiro's health experiences appeared to be immersed in nature. There are two meanings about nature: nature of a human child and nature of his environment. The immersed nature manifested in Jiro's responses as the appearance and disappearance of symptoms. The word *immersion* originated from Latin, *immergere*, meaning *dip or submerge in a liquid* (Oxford University Press, 2010).

On the other hand, the meaning of *nature* is twofold: (a) the phenomenon of the physical world collectively, including plants, animals, the landscape, and other features and products of the earth, and (b) the basic or inherent features of something (Oxford University Press, 2010). Thus, deeply immersed in nature as if under water, Jiro's inherent and environmental nature was fully saturated. This is the central phenomenon named "nature immersion."

Nature immersion is a budding concept to be examined for its applicability to other nursing practice situations. Importantly, the central phenomenon described by Liehr and Smith (2014) should be situated at a level of abstraction applicable to practice and research with different populations. As a result, an existing middle range theoretical lens was selected to provide a conceptually relevant link to integrative nursing. The theoretical lens is the *Theory of Integrative Nurse Coaching* (TINC; Dossey, 2015) that has healing as the central concept.

## ■ THEORETICAL LENS

The TINC is a middle range theory interwoven with the legacy of Florence Nightingale (1820–1910). Human–environment entanglements have long been noted through Nightingale's view about the effects of nature on human health and healing. She identified important aspects of nature in the human environment as fundamental elements essential to human development (Nightingale, 1860[1969]). A notion of manipulation or modification of human environments is niched originally in the work of Nightingale. Also, known as one of the first Bioneers, she prioritized the importance of *nature* not only to human health but also to vitality for all the species and ecosystems (Dossey, 2005).

Nurses as 21st century Nightingales, named in the TINC, are in a position to coach and cocreate persons', patients', or populations' environments to become integrated with nature. The TINC, as a midrange theoretical framework, produces philosophical yet pragmatic methods through coaching to integrate the human–environmental energy fields at the center of which a person may heal from within (Dossey, 2015, p. 30). Healing blooms from within the center of a person to peripherally penetrate all levels of being. It generates from within a core, like a flower bud blooming from within.

The nature–human process is an endless exchange in every moment with all the organic and inorganic parts of nature participating at the atomic through cosmic level. Nature immersion is a dance of the constant state of change and exchange between a unitary human being and the universe, birthing a whole new constellation and composition of body–mind–spirit–cultural–environmental connection. It is the unifying force of a person in connection with self, others, nature, and God or LifeForce (Dossey, 2008).

## ■ RELATED LITERATURE

Related literature addresses the question: "What core qualities describe the essence of the emerging concept?" (Liehr & Smith, 2014, p. 354). A search of Cumulative Index of Nursing and Health Literature (CINAHL), MEDLINE, and SearchWise databases and interlibrary loan with the key words nature immersion and holistic/integrative/integral nursing was conducted. The results were chronologically listed in a "literature matrix" set forth on a spreadsheet (Gerrard, 2011); see Table 18.1. Through related literature, nature immersion is widely defined as immersion in a natural environment, such as a forest or park. The definition of nature in this case is very broad from everything natural to virgin forest, as the word nature draws its etymological roots from *natura* (in Latin meaning *birth*) and *nasci* (*to be born*) (Louv, 2005, p. 8). Defined broadly, nature "might be sitting with a favorite plant or pet, lying in the grass cloud watching, visiting a neighborhood park or venturing further into forests or mountains, or taking a walk at the ocean shore" (Shields, Levin, Reich, Murnane, & Hanley, 2016). Thus, nature can be individualized and idealized to personal preference.

The literature related to the TINC provided theoretical insight into the emerging concept. The relation between the TINC and nature immersion is explored and elucidated for theoretical qualities of the phenomenon in the context of holistic nursing (Dossey & Keegan, 2016) and other supporting literature for the TINC.

Theoretically, there is a descriptive relationship between healing and nature that can be characterized as wholeness or oneness. "Healing, like nature, is the vibration of unity and wholeness" (Shields et al., 2016, p. 326). Within the nature of materials such as a stone or a seashell is a relationship to oneness that "gives us a sense of place within the whole" (Shields et al., 2016, p. 326). Healing is the position or path to wholeness (Quinn, 2016, p. 102). Wholeness is described as "harmony of body, mind, and spirit, while harmony is defined as an ordered or aesthetically pleasing set of relationships among the elements of the whole" (Quinn, 2016, p. 103). Healing is "an emerging pattern of relationships among the elements of the whole person that leads to greater integrity, connection, and cohesion of the whole system" (Quinn, 2016, p. 103). From the context of holistic nursing, nature immersion can therefore be seen as individually developing relationships to nature including both living and nonliving systems toward a wholeness or healing in the mind, body, and spirit.

Nature-deficit disorder (NDD), a neologism coined by Louv (2005), is defined as the human costs of alienation from nature (Louv, 2005, 2007). It is widely spreading among the public "hitting the younger generation particularly hard" (Louv, 2007, p. 71) as their daily physical contacts and intimacy with nature are fading (Louv, 2007). There is a trend of connection, disconnection, and reconnection between the child and nature leading to the rise of

(*text continues page on 385*)

**TABLE 18.1**  Literature Matrix for Nature Immersion Theory

| Reference | Core Qualities | Definition of Core Qualities Noted by the Author(s) | Other Relevant Thoughts | Key Words | Theory, Population, or Linguistics |
|---|---|---|---|---|---|
| Salzberg (1995) | Connecting with nature, *metta* | The ability to embrace all parts of ourselves as well as the world, as seen in the quality of mind during meditation, which is called *metta* meaning love in Pali, an Indo-European language | Finding a greater sense of connection with others and ourselves awakens the spiritual path and freedom in us | None | Linguistics |
| Wells (2000) | Connecting with nature, personal emergence | Proximity to nature nearby home environments enhances children's cognitive abilities with their attentional capacities increased | Higher levels of cognitive functioning links to relocation of home environments with more greenness among impoverished urban children | None | Population, Linguistics |
| Wells and Evans (2003) | Connecting with nature, personal emergence | As a buffer of the impact of stressful life events on rural children's psychological well-being | Children's cognitive abilities with the proximity to nature increases attention spans, abilities to focus, creative thought processes, problem-solving abilities, self-discipline, and self-regulation | Nature, restoration, children, stress, housing | Population |

*(continued)*

**TABLE 18.1** Literature Matrix for Nature Immersion Theory *(continued)*

| Reference | Core Qualities | Definition of Core Qualities Noted by the Author(s) | Other Relevant Thoughts | Key Words | Theory, Population, or Linguistics |
|---|---|---|---|---|---|
| Louv (2005) | *NDD* in children | The human costs of alienation from nature | Cutting-edge research shows direct exposure to nature is essential for healthy childhood development | None | Population |
| Louv (2007) | Connecting to nature | Nature stimulates cognition and creativity | Nature-connection is vitally important to health and it is dangerously threatened for today's generation | None | Population |
| Dossey (2008) | Grand theory | The innate natural phenomenon that comes from within a person and describes the indivisible wholeness, the interconnectedness of all people, all things | Theory of Integral Nursing, Florence Nightingale's philosophical foundation and legacy, healing and healing research | Global health, healing, integral nursing, meta-paradigm in a nursing theory, micro to macro, nonlocality, patterns of knowing, Theory of Integral Nursing, transpersonal, transdisciplinarian, transdisciplinary dialogues | Theory |

*(continued)*

**TABLE 18.1**   Literature Matrix for Nature Immersion Theory (*continued*)

| Reference | Core Qualities | Definition of Core Qualities Noted by the Author(s) | Other Relevant Thoughts | Key Words | Theory, Population, or Linguistics |
|---|---|---|---|---|---|
| Crede (2009) | Nature immersion, Nature Immersion Model of Education | A new model of education that involves outdoor leaning called sustainable pedagogical approach/sustainability education defined as learning about ecology/environment, ethics, economics, and education | Systems thinking; transformational teacher–student relationship; dialogue; teamwork; constructivism; Modern-Day Disconnection; Ecopsychology, Biophilia, Gaia, the great work, NDD, Nature/Mother Nature/the Natural World/Mother Earth, Nature Seven Generations Thinking, Sustainability, Sustainable Education | None | Linguistics |
| Driessnack (2009) | Connecting with nature, personal emergence | *"Green time"* as an adjunct in the treatment of children's mental health with advantages of wider accessibility, freedom from adverse side effects, nonstigmatization, and inexpensiveness, if not free | The studies on ADHD report the greener the natural setting, the greater the relief from symptoms | None | Population |

(*continued*)

377

**TABLE 18.1** Literature Matrix for Nature Immersion Theory *(continued)*

| Reference | Core Qualities | Definition of Core Qualities Noted by the Author(s) | Other Relevant Thoughts | Key Words | Theory, Population, or Linguistics |
|---|---|---|---|---|---|
| Keegan and Gilbert (2013) | Forest immersion | Immersion in the forest opens our senses, activates a biological response to our natural surroundings, and allows us to our inner guide | Fresh air; freedom from technology; absence of the ever present noise of contemporary society; simple whole foods; immersion in natural hot springs; olfactory stimulation of forest fragrance; escape from artificial light | None | Linguistics |
| Fukushima et al. (2014) | Connecting with nature, earthy materials, personal emergence | Immersion in the natural world heightens hypersonic alpha-wave amplitude to the thalamus and occipital lobe | The emergence of the *hypersonic effect*, known as a phenomenon where sounds with significant qualities of nonstationary high-frequency components activate the midbrain and diencephalon and evoke various physiological, psychological, and behavioral responses, depends on the frequencies above the human audible range (max. 20 kHz) | None | Linguistics |

*(continued)*

**TABLE 18.1**  Literature Matrix for Nature Immersion Theory *(continued)*

| Reference | Core Qualities | Definition of Core Qualities Noted by the Author(s) | Other Relevant Thoughts | Key Words | Theory, Population, or Linguistics |
|---|---|---|---|---|---|
| Kamioka et al. (2014) | Connecting with nature, personal emergence | Based on the evidence from RCTs on the effects of horticultural therapy, HT may be an effective treatment for mental and behavioral disorders | The levels of *phytoncides* released from trees meditate NK cell activity | Horticultural therapy, therapeutic horticulture, garden therapy, randomized controlled trial, rehabilitation effect | Linguistics |
| Blum (2015) | Connecting with nature (Shinrin-yoku and Sukiya-style gardens), earthy materials, personal emergence | Shinrin-yoku (forest bathing) reduces the level of cortisol in the body and is recognized as a traditionally preventive medicine; most Sukiya-style gardens are arranged to be viewed from a seated position inside the home, especially one that is individually tailored to be an idealized version of nature | The natural environment is embedded with a spirit and a soul | None | Linguistics |

*(continued)*

379

**TABLE 18.1** Literature Matrix for Nature Immersion Theory (*continued*)

| Reference | Core Qualities | Definition of Core Qualities Noted by the Author(s) | Other Relevant Thoughts | Key Words | Theory, Population, or Linguistics |
|---|---|---|---|---|---|
| Dossey (2015) | Midrange theory, Integrative Nurse Coach | A registered nurse as a 21st century Nightingale who views clients/patients as integrated whole beings; honors and emphasizes each person's unique history, culture, beliefs, and story; and recognizes each person's health and well-being as influenced by his or her internal and external environments | Theory of Integrative Nurse Coaching and its components: (1) Nurse coach self-development (self-reflection, self-awareness, self-evaluation, self-care), (2) Integral perspectives and change, (3) Integrative lifestyle, health, well-being, awareness, and choice—listening with HEART | None | Theory |
| Kobayash, Song, Ikei, Kagawa, and Miyazaki (2015) | Connecting with nature, earthy materials, personal emergence | Autonomic responses to urban and forest environments | Approximately 80% of the subjects showed an increase in the parasympathetic indicator; 64% of them exhibited decrease in the sympathetic indicator | None | Linguistics |

(*continued*)

**TABLE 18.1**  Literature Matrix for Nature Immersion Theory *(continued)*

| Reference | Core Qualities | Definition of Core Qualities Noted by the Author(s) | Other Relevant Thoughts | Key Words | Theory, Population, or Linguistics |
|---|---|---|---|---|---|
| Palomino, Taylor, Goker, Isaacs, and Warber (2015) | Social media relating to NDD | NDD, a journalistic term proposed to describe the ill effects of people's alienation from nature, is not yet formally recognized as a medical diagnosis but enthusiastically taken up by some segments of the public over the past decade | A Google search is known to produce more than 800,000 hits for NDD, while a search of PubMed produces only one | Nature-deficit disorder, sentiment analysis, Twitter, big data, nature–health | Linguistics |
| Warber, DeHudy, Bialko, Marselle, and Irvine (2015) | Nature immersion experiences on a wilderness camp | The wilderness camp experiences enhance well-being in youths, from the findings of a mixed method pilot study of youths attending a 4-week wilderness camp to investigate the impact of nature | Nature immersion is indicative of improving well-being of youth and preparing future environmental leaders | None | Population |

*(continued)*

**TABLE 18.1**  Literature Matrix for Nature Immersion Theory (*continued*)

| Reference | Core Qualities | Definition of Core Qualities Noted by the Author(s) | Other Relevant Thoughts | Key Words | Theory, Population, or Linguistics |
|---|---|---|---|---|---|
| Burkhardt and Nagai-Jacobson (2016) | Connecting with nature, earthy materials, personal emergence | A source of human empowerment and encouragement, both of which are attributes of spirituality; and indigenous spiritual traditions are acknowledged through a connectedness or conscious relationship with the Earth through the entire cosmos or other-than-human-beings of the world as a way of attuning to one's own soul and spirit | A feeling of connectedness with all things (the Earth and all of its creatures at an energetic level) is an experience of spirituality | None | Theory |
| Dossey (2016) | Holistic, integrative, and integral nursing | All nursing practice that has healing the whole person as its goal and honors relationship-centered care and the interconnectedness of self, others, nature, and spirituality; focuses on protecting, promoting, and optimizing health and wellness; and incorporates integrative modalities and CAM as appropriate | Healing is the goal of holistic nursing; caring is the context for holistic nursing | None | Theory |

(*continued*)

**TABLE 18.1** Literature Matrix for Nature Immersion Theory (*continued*)

| Reference | Core Qualities | Definition of Core Qualities Noted by the Author(s) | Other Relevant Thoughts | Key Words | Theory, Population, or Linguistics |
|---|---|---|---|---|---|
| James, Hart, Banay, and Laden (2016) | The prospective association between residential greenness and mortality | The data from the U.S.-based Nurses' Health Study prospective cohort show women living in the highest quintile of cumulative average greenness in the 250-m area around their home had a 12% lower rate of all-cause nonaccidental mortality | Higher levels of green vegetation are associated with decreased mortality, indicating planting vegetation may be used to improve health | None | Linguistics |
| Quinn (2016) | Wholeness, healing, personal emergence | Wholeness is defined as harmony of body, mind, and spirit while harmony is defined as an ordered or aesthetically pleasing set of relationships among the elements of the whole. The origin of the word heal is the Anglo-Saxon word *haelan*, which means to be or to become whole | Upon transpersonal human caring, a fact of human interaction is not an optional event but *caring occasions* termed by Jean Watson as in the field of consciousness, which is the potential to continue to heal the patient long after the physical separation of nurse and patient | None | Theory, Linguistics |

(*continued*)

**TABLE 18.1**  Literature Matrix for Nature Immersion Theory  (*continued*)

| Reference | Core Qualities | Definition of Core Qualities Noted by the Author(s) | Other Relevant Thoughts | Key Words | Theory, Population, or Linguistics |
|---|---|---|---|---|---|
| Shields, Levin, Reich, Murnane, and Hanley (2016) | Connecting with nature, earthy materials, personal emergence | Not only listening deeper into the inner rhythms and sounds of breaths, heartbeats, voices, etc., but also through imaging, smelling, writing, walking, storytelling or story-sharing, etc. | Healing is a holistic vibration consistent with a nature-process. | None | Theory, linguistics |

ADHD, attention deficit hyperactivity disorder; CAM, complementary and alternative modalities; HEART, Healing, Energy, Awareness, Resilience, Transformation; HT, horticultural therapy; NDD, nature-deficit disorder; NK, natural killer; RCT, randomized controlled trial.

reconnect-children-to-nature movements (Louv, 2008). Some of these movements (Louv, 2008) are: New Mexico's *Outdoor Classrooms Initiative* to increase outdoor education in the state, Washington's *Leave No Child Inside Initiative* with $1.5 million a year allocated to outdoor programs for underserved children, and California's *Sierra Club* for outdoor education/recreation programs serving at-risk youth. Louv (2005, 2007) claims that over the past decades, the outdoor-playing urban human child has become an endangered species (Louv, 2005, 2007). It is an unprecedented trend that children no longer spend much of their formative years in nature (Louv, 2005, 2007).

Nature immersion stimulates creativity and cognition among children (Louv, 2007). Proximity to nature environments enhances children's cognitive abilities and increases attentional capacities (Wells, 2000). The positive effects are also reported in emotional, biological, and/or behavioral situations, such as symptoms of attention deficit disorder (ADD; Wells & Evans, 2003). It was found that: higher levels of nearby nature buffer the impact of stressful life events on rural children's psychological well-being (Wells & Evans, 2003); and greater symptom relief occurred with greener spaces among children with ADD as young as age 5 (Louv, 2007).

However, in contrast to ADD, NDD is not formally recognized as a medical diagnosis (Driessnack, 2009; Warber, DeHudy, Bialko, Marselle, & Irvine, 2015). A Google search produced more than 800,000 hits for ADD, while a search of PubMed produced only 1 for NDD (Palomino, Taylor, Goker, Isaacs, & Warber, 2015). Despite the increasing awareness of *nature immersion* among the public, there are scarce resources and research on *nature immersion*. Emerging phases underlying nature's capacity to restore, bolster, and foster children have been little explored (Wells & Evans, 2003). In short, the phenomenon of *nature immersion* presents a new wave of consciousness that can impact biological, emotional, and behavioral symptoms among hard-hit children.

The importance of nature for health has begun to be recognized in the disciplines of education, medicine, and nursing. In these disciplines, there is beginning sensitivity to the nature–health connection, sometimes noted as biophilia. The word *biophilia*, which comes from Wilson (1984), is defined as humans' intrinsic and instinctive affinity for connecting to natural life forms. Biophilia postulates that this affinity is a biologically essential connection between humans and all other living species and systems (Wilson, 1984). It is based on the assumption that nature is integral to human development.

Likewise, integrality of humans and nature presents as emerging patterns of harmony in the person. Recent studies have shown that spending time immersed in nature has physical and psychological benefits to humans: (a) increasing parasympathetic activity (Keegan & Gilbert, 2013; Kobayashi, Song, Ikei, Kagawa, & Miyazaki, 2015); (b) heightening hypersonic alpha-wave amplitude to the thalamus and occipital regions of the brain (Fukushima, Yagi, Kawai, Honda, & Nishina, 2014); (c) increasing natural killer (NK) cell activity

(Kamioka et al., 2014); and (d) contributing to an epigenetic consequence of lowered mortality (James, Hart, Banary, & Laden, 2016).

Pedagogically, outdoor classroom settings offer personally transformative learning with ecological, ethical, and economic components (Crede, 2009). Forest immersion known as "forest bathing" promotes personal introspection and healing (Keegan & Gilbert, 2013). This is, in part, believed to be due to the effects from chemical properties such as phytoncides, secreted from trees like oak, cedar, and pine, and by plants like onions, garlic, and spices (Blum, 2015).

Through the related literature, two core qualities for nature immersion emerged; these are connecting with earthy material and personal emergence that enables health, healing, and well-being.

## Gather a Story

In contrast to the nursing practice story, which was retrospective and initiated the concept building process, the second story was prospective to deepen understanding and inquire into core qualities of the emerging concept (Liehr & Smith, 2014). For gathering a second story, questions to inquire about the core qualities that arise from the literature are formulated before the interview (Table 18.2). This story-gathering has two phases: the leading questions and the core qualities questions (Liehr & Smith, 2014). The leading questions are to explore the lived experience of the central phenomenon from the past to present to projected future, known as a story path approach (Liehr & Smith, 2014). Through the approach, nature immersion is reexplored anew from the perspective of the interviewee. The interviewee selected for this story-gathering is a parent whose child has lived nature immersion. The interview for this story-gathering was approved by the institutional review board (IRB) at Florida Atlantic University.

The reconstructed story, highlighting the core qualities, has a beginning, middle, and end (Liehr & Smith, 2014). Shared by the storyteller and reconstructed by the nurse, the story presents details about the emerging concept as shaped by the nurse in recounting the perspective of the mother of a child with nature immersion experiences. The story-gathering interview, lasting about 45 minutes, was recorded, transcribed, and reconstructed as follows.

Hana, the mother of a 10-year-old boy, Taro, recalls the days Taro showed signs of autism, at the age of 2. He was withdrawn inwardly. One day, he rampantly became febrile, without a known cause. He was given tablets of Baby-Tylenol prescribed by a pediatrician. His fever was rapidly quelled. He then appeared languid, listless, and lifeless. There was a mixed feeling in Hana if it was the only way to take care of him—to her, it appeared too allopathic and artificial for this little child. Taro's whole world split into parts inward, shutting off outward. Then, Hana looked for natural therapeutics with the hope that her child would grow up to be self-caring on his feet.

**TABLE 18.2**   Interview Questions

Leading questions

What is about nature that is therapeutic for your child?

How does your child experience these materials in everyday living?

When did you first learn about nature as therapeutic?

Since then to now, how does nature help your child's conditions?

What does healing mean to you and your child?

What are your hopes and dreams about healing outcomes that can occur as your child connects with nature?

Questions for the three core qualities

(1) Environment—earthy materials

What nature environments are provided for your child by program instructors?

What does the child call this (activity, material, etc., of nature) in his or her words?

(2) Experience—connection with nature

How often does your child come into contact with materials of nature during the day?

How does the child connect with the materials of nature?

(3) Emergence—personal health, healing, and well-being

What are the phases of your child's emerging good conditions and/or health in the mind and/or body through the contact with nature?

Soon Taro was enrolled in a school that enmeshes nature in education, called the *Early Childhood Program*. He started to spend more time touching and garnering pieces of wood, leaves, and pebbles, out of which toys were made at school. He brought home those made of nature that seemed just like junk but were a gem to him with true nature immanent within. He became more outwardly curious, with his spirit opening onward and upward. Also, his bouts of fever started to be taken care of by nature through minute doses of natural flower remedies in pellets. It eased him slowly and subtly, so that he looked allayed even in the midst of symptoms.

Nature applies to Hana in twofold elements: the internal and external nature of life. Healing emerges in the midst of nature immersion. Nature manifests in Taro's minigarden of toys, which are appealing, appeasing, and available for him anytime, anywhere. The healing emerges without force. Just like a flower comes into bloom without force but from within. Hana concludes that both sides of nature need to mix, mingle, and mesh inside and outside of the child.

## Minisaga

The reconstructed story was then distilled into a minisaga, "a short story that synthesizes the reconstructed story" (Liehr & Smith, 2014, p. 357) with "just fifty words long . . . no more, no less" (Pink, 2005, p. 119). It consists of a beginning, middle, and end, and just like the practice and reconstructed stories, it captures the core meaning of the phenomenon of interest and crystallizes the essence of the emerging concept to be readily shared with others (Liehr & Smith, 2014). It compresses "nature immersion" into a concise yet clear essence:

> Hana, the mother of 10-year-old Taro, recalls when he was withdrawn inwardly at the age of 2. Taro was enrolled in a school that enmeshes nature with education; he got more curious outwardly, and his spirit opened. Hana concludes healing emerged as nature inside and outside of Taro became one.

## Define the Core Qualities

"The core qualities are the defining properties of the emerging concept" (Liehr & Smith, 2014, p. 358). Nature immersion consists of the core qualities: personal emergence and connecting with earthy materials. Personal emergence is defined as personally developing relationships with any and all levels of the living and/or nonliving systems physically, psychologically, and spiritually. This is a guiding impulse and/or impetus generated from within an individual living system. It moves from chaos and disorder to order via self-organization leading to self-actualization and self-transcendence (Quinn, 2016). It cannot be coerced or controlled even by the person experiencing it but is a creative, unpredictable, and unfolding emergence into something new rather than something previous (Quinn, 2016). It can occur at any and all levels of the living and/or nonliving systems: cellular, physical, emotional, and spiritual (Quinn, 2016). For example, the new relationship emerges among the cells and tissues to patch the wound together, transcending past and present memories to let go of emotions, and harness the life force, to dance in cosmic rhythms and move beyond existing limits.

Connecting with earthy materials is defined as an act of integrating rhythms of nature in two environments: internal and external. It is cultivated through not only listening deeper into the inner rhythms and sounds of breaths, heartbeats, and voices, but also through imaging, smelling, writing, walking, and storytelling (Shields et al., 2016). In addition, there are also outer rhythms, like the ever-changing seasons and the pull of the moon to alter tides. There is one symphony or song between the internal and external sides of nature intricately interwoven in oneness; internal and external are in unison and synchronized.

Connecting is to sink gently into the center (Shields et al., 2016, p. 334), a place of openness to receive (Shields et al., 2016, p. 334) inner wisdom and grace. Immersing oneself in a liquid epitomizes the sort of connecting and embracing all (Salzberg, 1995), which is intended in describing nature immersion. Indigenous spiritual traditions that draw on sacred rituals are exemplary of connecting or sinking gently into Mother Earth's embrace as a way of attuning to one's own soul and spirit (Burkhardt & Nagai-Jacobson, 2016, p. 139). Earthy constituents of nature including the organic and inorganic exist in harmony even with disharmonious environments. Encouraging the capacity of nature enables arriving at a new harmony. It affirms Nightingale's notion of nature as acting on a person, enabling a new harmony to emerge from within.

Earthy materials are all the constituents both organic and inorganic on Mother Earth. These can be visible as the sunlight, invisible as sounds, tangible as stones, and intangible as scent. Earthy materials can also be pictures or illustration of creatures (Shields et al., 2016), including animals, plants, or landscapes, expressive of features like sounds, silence, or even stillness.

There are cycles of connection and reconnection between earthy materials and a person as he or she reflects or resonates to a rhythm of nature. Each time it cycles, the personal emergence also cycles to radiate differently in rhythm and relationship with all inner and outer dimensions of a person.

## ■ DEFINE THE WORKING CONCEPT

The concept, nature immersion, is defined through its two core qualities. Nature immersion is personal emergence occurring through connecting with earthy materials.

### Model

The model (Figure 18.1) represents a structural representation of relationship among the core qualities with an understanding that the emerging concept is grounded in the theoretical niche of the TINC.

The personally emerging phases of health and wellness are noted in circular, nonlinear directions of flow. Each component of "person," "person and earthy material," and "personal emergence" occurs both consequently and simultaneously. It flows in a round rather than in a linear, single direction. At the "person and earthy material" phase, the "person" and "earthy material" interact in a new and/or renewed level of immersions, in terms of the cycle of human–nature connection. It reminds one to "remember" how to listen with the heart and soul in "reconnection" to nature. It is a form of communication with the energies of all living and nonliving earthy materials.

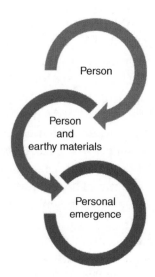

**FIGURE 18.1**   Model of Nature Immersion.

## Minisynthesis

The minisynthesis is composed of three sentences with the significance of the phenomenon in the first sentence, the definition in the second sentence, and suggestion for research in the third sentence (Liehr & Smith, 2014).

Positive effects of nature to develop mental, physical, and/or spiritual health and wellness have been significantly noted, especially in children. Nature immersion is personal emergence occurring through connecting with earthy materials. Researching the personal change that occurs when children connect with earthy materials may provide information to support the power of nature to promote health and wellness.

## ■ CONCLUSION

This chapter presents the concept building process guided by Liehr and Smith (2014). Born from a story occurring during integrative nursing practice, niched by a holistic theoretical framework, and evidenced by literature from various disciplines, this nascent phenomenon is gradually shaped, sophisticated, and solidified into multidimensional facets of a clearer crystal. It has now advanced to enable identification of a research question. Conducting the research study among individuals who have lived the concept of nature immersion is necessary to gain more insights into nature immersion. Increased understanding of the impact of nature deficit and the experiences of being immersed in nature will better equip nurses to recognize nature deficit as a possible factor contributing to compromised health and wellness. Likewise, approaches that may be used to treat the deficit could inform integrative nursing practice.

## ■ REFERENCES

Blum, H. (2015). A walk in the woods. *Sukiya Living Magazine, 108*, 26–19.

Burkhardt, M. A., & Nagai-Jacobson, M. G. (2016). Spirituality and health. In B. M. Dossey & L. Keegan (Eds.), *Holistic nursing: A handbook for practice* (7th ed., pp. 135–163). Burlington, MA: Jones & Bartlett.

Crede, J. L. (2009). *Nature immersion: A model of sustainability education* (Doctoral Dissertation). Retrieved from ProQuest Dissertations Publishing.

Dossey, B. M. (2005). Florence Nightingale's tenets: Healing, leadership, global action. In B. M. Dossey, L. C. Selanders, D. Beck, & A. Attewell (Eds.), *Florence Nightingale today: Healing leadership global action* (pp. 1–28). Silver Spring, MD: American Nurses Association.

Dossey, B. M. (2008). Theory of integral nursing. *Advances in Nursing Science, 31*(1), E52–E73.

Dossey, B. M. (2015). Theory of integrative nurse coaching. In B. M. Dossey, S. Luck, & B. G. Schaub (Eds.), *Nurse coaching: Integrative approaches for health and well-being* (pp. 29–49). Miami, FL: International Nurse Coach Association.

Dossey, B. M. (2016). Nursing: Holistic, integral, and integrative–local to global. In B. M. Dossey & L. Keegan (Eds.), *Holistic nursing: A handbook for practice* (7th ed., pp. 3–52). Burlington, MA: Jones & Bartlett.

Driessnack, M. (2009). Children and nature-deficit disorder. *Journal of Specialists in Pediatric Nursing, 14*(1), 73–75.

Fukushima, A., Yagi, R., Kawai, N., Honda, M., Nishina, E., & Oohashi, T. (2014). Frequencies of inaudible high-frequency sounds differentially affect brain activity: Positive and negative hypersonic effects. *PLOS ONE, 9*(4), e95464. doi:10.1371/journal.pone.0095464

Gerrard, J. (2011). *Health sciences literature review made easy*. Sudbury, MA: Jones & Bartlett.

James, P., Hart, J. E., Banay, R. F., & Laden, F. (2016). Exposure to greenness and mortality in a nationwide prospective study of women. *Environmental Health Perspectives, 124*(9), 1344–1352.

Kamioka, H., Tsutani, K., Yamada, M., Park, H., Okuizumi, H., Honda, T., . . . Okada, S. (2014). Effectiveness of horticultural therapy: A systematic review of randomized controlled trials. *Complementary Therapies in Medicine, 22*, 930–943.

Keegan, L., & Gilbert, T. (2013). Forest immersion experience: Mother nature promotes introspection and healing. *Beginnings, 33*(3), 10–12.

Kobayashi, H., Song, C., Ikei, H., Kagawa, T., & Miyazaki, Y. (2015). Analysis of individual variations in autonomic responses to urban and forest environments. *Evidence Based Complementary and Alternative Medicine, 2015*, 1–7. doi:10.1155/2015/671094

Liehr, P. R., & Smith, M. J. (2014). Concept building for research. In M. J. Smith & P. R. Liehr (Eds.), *Middle range theory for nursing* (3rd ed., pp. 349–360). New York, NY: Springer Publishing.

Louv, R. (2005). *Last child in the woods: saving our children from nature-deficit*. Chapel Hill, NC: Algonquin Books.

Louv, R. (2007). In the garden of childhood. *Organic Gardening, 54*(2), 70–71.

Louv, R. (2008). Paul F-Brandwein Lecture 2007: A brief history of the children & nature movement. *Journal of Science and Technology, 17,* 217–218.

Nightingale, F. (1860 [1969]). *Notes on nursing: What it is and what it is not.* New York, NY: Dover.

Oxford University Press. (2010). *New Oxford American Dictionary* (3rd ed.). Oxford, UK: Oxford University Press.

Palomino, M., Taylor, T., Goker, A., Isaacs, J., & Warber, S. (2015). Concepts: Lessons from sentiment analysis of social media relating to "Nature-Deficit Disorder". *International Journal of Environmental Research and Public Health, 13,* 1–23.

Pink, D. H. (2005). *A whole new mind: moving from the information age to the conceptual age.* New York, NY: Penguin Group.

Quinn, J. F. (2016). Transpersonal human caring and healing. In B. M. Dossey & L. Keegan (Eds.), *Holistic nursing: A handbook for practice* (7th ed., pp. 101–110). Burlington, MA: Jones & Bartlett.

Salzberg. (1995). *Lovingkindness: the revolutionary art of happiness.* Boston, MA: Shambhala.

Shields, D. A., Levin, J., Reich, J., Murnane, S., & Hanley, M. A. (2016). Creative expressions in healing. In B. M. Dossey & L. Keegan (Eds.), *Holistic nursing: A handbook for practice* (7th ed., pp. 321–343). Burlington, MA: Jones & Bartlett.

Warber, S. L., DeHudy, A. A., Bialko, M. F., Marselle, M. R., & Irvine, K. N. (2015). Addressing "Nature-Deficit Disorder": A mixed methods pilot study of young adults attending a wilderness camp. *Evidence-Based Complementary Alternative Medicine,* 1–13. doi:10.1155/2015/651827

Wells, N. (2000). At home with nature effects of "greenness" on children's cognitive functioning. *Environment and Behavior, 32*(6), 775–795.

Wells, N., & Evans, G. (2003). Nearby nature: A buffer of life stress among rural children. *Environment and Behavior, 35*(3), 311–330.

Wilson, E. O. (1984). *Biophilia.* Cambridge, MA: Harvard University Press.

# CHAPTER 19

## Sheltering-in-Place: A Concept for Nursing Research

Kimberly Ann Wallace

The evolution of nursing science occurs gradually over time as new phenomena are identified and explored. These phenomena are rooted in nursing practice and can be identified as demonstrations of caring in the human health experience (Newman, Sime, & Corcoran-Perry, 1991). Sheltering-in-place is a concept that identifies a phenomenon in which women delay medical evaluation after identification of a breast abnormality in order to preserve normalcy in their lives. Delay in seeking healthcare by women with self-identified breast abnormalities is prevalent in the United States (SEER, 2012). Delay is identifiable with overall breast cancer outcomes and is recognizable in inpatient, outpatient, and particularly community nursing practice. The purpose of this chapter is to detail the concept building process as developed by Liehr and Smith (2014) describing how this process was utilized to guide the development of the concept sheltering-in-place.

The phenomenon of sheltering-in-place has been seen often in my own practice. Commonly, women present for a surgical procedure many months after self-identification of a breast abnormality. Consistently, women choose treatment delay despite access to insurance, resources, and sufficient knowledge, factors commonly attributed to delay in this population. After identification of this perceived discrepancy in my practice, further inquiry was deemed necessary. Gaining a better understanding of the human health experience in this population required the development of the concept sheltering-in-place.

## ■ CONCEPT DEVELOPMENT

Concept building is a skill set required for any researcher. The practiced ability to navigate the ladder of abstraction through induction, deduction, and abduction as well as analysis and synthesis of information is required for this process. Concepts are used to guide and mold research. As proposed by Liehr and Smith (2014), the systematic approach consists of 10 phases: (1) write a meaningful practice story, (2) name the central phenomenon in the practice story, (3) identify a theoretical lens for viewing the emerging concept, (4) link the emerging concept to existing literature, (5) gather a story from a person who has experienced the central idea of the emerging concept, (6) write a reconstructed story using what was shared in phase 5 and create a minisaga that captures the message of the reconstructed story, (7) identify core qualities of the emerging concept, (8) formulate a definition that integrates the core qualities, (9) draw a model that depicts relationships between core qualities of the working concept, and (10) create a minisynthesis that integrates the working concept definition with a population to suggest a research direction. Throughout this chapter, each of these phases is discussed in detail to outline the development of the concept sheltering-in-place. Exemplars serve as a point of reference to increase understanding.

## ■ PRACTICE STORY AND CENTRAL PHENOMENON

The systematic concept development approach begins with the writing of a meaningful practice story. The story, rooted in nursing practice, outlines a critical incident that is related to caring in the human health experience. Practice stories are often identified by clinical personnel, but can be gathered by anyone with an interest and access to a particular phenomenon. The exercise begins the process of understanding the link between empirical and conceptual understanding. The practice story will serve as a standard by which to analyze the phenomenon during the developmental phase. The practice story of Beverly that follows does not truly represent one individual patient, but is a summation of the researcher's experience with the phenomenon—a synthesis of many pertinent patient situations.

### Practice Story

Beverly was a mother, a daughter, a sister, and a secretary for her husband's company. The day I met her, she was exhausted. She had completed multiple medical appointments already and the extended drive to and from the healthcare facility further complicated her experience. She mentioned difficulty in finding coverage at work. She was alone in the clinic and seemed eager to be finished.

While discussing her history, Beverly shared that she had known of her breast cancer diagnosis for a couple of weeks and she still seemed to be in shock. She was tearful on occasion and cycled through multiple emotions in a short time: shock, grief, fear, and isolation. Sometimes, she voiced these feelings aloud, but there was also nonverbal communication. She was in uncharted territory and processing her new situation before my eyes.

Her appearance and demeanor prompted a more personal conversation, providing an opportunity to tell her story. Beverly shared that she had learned her tumor was "big" and that she "couldn't believe she waited so long" to seek treatment. I discussed with her that her new diagnosis brought a lot of emotions along with it and I questioned whether she had support and resources available to her. She was happy to share that, while she was alone today, she was "blessed" to have a wonderful husband and two children who were eager to help in any way.

Beverly opened up about her current situation. She discussed that she felt the lump "many months ago" and that she couldn't "even really remember how long it had been." Time had passed quicker than she realized. She remembered "worrying about it over Thanksgiving and Christmas," so according to her, it must have been "a while." Beverly shared that while she had a strong support system in her family and "good insurance" that she chose not to seek healthcare even after she felt it was "probably necessary." After months of "back and forth" and telling no one of her suspicions, she made an appointment with her physician. After weeks of appointments, she was sitting in the clinic only days before her scheduled mastectomy, still unsure of her stage of cancer or plan for chemotherapy and radiation. After more discussion, Beverly shared that she could not really "put her finger on" why she waited so long to seek help. She stated that "it just seemed easier" to leave everything "the way it was."

For days after her visit, I wondered: Why? Why did she not seek care if she had the insurance? Why did she not tell anyone of her suspicions? Why wait so long once you start to worry that it might be cancer?

## Central Phenomenon

Deliberation on Beverly's situation heightened my awareness during visits with other women scheduled for mastectomy. I began to suspect that Beverly's case was not an isolated event. Many women were making the choice to shelter in place, most with the similar inability to provide explanation as to why delay occurred. Reflecting on the stories provided by these women led to an understanding that this phenomenon was more than simple denial. Instead, it was an intentional desire to maintain normalcy in their lives. With a common theme among patients and a desire to better understand this phenomenon, the process of discovery through concept development began.

## ■ THEORETICAL FOUNDATION

A developing concept must be viewed from the perspective of a theory. This theoretical perspective provides guidance and assigns meaning to the emerging concept. This theoretical niche provides a suitable position essential in concept development. Concept developers are encouraged to find a theory that "fits like a glove" (Liehr & Smith, 2014, p. 354). Choosing a theory at the middle range level of abstraction is a step in the concept building process and is vital to provide a foundation on which to further build a conceptual structure.

## Middle Range Theory: Moral Reckoning

For development of this concept, the Theory of Moral Reckoning (2003) was applied. It is proposed that sheltering-in-place is a process of moral reckoning. The Theory of Moral Reckoning is composed of the concepts of ease, situational binds, resolution, and reflection. These concepts describe stages of moral reckoning that occur over a period of time (Nathaniel, 2003).

### EASE

"Ease is a state of naturalness, a sense of comfort" (Nathaniel, 2003, p. 332). Ease implies a period of calm and lack of worry or concern. Any event that disrupts a person's self-defined state of ease can be understood as a situational bind. The concept of ease in Nathaniel's Theory of Moral Reckoning is readily relatable to the sense of normalcy found in the concept sheltering-in-place. Ease is viewed as a normal routine and life—an individualized definition of normalcy. This state of ease can last varying amounts of time during which a sense of normalcy is defined and strengthened. This will continue until there is disruption in the state of ease.

### SITUATIONAL BINDS

Situational binds are serious conflicts that force a person to question "his or her central purpose, asking to what, for what, or to whom she is committed. The person experiences turmoil and inner dialogue that leads to a decision" (Nathaniel, 2003, p. 333). The concept of situational binds represents any occurrence that disrupts the state of ease. In application to the concept of sheltering-in-place, situational binds represent the uncertainty felt with the presence of a new threat. According to Nathaniel (2003), each individual must choose to "make a stand" or "give up." Many feel a desire, at least initially, to continue living as normally as possible. While the state of ease has unquestionably been disrupted, the sense of normalcy is not easily sacrificed. According to the Theory of Moral Reckoning, the chosen path most closely aligns with "giving up." However, in the population of women with breast cancer, there is a deliberate choice to avoid a threat; it is different than "giving up." Very often, these women change their response after a period of time and seek care. After the initial threat and subsequent response, the women move to the stages of resolution and reflection.

### RESOLUTION AND REFLECTION

The concept of resolution is the stage during which the individual seeks a solution to the problem. Reflection is the stage in which a person considers past events. During the stage of reflection, the person progresses through remembering, telling the story, examining conflicts, and living with the consequences of previously made choices (Nathaniel, 2003). Resolution and reflection, as applied to the concept of sheltering-in-place, are an individual's way of making sense of recent events and returning structure to his or her life. This stage is one way in which to provide self-protection. During this stage, the women come to terms with what really happened, who was to blame, and what will now happen in the future as a result of those decisions. While the initial threat has been addressed, the uncertainty of future threats—diagnosis, prognosis, and possible recurrence—may present a new set of challenges resulting in a repeat of the process.

## ■ EMPIRICAL FOUNDATION

Exploration of existing literature ensures that the phenomenon has a current place in nursing science. After theoretical and conceptual structures have been established in the previous phase, evaluating literature for identified themes and concepts moves the scholar down the ladder of abstraction to solidify the concept empirically. The literature review begins with exploration of the identified phenomenon, then further seeks to include the population of interest. This process allows for the emergence of core qualities that have strong foundations in existing knowledge.

A literature search using Cumulative Index of Nursing and Health Literature (CINAHL) with full text, MEDLINE, PsycInfo, and PsycARTICLES databases was completed using the key words breast, breast cancer, uncertainty, protect self, self-protection, familiar, and normalcy. Identified literature included many qualitative and quantitative studies as well as dissertations, book chapters, and theories. All included articles show a relationship to one of the core qualities. The literature search results can be found in Table 19.1, organized chronologically.

### Gathering a Story, Reconstruction of the Story, and Minisaga

A story is gathered from someone who has personally experienced the emerging concept. During this stage of the process, questions are posed to elicit the individual's assigned meaning to the phenomenon, not biased by the interviewer's assumptions. This part of the process serves to uphold or oppose the core qualities as identified. Making an effort to identify a story from a person with lived experience further validates the phenomenon of interest and the supporting qualities identified thus far. Initially, the gathered story will be a collection of quotes and thoughts from the selected person. The story will be told beginning with the present, going to the past, and then to the future. To better understand the thought processes and qualities in this story, the gathered story will be reconstructed. The purpose of the reconstructed story is to transform the shared information into a coherent story, one with a beginning,

(*text continues page on 404*)

**TABLE 19.1**  Literature Matrix for the Theory of Sheltering-in-Place

| Author | Year | Journal | Title | Core Quality | Definition | Nursing Substantive Foundation | Key Words |
|---|---|---|---|---|---|---|---|
| Brashers et al. | 2003 | *Issues in Mental Health Nursing* | The medical, personal, and social causes of uncertainty in HIV illness | Uncertainty | Important stressor in both acute and chronic illness; ambiguity of diagnosis | Important part of illness experience; medical forms of uncertainty typically involve issues of diagnosis, symptom patterns, systems of treatment and care, and disease progression and prognosis | Use of Lazarus and Folkman's Stress and Coping Theory |
| Clutton, Buckley, & Pakenham | 1999 | *Psychology and Health* | Predictors of emotional well-being following a false positive breast cancer screening result | Uncertainty | Effectiveness of coping strategies vary dependent on controllability of the situation | | Controllability; use of Lazarus and Folkman's Stress and Coping Theory |
| Demir et al. | 2008 | *Journal of Clinical Nursing* | Patients' lived experiences of excisional breast biopsy: A phenomenological study | Uncertainty | Fear, need for information, spiritual needs; strong desire to remove the uncertainty | Three themes identified:<br>• Fear<br>• Need for information<br>• Spiritual needs | None |

(continued)

**TABLE 19.1** Literature Matrix for the Theory of Sheltering-in-Place *(continued)*

| Author | Year | Journal | Title | Core Quality | Definition | Nursing Substantive Foundation | Key Words |
|---|---|---|---|---|---|---|---|
| Denford, Harcourt, Rubin, & Pusic | 2010 | *Psycho-Oncology* | Understanding normality: A qualitative analysis of breast cancer patients' concepts of normality after mastectomy and reconstructive surgery | Normalcy | Looking normal, being able to fulfill everyday activities, adapting to a new normal, and not being ill | Four main concepts of normality:<br>• Appearance<br>• Behavior<br>• Feelings<br>• Health | Normality |
| Drageset, Lindstrom, Giske, & Underlid | 2011 | *Journal of Advanced Nursing* | Being in suspense: Women's experience awaiting breast cancer surgery | Uncertainty | Appraised as "danger"; need for knowledge; major stressor that influences experiences during breast cancer trajectory | Attempts to reduce feelings of uncertainty by focusing on the present | Mentions Mishel's Uncertainty in Illness Theory; losing control |
| Hall, Mishel, & Germino | 2014 | *Supportive Care in Cancer* | Living with cancer-related uncertainty associations with fatigue, insomnia, and affect in younger breast cancer survivors | Uncertainty | Conceptualized to be a cognitive state generated by a patient's or survivor's inability to determine the outcome of cancer-related stimuli | | Mentions Mishel's Uncertainty in Illness Theory |

*(continued)*

**TABLE 19.1** Literature Matrix for the Theory of Sheltering-in-Place *(continued)*

| Author | Year | Journal | Title | Core Quality | Definition | Nursing Substantive Foundation | Key Words |
|---|---|---|---|---|---|---|---|
| Hilton, Crawford, & Tarko | 2000 | *Western Journal* | Men's perspectives on individual and family coping with their wives' breast cancer and chemotherapy | Protecting self, normalcy | Not expressing feelings, trying to be positive, and maintaining normal routines and activities | Major themes on ways of coping:<br>• Being there<br>• Relying on health-care professionals for quality care<br>• Being informed and contributing to decision making<br>• Trying to keep patterns normal<br>• Helping out and relying on others<br>• Trying to be positive<br>• Putting self on hold<br>• Adapting work life<br>• Managing finances<br><br>Protective talk interfered with effective communication, increased energy expenditure, and added stress | |

*(continued)*

**TABLE 19.1** Literature Matrix for the Theory of Sheltering-in-Place *(continued)*

| Author | Year | Journal | Title | Core Quality | Definition | Nursing Substantive Foundation | Key Words |
|---|---|---|---|---|---|---|---|
| Howard, Balneaves, Bottorff, &Rodney | 2011 | *Qualitative Health Research* | Preserving the self: The process of decision making about hereditary breast cancer and ovarian cancer risk reduction | Protecting self | | Development of Preserving the Self Theory | |
| Lebel et al. | 2003 | *Journal of Psychosomatic Research* | Waiting for a breast biopsy: Psychosocial consequences and coping strategies | Uncertainty | Use of cognitive-avoidant coping strategies | High levels of distress at the beginning and end of waiting period for biopsy; levels of intrusion and avoidant thoughts | Mentions Lazarus and Folkman's Stress and Coping Theory |
| Liao, Chen, Chen, & Chen | 2008 | *Cancer Nursing* | Uncertainty and anxiety during the diagnostic period for women with suspected breast cancer | Uncertainty | A cognitive state in which a person is unable to determine the meaning of illness-related events | | Mentions Mishel's Uncertainty in Illness Theory |
| Logan, Hackbusch-Pinto, & De Grasse | 2006 | *Oncology Nursing Forum* | Women undergoing breast diagnostics: The lived experience of spirituality | Protecting self | Physical withdrawal and emotional barrier | Reflection on personal self and spirituality that occurred during the period of isolation supported women and helped them to cope with the uncertainty of diagnosis | |

*(continued)*

**TABLE 19.1** Literature Matrix for the Theory of Sheltering-in-Place *(continued)*

| Author | Year | Journal | Title | Core Quality | Definition | Nursing Substantive Foundation | Key Words |
|---|---|---|---|---|---|---|---|
| Montgomery | 2010 | *Oncology Nursing Forum* | Uncertainty during breast diagnostic evaluation: State of the science | Uncertainty | Inability to determine the meaning of an illness-related event and occurs when an individual is unable to predict outcomes accurately | High levels of anxiety, fear. Optimism and hope correlate with lower anxiety levels | |
| Miller | 2012 | *Journal of Cancer Survivorship* | Sources of uncertainty in cancer survivorship | Uncertainty | Cognitive processing of illness-related events | • Medical<br>• Personal<br>• Social | Mentions Mishel's Uncertainty in Illness Theory |
| Schmid-Buchi, Halfens, Dassen, & van der Borne | | *Journal of Clinical Nursing* | A review of psychosocial needs of breast-cancer patients and their relatives | Protecting self | Keep life going, fulfill wife's needs and may subordinate their own difficulties | Conceptual framework with four main dimensions:<br>• Breast cancer and its treatment<br>• The needs of women suffering from breast cancer<br>• The needs of the women's partners<br>• The interaction between the women and their partners | |

*(continued)*

**TABLE 19.1**  Literature Matrix for the Theory of Sheltering-in-Place (*continued*)

| Author | Year | Journal | Title | Core Quality | Definition | Nursing Substantive Foundation | Key Words |
|---|---|---|---|---|---|---|---|
| Shaha, Cox, Talman, & Kelly | 2008 | *Journal of Nursing Scholarship* | Uncertainty in breast, prostate, and colorectal cancer: Implications for supportive care | Uncertainty | A lack of certainty about the long-term future; sensation of feeling unsure about the best action or choice in a given situation | • Information-related issues<br>• Decisions about treatment and the effect of cancer-related uncertainty | Mishel's Uncertainty in Illness Theory |
| Strickland, Wells, & Porr | 2015 | *Oncology Nursing Forum* | Safeguarding the children: The cancer journey of young mothers | Normalcy | | • Customizing exposure<br>• Finding new ways to be close<br>• Increasing vigilance<br>• Reducing disruption to family life | Utilizes Glaser and Strauss's Grounded Theory |
| Wonghongkul, Dechaprom, Phumivichuvate, & Losawatkul | 2006 | *Cancer Nursing* | Uncertainty appraisal coping and quality of life in breast cancer survivors | Uncertainty | When persons are unable to understand the meaning of an event because of its complexity, ambiguity, or mismatch between their own expectation and the realistic world | | Utilizes Mishel's Uncertainty in Illness scale, Lazarus and Folkman's Stress and Coping Theory |

middle, and end. The reconstructed story will further be synthesized into a shorter story—the minisaga. Pink (2005) describes minisagas as "extremely short stories—just fifty words long. . . no more, no less" (p. 117). A reader of the minisaga should be able to extrapolate the core meaning of the individual's story from the perspective of the individual.

## RECONSTRUCTED STORY

Phyllis is a 49-year-old mother. She is employed as an elementary education teacher with long hours and many commitments. She was diagnosed with breast cancer after a substantial delay in seeking medical evaluation. She reports that she first noticed the lump 9 months ago while taking a shower. She described the first time she noticed the lump. She shared that she spent several minutes examining her breast the way she had been instructed to in the past by her doctor. By the time she stepped out of the shower, however, she said, "I had already convinced myself it wasn't really there." Phyllis could describe the first few weeks with only one word: "scary." In the days and weeks that followed, she explained that her thoughts went "back and forth." She would alternate between acceptance and denial. She found comfort in "putting it off." She shared, "It was easier to convince myself I was too busy to have it checked anyway." Her thoughts were centered on her family and their current financial situation. She shared that she always felt that the majority of her concerns were financial. She stated "I knew I had insurance, but I didn't figure it was good enough to cover something like this."

Phyllis admits that she endured this alone. She did not share the knowledge of the lump with anyone, not even her husband. She said, "I didn't want to worry him for no reason. It just seemed better to wait." During this time period, she had many conversations with herself. This usually occurred during the rare time that she was alone and not overwhelmed with other commitments. She shared that it was easy to stay distracted and ignore the lump due to her hectic schedule. When she was dressing or in the shower, she was always reminded. At that time, she says she often thought "What if?" She stated, "I was so scared that it would be what I now know it is." When asked directly about how it felt to face the unknown and unfamiliar, she became tearful after a brief pause. She stated, "I haven't talked about it like this in a little while. It's hard to talk about. It's hard."

On many occasions, Phyllis mentioned what she held dear and how important it was to maintain that stability throughout the entire process. She shared that her biggest initial concern was to "uproot the family" and incur unexpected costs. Even after she had agreed to seek medical evaluation, she says that she waited to tell her husband until merely days before the biopsy. She said "I knew he would just worry and he had so much going on at work." She did not inform her son until just before the first round of chemotherapy and only because she feared losing her hair would "frighten him."

At the conclusion of the interview, Phyllis was asked one final question. I asked her, in the context of what had been discussed, could she relate to the thought of "sheltering-in-place?" She paused for a moment and then responded:

> When I hear that, I think of preparation. Preparing to fight, maybe? I don't know. I guess that's what I was doing. I guess that's what we all do. We prepare in any way that we know how to face whatever is threatening us or our family. Yeah. I guess I can relate to that.

### MINISAGA

Long after the first time it was felt, she convinced herself that it was not really there. Fearing the worst, and unsure of the consequences, she delayed evaluation for over 9 months. Preserving personal and family normalcy was her only known response to the lump.

## ■ CORE QUALITIES AND CONCEPT CLARIFICATION

Throughout the concept development process, core qualities will emerge and must subsequently be defined. The process should reveal two to four core qualities. Each core quality should be supported in previously identified literature. These core qualities ground the concept in nursing science. The link between these core qualities, or the definition, will explain the relationship and provide the reader with clarification of the conceptually and empirically supported concept.

### Core Qualities

#### PROTECTING SELF

Protecting self represents any act or effort toward self-protection for an individual or family. A person's choice regarding the manner in which to self-protect is based on each individual's rationalization of the best available option. Based on family and personal history and current circumstances, each person arrives at a unique decision. Women make a deliberate choice of avoidance (Nonzee et al., 2015). This decision is different from denial because it is an active choice made after at least some acknowledgment of risk.

In the literature, there are multiple definitions to the concept of protecting self. Hilton, Crawford, and Tarko (2000) identified an individual's attempt at being positive and continuation of regular routines as an act of self-protection. Logan, Hackbusch-Pinto, and DeGrasse (2006) identified physical withdrawal and the construction of an emotional barrier as another strategy to protect self. Schmid-Buchi, Halfens, Dassen, and van der Borne (2008) described the process as to "keep life going" (p. 2906).

## UNCERTAINTY

Uncertainty is the inability of an individual to assign meaning to illness-related events (Mishel, 1988). Uncertainty creates doubt in the person's mind about which response is the correct response to a threat. Women often wonder if the risk is great enough to alter their routine and disrupt family processes. This presents a situation during which many difficult decisions must be made. The felt threat impacts multiple areas of one's life regarding health consequences, financial ramifications, and other areas of concern specific to each individual.

There is an abundance of literature on uncertainty and many specific to breast cancer. Uncertainty can be defined as a stressor in acute and chronic illness (Brashers et al., 2003), a lack of certainty about long-term future (Shaha, Cox, Talman, & Kelly, 2008), a need for information (Demir, Donmez, Ozsaker, & Diramali, 2008; Drageset, Lindstrom, Giske, & Underlid, 2011), or a cognitive state in which a person is unable to determine the meaning of illness-related events (Hall, Mishel, & Germino, 2014; Miller, 2012; Mishel, 1988; Montgomery, 2010; Wonghongkul, Dechaprom, Phumivichuvate, & Losawatkul, 2006). Wonghongkul et al. (2006) further describe uncertainty as a mismatch between an individual's expectations and the real world.

## NORMALCY

Normalcy is that which provides a sense of normal and comfort. The manner in which each individual defines normalcy is specific and individualized. A strong desire to preserve this sense of normalcy can result in difficult choices with unknown and unexpected outcomes. In the literature, the term normalcy was defined in multiple ways. There were references to normal, normalcy, and normality. According to one study, normalcy is "looking normal, being able to fulfil everyday activities, adapting to a new normal, and not being ill" (Denford, Harcourt, Rubin, & Pusic, 2011, p. 555). Hilton, Crawford, and Tarko (2000) also include maintenance of normal routines as important to individuals facing breast cancer and chemotherapy. Strickland, Wells, and Porr (2015) identified an effort to reduce "disruption to family life" and "maintaining routines" (p. 537).

Initially in the concept development process, I was confident that the three core qualities best suited to relay meaning to this phenomenon were protecting self, uncertainty, and familiarity. In the beginning, I thought that women were preserving familiarity within their lives. However, upon review of the literature, it became obvious that the concept of familiarity was not well studied nor well understood. However, the concept of normalcy was identified often throughout the literature and was well-documented in my population of interest. From this, I learned that assigning meaning without support of the literature only shares my own perceptions and definition of the phenomenon, but does not empirically ground the concept in existing science. As intended,

I allowed the 10-step process to guide me and I quickly realized that the core quality should be normalcy rather than familiarity.

## Concept Definition

Forming a definition that explains the relationship between the core qualities is extremely important to the concept building process. The definition should contain the concept name and the identified core qualities. Careful consideration should be placed on the order of the core qualities as wording in the definition could imply an unintended relationship. For this concept, the definition is as follows: Sheltering-in-place is protecting self in the face of uncertainty in order to preserve normalcy. Climbing the ladder of abstraction from theoretical underpinnings, the concept definition describes the process of moral reckoning that is occurring in the lives of these individuals.

## ■ MODEL: VISUAL REPRESENTATION OF THE RELATIONSHIP BETWEEN CORE QUALITIES

After definition development, a visual and structural depiction of the association between the concept and the core qualities is created. The model displays an easily followed structure that depicts the concept definition. The model for the concept sheltering-in-place can be found in Figure 19.1.

The structure of the model was developed with careful thought on the core qualities and the relationship between them. In the concept sheltering-in-place, preserving normalcy is the ultimate goal for most women. In this phenomenon, all steps taken by the individual are completed with the goal of maintaining normalcy in their lives. Because of this, it was determined that normalcy should be placed on the highest level of this visual model. The qualities of

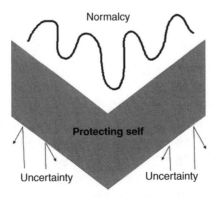

**FIGURE 19.1** Model of Sheltering-in-Place.

protecting self and normalcy have a fluid relationship. This is depicted in the model with a curved line between the two core qualities. The "self" that is being preserved consists of qualities and behaviors that the individual identifies as normal. However, the distinguishing factor between self and normalcy is that protecting self is an action that the individual performs. This action of protecting self provides a barrier in order to prevent uncertainty from impacting the woman's definition of normalcy. This is pictured by a thick line, which deflects uncertainty. If the barrier of protecting self was not present, the threat of uncertainty would impact normalcy.

The charge of clearly demonstrating a multidimensional, multifaceted phenomenon in a two-dimensional manner was challenging. Multiple drafts of this chapter, and gaining a better understanding of the concept development process and my own concept, allowed for an improved model with each edit. It is doubtful that the model shared in this chapter will be the final model. It is also helpful to share the model with colleagues to receive constructive criticism about what an unbiased reader perceives from the model. For classroom instruction, model development is a good group activity. This allows for brainstorming and consistent feedback during the early stage of development.

## ■ MINISYNTHESIS

The minisynthesis is a three-sentence representation of the concept building process as it relates to the phenomenon. Each sentence in the minisynthesis has a specific purpose. The first sentence serves to explain the significance of the phenomenon in the context of the population in question. The second sentence defines the working concept as it is developing. The third sentence provides suggestion for further development toward a research question. Example: Women significantly delay medical evaluation upon self-identifying breast abnormalities. Sheltering-in-place is protecting self in the face of uncertainty in order to preserve normalcy. A qualitative study exploring this phenomenon may provide insight into the lived experience of protecting self.

## ■ CONCLUSION

Concept development is a time-intensive process through which the phenomenon, identified in practice, is lifted up the ladder of abstraction in order to analyze from a scholarly perspective. Analysis is completed in order to better understand the human health experience of those living the situation, but also to better understand ways in which research may impact and ultimately improve patient outcomes. Viewing a concept from empirical, theoretical, and philosophical perspectives ensures both tacit and explicit understanding of a concept.

Induction from an empirical to a theoretical understanding is of paramount importance for successful concept building. The theory provides the meaning through which the concept and its core qualities are understood. Theory selection takes careful consideration and consists of much thought in order to find the theory that "fits like a glove" into the required niche.

Gaining insight into the concept from a person with the lived experience ensures that the concept is validated through an individual who understands the core qualities on a personal level. This ensures that the foundation of the concept is directed by true experiences and not an outside perception of the experience. In this way, word choice and definitions are carefully extracted from the individual's answers to carefully and simply stated questions. Further transitioning this story to a minisaga, and subsequently a minisynthesis, allows for a succinct explanation of the concept and core qualities from the perspective of the storyteller. This story must then be identified in the available literature to support the concept and core qualities. The literature roots the phenomenon empirically in science.

The concept sheltering-in-place is applicable to a population of women making a choice in response to a threat to preserve normalcy in their lives, even though the choice could result in poor outcomes. When faced with uncertainty in the form of a breast abnormality, these women must make a choice about what is best for them and their families. The risk is weighed and, often, a choice is made to delay treatment.

When viewing this phenomenon through the perspective of the Moral Reckoning Theory, one can better understand the difficult situation in which these women find themselves. The theory provides an avenue for relatability and understanding. With the state of ease disrupted, a choice is made to protect self in the face of uncertainty and without a thorough understanding of the long-term consequences. The theory explains that after these decisions, the person will ultimately resolve the threat and reflect on this time period of their life.

With a thorough grasp of the concept as defined, and viewed through the lens of the Moral Reckoning Theory, generalizability to other situations and demographics may be made. While the literature supports the obstacle of uncertainty related to breast cancer, research based on the concept as defined may offer a fresh look at sheltering-in-place.

## ■ REFERENCES

Brashers, D., Neidig, J., Russell, J., Cardillo, L., Haas, S., Dobbs, L., & Nemeth, S. (2003). The medical, personal, and social causes of uncertainty in HIV illness. *Issues in Mental Health Nursing*, 24(5), 497–522.

Clutton, S., Buckley, B., & Pakenham, K. (1999). Predictors of emotional well-being following a false positive breast cancer screening result. *Psychology and Health*, 14(2), 263. Retrieved from http://linkinghub.elsevier.com/retrieve/pii/S0022399901002276

Demir, F., Donmez, Y., Ozsaker, E., & Diramali, A. (2008). Patients' lived experiences of excisional breast biopsy: A phenomenological study. *Journal of Clinical Nursing*, *17*(6), 744–751. doi:10.1111/j.1365 -2702.2007.02116.x

Denford, S., Harcourt, D., Rubin, L., & Pusic, A. (2011). Understanding normality: A qualitative analysis of breast cancer patients' concepts of normality after mastectomy and reconstructive surgery. *Psycho-Oncology*, *20*(5), 553–558.

Drageset, S., Lindstrom, T., Giske, T., & Underlid, K. (2011). Being in suspense: Women's experiences awaiting breast cancer surgery. *Journal of Advanced Nursing*, *67*(9), 1941–1951. doi:10.1111/j.1365-2648.2011.05638.x

Hall, D., Mishel, M., & Germino, B. (2014). Living with cancer-related uncertainty: Associations with fatigue, insomnia, and affect in younger breast cancer survivors. *Supportive Care in Cancer: Official Journal of the Multinational Association of Supportive Care in Cancer*, *22*(9), 2489–2495. doi:10.1007/ s00520-014-2243-y

Hilton, B., Crawford, J., & Tarko, M. (2000). Men's perspectives on individual and family coping with their wives' breast cancer and chemotherapy. *Western Journal of Nursing Research*, *22*(4), 438–459.

Howard, A., Balneaves, L., Bottorff, J., & Rodney, P. (2011). Preserving the self: The process of decision making about hereditary breast cancer and ovarian cancer risk reduction. *Qualitative Health Research*, *21*(4), 502–519.

Lebel, S., Jakubovits, G., Rosberger, Z., Loiselle, C., Seguin, C., Cornaz, C., . . . Lisbona, A. (2003). Waiting for a breast biopsy: Psychosocial consequences and coping strategies. *Journal of Psychosomatic Research*, *55*(5), 437. Retrieved from http://linkinghub.elsevier.com/retrieve/pii/S0022399903005129

Liao, M., Chen, M., Chen, S., & Chen, P. (2008). Uncertainty and anxiety during the diagnostic period for women with suspected breast cancer. *Cancer Nursing*, *31*(4), 274–283.

Liehr, P., & Smith, M. (2014). Concept building for research. In M. Smith & P. Liehr (Eds.), *Middle range theory for nursing* (3rd ed., pp. 349–360). New York, NY: Springer Publishing.

Logan, J., Hackbusch-Pinto, R., & De Grasse, C. (2006). Women undergoing breast diagnostics: The lived experience of spirituality. *Oncology Nursing Forum*, *33*(1), 121–126. doi:10.1188/06.ONF.121-126

Miller, L. (2012). Sources of uncertainty in cancer survivorship. *Journal of Cancer Survivorship*, *6*(4), 431–440. doi:10.1007/s11764-012-0229-7

Mishel, M. (1988). Uncertainty in illness. *Journal of Nursing Scholarship*, *20*(4), 225–232.

Montgomery, M. (2010). Uncertainty during breast diagnostic evaluation: State of the science. *Oncology Nursing Forum*, *37*(1), 77–83.

Nathaniel, A. (2003). *A grounded theory of moral reckoning in nursing* (Doctoral dissertation). West Virginia University, Morgantown, WV.

Newman, M., Sime, A., & Corcoran-Perry, S. (1991). The focus of the discipline of nursing. *Advances in Nursing Science*, *14*(1), 1–6. Retrieved from http:// journals.lww.com/advancesinnursingscience/Citation/1991/09000/ The_focus_of_the_discipline_of_nursing_.2.aspx

Nonzee, N., Ragas, D., Ha Luu, T., Phisuthikul, A., Tom, L., Dong, X., & Simon, M. (2015). Delays in cancer care among low-income minorities despite access. *Journal of Women's Health*, 24(6), 506–514.

Pink, D. (2005). *A whole new mind: Moving from the information age to the conceptual age.* New York, NY: Penguin Group.

Schmid-Büchi, S., Halfens, R. J., Dassen, T., & Van Den Borne, B. (2008). A review of psychosocial needs of breast-cancer patients and their relatives. *Journal of Clinical Nursing*, 17(21), 2895–2909.

SEER. (2012). *Cancer stat facts: Female breast cancer.* Retrieved from https://seer.cancer.gov/statfacts/html/breast.html

Strickland, J., Wells, C., & Porr, C. (2015). Safeguarding the children: The cancer journey of young mothers. *Oncology Nursing Forum*, 42(5), 534–541.

Shaha, M., Cox, C. L., Talman, K., & Kelly, D. (2008). Uncertainty in breast, prostate, and colorectal cancer: Implications for supportive care. *Journal of Nursing Scholarship*, 40(1), 60–67.

Wonghongkul, T., Dechaprom, N., Phumivichuvate, L., & Losawatkul, S. (2006). Uncertainty appraisal coping and quality of life in breast cancer survivors. *Cancer Nursing*, 29(3), 250–257.

# CHAPTER 20

## Yearning for Sleep While Enduring Distress: From Concept Building to Research Proposal Development

**April L. Shapiro**

The purpose of this chapter is to discuss the progression of a phenomenon from the concept building stage through research proposal development. Employing a rigorous process and continued study, my initial concept, Yearning for Sleep While Enduring Distress (Shapiro, 2014), led to testing an intervention for dissertation study, entitled *Effect of the CPAP-SAVER Intervention on Adherence Among Adults With Newly Diagnosed Obstructive Sleep Apnea* (Shapiro, 2017). The evolution of a sleep-related concept to an intervention study is described.

## ■ REVIEW OF THE CONCEPT BUILDING PROCESS

Building the concept for research, Yearning for Sleep While Enduring Distress (Shapiro, 2014), involved an iterative, reflective process and was guided by the 10 phases proposed by Liehr and Smith (2008). The concept development process was detailed in the previous edition of this book (M. J. Smith & Liehr, 2014) and is summarized here for the reader. The first step involved writing a practice story about Mark and his daily struggles with obstructive sleep apnea (OSA) to capture the phenomenon in a practice situation and to begin to name the phenomenon. Examining the phenomenon through a theoretical lens, the Symptom Management Theory (Dodd et al., 2001; Humphreys et al., 2008), established a conceptual link to ground the concept in nursing theory. Exploring the concept in the existing knowledge base through development of a literature matrix (Garrard, 2011) served to ground the concept in nursing science. A reconstructed story and minisaga about Jenny's chronic problems with insomnia clarified the concept and the theoretical perspective, provided empirical evidence, and crystallized the essence of the Yearning for Sleep While Enduring Distress concept. Subsequently, three core qualities were identified that defined the concept of Yearning for Sleep While Enduring Distress; these qualities—suffering, longing, and comfort—were defined and modeled

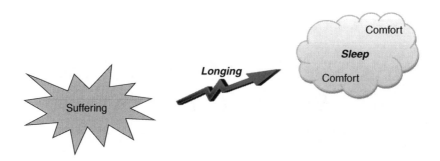

**FIGURE 20.1** Model of Yearning for Sleep While Enduring Distress.

Yearning for sleep while enduring distress is. . . *Suffering yet longing for comfort (in the form of sleep).*

for visual representation (Figure 20.1). The last phase of the concept building process, the minisynthesis, highlighted the impact of sleep disturbances for persons who are OSA sufferers. The process of building the research concept, Yearning for Sleep While Enduring Distress, and its outcomes provided the foundation for the dissertation study.

## ■ PROGRESSION FROM CONCEPT BUILDING TO RESEARCH PROPOSAL DEVELOPMENT

Upon development of the concept, I took further steps to transition the concept into a proposal for research. First, I examined the literature related to the adult population with OSA who were prescribed with continuous positive airway pressure therapy (CPAP) and found that difficulty adhering to the treatment was a common problem for many people. To further understand the problem, I observed four persons with OSA during in-lab sleep studies over two nights and followed them through the OSA–CPAP trajectory from diagnosis to treatment. I also conducted a small focus group to identify CPAP problems with adherence among middle-aged and older men with OSA (Shapiro & McCrone, 2017).

In addition, I had discussions with my dissertation chairperson and committee members and made contacts with individuals who were involved in nursing and sleep-related research. I made email contact with sleep researchers, CPAP-related instrument developers, and intervention-related theorists. These discussions and contacts guided me in establishing the foundation for the theory-based CPAP adherence intervention. I began to make connections between the research already completed in the area of CPAP adherence science and the gaps in knowledge. I developed an intervention, named CPAP-SAVER, and tested it in an adult sample.

The CPAP-SAVER intervention components were:

| | | |
|---|---|---|
| **S** | Support calls | Supportive calls made at midweek one and midweek two |
| **A** | Airway model | Demonstration of the OSA airway–brain mechanism |
| **V** | Video | Reinforcement of the OSA airway–brain mechanism using *How CPAP Works* |
| **E** | Education sheet | Education about OSA risks and CPAP benefits using *The Risks of Obstructive Sleep Apnea & the Benefits of CPAP* sheet |
| **R** | Report card | Documentation of the OSA–CPAP progress |

# ■ EXEMPLAR PROPOSAL

## Introduction

OSA is the most common form of sleep-disordered breathing, affecting at least 25 million adults in the United States (American Academy of Sleep Medicine, 2014). The gold standard treatment for OSA is CPAP (Epstein et al., 2009; Qaseem et al., 2013; Rakel, 2009); however, CPAP adherence is poor (Aloia, Arnedt, Riggs, Hecht, & Borrelli, 2004; Olsen, Smith, & Oei, 2008), with rates varying from 30% to 60% (Weaver & Sawyer, 2010). In addition, about 25% of all users discontinue CPAP use within the first year; those who continue to use CPAP do so inconsistently and/or improperly (Aloia et al., 2004; Olsen et al., 2008). To compound the problem, night-to-night variability is high among CPAP users, with early patterns of use predicting long-term adherence patterns (Aloia, Arnedt, Stanchina, & Millman, 2007; Budhiraja et al., 2007; Gay, Weaver, Loube, & Iber, 2006). Poor CPAP adherence impacts morbidity, mortality, and quality of life among those with OSA. Previous CPAP adherence interventions tended to focus on CPAP use, typically were not theory based, and tended to involve lengthy, costly behavioral and/or cognitive therapy sessions. A theory-based, multidimensional, time- and cost-effective CPAP adherence nursing intervention was warranted.

Addressing CPAP adherence issues may result in improved patient health outcomes. It has been noted that adherence may have a greater impact on health than improvements in specific medical treatments; thus, healthcare professionals should be trained in issues regarding adherence and deliver interventions to optimize it (Sabate, 2003). Improved CPAP adherence may have implications for improved morbidity, decreased mortality, decreased healthcare burden, and decreased healthcare costs, as well as improved quality of life for adults with OSA. Improved CPAP adherence and subsequent OSA management may impact other chronic diseases, especially those affecting the cardiovascular, cerebrovascular, neurological, and endocrine systems, since OSA has been shown to be an independent risk factor for these morbidities (Park, Ramar, & Olson, 2011). In addition, management of these comorbidities may improve with CPAP adherence and result in enhanced quality of life for adults with OSA.

## Theoretical Framework

The overall purpose of this study was to determine the effect of a theory-based, multidimensional, time- and cost-effective nursing intervention, referred to as CPAP-SAVER, on 1-month CPAP adherence in a sample of adults (aged 18 or older) with newly diagnosed OSA receiving CPAP treatment for the first time (CPAP naïve). The CPAP-SAVER intervention was based on the constructs of the Theory of Planned Behavior (TPB; Ajzen, 1985, 1991, 2005, 2011). The theory postulates that personal (attitude), social (subjective norm), and internal/environmental (perceived behavioral control) factors guide the process of behavioral intention and eventual action (Ajzen, 2011). The proposed CPAP-SAVER intervention was designed to: (a) promote a favorable CPAP attitude by educating the intervention participants about the OSA airway–brain mechanism and OSA risks–CPAP benefits through the use of an airway model, video, and education sheet; (b) promote a favorable subjective norm regarding CPAP adherence by providing support telephone calls; and (c) improve perceived behavioral control (perceived controllability and self-efficacy) by implementing an OSA–CPAP report card. Most of the CPAP-SAVER intervention was initiated within the first week of the participant's CPAP use, a critical time for CPAP users. The first week of CPAP therapy is a critical time for users because adherence patterns are reported to be established within this time frame (Gay et al., 2006); in fact, a stable pattern of first-week CPAP use has been shown to be predictive of longer term CPAP adherence, as far out as 6 months (Aloia et al., 2007; Budhiraja et al., 2007). In addition, a successful CPAP intervention should consider the typologies of adherers and nonadherers (Sawyer, Deatrick, Kuna, & Weaver, 2010), as well as behavior change techniques (Abraham & Michie, 2008). The CPAP-SAVER intervention study was designed around these concepts, with the intent to advance nursing science in the area of CPAP adherence intention and CPAP adherence behavior among adults with OSA.

## Research Questions

The research questions guiding the study were:

1. What is the effect of the CPAP-SAVER intervention (compared to standard care) on 1-month CPAP adherence behavior? It was hypothesized that the CPAP-SAVER intervention group will demonstrate higher 1-month CPAP adherence behavior rates than the standard care (control) group.

2. What is the effect of the CPAP-SAVER intervention on anxiety as a background factor? It was hypothesized that the CPAP-SAVER

intervention group will demonstrate a decrease in anxiety scores over time compared to the standard care (control) group.

3.  What is the effect of the CPAP-SAVER intervention on CPAP adherence beliefs? It was hypothesized that the CPAP-SAVER intervention group will demonstrate an increase in CPAP adherence belief scores over time compared to the standard care (control) group.

4.  What is the effect of the CPAP-SAVER intervention on CPAP adherence attitude? It was hypothesized that the CPAP-SAVER intervention group will demonstrate an increase in CPAP adherence attitude scores over time compared to the standard care (control) group.

5.  What is the effect of the CPAP-SAVER intervention on CPAP adherence subjective norm? It was hypothesized that the CPAP-SAVER intervention group will demonstrate an increase in CPAP adherence subjective norm scores over time compared to the standard care (control) group.

6.  What was the effect of the CPAP-SAVER intervention on CPAP adherence perceived behavioral control? It is hypothesized that the CPAP-SAVER intervention group will demonstrate an increase in CPAP adherence perceived behavioral control scores over time compared to the standard care (control) group.

7.  What is the effect of the CPAP-SAVER intervention on CPAP adherence intention? It was hypothesized that the CPAP-SAVER intervention group will demonstrate an increase in CPAP adherence intention scores over time compared to the standard care (control) group.

8.  Are 1-month CPAP adherence attitude, CPAP adherence subjective norm, and/or CPAP adherence perceived behavioral control predictive of 1-month CPAP adherence intention? It was hypothesized that 1-month CPAP adherence attitude, CPAP adherence subjective norm, and CPAP adherence perceived behavioral control will be predictive of 1-month CPAP adherence intention.

9.  Is 1-month CPAP adherence intention predictive of 1-month CPAP adherence behavior? It was hypothesized that 1-month CPAP adherence intention will be predictive of 1-month CPAP adherence behavior.

## Method

### DESIGN

The CPAP-SAVER intervention study used a randomized controlled trial (RCT) design. This type of design was suitable for testing the effect of an intervention

(Polit & Beck, 2012), such as the CPAP-SAVER, and examining relationships among variables, including the TPB constructs, CPAP adherence intention, and CPAP adherence behavior. There was random assignment of subjects to either the intervention or standard care group. In this design, there was no random selection of a sample; a convenience sample was enrolled in the study.

### POPULATION, RECRUITMENT, AND SETTING

Based on G*Power 3.1 (Faul, Erdfelder, Lang, & Buchner, 2007) a priori power analysis results, a convenience sample of 66 adults (aged 18 and over) newly diagnosed with OSA and prescribed CPAP for the first time (CPAP naïve) was recruited from two home medical supply facility customer lists over 10 months. Flyers, posters, and word of mouth were strategies used for recruitment. The flyers and posters included information about the study's purpose, inclusion/exclusion criteria, and voluntary nature.

Inclusion and exclusion criteria guided the recruitment and delimitation of the accessible population of participants.

Inclusion criteria:

- Age 18 or older
- Able to read, understand, write, and speak English
- Newly diagnosed with OSA by overnight, in-lab polysomnogram
- Commencing OSA treatment for the first time
- Prescribed CPAP for OSA treatment
- Using a CPAP machine with smart card technology
- Using one of the home medical supply facilities participating in the study
- Provided informed consent

Exclusion criteria:

- Requires bilevel ventilation
- Has significant craniofacial abnormalities
- Diagnosed with Down syndrome
- Diagnosed with a cognitive delay
- Diagnosed with hypotonia
- Diagnosed with a neuromuscular degenerative disorder
- Taking medication for anxiety
- Pregnant

Upon informed consent, participants were randomly assigned to either the intervention ($n = 33$) or control ($n = 33$) group, and were masked as to group assignment.

### INTERVENTION

The intervention group received the CPAP-SAVER intervention in addition to standard care; the control group received standard care only. In this study, the intervention components were implemented by three respiratory therapist research assistants in the home medical supply facilities and a single nurse investigator. Each component was scripted, printed, and compiled into the *CPAP-SAVER Intervention Protocol Training Manual*.

The total amount of time it took to implement the 1-month CPAP-SAVER intervention was approximately 22 minutes per intervention participant. Of the 22 minutes, 12 of the minutes were added to the research assistant's time with the participant (airway model/video/education sheet time and report card initiation and maintenance) and 10 of the minutes were nurse (investigator) time with the participant (two telephone calls focused on support and review of the report card). The order of the components was based on educational principles, the intervention protocol, and standard care provision.

## STANDARD CARE

Standard care was operationalized in the study as a control group. Standard care was defined as the usual, basic OSA–CPAP teaching and follow-up provided by the respiratory therapist employed by the home medical supplier. Standard care focused on CPAP machine setup, use, and maintenance; resolving side effects; machine problem solving/technical issues; and CPAP adjustments based on smart card readings.

## INSTRUMENTS

After consent, data were collected from participants using a demographic survey; the Beck Anxiety Inventory (BAI; Beck & Steer, 1993); the Apnea Beliefs Scale (ABS; S. Smith, Lang, Sullivan, & Warren, 2004); TPB questionnaires (Francis et al., 2004) tailored to measure the constructs of CPAP adherence attitude, CPAP adherence subjective norm, CPAP adherence perceived behavioral control, and CPAP adherence intention; the sleep study report; and CPAP smart card readings for CPAP adherence behavior.

**Beck Anxiety Inventory.** Anxiety (as a background factor) was measured using the BAI (Beck & Steer, 1993). The instrument was composed of 21 items (symptoms) on which participants rated themselves on their experience over the past 2 weeks on items such as *unable to relax* and *fear of the worst happening*, using a Likert scale from 0 (not at all) to 3 (severely—I could barely stand it). The total score ranged from 0 to 63 and was interpreted as: 0 to 7—minimal anxiety, 8 to 15—mild anxiety, 16 to 25—moderate anxiety, and 26 to 63—severe anxiety. In initial testing of the instrument ($N = 1,086$), the inventory demonstrated high internal consistency (coefficient alpha of .92) and 1-week test–retest reliability (0.75). In a sample of OSA patients ($N = 303$), Cronbach's alpha levels of .92, .91, and .92 for the total sample, men, and women, respectively, were reported (Sanford, Bush, Stone, Lichstein, & Aguillard, 2008). The BAI was written at the fifth-grade reading level, took about 10 minutes to complete and about 10 minutes to score manually, and was used in paper format. The cost for the scoring manual and 25 forms was $128, and $56.40 for each additional 25 forms (purchased through Pearson's Assessments).

**Apnea Beliefs Scale.** The ABS (S. Smith et al., 2004) is a scale composed of 24 items designed to assess OSA–CPAP-related beliefs related to perceived impact of OSA, trust in medical staff, outcome expectations, CPAP acceptance, openness to new experiences, commitment to change, willingness to ask for help, attitude toward health, and self-confidence. Participants completing the instrument rated themselves on items, such as *Sleep apnea has no effect on my life* and *If things become too much I generally don't go through with them*, using a Likert scale from 1 (strongly disagree) to 5 (strongly agree); 10 of the items were negatively worded and were reverse-coded upon scoring. The total ABS score ranged from 24 to 120, with higher scores indicating more positive attitude and beliefs toward CPAP adherence (S. Smith et al., 2004). In initial testing of the instrument in a sleep apnea sample ($N = 81$), the scale demonstrated moderate internal consistency (coefficient alpha of .75) and validity in clinical and nonclinical samples ($t[41.79] = 6.43, p < .01$; S. Smith et al., 2004). In a subsequent intervention study testing psychological variables as predictors of CPAP adherence in a sample of adults with OSA ($N = 120$), discriminant validity was evident; participants with maladaptive beliefs (total ABS score less than 84.5) were 2.21 times more likely to be nonadherent to CPAP (CI: 1.03–4.72, $p = .04$), differentiating adherers from nonadherers (Poulet et al., 2009). The ABS was written at the sixth-grade reading level (S. Smith et al., 2004), took about 10 minutes to complete and about 10 minutes to score manually, and was used in paper format. There was no cost to use the instrument.

**Theory of Planned Behavior Questionnaires.** The TPB-based questionnaires to measure attitude, subjective norm, perceived behavioral control, and intention were tailored to measure these constructs in this OSA–CPAP sample from recommendations provided by Francis et al. (2004). For each construct, direct-measure questions were used to ask participants to rate themselves on seven-point, bipolar adjective scales. To collect the total score for each construct, the negatively worded adjectives were reverse-coded and the mean of the item scores calculated to determine the overall score. The mean score was interpreted as the higher the mean, the more positive the construct toward intention/behavior. No permission was needed and no costs were involved to use the questionnaires. The instrument was written at the seventh-grade reading level, took about 10 minutes to complete and about 10 minutes to score manually, and was used in paper format.

Although the direct-measure questions for attitude, subjective norm, perceived behavioral control, and intention have not been tested in the OSA–CPAP population, they have demonstrated adequate reliability and validity in other samples. In a study of a TPB-based intervention designed to promote healthy eating and physical activity in older adults with type 2 diabetes or cardiovascular disease (White et al., 2012; $N = 183$), the direct-measure attitude questions yielded Cronbach's alphas of .81 to .89. Internal consistency for direct-measure subjective norm questions was reported between .67 in a study to predict postanterior cruciate ligament rehabilitation intention among 87 athletes (Niven, Nevill, Sayers, & Cullen, 2012) to .85 in a study to predict the maintenance of physical activity among 94 people enrolled in a gym for the first time (Armitage, 2005). In an intervention study designed to promote fruit and vegetable intake among undergraduate college students in a first-year psychology course ($N = 194$), Kothe, Mullan, and Butow (2012) reported a Cronbach's alpha of .72 for the direct-measure perceived behavioral control questionnaire, with similar results (Cronbach's alpha = .71) reported in a pilot intervention study designed to increase chlamydia testing among college students living in deprived areas ($N = 253$; Booth, Norman, Goyder, Harris, & Campbell, 2014). Internal consistency for the direct-measure intention scale was reported between .63 in a study to predict postanterior cruciate ligament rehabilitation intention among 87 athletes (Niven et al., 2012) and .72 in a study to predict treatment adherence among 117 South Africans living with diabetes and hypertension (Kagee & Merwe, 2006). Other studies have reported similar numbers for these direct-measure questions.

**OSA Severity, CPAP Setup, and CPAP Use/Adherence.** Initial OSA severity data (apnea–hypopnea index [AHI] and oxygen saturation nadir) were collected from the sleep study report; subsequent OSA severity and CPAP use/adherence data (including AHI and mask-on time) were collected from the CPAP machine's smart card. AHI and mask-on time were the two data points that were collected from the smart card to be recorded on the intervention report card. AHI was measured as the average number of events per hour, and was categorized as: 5 to 15 = mild, over 15 to 30 = moderate, and over 30 = severe (American Academy of Sleep Medicine, 2008). Mask-on time indicated adherence or not; adherence was defined as mask-on time at the prescribed pressure for at least 4 hours per night for 70% of the nights (Centers for Medicare and Medicaid Services, 2013; for week one: 7 × 70% = five nights; for month one: 30 × 70% = 21 nights). CPAP machine humidification and pressure settings, as well as the type of mask the participant was wearing (full, nasal, or nasal pillows), were also noted.

## DATA COLLECTION AND ANALYSIS

As data were collected, it was entered twice into the Double Data Entry Spreadsheet (DeCoster & Iselin, 2006) and then checked for errors; the researcher referred to the source data to resolve errors. Data were imported into and analyzed using Statistical Package for the Social Sciences (SPSS), version 24 (IBM, 2016). Alpha was set at .05 for all analyses. The SPSS Survival Manual (Pallant, 2016) was used as an instructional guide for the statistical analyses. Assumptions testing was performed, as appropriate (homogeneity of intercorrelations, homogeneity of variance, multicollinearity, singularity, outliers, normality, linearity, homoscedasticity, and independence of residuals). Univariate analyses (frequencies and descriptives) were conducted on all variables at baseline for the entire sample. Univariate analyses (frequencies and descriptives) were conducted on all variables at baseline for participants by group (intervention and control) to determine homogeneity of the groups.

### FIDELITY, RIGOR, AND HUMAN RIGHTS

Training of the research assistants was conducted in initial and booster sessions, using the *CPAP-SAVER Intervention Protocol Training Manual*. Fidelity checks were commenced after two participants had been enrolled at a site and were completed monthly, following the *CPAP-SAVER Intervention Fidelity Checklist*. Upon completion of the study (at 1 month), the researcher evaluated each intervention participant's perception of the intervention using an Intervention Effectiveness Survey.

A priori power analysis, randomization, intervention fidelity checks, and reliable instrumentation were implemented to enhance the CPAP-SAVER intervention study rigor. A priori power analysis was conducted with G*Power 3.1 (Faul et al., 2007). Participants were randomized to either the intervention or control group to improve the chance of homogeneous groups and equally distributed potential confounding variables. The investigator conducted extensive training and booster sessions with the research assistants, and supplemented the training with the use of a protocol manual and monthly fidelity checks.

The Belmont Report Principles (National Commission for the Protection of Human Subjects of Biomedical and Behavioral Research, 1979), including respect for persons, beneficence, and justice, were upheld throughout the study. Before data collection began, institutional review board approval was obtained. Each research assistant completed research ethics training as per the Collaborative Institutional Training Initiative (CITI) protocol; the investigator was current with CITI training. Privacy, confidentiality, and anonymity were maintained. Participants were reminded that they could withdraw from the study at any time without any recourse or effect on their CPAP treatment. If a study participant expressed any physical or emotional distress related to the study or demonstrated a moderate-to-severe anxiety level (BAI score of 16–63), the investigator referred the participant to his or her primary care provider.

# ■ EVALUATION OF THE STRUCTURE BUILDING PROCESS FOR PROPOSAL DEVELOPMENT

From personal and professional experiences with patients, the concept of *Yearning for Sleep While Enduring Distress* (Shapiro, 2014) evolved. My experiences and the concept building process served as the impetus for further doctoral study and catalyzed development of my dissertation proposal. The 10-phase structure building process (Liehr & Smith, 2008) has guided me in explicating meaning from human health experiences of individuals who face the challenge of sleep-disordered breathing. In essence, the process served as a road map to get me started on my research trajectory. As the phenomenon unfolded, every step of the process served as a critical juncture. However, I learned that the process could not be rushed—it involved much reflection, iteration, and time, and required both inductive and deductive reasoning. Having this guide was invaluable, especially for a novice scientist such as me.

Nursing's presence in OSA–CPAP research is critically needed. OSA affects millions of adults and is expected to become more prevalent in upcoming years. Even though CPAP is the gold standard treatment, adherence is poor; this presents a major problem with many health, research, and policy implications. Poorly or undertreated OSA (and the disordered sleep and breathing patterns that result) potentially leads to morbidity and mortality outcomes that subsequently impact quality of life (distress) and place burden on the healthcare system. I believe that further intervention study in this area, especially through a nursing lens, can impact patient outcomes. With the strong foundation provided by the structure building process, and testing and further work on the CPAP-SAVER intervention, I believe the intervention may provide groundwork for the eventual development of a clinical guideline for OSA–CPAP management. In addition, the CPAP-SAVER study may serve to highlight nursing's contribution to sleep implementation science. At this time, the dissertation study has been completed and findings are being compiled in a manuscript for publication.

# ■ REFERENCES

Abraham, C., & Michie, S. (2008). A taxonomy of behavior change techniques used in interventions. *Health Psychology, 27,* 379–387. doi:10.1037/0278-6133.27.3.379

Ajzen, I. (1985). From intentions to action: A theory of planned behavior. In J. Kuhl & J. Beckman (Eds.), *Action-control: From cognition to behavior* (pp. 11–39). Heidelberg, Germany: Springer.

Ajzen, I. (1991). The theory of planned behavior. *Organizational Behavior and Human Decision Processes, 50,* 179–211. doi:10.1016/0749-5978(91)90020-T

Ajzen, I. (2005). *Attitudes, personality and behavior* (2nd ed.). Maidenhead, UK: Open University Press.

Ajzen, I. (2011). Behavioral interventions: Design and evaluation guided by the Theory of Planned Behavior. In M. M. Mark, S. I. Donaldson, & B. Campbell (Eds.), *Social psychology and evaluation* (pp. 74–100). New York, NY: Guilford Press.

Aloia, M. S., Arnedt, J. T., Riggs, R. L., Hecht, J., & Borrelli, B. (2004). Clinical management of poor adherence to CPAP: Motivational enhancement. *Behavioral Sleep Medicine, 2*, 205–222. doi:10.1207/s15402010bsm0204_3

Aloia, M. S., Arnedt, J. T., Stanchina, M., & Millman, R. P. (2007). How early in treatment is PAP adherence established? Revisiting night-to-night variability. *Behavioral Sleep Medicine, 5*, 229–240. doi:10.1080/15402000701264005

American Academy of Sleep Medicine. (2008). *Obstructive sleep apnea*. Darien, IL: Author.

American Academy of Sleep Medicine. (2014). Rising prevalence of sleep apnea in U.S. threatens public health. Retrieved from http://www.aasmnet.org/articles .aspx?id=5043

Armitage, C. J. (2005). Can the theory of planned behavior predict the maintenance of physical activity? *Health Psychology, 24*, 235–245. doi:10.1037/0278-6133.24.3.235

Beck, A. T., & Steer, R. A. (1993). *Beck anxiety inventory* (1993 ed.). San Antonio, TX: The Psychological Corporation.

Booth, A. R., Norman, P., Goyder, E., Harris, P. R., & Campbell, M. J. (2014). Pilot study of a brief intervention based on the theory of planned behaviour and self-identity to increase chlamydia testing among young people living in deprived areas. *British Journal of Health Psychology, 19*, 636–651. doi:10.1111/bjhp.12065

Budhiraja, R., Parthasarathy, S., Drake, C. L., Roth, T., Sharief, I., Budhiraja, P., . . . Hudgel, D. W. (2007). Early CPAP use identifies subsequent adherence to CPAP therapy. *Sleep, 30*, 320–324.

Centers for Medicare and Medicaid Services. (2013). *Continuous and bi-level positive airway pressure (CPAP/BPAP) devices: Complying with documentation & coverage requirements*. Retrieved from http://www.cms.gov/Outreach-and-Education/ Medicare-Learning-Network-MLN/MLNProducts/downloads/PAP_DocCvg_ Factsheet_ICN905064.pdf

DeCoster, J., & Iselin, A.-M. (2006). *Double data entry* [Computer Software]. Charlottesville, VA: Author.

Dodd, M., Janson, S., Facione, N., Faucett, J., Froelicher, E. S., Humphreys, J., . . . Taylor, D. (2001). Advancing the science of symptom management. *Journal of Advanced Nursing, 33*(5), 668–676.

Epstein, L. J., Kristo, D., Strollo, P. J., Jr., Friedman, N., Malhotra, A., Patil, S. P., . . . Weinstein, M. D. (2009). Clinical guideline for the evaluation, management and long-term care of obstructive sleep apnea in adults. *Journal of Clinical Sleep Medicine, 5*, 263–276.

Faul, F., Erdfelder, E., Lang, A. G., & Buchner, A. (2007). G*Power 3: A flexible statistical power analysis program for the social, behavioral, and biomedical sciences. *Behavior Research Methods, 39*, 175–191.

Francis, J., Eccles, M. P., Johnston, M., Walker, A. E., Grimshaw, J. M., Foy, R., . . . Bonetti, D. (2004). *Constructing questionnaires based on the theory of planned behaviour: A manual for health services researchers.* Newcastle upon Tyne, UK: Centre for Health Services Research, University of Newcastle upon Tyne.

Garrard, J. (2011). *Health sciences literature review made easy: The matrix method* (3rd ed.). Sudbury, MA: Jones & Bartlett.

Gay, P., Weaver, T., Loube, D., & Iber, C. (2006). Evaluation of positive airway pressure treatment for sleep related breathing disorders in adults. *Sleep, 29,* 381–401.

Humphreys, J., Lee, K. A., Carrieri-Kohlman, V., Puntillo, K., Faucett, J., Janson, S., . . . The UCSF School of Nursing Symptom Management Faculty Group. (2008). Theory of symptom management. In M. J. Smith & P. R. Liehr (Eds.), *Middle range theory for nursing* (2nd ed., pp. 145–158). New York, NY: Springer Publishing.

IBM. (2016). *IBM SPSS statistics version 24* [Computer Software]. Armonk, NY: Author.

Kagee, A., & Merwe, M. (2006). Predicting treatment adherence among patients attending primary health care clinics: The utility of the Theory of Planned Behaviour. *South African Journal of Psychology, 36,* 699–714.

Kothe, E. J., Mullan, B. A., & Butow, P. (2012). Promoting fruit and vegetable intake: Testing an intervention based on the Theory of Planned Behavior. *Appetite, 58,* 997–1004. doi:10.1016/j.appet.2012.02.012

Liehr, P. R., & Smith, M. J. (2008). Building structures for research. In M. J. Smith & P. R. Liehr (Eds.), *Middle range theory for nursing* (2nd ed., pp. 33–54). New York, NY: Springer Publishing.

National Commission for the Protection of Human Subjects of Biomedical and Behavioral Research. (1979). *The Belmont Report: Ethical principles and guidelines for the protection of human subjects of research.* Washington, DC: Department of Health, Education, and Welfare. Retrieved from http://www.hhs.gov/ohrp/humansubjects/guidance/belmont.html

Niven, A., Nevill, A., Sayers, F., & Cullen, M. (2012). Predictors of rehabilitation intention and behavior following anterior cruciate ligament surgery: An application of the Theory of Planned Behavior. *Scandinavian Journal of Medicine & Science in Sports, 22,* 316–322. doi:10.1111/j.1600-0838.2010.01236.x

Olsen, S., Smith, S., & Oei, T. P. S. (2008). Adherence to continuous positive airway pressure therapy in obstructive sleep apnea sufferers: A theoretical approach to treatment adherence and intervention. *Clinical Psychology Review, 28,* 1355–1371. doi:10.1016/j.cpr.2008.07. 004

Pallant, J. (2016). *SPSS survival manual: A step by step guide to data analysis using IBM SPSS* (6th ed.). Berkshire, England: McGraw-Hill.

Park, J. G., Ramar, K., & Olson, E. J. (2011). Updates on definition, consequences, and management of obstructive sleep apnea. *Mayo Clinic Proceedings, 86,* 549–555. doi:10.4065/mcp.2010.0810

Polit, D. F., & Beck, C. T. (2012). *Nursing research: Generating and assessing evidence for nursing practice* (9th ed.). Philadelphia, PA: Walters Kluwer Health/Lippincott Williams & Wilkins.

Poulet, C., Veale, D., Arnol, N., Lévy, P., Pepin, J. L., & Tyrrell, J. (2009). Psychological variables as predictors of adherence to treatment by continuous positive airway pressure. *Sleep Medicine, 10*, 993–999. doi:10.1016/j.sleep.2009.01.007

Qaseem, A., Holty, J. E. C., Owens, D. K., Dallas, P., Starkey, M., & Shekelle, P. (2013). Management of obstructive sleep apnea in adults: A clinical practice guideline from the American College of Physicians. *Annals of Internal Medicine, 159*, 471–483.

Rakel, R. E. (2009). Clinical and societal consequences of obstructive sleep apnea and excessive daytime sleepiness. *Postgraduate Medicine, 121*, 86–95. doi:10.3810/pgm.2009.01.1957

Sabate, E. (2003). *Adherence to long-term therapies: Evidence for action*. Geneva, Switzerland: World Health Organization.

Sanford, S. D., Bush,A. J., Stone, K. C., Lichstein, K. L., & Aguillard, N. (2008). Psychometric evaluation of the Beck Anxiety Inventory: A sample with sleep-disordered breathing. *Behavioral Sleep Medicine, 6*, 193–205. doi:10.1080/15402000802162596

Sawyer, A. M., Deatrick, J. A., Kuna, S. T., & Weaver, T. E. (2010). Differences in perceptions of the diagnosis and treatment of obstructive sleep apnea and continuous positive airway pressure therapy among adherers and nonadherers. *Qualitative Health Research, 20*, 873–892. doi:10.1177/1049732310365502

Shapiro, A. L. (2014). Yearning for sleep while enduring distress: A concept for nursing research. In M. J. Smith & P. R. Liehr (Eds.), *Middle range theory for nursing* (3rd ed., pp. 361–381). New York, NY: Springer Publishing.

Shapiro, A. L. (2017). *Effect of the CPAP-SAVER intervention on adherence among adults with newly diagnosed obstructive sleep apnea* (Doctoral dissertation). Retrieved from ProQuest Dissertations and Theses database. (Publication No. 10266828)

Shapiro, A. L., & McCrone, S. (2017). CPAP nonadherence issues in a small sample of men with obstructive sleep apnea. *Applied Nursing Research, 36*, 81–83. doi:10.1016/j.apnr.2017.06.001

Smith, M. J., & Liehr, P. R. (Eds.). (2014). *Middle range theory for nursing* (3rd ed.). New York, NY: Springer Publishing.

Smith, S., Lang, C., Sullivan, K., & Warren, J. (2004). Two new tools for assessing patients' knowledge and beliefs about obstructive sleep apnea and continuous positive airway pressure therapy. *Sleep Medicine, 5*, 359–367. doi:10.1016/j.sleep.2003.12.007

Weaver, T. E., & Sawyer, A. M. (2010). Adherence to continuous positive airway pressure treatment for obstructive sleep apnea: Implications for future interventions. *Indian Journal of Medical Research, 131*, 245–258.

White, K. M., Terry, D. J., Troup, C., Rempel, L. A., Norman, P., Mummery, K., . . . Kenardy, J. (2012). An extended theory of planned behavior intervention for older adults with type 2 diabetes and cardiovascular disease. *Journal of Aging and Physical Activity, 20*, 281–299.

# CHAPTER 21

## Reconceptualizing Normal: From Concept Building to Proposal Development

**Shelley J. Greif**

The idea of studying and understanding challenges faced by parents caring for a child after traumatic brain injury (TBI) grew directly out of my work providing care coordination, education, and support caring for children and families who had recently sustained TBI. This practice was within a state program for children with special healthcare needs as well as brain and spinal cord injury. I worked for many years with the broad population of children with special healthcare needs and families. However, I found when working with TBI survivors and families there was a unique depth of parental involvement and commitment that was different from previous experience. I wanted to better understand the experience of those parents in order to inform and improve practice in the field. The structure and process that was used in the development of this concept is described in detail in Reconceptualizing Normal (Greif, 2014). This chapter briefly summarizes the concept development and then describes the process used in moving from concept building to proposal development for my doctoral dissertation.

## ■ FOUNDATION OF CONCEPT BUILDING

The concept reconceptualizing normal was derived from practice. The practice story situation was about Maria, who sustained a severe TBI at the age of 16, when she was struck and dragged by a truck while riding a bicycle. The story describes the experience of Maria and her mother as they moved through trauma care, inpatient rehabilitation, and outpatient services, including integration into educational and community settings.

## ■ THEORETICAL LENS

The Theory of Uncertainty in Illness (Mishel & Clayton, 2008) was used as a lens to shape reconceptualizing normal. This theory describes uncertainty in situations where the impact of illness is unpredictable or there is insufficient information to determine the meaning of the event. In a study on adjustment of families with members who had heart transplants, Mishel and Murdaugh (1987) found that adjustments were continually being made and belief of return to normal was gradually eroded. They described the process of adjustment as one which includes an awareness of the need to redefine what is normal.

# ■ LITERATURE REVIEW

TBI is frequently referred to as the "silent epidemic" because the complications from TBI, such as changes affecting thinking, sensation, language, or emotions, may not be readily apparent. Each year, TBIs contribute to a substantial number of deaths and cases of permanent disability. Recent data show that, on average, approximately 1.7 million people sustain a TBI annually (Faul, Xu, Wald, & Coronado, 2010). Children from birth to 4 years of age, teenagers 15 to 19, and adults over the age of 65 are most likely to sustain a TBI. Furthermore, almost half a million emergency department visits are made annually by children from birth to 14 years.

Consistent throughout the literature is the importance of family functioning. Review of qualitative research suggests that what is central to successful adaptation and community reintegration is the family's ability to reconceptualize what is normal to change expectations about how they and their child will live and experience daily activities (Duff, 2002, 2006; Kao & Stuifbergen, 2004; Mishel & Murdaugh, 1987; Roscigno, 2008; Wongvatunyu & Porter, 2008a, 2008b).

# ■ CORE QUALITIES/CONCEPT DEFINITION/MODEL

There is persistent uncertainty associated with how a child will recover from brain injury. Families develop basic competencies and patterns that foster growth, protect their child, and enable recovery. In coping with uncertainty, they demonstrate flexibility and draw on unconditional love that enables them to get to know their child again and to develop new approaches for everyday living. Willing openness to know anew (Roscigno, 2008; Wongvatunyu & Porter, 2008b), intentional flexibility (Duff, 2002, 2006; Kao & Stuifbergen, 2004), and unconditional love (Kao & Stuifbergen, 2004; Wongvatunyu & Porter, 2008b) are the core qualities of reconceptualizing normal. Reconceptualizing normal is willing openness to know anew through intentional flexibility and unconditional love (Greif, 2014).

Figure 21.1 illustrates the process of reconceptualizing normal after TBI.

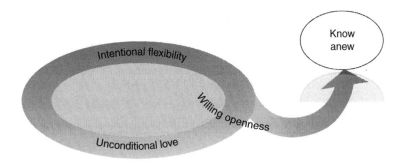

**FIGURE 21.1**   Model of Reconceptualizing Normal.

## ■ RELATIONSHIP OF THE MODEL TO THE RESEARCH PROPOSAL

In continuing to develop and refine the concept of reconceptualizing normal, Story Theory provided an approach that intuitively resonated with exploring and understanding the phenomenon. Story Theory was developed by Smith and Liehr to provide a story-centered structure for guiding nursing practice and research (Smith & Liehr, 2014). The theory recognizes that listening to persons' stories about their health experience is a fundamental nursing process that allows people to express what matters to them. Smith and Liehr (2014) describe story as the "narrative happening of connecting with self-in-relation through intentional dialogue to create ease." In this description story incorporates narration of events as remembered and infuses unique personal perspectives that shape meaning and guide choices in the moment.

## ■ EXEMPLAR PROPOSAL

The purpose of this study is to understand how parents manage the care and community reintegration of their child who has experienced a TBI over time. This study uses a mixed-method approach, exploring critical turning points for parents as they move from "normalcy" prior to and then an altered health trajectory following their child's TBI. Health challenges that parents experience and their approaches for resolving health challenges are also explored.

The population of interest is parent caregivers of children who had a moderate or severe TBI (at least 2 years ago) when they were between the ages of 12 and 18 years. This population is selected for several reasons. It is the age group most at risk and is the largest percentage of children referred for TBI. Adolescents and young adults, who have already begun the developmental processes of independence, are beginning to gain the skills for transition to adulthood. The significant change in their needs following TBI, including dependence and behavioral and cognitive needs, puts them and their families at high risk for dysfunction, stress, and depression.

The research questions for the qualitative component are:

- What are the dimensions of the health challenge of caring for a child who has had a moderate-to-severe TBI?
- What are the turning points that mark change over time for parents of children who have experienced a TBI?
- How have parents managed the challenges they face?

The research questions for the quantitative component are:

- How do parents assess the quality of life for their child who has experienced a TBI?
- How do parents self-appraise management of everyday living following their child's TBI?

## ■ BACKGROUND AND SIGNIFICANCE

Studies of children's cognitive and functional recovery following TBI identify factors that influence outcomes, including pretrauma profile, family characteristics, and severity of injury. None of these factors or variables exists in isolation. Lack of recognition of need by parents or caregivers has been identified as one barrier to improved outcomes, with the recommendation that primary care providers be alert to unrecognized need and provide appropriate referrals (Slomine et al., 2006). Children with preexisting psychosocial conditions such as learning disabilities, behavior disorders, and/or low socioeconomic status are more likely to report unmet needs. It has been suggested that intensive nurse visiting to assess needs and provide support for cognitive and social interventions may improve outcomes for both the family and the child (Keenan, Runyan, & Nocera, 2006). Findings from quantitative research on children's TBI suggest the importance of inquiring into the care and experience of children who have had TBIs. In addition, the experience of families is warranted, given the role that families play in their child's outcomes.

This research is an attempt to understand and appreciate the impact of pediatric TBI through the lens of Story Theory, using a mixed-method design for data collection and analysis. It is expected that this research will: (a) inform nursing practice with respect to understanding the experience for families in managing the care and community reintegration of their child; and (b) highlight opportunities to support family management and strengthening.

## ■ THEORETICAL FRAMEWORK

Story Theory was developed to provide a story-centered structure for guiding nursing practice and research, recognizing that stories are a fundamental dimension of the human experience. Smith and Liehr (2014) identified three interrelated concepts of the theory: intentional dialogue, connecting with self-in-relation, and creating ease. Intentional dialogue is "purposeful engagement with another to summon the story of a complicating health challenge" (p. 230). It is the nurse's intentional presence as a way of coming to know the other person. Connecting with self-in-relation is "the active process of recognizing self as related with others in a story plot" (p. 231), and in Story Theory, connecting with self-in-relation incorporates personal history and reflective awareness. Creating ease is a "release experienced as the story comes together in a movement toward resolving" (p. 232). These three concepts interrelate with each other in a dynamic way to describe story as "a narrative happening of connecting with self-in-relation through intentional dialogue to create ease" (p. 234). The theory proposes concept-related processes named as components of the theory method: intentional dialogue about a complicating health challenge, connecting with self-in-relation through developing story plot (high points, low points, turning points), and creating ease through movement toward resolving the complicating health challenge. The gathering of stories is relevant to both nursing practice and research. The development of Story Theory and method offers an opportunity to embrace story-gathering as an intentional intervention as well as a tool for research expanding nursing knowledge and wisdom.

## ■ METHOD

### Design

This study utilizes a mixed-method approach. In the qualitative component, the following experiences were explored: (a) dimensions of the health challenges faced by parents caring for a child after a TBI; (b) critical turning points for parents as they face the health challenges; and (c) approaches for movement toward resolving health challenges. In the quantitative component, parents' perceptions of their child's quality of life and their own ability to manage their child's health challenge are also explored. Mixed methods refers to the combination of qualitative and quantitative research, and is used when the two approaches complement one another and lead to a more comprehensive understanding of the phenomenon than one or the other could do alone.

Story inquiry method is used to gather and analyze data about health challenges, approaches for resolving health challenges, and turning points as parents move along to reconceptualize normal. These qualitative data are enhanced with a quantitative study component. The Pediatric Quality of Life Inventory (PedsQL) Measurement Model is used to assess the child's quality of life and the Family Management Measure (FaMM) is used to assess parents' ability to manage their child's health challenge.

## Qualitative Approach

According to Creswell (2007), "narrative research is best for capturing the detailed stories or life experiences of a single life or the lives of a small number of individuals" (p. 55). Narrative research draws from the humanities, including anthropology, literature, psychology, sociology, and history, and is well suited for telling the stories of individual experiences. The procedures for conducting narrative research include collecting information about the context of the stories, which are situated within the participants' personal experiences, their culture, and their historical contexts; analyzing the participants' stories; and then "restorying" them into an organized framework. It also calls for collaborating with participants by actively involving them in the research. Creswell noted that in narrative research, there is a relationship between the researcher and the researched in which both parties learn and change in the encounter. This relationship allows the parties to negotiate the meaning of the stories, adding a validation check to the analysis (Creswell, 2007).

Story narrative encourages and allows the participant to articulate experiences that are meaningful, offering the researcher an opportunity to fully understand. In this case, how families moved through the experience of having a child with a TBI is the focus of inquiry. This approach is particularly valuable in uncovering the life-changing dimensions of being thrust unexpectedly into an intensive and complex system of health and related care needs. Engaging in dialogue and eliciting stories that are meaningful to participants allows for the expression of whatever is most important and vital for the care of their child, and allows for consideration of ways to incorporate care into their daily lives.

### STORY INQUIRY METHOD

Story inquiry method is used to gather and analyze data about health challenges, turning points, and movement toward resolving health challenges. Story inquiry method derives from Story Theory and is an approach for systematically gathering and analyzing stories with the intention of informing nursing knowledge development (Liehr & Smith, 2007). Liehr and Smith (2007) proposed five inquiry processes: (a) gathering stories about a complicating health challenge, (b) deciphering dimensions of the complicating health challenge, (c) describing the developing story plot (turning points), (d) identifying movement toward resolving, and (e) synthesizing findings to address the research question. Each phase of the story inquiry method is used in this study.

## Quantitative Approach

Several existing tools were examined to determine feasibility of use with this population. The challenge was to identify tools that adequately measure family management and how it influences outcomes in quality of life for children with TBI.

## FAMILY MANAGEMENT MEASURE

The FaMM was created to assess families' strategies for managing caring for children with chronic illness and the extent to which they incorporate condition management into everyday life (Knafl et al., 2011). The eight dimensions of the *Family Management Style Framework* (FMSF; Child Identity, Illness View, Management Mindset, Parental Mutuality, Parenting Philosophy, Management Approach, Family Focus, and Future Expectations) were used to generate the initial set of items for the FaMM (Knafl et al., 2011). The current version of the FaMM has 65 items with 7 to 9 items/subscale. The final set of items of the measure comprises the Parent Mutuality subscale for partnered parents only. Alpha reliability for mothers/fathers for each of the subscales were acceptable: Child's Daily Life (.76/.79), Condition Management Ability (.72/.73), Condition Management Effort (.74/.78), Family Life Difficulty (.90/.91), View of Condition Impact (.73/.77), and Parental Mutuality (.79/.75); test–test reliability for the subscales ranged from .71 to .94 (Knafl et al., 2011). Knafl et al. (2011) also reported construct validity testing that indicated consistency with established measures.

## PEDIATRIC QUALITY OF LIFE INVENTORY

The PedsQL (Varni, Seid, & Kurtin, 1999) is a 23-item self-report instrument for children and proxy report for parents that includes physical functioning (8 items), emotional functioning (5 items), social functioning (5 items), and school functioning (5 items). The measure includes developmentally appropriate report forms for different age ranges, as well as condition-specific modules to complement the generic scales. It is designed to be used for healthy populations as well as children with acute and chronic health conditions. The tool has been used in numerous studies of health-related quality of life for both typically developing children and children with special healthcare needs. Internal consistency reliability for the full 23-item scale approaches .90 for both reports. Validity has been demonstrated through correlation with other measures of disease burden. In this study, the PedsQL Measurement Model proxy report for parents will be used to enhance understanding about how parents assess the quality of life for their child who has had a TBI.

## ■ SAMPLE AND RECRUITMENT

The sample for this study is a purposive sample of parents who have cared for a child after a TBI. Participants will be identified from a population of individuals who had been referred to the Florida Department of Health—Brain and Spinal Cord Injury Program. Florida statute requires trauma centers to report all moderate-to-severe traumatic brain and spinal cord injuries through a central registry. Individuals identified through the registry are referred to local case managers in their community or region to contact for education, resources, and assistance with coordination of inpatient and/or rehabilitation discharge plans with the goal of community reintegration. Participation in the program is voluntary.

## Procedure

Invitations to participate will be sent by the Regional Children's Medical Services Nursing Director to all families who meet the inclusion criteria, with request to contact the researcher if they are interested in and willing to participate. While it is hypothesized that there may be similarities and differences in culture care beliefs and how families reconceptualize normal and manage care of a child who has had a TBI, families who do not speak or read English will be excluded due to the difficulties of translating and effectively understanding the nuances of language in their stories.

## Sample Size Consideration

Stories will be collected from 10 to 15 parent caregivers of a child who has sustained a TBI. The maximum of 15 participants was chosen with the expectation that it will be a sufficient number to reach saturation. Saturation in qualitative research occurs when there is no longer additional information that adds to the understanding of the area of study. In this mixed-method approach the qualitative dimension of the study is guiding sample size determination. Creswell (2007) suggests that in narrative research, as few as one or two individuals can be sampled unless a larger pool is used to develop a collective story. In this proposed research, a larger pool is indicated to understand the collective story of parenting a child with TBI. In phenomenology, recommendations are to study 3 to 10 subjects, and for Grounded Theory, 20 to 30 individuals (Creswell, 2007). Analysis of the quantitative data is conceptualized as descriptive, and is intended to enhance understanding of the qualitative data.

Stories will be audiotaped and transcribed for analysis. Stories will be analyzed to identify the dimensions of what matters most about the complicating health challenge for the parent caregiver. Descriptive statements will be grouped and labeled with the themes that reflect the complex dimensions of the health challenge. Stories will be examined to identify the turning points that contribute to management of the care of their child with TBI. An additional step in the inquiry process will be to identify approaches used by parents to move toward resolving the health challenge of parenting a child with TBI.

Story-gathering will begin by asking the participant to share their "Story of Parenting a Child Who Has Had a Traumatic Brain Injury." The participant will be provided with a piece of paper with the title and a horizontal line drawn on it. They will be asked to identify the date of the circumstance that resulted in the TBI and it will be noted near the left end of the line. Then the date that the story is being gathered will be noted on the line. Story-gathering will follow a story path approach (Smith & Liehr, 2014). The researcher will begin the dialogue in the present. Participants will be asked to describe challenges that they are facing in the present and how they are managing those challenges. Then, participants will be asked to think about the time before the TBI and tell the researcher what they remember about what life was like for them and their child. They will then be asked to think about and describe the time between the injury and now, and how they got from the time of the injury to the present point in time. Finally, the last inquiry will ask participants to describe their hopes and dreams for the future.

## Analysis Plan

### ANALYZING THE HEALTH CHALLENGE

Deciphering the dimensions of the complicating health challenge involves engaging with the stories to figure out "what matters most." Dimensions are unique descriptions shared by the storyteller about his or her personal experience of the complicating health challenge (Liehr & Smith, 2011). Multiple themes will reflect the different and complex dimensions of the health challenge. An inductive approach will be used. Stories will be read and reread to ascertain meaning. Passages related to the health challenge description will be identified. Like passages will be grouped and themes that address the dimensions of the health challenge will be named.

### ANALYZING MOVEMENT TOWARD RESOLVING

Movement toward resolving refers to action taken to resolve the health challenge. Stories will be examined to evaluate movement toward resolving the health challenge of caring for a child who has suffered a TBI. It is expected that there will be stories along the continuum from nearly complete resolution to little or no resolution. Once again, an inductive approach will be used as previously described. At the completion of this process, there will be a set of health challenge themes, and a second set of themes descriptive of approaches used to resolve the health challenge of parenting a child who has experienced a TBI.

### ANALYZING TURNING POINTS

Finally, stories will be analyzed to identify the turning points that are integral to the health challenge. Turning points are defined as issues that have importance for moving through the health challenge being faced, in this case caring for a child who has had a TBI. Turning points are important decisions or shifts in the story of the unfolding health challenge, and may interplay with movement toward resolving. An inductive approach will, once again, be used, grouping similar descriptions of transition shared by parents. Themes will be identified for each set of turning point descriptions.

Results of the PedsQL and the FaMM will be analyzed using descriptive statistics (means and standard deviations) to address the quantitative research questions: (a) How do parents assess the quality of life for their child who has experienced a TBI? and (b) How do parents self-appraise management of everyday living following their child's TBI? The small sample size prohibits inferential statistics but these descriptive data may shed light on the qualitative findings by providing another perspective regarding how caregivers are managing their challenges in relation to the circumstance of having a child who suffered a TBI.

This parallel mixed-method design results in two sets of inferences, one qualitative and one quantitative, each developed from independent analysis (Chiang-Hanisko, Newman, Dyess, Piyakong, & Liehr, 2016). At the completion of independent data analysis, the inferences will be examined together to identify areas of consistency and discrepancy, thereby enabling identification of guidance for both practice and research.

## Study Rigor

Sandelowski (1986) addresses the issue of rigor in qualitative research, noting that qualitative research emphasizes the meaningfulness of the research product rather than control of the process. Guba and Lincoln (1981) suggest that credibility of a qualitative study is the measure of its truth value, and is evident when the study presents such faithful descriptions of the experience that people immediately recognize it from description or interpretation as their own.

Tappen (2011) identifies a number of ways to ensure trustworthiness of qualitative research. Credibility is established through prolonged engagement and observation, member checking, peer debriefing, negative case analysis, and triangulation. Two of these approaches will be used: prolonged engagement and peer debriefing.

Prolonged engagement and persistent observation allow time and opportunity to test possible explanations and develop emerging explanations. Length of engagement is influenced by how well you already know the language and culture. This researcher has worked directly with children and families of children with TBIs for more than 5 years and is familiar with what families experience. Story-gathering is intended to provide a structure and framework for enhancing understanding of the multiple dimensions of the health challenge. During the interview the researcher will ask participants to clarify information that has been shared as part of story-gathering, to be sure that an accurate reflection of their intention has been heard.

Peer debriefing, seeking feedback from individuals with expertise on the subject and methodology, is another strategy for ensuring trustworthiness of qualitative research. The doctoral candidate's dissertation committee chair will serve as the expert, and will be asked to review 20% of the sample for assessment of analysis. Feedback will be elicited from other committee members who are subject matter experts.

Cases will be examined after the initial analysis is completed to see whether the dimensions of the health challenge, movement toward resolving, and turning points are applicable to all cases. Negative cases (those that differ from the prevailing themes), if identified, will also be included for analysis. It is important to consider divergent meaning and incorporate this consideration into conclusions.

The dependability of qualitative research is equivalent to reliability in quantitative research. Lincoln and Guba address the importance of an audit trail, a careful compilation of material. The researcher will keep careful records of raw data (field notes, audio recordings, documents), data analysis products (summaries or ideas that occur to the researcher during study), coding schemes, process notes (descriptions of how data were obtained and how analysis done), reflections of the investigator (personal notes and reflective journal), and surveys or questionnaire guides (forms used to collect information on participants, interview guides).

## Ethics and Institutional Review Board

Because this is research involving human subjects, institutional review board approval will be necessary. Institutional review board approval will need to be obtained from the Florida Department of Health as well as Florida Atlantic University. Invitations will be sent by the Regional Nursing Director for Children's Medical Services, in order to protect the confidentiality of clients. Subjects who express interest in the study will be informed that their participation is voluntary, and their decision about participation will not affect the services they receive through the Brain and Spinal Cord Injury Program. Also, refusal to participate will involve no penalty or loss of benefits, and they may stop participating at any time. The purpose of the research will be explained to participants both verbally and in writing, to ensure understanding of participation.

It is possible that in the process of sharing stories about managing care of their child with TBI, parents may identify unmet needs. They will be provided with contact information for the Brain Injury Association of Florida, which provides family support to survivors and caregivers of survivors of TBI, information, and educational resources. They will also be provided contact information as appropriate for their local community health and/or community mental health center.

## Data Collection Protocol

Parents who respond to the invitation to participate will be contacted by the researcher to further explain the study and to set up an appointment. The total time allocated for the appointment will be 1.5 to 2 hours. The consent form will be introduced and explained. Time for story-gathering will be 45 minutes to 1 hour, with additional time for introduction, demographic and health data, and completion of quantitative measures.

Demographic and health data will be collected in an interview format, in order to establish rapport and get to know the participant. These data will include caregiver and child information. Caregiver information will include: age, gender, ethnic background, marital status, duration of marriage, education, occupation, and parent perception of severity of injury. Child information will include: age, gender, ethnic background, age at time of injury, and preexisting conditions (e.g., attention deficit hyperactivity disorder [ADHD], behavioral or learning disabilities).

Stories will be collected as previously described using a story path approach (Smith & Liehr, 2014), beginning with the present experience, life before the TBI, time from the TBI to the present, and future hopes and dreams. Stories will be audiotaped for accuracy and to facilitate the analysis process.

Parents will be asked to complete the PedsQL and FaMM immediately after the story is completed. If they are unable to complete these due to time constraints or other factors at that time, they will be offered the option to complete the measures within 48 hours and then mail back to the researcher. The researcher will telephone participants after 48 hours to see if there is anything they want to add to the story that might not have been included, and to remind them to mail back the measures.

## ■ EVALUATION OF THE STRUCTURE BUILDING PROCESS

The process of moving from concept development to the proposal and implementation of research was guided by the concept of reconceptualizing normal after TBI. The foundational understanding of this idea emerging during concept building set in motion a proposal development process that integrated qualitative and quantitative approaches for data gathering and analysis.

This study used a parallel mixed-method approach to understand how families manage the care of a child with TBI. The qualitative inquiry was guided by Story Theory and story inquiry method. This narrative approach was selected because of its essential congruence with nursing practice and research and my understanding about the importance of knowing the stories of these families, based on years of nursing practice experience. Quantitative data was collected using the PedsQL and the FaMM to provide descriptive data with the potential to enhance understanding of the complexity of the health challenge of parenting a child who had suffered a TBI.

One of the qualities essential for both concept building and proposal development was adherence to a systematic scholarly process. The skills that were developed during concept building, like thoughtful reflection to synthesize ideas and determine next directions, were critical to proposal development. Each step from beginning with the practice story in concept building to preparation of a three-chapter dissertation proposal was built upon the learning that has come before it. From my perspective, concept building and dissertation proposal development are parts of a whole for scholars on a path to complete dissertation research.

## ▪ REFERENCES

Chiang-Hanisko, L., Newman, D., Dyess, S., Piyakong, D., & Liehr, P. (2016). Guidance for using mixed methods design in nursing practice research. *Applied Nursing Research, 31,* 1–5.

Creswell, J. W. (2007). *Qualitative inquiry & research design: choosing among five approaches.* Thousand Oaks, CA: Sage.

Duff, D. (2002). Family concerns and responses following a severe traumatic brain injury: A grounded theory study. *Axon, 24*(2), 14–22.

Duff, D. (2006). Family impact and influence following severe traumatic brain injury. *Axon, 27*(2), 9–23.

Faul, M., Xu, L., Wald, M. M., & Coronado, V. G. (2010). *Traumatic brain injury in the United States: Emergency department visits, hospitalizations, and deaths.* Atlanta, GA: Centers for Disease Control and Prevention, National Center for Injury Prevention and Control.

Greif, S. J. (2014). Reconceptualizing normal. In M. J. Smith & P. R. Liehr (Eds.), *Middle range theory for nursing* (3rd ed., pp. 383–396). New York, NY: Springer Publishing.

Guba, E. G., & Lincoln, Y. S. (1981). *Effective evaluation.* San Francisco, CA: Jossey-Bass.

Kao, H.-F. S., & Stuifbergen, A. K. (2004). Love and load–the lived experience of the mother-child relationship among young adult traumatic brain-injured survivors. *Journal of Neuroscience Nursing, 36*(2), 73–81.

Keenan, H.T., Runyan, D.K., & Nocera, M. (2006). Longitudinal follow-up of families and young children with traumatic brain injury. (Disease/Disorder overview). *Pediatrics 117*(4), 1291.

Knafl, K., Deatrick, J. A., Gallo, A., Dixon, J., Grey, M., Knalt, G., & O'Malley, J. (2011). Assessment of the psychometric properties of the Family Management Measure. *Journal of Pediatric Psychology, 36*(5), 494–505.

Liehr, P., & Smith, M. J. (2007). Story inquiry: A method for research. *Archives of Psychiatric Nursing, 21*(2), 120–121.

Liehr, P., & Smith, M. J. (2011). Refining story inquiry as a method for research. *Archives of Psychiatric Nursing, 25*(1), 74–75.

Mishel, M. H., & Clayton, M. F. (2008). Theories of uncertainty in illness. In M. J. Smith & P. R. Liehr (Eds.), *Middle range theory for nursing* (2nd ed., pp. 55–84). New York, NY: Springer Publishing.

Mishel, M. H., & Murdaugh, C. L. (1987). Family adjustment to heart transplantation: redesigning the dream. *Nursing Research, 36,* 332–336.

Roscigno, C. (2008). *Children's and parents' experiences following children's moderate to severe traumatic brain injury* (Unpublished doctoral dissertation). University of Washington, Seattle, WA.

Sandelowski, M. (1986). The problem of rigor in qualitative research. *Advances in Nursing Science, 8*(3), 27–37.

Slomine, B. S., McCarthy, M. L., Ding, R., MacKenzie, E. J., Jaffe, K. M., Aitken, M. E., . . . Paidas, C. N. (2006). Health care utilization and needs after pediatric traumatic brain injury. *Pediatrics, 117*(4), e663–e674. doi:10.1542/peds.2005-1892

Smith, M. J., & Liehr, P. (2014). Story theory. In M. J. Smith & P. R. Liehr (Eds.), *Middle range theory for nursing* (3rd ed., pp. 225–251). New York, NY: Springer Publishing.

Tappen, R. M. (2011). *Advanced nursing research, from theory to practice.* Sudbury, MA: Jones & Bartlett.

Varni, J. W., Seid, M., & Kurtin, P. S. (1999). Pediatric health-related quality of life measurement technology: A guide for health care decision makers. *Journal of Clinical Outcomes Management,* (6), 33–40.

Wongvatunyu, S., & Porter, E. J. (2008a). Changes in family life perceived by mothers of young adult TBI survivors. *Journal of Family Nursing, 14*(3), 314–332.

Wongvatunyu, S., & Porter, E. J. (2008b). Helping young adult children with traumatic brain injury: the life-world of mothers. *Qualitative Health Research, 18*(8), 1062–1074.

# SECTION FOUR

## Current State of Middle Range Theory

Scholarly endeavors often emerge in connection with each other, shaping and spurring direction over time. We first wrote about middle range theory in 1999 when Story Theory was published in Scholarly Inquiry for Nursing Practice (now, Research and Theory for Nursing Practice). At that time, spawned by our own theory-development efforts, we began to consider explicating the state of the science for middle range theory.

In order to move middle range theory state of the science ideas forward, we responded to a call in Advances in Nursing Science (ANS) for manuscripts focused on Nursing Theory for the 21st Century. In the editorial for this issue, the editor Dr. Peggy Chinn noted: "The time has come to claim and proclaim the insights that come from our theoretical ideas, and shape the ideas into substantive action toward health and healing." The first paper in this section, published in 1999 titled "Middle Range Theory: Spinning Research and Practice to Create Knowledge for the New Millennium," focused on insights that characterized approaches for generating middle range theory, how middle range connected with grand theory, and future directions for middle range theory. This paper also included an inductive analysis of middle range theory names to identify two disciplinary themes: caring–healing process and transforming struggle–growth.

The first paper in this section catalyzed action to write this book, which would help nurse scholars in coming to know a body of middle range theory and how to use it to guide practice and research. The first edition of Middle Range Theory for Nursing was published in 2003 and the current version is the fourth edition of the book. We have continued to develop and test Story Theory since 1999 and have continued our interest in the state of the science, noting an increase in the appearance of theories identified as middle range over the years.

In 2017, again in response to a call in ANS for papers that replicated or built on previously published articles in the journal, we wrote the second paper in this section titled "Middle Range Theory: A Perspective on Development and Use." This paper focused on evaluation of middle range theories with ongoing use based on reconsideration of the recommendations from the 1999 paper by noting how the current literature stacks up in relation to each recommendation. In the conclusion, we emphasized the importance of: (a) staying with a theory by developing it over time; (b) selecting a theory name that positions it solidly within the disciplinary perspective of nursing; (c) moving middle range theory to the empirical level through *both practice and research; and (d) establishing a comfortable footing within a specific middle range theory to enable meaningful inclusion when participating at the interdisciplinary table.*

*This section of the book presents a historical perspective inclusive of critique of knowledge about middle range theory via the 1999 and 2017 papers. These offerings serve as sources of synthesis that can inform ongoing theory development through testing in research and use in practice.*

# Middle Range Theory: Spinning Research and Practice to Create Knowledge for the New Millennium

The foundation of middle range theory reported during the past decade was described and analyzed. A CINAHL search revealed 22 middle range theories that met selected criteria. This foundation is a firm base for new millennium theorizing. Recommendations for future theorizing include: clear articulation of theory names and approaches for generating theories; clarification of concept linkages with inclusion of diagrammed models; deliberate attention to research-practice connections of theories; creation of theories in concert with the disciplinary perspective; and, movement of middle range theories to the front lines of nursing research and practice for further analysis, critique, and development. Key words: *middle range theory, theory, 21st century perspective*

*Patricia Liehr, PhD, RN*
*Associate Professor, School of Nursing*
*The University of Texas—Houston Health*
  *Science Center*
*Houston, Texas*

*Mary Jane Smith, PhD, RN*
*Professor, School of Nursing*
*West Virginia University—Robert C. Byrd*
  *Health Science Center*
*Morgantown, West Virginia*

A SPINNER prepares wool by combing, to discard debris and align the strands of a matted mass in much the same way as content is sifted to tease central ideas out of extraneous ones. Just as the spinner twirls strands to compose a single thread; the nurse theorist spins central ideas into a synthesized thread for research and practice. Twisting single threads with each other enhances the strength of the product; as does the crafting of research-practice links in the creation of strong middle range theory. The beauty of any woven article is dependent on its warp and weft; likewise, the esthetics of the discipline is dependent on its theories. Spinning, like theorizing, is rigorous work aimed at creating esthetic, useful products. This article describes and analyzes a decade of middle range theory products that establish a foundation for the new millennium. This foundation highlights the current structure of middle range theory and offers direction for 21st century spinning.

*Adv Nurs Sci* 1999;21(4):81–91
© 1999 Aspen Publishers, Inc.

## THE HISTORICAL CONTEXT OF MIDDLE RANGE THEORY

Modernism, postmodernism, and neo-modernism are historical descriptors that represent change in the course of a developing discipline by influencing thinking and scholarship. Modernism espouses beliefs about human beings that affirm a unidimensional and stable existence, while post modernism adheres to views that affirm multidimensional, ever-changing, and complex human unfolding existence.[1] Watson[2] identified the postmodern for nursing as reconnecting with "the truths of unfoldment, an expansion and fusing of horizons of meaning, an attending to the authenticity, ethos, and ethic of caring relations, context, continuity, connections, aesthetics, interpretation and construction."[2(p63)] She concludes that these postmodern dimensions tie directly to developing the art and science of nursing as a caring-healing transformative praxis paradigm. Reed[3] moves beyond postmodernism to neomodernism and calls for a synthesis of modernism and postmodernism. She describes the synthesis as a metanarrative reflecting the human development potential, transformation, and self-transcendent capacity for health and healing, including a recognition of the development histories of persons and their contexts.[3] It is expected that theories that offer direction for the new millennium will emerge from the historical context that defines the time. The current context urges a focus on the human development potential of health and healing and supports a nursing knowledge base that synthesizes art and science; practice and research. Theories at the middle range level of discourse are in keeping with the historical context launching the new millennium.

Merton describes theories of the middle range as those

that lie between the minor but necessary working hypotheses that evolve in abundance during day-to-day research and the all-inclusive systematic efforts to develop unified theory that will explain all the observed uniformities of social behavior, social organization and social change.[4(p39)]

He goes on to describe the principle ideas of middle range theory as relatively simple. Simple, in this sense, means rudimentary straightforward ideas that stem from the perspective of the discipline. An example of such an idea is that when individuals tell their story to one who truly listens, a change takes place. This idea is central to the middle range theory of attentively embracing story.[5] The ideas of middle range theory are simple yet general and are more than mere empirical generalizations.

In keeping with the views of Merton,[4] the following descriptions of middle range theory are found in the nursing literature: testable and intermediate in scope,[6] adequate in empirical foundations,[7] neither too broad nor too narrow,[8] circumscribed and substantively specific,[9] and more circumscribed than grand theory but not as concrete as practice theory.[10] In 1974, Jacox[11] described middle range theories as those including a limited number of variables and focused on a limited aspect of reality. Each of these descriptions highlights a scope somewhere in the middle, allowing for broad definitions. Lenz[12] addresses the issue of definitional clarity and believes that although the definitions of middle range theory are consistent, theories of varying scope have been labeled middle-range and the discipline may be well served by recognizing levels of theory within the middle range. She states the challenge for the discipline will be to not generate a plethora of middle range theories, but to develop a few that are empirically sound, coherent, meaningful, useful, and illuminating.[12] To meet the challenge set by Lenz in the next century, it is essential that middle range theories emerge from the twisting of research and practice threads by nurse scholars who are building on the work of others and creating the future direction of the discipline. The spinning of middle range theory in the next century will be guided by the existing middle range theory foundation.

## THE EXISTING MIDDLE RANGE THEORY FOUNDATION

To assess the current foundation of middle range theory, a CINAHL search of the past 10 years of nursing literature was done entering middle range theory, mid-range theory, and nursing as search terms. The search was conducted independently in two institutions. All papers written in English that surfaced from the combined search were evaluated for inclusion in the foundation list of middle range theories (Table 1). Criteria for inclusion were

1. the theory was identified as middle range by its author;
2. the theory name was accessible in the paper;
3. concepts of the theory were explicitly identified or implicitly identified in propositions; and
4. the development of the theory was the major focus of the paper.

These criteria represent an intent to be inclusive, providing the broadest view of available middle range nursing theory.

However, some papers excluded were primarily methodological in focus.[13,14] These were identified in the literature search but did not meet the criteria. Table 1 describes the middle range theory foundation that has emerged during the past decade. Along with including identifying and locating information about the theory, it notes the inclusion of a diagrammed model and the approaches for theory generation identified by the author.

## ANALYSIS OF THE MIDDLE RANGE THEORY FOUNDATION

### The middle range theories

There are 22 middle range theories proposed as the current foundation. Two theories, Unpleasant Symptoms[7,15] and Balance between Analgesia and Side Effects,[16,17] are accompanied by two citations. Unpleasant Symptoms is the only theory to have documented, ongoing development in the past decade. The second citation for Balance between Analgesia and Side Effects provides examples of use of the theory for research but does not alter its original structure. Powell-Cope,[18] using Swanson's[19] theory of Caring-with the intent of extending it-derived yet another theory, Negotiating Partnerships. This was the only instance of one middle range nursing theory generating another. However, Levesque et al.[20] report that a foundation of middle range theories from other disciplines was the basis of their work.

Several theories that have been labeled middle range by persons who are not the primary author of the theory do not appear in the middle range foundation list. For instance, Fawcett[9] labels Orlando's Deliberative Nursing, Peplau's

**Table 1.** Middle range theories over the decade: 1988–1998

| Year published | Author(s), journal | Name of theory | Inclusion of model | | Theory generating approach |
|---|---|---|---|---|---|
| | | | Yes | NO | |
| 1988 | Mishel *Image* | Uncertainty in Illness | X | | Empirical research, literature synthesis from nursing and other disciplines |
| 1989 | Thompson, et al. *Journal of Nurse Midwifery* | Nurse Midwifery Care | | X | Philosophy of nurse-midwifery profession , survey data, patient-nurse practice videotapes, empirical research |
| 1990 | Kinney *Issues in Mental H ealth Nursing* | Facilitating Growth and Development | | X | Middle range model from Erickson's Modeling and Role Modeling theory, practice |
| 1991 | Reed *ANS* | Self-Transcendence | | X | Literature reviews, clinical experience, empirical research, deductive reformulation of life span theories from developmental psychology with Rogers Conceptual System |
| 1991 | Burke, Kauffmann, Costello, Dillon *Image* | Hazardous Secrets and Reluctantly Taking Charge | X | | Grounded theory |
| 1991 | Thomas *Issues in Mental Health Nursing* | Women 's Anger | X | | Existential and cognitive- behavioral theories, literature review, clinical know ledge, intuition , logic |
| 1991 | Swanson *Nursing Research* | Caring | | X | Phenomenological studies |
| 1994 | Powell-Cope *Nursing Research* | Negotiating Partnership | | X | Extending Swanson's Caring theory using grounded theory |
| 1995, 1997 | Lenz, et al. *ANS* | Unpleasant Symptoms | X | | Empirical research, clinical observation, concept analysis, collaboration Concept analysis, ethnography, grounded theory, practice |
| 1995 | Jezewski *ANS* | Cultural *Brokering* | X | | Concept analysis, ethnography, grounded theory, practice experience, literature synthesis |
| 1996, 1998 | Good, Moore, Good *Nursing Outlook* | Balance between Analgesia and Side Effects | X | | Clinical practice guidelines; empirical research |
| 1997 | Auvil-Novak *Nursing Researc/1* | Chronotherapeutic Intervention for Post-surgical Pain | X | | Chronobiologic theory, literature synthesis, empirical research |
| 1997 | Olson, Hanchett *Image* | Nurse-Expressed Empathy and Patient Distress | X | | Orlando's nursing model, empirical research |
| 1997 | Brooks, Thomas *ANS* | Interpersonal Perceptual Awareness | X | | Concept analysis to extend King's Interactin g System framework |
| 1997 | Polk *ANS* | Resilience | X | | Concept synthesis u sing literature from other disciplines, Roger's Science of Unitary Beings |
| 1997 | Gerdner | Individualized Music Intervention for Agitation | X | | Clinical practice, literature review, pilot study |
| 1997 | Acton *Journal of Holistic* | Affiliated Individuation as a Mediator of Stress | X | | Middle range model from Erickson's Modeling and Role Modeling theory, Empirical research |
| 1998 | Eakes, Burke, Hain sworth *Image* | Chronic Sorrow | X | | Concept analysis, literature review, qualitative research |

**Table 1.** (*continued*)

| Year published | Author(s), journal | Name of theory | Inclusion of model | | Theory generating approach |
|---|---|---|---|---|---|
| | | | Yes | NO | |
| 1998 | Huth, Moore *Journal of the Society of Pediatric Nurses* | Acute Pain Management | X | | Clinical practice guidelines |
| 1998 | Levesque, et al. *Nursing Science* | Psychological Adaptation | X | | Middle range theories from other disciplines, empirical research, collaboration, Roy's Adaptation Model |
| 1998 | Ruland, Moore *Nursing Outlook* | Peaceful End of Life | X | | Standards of care |

Interpersonal Relations, and Watson's Human Caring theory as middle range; however, none of these came up in the literature search for middle range theory. Nolan and Grant[21] labeled Chenitz's theory of Entry into a Nursing Home as Status Passage as middle range and reported a test of the theory with a respite care sample. Review of Chenitz's theory[22] indicated that it was labeled practice theory by the author even though it may be at the middle range level of discourse. There are other theories that seem to be at the middle range level of discourse but have not been so identified by the primary author. One example is the work of Beck, who has developed a theory of postpartum depression that includes initial quantitative inquiry[23] followed by qualitative study.[24-26] Although this body of work is at the middle range level of discourse, Beck has not labeled it as middle range theory.

Based on the identified foundation of middle range theory, as the decade unfolded, there appeared to be increased willingness to label theory as middle range. Seven of the theories in Table 1 were proposed in the 4-year span between 1988 and 1992 and 15 were proposed in the most recent 4 years of the decade, since 1994, with six middle range theory papers published in 1997 alone. Some of the 1997 proliferation can be attributed to an issue of *Advances in Nursing Science* devoted to middle range theory. Three of the middle range theories listed in 1997 were published in this issue. In her editorial for the issue, Chinn[27] highlighted a shift in nurses' scholarly endeavors to create possibilities for healing science-art as evidenced by the issue's middle range theories, which, she noted, defy a single, limited perspective definition. The question about what constitutes theory at the middle range is not a black and white issue for which a precise and clear definition can be offered. Middle range theory holds to a given level of abstraction. It is not too broad nor too narrow, but somewhere in the middle. It is expected that finding the middle will come as theory in the middle range is spun in the next millennium.

*Based on the indentified foundation of middle range theory, as the decade unfolded, there appeared to be increased willingness to label theory as middle range.*

## Naming the theory

Theory, especially at the middle range, is known to practitioners and researchers by the way it is named. It is essential that theories at the middle range be named in the context of the disciplinary perspective and at the appropriate level of discourse. Figuring out the name is a process of creative conceptualization that moves back and forth between putting together and pulling apart until the right name is found. Implicit in naming is a search for a conceptual structure as the theorist remembers and relives practice and research experiences, reflecting on the author's proposed meaning in relation to the literature. This is a creative, energy-demanding process intended to uncover the heart of the theory. The central theory core is molded by the conceptual structure that exposes it and is articulated at the middle range level of abstraction as the name of the theory.

A theory name was accessible in each of the papers in Table 1, although some names were more accessible than others. A few theorists announced the presentation of a middle range theory and provided a name in the title of the paper,[7,15,28-31] while others were embedded the name in the body of the paper. Facilitating Growth and Development[32] and Affiliated Individuation[33] both emerge from Modeling and Role-Modeling theory.[34] While each is described as a model at the middle range level of abstraction, distinguishing the unique name from the parent theory was difficult. The challenge of naming a middle range theory resides in determining the middle as sufficiently abstract to allow a breadth of application yet narrow enough to permit guidance in research and practice. Table 2 organizes the existing middle range

**Table 2.** Middle range nursing theories by level of abstraction

| High middle | Middle | Low middle |
|---|---|---|
| Caring | Uncertainty in Illness | Hazardous Secrets and Reluctantly Taking Charge |
| Facilitating Growth and Development | Unpleasant Symptoms | Affiliated Individuation as a Mediator of Stress |
| Interpersonal Perceptual Awareness | Chronic Sorrow | Women's Anger |
| Self-Transcendence | Peaceful End of Life | Nurse Midwifery Care |
| Resilience | Negotiating Partnerships | Acute Pain Management |
| Psychological Adaptation | Cultural Brokering | Balance between Analgesia and Side Effects |
| | Nurse-Expressed Empathy and Patient Distress | Homelessness-Helplessness |
| | | Individualized Music Intervention for Agitation |
| | | Chronotherapeutic Intervention for Post-Surgical Pain |

theories into the high-middle, middle, and low-middle level of abstraction, using the theory name. The theories were grouped, relative to each other, based on the generality or scope of the theory indicated by the name. Using the theory name to distinguish the level of abstraction has inherent limitations because the name may not reflect theory content. However, the theory name is its guiding label and this analysis highlights the importance of the theory name. It also highlights the existence of multiple levels of abstraction within the middle range, a fact introduced by Lenz,[12] for further recognition and development. To name a middle range theory is to locate it at an appropriate level of abstraction and to commit to a conceptual structure. Capturing a conceptual structure and expressing theory at the middle range level of abstraction will enable 21st century scholars to recognize, use, and critique the theory for practice and research applications.

### Inclusion of a model

Chinn and Kramer[35] define theory as "a creative and rigorous structuring of ideas that projects a tentative, purposeful, and systematic view of phenomena."[35(p106)] They include purpose, concepts, definitions, relationships, structure, and assumptions as components of theory suggested by their definition, noting that purpose and assumptions may be implicit rather than explicit. So, concepts with their definitions-and relationships expressed as structure-are the core components expected to be made explicit regardless of the theory's level of abstraction. One of the criteria for theories in the foundation list was the presentation of concepts. The relationship and structure components were evaluated by determining whether the theorist included a diagrammed model in the paper. Of the

22 theories in the foundation list, only 5 did not diagram a model.[18,19,32,36,37] Three[18,19,36] did not explicitly address relationships between concepts. One[37] specified relationships through propositions; one[32] described middle range relationships between concepts of a parent theory. All middle range theories since 1995 have included a diagrammed model.

## APPROACHES FOR GENERATING MIDDLE RANGE THEORY

Lenz[12] has identified six approaches for generating middle range theory; these were used to categorize the methods used by the creators of the 22 theories identified in the foundation. The categories are not mutually exclusive because theorists often used more than one approach. Lenz's approaches are

1. inductive theory building through research,
2. deductive theory building from grand nursing theories,
3. combining existing nursing and non-nursing theories,
4. deriving theories from other disciplines,
5. synthesizing theories from published research findings, and
6. developing theories from clinical practice guidelines.

A review of the foundation theories indicates that fourteen* appeared to use inductive theory building through research. Three derived the theory from grand nursing theory,[20,29,43] two combined nursing and non-nursing theories,[30,37] four derived theories from those of other disciplines,[20,28,37,44] and two[16,45] developed theory from practice guidelines. The approach of synthesizing

_____

*References 7,15,18–20,28,29,31,33,36,38–42

theories from published research identified by Lenz was difficult to determine when categorizing the theories. No middle range theory was cited that was generated only by published research. Even when not stated explicitly, there were implicit indications that every theory had referred to published research when generating the theory. Two theories[32,46] fit into none of the approaches described by Lenz. Ruland and Moore[46] recently have proposed using standards of care to generate middle range theory and Kinney[32] describes a practice example to demonstrate a middle range model. Including Kinney, seven theories[7,15,32,36,37,40,42,44] explicitly cited personal practice experiences as contributing to middle range theory development. Only four[7,15,36,40,42] of the seven also described research threads, thus enabling the spinning of research with practice in the building of middle range theory.

The analysis of approaches for generating middle range theory suggests that Lenz's listing generally is comprehensive. The elimination of the approach noting synthesis from published research findings may be appropriate, and an expansion of "clinical practice guidelines" to "practice guidelines and standards" will cover the recent work by Ruland and Moore.[46] Inclusion of the practice thread is critical for 21st century spinning. Therefore, the following five approaches are proposed for middle range theory generation in the new millennium:

1. induction through research and practice;
2. deduction from research and practice applications of grand theories;
3. combination of existing nursing and non-nursing middle range theories;
4. derivation from theories of other disciplines that relate to nursing's disciplinary perspective; and

5. derivation from practice guidelines and standards rooted in research.

It is unlikely that any of these theory generation approaches will stand alone as nursing moves into the next century. Each will need to be combined to most effectively guide the discipline. Guidance for the new millennium is most likely to emerge from theories that spin research and practice to focus on the human developmental potential of health and healing.

## JUXTAPOSITION WITH GRAND NURSING THEORY

As middle range theory is generated for the new millennium, it is essential that it move beyond the polarities often created between it and grand theories. The all-embracing grand theories were espoused by individuals who attempted to create a view of the whole of nursing. Groups have developed into small circles of schools of thought in which an all-or-nothing adherence to the perspective is advocated strongly. This approach has advanced the discipline through generation of scholarly pursuits and offers a grounding for middle range theory. It is not separate nor antithetical to middle range theory development. Merton[4] identifies the following criticisms of middle range theory leveled by those who advocate grand approaches: (1) conceptualizing middle range theory is low in intellectual ambitions; (2) it completely excludes grand theory; (3) it will fragment the discipline into unrelated special theories; and (4) a positivist conception of theory will be the result. There is no evidence that these criticisms have been realized. Nursing's current middle range theory foundation: reflects scholarly work conceptualized at a lower level of abstraction that rises to intellectual challenge; builds on' grand theory that continues to offer a foundation for development; and projects a historical context to begin the millennium with theories at the middle range in the perspective of the discipline.

## DISCIPLINARY PERSPECTIVE OF THE MIDDLE RANGE THEORY FOUNDATION

An association between the existing middle range theory foundation and the disciplinary perspective synthesized as a caring, healing process in which the human developmental potential for health and transformation emerge[2,3] is depicted in Table 3. Through the reflective process of dwelling with the essence of the disciplinary perspective and the middle range theories as named, two themes surfaced. These themes were caring-healing processes

and transforming struggle-growth. These themes offer a view of the existing middle range theory foundation in the context of a disciplinary perspective as well as an integrated paradigm for spinning middle range theory in the new millennium.

## THE FUTURE: WHERE DOES NURSING THEORY GO FROM HERE?

In conclusion, a lot of thoughtful spinning of middle range theory has been done in the past decade; and although knots and tangles have been created along the way, one must remember that spinning theory is a creative human endeavor that can best be described as a work in progress. It is expected that the knots and tangles will be sorted out with the spinner's persistence and careful attention to creating and combining fibers. Based on the description and

**Table 3.** Middle range theories by disciplinary themes

| Caring-healing process | Transforming struggle-growth |
| --- | --- |
| Caring | Self-Transcendence |
| Facilitating Growth and Development | Resilience |
| Interpersonal Perceptual Awareness | Psychological Adaptation |
| Cultural Brokering | Uncertainty in Illness |
| Nurse-Expressed Empathy and Patient Distress | Unpleasant Symptoms |
| Nurse Midwifery Care | Chronic Sorrow |
| Acute Pain Management | Peaceful End of Life |
| Balance between Analgesia and Side Effects | Negotiating Partnerships |
| Individualized Music Intervention for Agitation | Hazardous Secrets and Reluctantly Taking Charge |
| Chronotherapeutic Intervention for Post-Surgical Pain | Affiliated Individuation as a Mediator of Stress |
| | Women's Anger |
| | Homelessness-Helplessness |

analysis of the current middle range theory foundation, several recommendations are presented for developing middle range theory in the future. The recommendations are that the creators of middle range theory:

1. take care to clearly articulate the theory name and approach used for generating the theory;
2. strive to clarify the conceptual linkages of the theory in a diagrammed model;
3. give deliberate attention to articulating the research-practice links of the theory;
4. create an association between the proposed theory and a disciplinary perspective in nursing; and
5. move middle range theory to the front lines of nursing practice and research for further analysis, critique, and development.

Twenty-first century theorists are offered the challenge of these recommendations. The challenge is to move nursing theory forward by spinning research and practice in the creation of middle range theories congruent with the current historical context. It is this forward movement that will give substance and direction to the discipline. Middle range theory will create the disciplinary fabric of the new millennium as nurse theorists spin and twist fibers from the past-present into the future.

## REFERENCES

1. Anderson TA. Post modern person. *Noetic Sciences Review*. 1998;45:28-33.
2. Watson J. Postmodernism and knowledge development in nursing. *Nurs Sci Quarterly*. 1994;8:60-64.
3. Reed PG. A treatise on nursing knowledge development for the 21st century: Beyond postmodernism. *ANS*. 1995;17:70-84.
4. Merton RK. On sociological theories of the middle range. In: *Social Theory and Social Structure*. New York: Free Press; 1968.
5. Smith MJ, Liehr P. Attentively embracing story: Derivation of a middle range theory with practice and research implications. *Sch Ing Nurs Prac*. In press.
6. Suppe F. Middle range theory-Role in nursing theory and knowledge development. In: *Proceedings of the Sixth Rosemary Ellis Scholar's Retreat, Nursing Science Implications for the 21st century*. Cleveland, OH: Frances Payne Bolton School of Nursing, Case Western Reserve University; 1996.
7. Lenz ER, Suppe F, Gift AG, Pugh LC, Milligan RA. Collaborative development of middle-range nursing theories: toward a theory of unpleasant symptoms. *ANS*. 1995;17:1-13.
8. Reed P. Toward a nursing theory of self-transcendence: deductive reformulation using developmental theories. *ANS*. 1991;12:64-74.
9. Fawcett J. *Analysis and Evaluation of Nursing Theories*. Philadelphia, PA: F.A. Davis; 1993.
10. Morris D. Middle range theory role in education. In: *Proceedings of the Sixth Rosemary Ellis Scholar's Retreat, Nursing Science Implications for the 21st century*. Cleveland, OH: Frances Payne Bolton School of Nursing, Case Western Reserve University; 1996.
11. Jacox A. Theory construction in nursing: an overview. *Nurs Res*. 1974;23:4-12.
12. Lenz E. Middle range theory-Role in research and practice. In: *Proceedings of the Sixth Rosemary Ellis Scholar's Retreat, Nursing Science Implications for the 21st century*. Cleveland, OH: Frances Payne Bolton School of Nursing, Case Western Reserve University; 1996.
13. Dluhy NM. Mapping knowledge in chronic illness. *J Adv Nurs*. 1995;21:1051-1058.
14. Jenny JJ, Logan J. Caring and comfort metaphors used by patients in critical care. *Image*. 1996;28:349-352.
15. Lenz ER, Pugh LC, Milligan RA, Gift AG, Suppe F. The middle range theory of unpleasant symptoms: an update. *ANS*. 1997;19:14-27.
16. Good M, Moore SM. Clinical practice guidelines as a new source of middle range theory: focus on acute pain. *Nurs Outlook*. 1996;44:74-79.
17. Good M. A middle range theory of acute pain management: use in research. *Nurs Outlook*. 1998;46:120-124.
18. Powell-Cope GM. Family caregivers of people with AIDS: negotiating partnerships with professional health care providers. *Nurs Res*. 1994;43:324-330.

19. Swanson KM. Empirical development of a middle range theory of caring. *Nurs Res.* 1991;40:161-166.

20. Levesque L, Ricard N, Ducharme F, Duquette A, Bonin J. Empirical verification of a theoretical model derived from the Roy Adaptation Model: Findings from five studies.*Nurs Sci Q.* 1998;11:31-39.

21. Nolan M, Grant G. Mid-range theory building and the nursing theory-practice gap: A respite care case study. *J Adv Nurs.* 1992;17:217-223.

22. Chenitz WC. Entry into a nursing home as status passage: A theory to guide nursing practice. *Geriatric Nurs.* 1983; Mar/Apr:92-97.

23. Beck CT, Reynolds MA, Rutowksi P. Maternity blues and postpartum depression. *JOGNN.* 1992;21:287-293.

24. Beck CT. The lived experience of postpartum depression: A phenomenological study. *Nurs Res.* 1992;41:166-170.

25. Beck CT. Teetering on the edge: A substantive theory of postpartum depression. *Nurs Res.* 1993;42:42-48.

26. Beck CT. Postpartum depressed mothers' experiences interacting with their children. *Nurs Res.* 1996;45;98-104.

27. Chinn P. Why middle range theory? *ANS.* 1997;19:viii.

28. Auvil-Novak SE. A mid-range theory of chronotherapeutic intervention for postsurgical pain. *Nurs Res.* 1997;46:66-71.

29. Olson J, Hanchett E. Nurse-expressed empathy, patient outcomes, and development of a middle-range theory. *Image.* 1997;29:71-76.

30. Polk LV. Toward a middle range theory of resilience. *ANS.* 1997; 19:1-13.

31. Eakes GG, Burke ML, Hainsworth MA. Middle-range theory of chronic sorrow. *Image.* 1998;30:179-184.

32. Kinney CK. Facilitating growth and development: A paradigm case for modeling and role-modeling. *Issues Ment Health Nurs.* 1990;11:375-395.

33. Acton GJ. Affiliated-individuation as a mediator of stress and burden in caregivers of adults with dementia. *J Holistic Nurs.* 1997;15:336-357.

34. Erickson HC, Tomlin EM, Swain MAP. *Modeling and Role-Modeling: A Theory and Paradigm for Nursing.* Englewood Cliffs, NJ: Prentice-Hall; 1983.

35. Chinn PL, Kramer MK. *Theory and Nursing: A Systematic Approach.* St. Louis, MO: Mosby; 1995.

36. Thompson JE, Oakley D, Burke M, Jay S, Conklin M. Theory building in nurse-midwifery: the care process. *J Nurs-Midwifery.* 1989;34:120-130.

37. Reed PG. Toward a nursing theory of self-transcendence: deductive reformulation using developmental theories. *ANS.* 1991;13:64-77.

38. Mishel MH. Uncertainty in illness. *Image.* 1988;20:225-232.

39. Burke SO, Kauffmann E, Costello EA. Dillon MC. Hazardous secrets and reluctantly taking charge: parenting a child with repeated hospitalizations. *Image.* 1991;23:39-45.

40. Jezewski MA. Evolution of a grounded theory: conflict resolution through culture brokering. *ANS.* 1995;17:14-30.

41. Tollett JH, Thomas SP. A theory-based nursing intervention to instill hope in homeless veterans. *ANS.* 1995;18:76-90.

42. Gerdner L. An indiviualized music intervention for agitation. *J Am Psych Nurs Assoc.* 1997;3:177-184.

43. Brooks EM, Thomas S. The perception and judgment of senior baccalaureate student nurses in clinical decision making. *ANS.* 1997;19:50-69.

44. Thomas SP. Toward a new conceptualization of women's anger. *Issues Ment Health Nurs.* 1991; 12:31-49.

45. Huth MM, Moore SM. Prescriptive theory of acute pain management in infants and children. *JSPN.* 1998;3:23-32.

46. Ruland CM, Moore SM. Theory construction based on standards of care: A proposed theory of the peaceful end of life. *Nurs Outlook.* 1998;46:169-175.

*Advances in Nursing Science*
Vol. 40, No. 1, pp. 51–63

# Middle Range Theory

## A Perspective on Development and Use

*Patricia Liehr, PhD, RN; Mary Jane Smith, PhD, RN, FAAN*

This replication and critique addresses ongoing development and use of middle range theory since considering this body of nursing knowledge 18 years ago. Middle range theory is appreciated as essential to the structure of nursing knowledge. Nine middle range theories that demonstrate ongoing use by the theory authors are analyzed using the criteria of theory name, theory generation, disciplinary perspective, theory model, practice use and research use. Critique conclusions indicate the importance of staying with the theory over time, naming and development consistent with the disciplinary perspective, movement to an empirical level, and bringing middle range theory to the interdisciplinary table. **Key words:** *disciplinary perspective, literature analysis/synthesis, middle range theory, theory use in practice and research*

It has been nearly 2 decades since *Advances in Nursing Science* published a description of spinning research and practice to create knowledge for the 21st century.[1] So, it is time for critique and reworking the knowledge tapestry. In a 1999 analysis of the existing body of middle range theories, Liehr and Smith[1] focused on describing a decade (1988-1998) of middle range theory publications with the intention of proposing direction for the future. The authors concluded with recommendations for ongoing development of middle range theory that necessitated (1) description of

the theory name and approach for generating the theory, (2) delineation of conceptual links in a diagramed model, (3) articulation of research-practice connections, (4) explicit description of the association between the theory and a disciplinary perspective in nursing, and (5) movement of middle range theory to the front lines of practice and research. The purpose of this article was to replicate the 1999 literature search process, state the recommendations as criteria to critique ongoing development and use of middle range theory, and identify approaches for moving on.

*Author Affiliations: Christine E. Lynn College of Nursing, Florida Atlantic University, Boca Raton (Dr Liehr); and School of Nursing, West Virginia University, Morgantown (Dr Smith).*

*The authors thank Manika Petcharat, who supported the literature search for this publication.*

*The authors have disclosed that they have no significant relationships with, or financial interest in, any commercial companies pertaining to this article.*

*Correspondence: Patricia Liehr, PhD, RN, Christine E. Lynn College of Nursing, Florida Atlantic University, 777 Glades Rd #330, Boca Raton, FL 33431 (pliehr@fau.edu).*

DOI: 10.1097/ANS.0000000000000162

## MIDDLE RANGE THEORY: HISTORICAL CONTEXT

Theories at the middle range level of discourse are described by the sociologist, Merton, as "those between the minor hypotheses of day to day research and unified theory."[2(p39)] Thus, the middle range level is below the more philosophical or grand theories and above empirical generalizations framed as hypotheses. Following the guidance of Merton,[2] Jacox[3] and Lenz[4,5] were instrumental in transporting middle range theory to nurse scholars who were

**Statements of Significance**

**What is known:**

We know that middle range theory is a dimension of nursing knowledge with promise for guiding practice and research. Although effort has been directed in the past to describe the processes related to middle range theory development, there has been little effort directed to consider ongoing use after development. Many middle range theories have been published over recent decades and there is a need to critique the ongoing development and use of middle range theory to enhance potential for contributing to knowledge development in the decades ahead.

**What this article adds:**

As a discipline, we have seldom looked at the body of middle range theory to consider ongoing development and use over time. This article adds a perspective regarding ongoing development and use. It replicates a literature search process from 18 years ago and applies previous recommendations to arrive at guidance for theory authors including staying with the theory over time; naming and development consistent with the disciplinary perspective; movement to an empirical level, with added attention to nursing practice; and bringing middle range theory to the interdisciplinary table.

interested in theory development for research and practice. More recently, this movement to middle range theory development has been energized by the growth of doctor of nursing practice programs[6] that emphasize guidance for evidence-based practice projects and by hospital emphasis on achieving Magnet status that requires consideration of a "schematic description" such as theory to guide practice.[7(p41)] Each of these contextual dimensions has

contributed to pursuit of disciplinary guidance at a level of discourse that lends itself to practice application.

Today, middle range theories are part of the structure of the knowledge base of nursing, standing with grand theories as expressions of disciplinary roots for guiding practice and research. Ongoing use of middle range theory offers potential for testing and shaping to enhance relevance and optimize the contribution to nursing knowledge development over the next decades.

## RECONSIDERING THE 1999 RECOMMENDATIONS

The recommendations that were described in the conclusion of the 1999 article are stated as criteria to be used in critiquing current middle range theories. The criteria include (1) identification of the theory name, (2) description of the theory-generating approach, grounding in the disciplinary perspective, inclusion of a diagramed model, (5) description of use to guide practice, and (6) description of use to guide research. While the second criterion, focused on theory generation, may have resulted in publications that were available before the original publication introducing the middle range theory, the fifth (testing in practice) and sixth (testing in research) criteria refer to documentation of theory use after the introduction of the middle range theory in a professional paper. The fifth and sixth criteria were particularly important to the selection of theories for this review, which proposes to address ongoing development *and* use of middle range theory over the past 18 years. Each of the criteria is briefly addressed before applying the criteria to the 9 current middle range theories whose authors have demonstrated continued use.

## CRITERION 1: NAMING

Naming a theory can be evaluated with 2 criteria: assessing consistency between the name and the theory central ideas presented in the description and identifying the name as one that is at the middle range level of abstraction. Naming without thoughtful reflection can lead to a name that does not capture the nature of the theory and/or a name that is at a level of abstraction that is not consistent with the middle range, being either too abstract or too concrete. Starting abstractly can lead to a name that moves toward the grand theory or philosophical level, resulting in application challenges when taken to practice and research. Starting concretely can lead to naming the theory at the micro level, limiting application across populations and health circumstances. Generally, the name of a middle range theory does not include a population or a disease experience. An exception may be a name that includes a broad population, such as the middle range theory of women's anger[8] or a broad health experience such as the middle range theory of self-care of chronic illness.[9]

## CRITERION 2: THEORY GENERATING APPROACH

In the 1999 article,[1] theory-generating approaches were synthesized with guidance from Lenz.[4,5] The view nearly 2 decades later adheres to the original set of approaches with attention to those highlighted in current literature. For instance, although practice standards and guidelines were identified in 1999, this approach has not persisted in recent years. As noted in 1999, there is not a middle range theory that does not have a foundation of synthesized literature, making this an implicit expectation for all theory generation. Given where we are now, we propose the following specific theory-generating approaches: (1) induction from practice; (2) induction from research; (3) concept building followed by testing in research and practice; (4) deduction from theories at a higher level of abstraction, including grand theories; and (5) derivation from theories of other disciplines that have foundations consistent with nursing's disciplinary perspective. Each of these approaches is briefly discussed.

### Induction through practice

As a practice discipline, it is logical that nursing theory is inextricably linked to practice as noted by Donaldson and Crowley in 1978: " . . . .both the discipline and the practice evolved interdependently in response to societal needs."[10(p117)] Even when not explicitly noted, it is often the case that generation of middle range theory came with the theory author's footing in nursing practice.

### Induction through research

The most obvious situation in which theory emerges by induction through research is related to the grounded theory method that has as its final product a theoretical structure that depicts the relationship between the major dimensions of the phenomenon under study. Polit and Beck note that grounded theory methods have contributed to the development of many middle range theories proposed by nurses.[11] However, this is not the only approach for generating theory from research and even doctoral dissertation research can supply direction for middle range theory development as it did for Covell, who proposed a middle range theory of intellectual capital.[12]

### Concept building

Concept building has been described as a critical thought process inclusive of a systematic approach to developing and modeling ideas that begin with a foundation in nursing practice and culminate with a model that can be tested in research and practice.[13] Sometimes concept models after testing and further development emerge as middle range theories, such as the middle range theory of cultural marginality,[14] but this is not always the case. Regardless of which process a scholar uses to build, analyze or synthesize concepts, the culminating model is, at most, a start for theory development. Although the concept building process alone is inadequate as an approach for theory generation, it can serve as a starting point.

**Grand theories**

Middle range theories are often generated from grand theories and *Nursing Science Quarterly,* as a publication that emphasizes the relevance of this approach,[15] has published multiple examples in recent years. In addition to generation from grand theories, it is possible that middle range theory develops from higher-level discourse theories that are not necessarily grand theories. For instance, Meleis and colleagues[16] introduced transitions as an emerging middle range theory in 2000; multiple situation-specific theories have emerged from this middle range theory.[17] While situation-specific theories could be judged at the micro level of abstraction, their authors envelope them within the middle range level of abstraction.

**Derivation of theories from other disciplines**

There is controversy about the wisdom of using theories from other disciplines as structures enabling derivation of middle range theories for nursing.[18] However, to eliminate this theory-generating approach is to turn away from existing interdisciplinary knowledge that has merit for guiding practice and research. When a scholar chooses to use this theory-generating approach, it is imperative that consistency with a nursing disciplinary perspective is clearly articulated. Thorne suggests that nurses do not simply "borrow" theories from other disciplines but "twist and bend" them to serve the disciplinary purpose of nursing.[18(p85)]

**CRITERION 3: DISCIPLINARY PERSPECTIVE**

In the current research climate where team science is advanced as a preferred modality for scholarly advancement, the disciplinary perspective can fade into a background that becomes barely discernable, thereby threatening the identity of the discipline.[18,19] The disciplinary perspective is critical for nursing knowledge building and as such it is an inherent foundation for generating middle range theory for nursing. Grace and colleagues[20] emphasize the importance of the "balance among the philosophical, conceptual/theoretical and empirical" dimensions of knowledge building as an essential criterion for disciplinary advancement that serves society in the decades ahead.

**CRITERION 4: MODELING**

To model a theory is to create meaning through design. Pink refers to design as creating something that transmits ideas that words alone cannot convey.[21(p70)] The model design represents relationships among the theory concepts as simply but comprehensively as possible. Root-Bernstein describes modeling as the imitation of one thing by another.[22(p481)] Both Pink and Root-Bernstein emphasize the creative nature of modeling. When, as often is the case, the theory being modeled represents dynamic interplay between and among concepts, the theory author is challenged to depict patterning in a 2-dimensional space. The mind's eye recognizes the complexity but the portrayed image is static.[23] Making what is static, dynamic, demands creative effort that captures complexity with simplicity.

**CRITERION 5: THEORY GUIDANCE FOR PRACTICE**

As noted by our ancestors and contemporaries, nursing is a practice discipline with a mandate to make a difference in quality living for society.[10,18,24-26] While making a difference in quality living for society as a whole rests in a community imperative with strong policy threads, application of middle range theory to practice often begins with an individual focus. At this point in the disciplinary history of nursing, explicit descriptions of using middle range theory to guide practice promise a substantive step toward meeting the mandate for making a difference for society through theory guidance.

## CRITERION 6: THEORY GUIDANCE FOR RESEARCH

Moving a theory on to research involves immersing self in the theory and related literature to have a clear and substantive grasp of the ontological and epistemological foundations. The authors of middle range theory are steeped in the essence of their ideas expressed as middle range theory. It is critical that they move their theories forward for testing through research, articulating research questions reflective of theory substance. To borrow an idea from Paley,[27] theory creates a niche that in this case guides research questions, methods, and analyses. When middle range theory is applied in this way, the potential for knowledge building is enhanced; guidance for the next steps in research arises within the theoretical context; and the context-relative findings enable systematic application and evaluation in practice.

### Middle range theory: Replication and critique

To address the 6 criteria that create the structure for critique, we identified middle range theories by replicating the 1999 literature search using CINAHL and searching with the terms middle range theory *and* nursing and then mid-range theory *and* nursing. This resulted in a total of 75 middle range theories published since 1988 (inclusive of those reported in the 1999 paper). Because we were interested in ongoing development *and* use, we selected an approach that prioritized effort by the theory author to grow the theory with research and practice application. Another wave of CINAHL searching was undertaken. In this wave, each of the 75 theory names was entered (one by one), and the theory author name was entered designated as "author"; and the word "theory"

was entered. Only theories where there were at least 3 English-language articles beginning with the article that introduced the theory as "middle range" are reported in the tables. It is interesting to note that 5 (uncertainty, self-transcendence, women's anger, caring, and unpleasant symptoms) of the 9 middle range theories reported in the tables were noted in the original 1999 paper. At that time, the 5 theories comprised only 23% of the total number of theories generated in the decade from 1988 to 1999. In this current analysis of ongoing development and use, they represent 55%. Table 1 summarizes information about each theory relative to the criteria and Table 2 provides a description of each theory.

The number of published articles for each of the theories in Table 1 ranges from 3 to 15. All but 2 of the theories[16,28] in the table have CINAHL-identified publications, documenting use within the last 5 years. It is important to note that the authors of these 2 theories[16,28] continue to publish updates of their respective theories in books,[29,30] another venue contributing to documentation of ongoing development and use. There are currently 2 nursing textbooks dedicated to middle range theory in nursing[31,32] and another, focused on nursing practice that includes a substantial section on middle range theory.[33] When the 1999 manuscript was published, there were no books dedicated to middle range theory for nursing; so textbooks specifically addressing middle range theory are a new development in the past 18 years.

In 1999, we found that there was an increasing propensity over the previous decade to propose models when introducing middle range theory[1] and this pattern has persisted. Because all theories in Table 1 included a model, this criterion was eliminated from the forthcoming description. The other criteria are noted to enable critique and provide a perspective about ongoing development and use of middle range nursing theories.

**Table 1.** Addressing Evaluation Criteria for Middle Range Theories With Ongoing Use

| Date | Author/Journal | Name | Theory Generation | Disciplinary Perspective | Practice | Research |
|---|---|---|---|---|---|---|
| 1988 | Mishel MH. *Image J Nurs Scholarsh, 20*(4), 225-231. | Uncertainty in illness (acute) | Literature synthesis from nursing and other disciplines including ideas from cognitive psychology and stress/adaptation; practice | Human health focus: transforming struggle—growth | | X |
| 1990 | Mishel MH. *Image: Journal of Nursing Scholarship, 22*(4), 256-262. | Uncertainty in illness (chronic) | | | | |
| 1991 | Reed PG. *Advances in Nursing Science, 13*(4), 64-77. | Self-transcendence | Nursing literature synthesis incorporating lifespan development from psychology; grand theory foundation (Rogers) | Human health focus: transforming struggle—growth | | X |
| 1991 | Thomas SP. *Issues in Mental Health Nursing, 12,* 31-49. | Women's anger | Literature synthesis with psychological/psychiatric/cognitive/behavioral focus; practice | Human health focus: transforming struggle-growth | | X |
| 1991 | Swanson KM. *Nursing Research, 40*(3), 161-166. | Caring | Nursing literature synthesis inclusive of multidisciplinary ethical perspective; qualitative study | Nurse-caring focus | X | X |
| 1995 | Lenz ER, Suppe F, Gift AG, Pugh LC, Milligan RA. *Advances in Nursing Science, 17*(3), 1-13. | Unpleasant symptoms | Nursing literature synthesis incorporating sociological perspective: concept analysis; research | Human health focus: transforming struggle—growth | X | |
| 2000 | Meleis AI, Sawyer LM, Im E, Messias DKH, Schumacher K. *Advances in Nursing Science, 23*(1), 12-28. | Transitions | Nursing literature synthesis beginning with a sociological perspective; concept analysis; qualitative study | Human health focus: transforming struggle—growth | | X |
| 2001 | Kolcaba K. *Nursing Outlook, 49*(2), 86-92. | Comfort | Nursing literature synthesis grounded in an appreciation of "basic human needs"; concept analysis; practice; research | Nurse-caring focus | X | X |
| 2002 | Roux G, Dingley CE, Bush HA. *Journal of Theory Construction and Testing, 6*(1), 86-93. | Inner strength | Nursing literature synthesis noting importance of psychological well-being and human health potential; qualitative study | Human health focus: transforming struggle—growth | | X |
| 2008 | Covell CL. *Journal of Advanced Nursing, 63,* 94-103. | Intellectual capital | Literature synthesis originating in economics, accounting and organizational learning; Concept analysis | Systems focus | | X |

**Table 2.** Concepts From Middle Range Theories With Ongoing Use

| Middle Range Theories | Theory Concepts |
| --- | --- |
| Uncertainty | Uncertainty in illness (acute) encompasses 3 themes including **antecedents** of uncertainty, **appraisal** of uncertainty, and **coping** with uncertainty. Antecedents are stimuli frame, cognitive capacity, and structure providers; appraisal includes inference and illusion; and coping includes the concepts of danger, opportunity, coping, and adaptation.[35] |
| | A reconceptualized theory of uncertainty was introduced for chronic illness. In this version of the theory the process of moving from uncertainty appraised as **danger**, to uncertainty appraised as **opportunity** is described. Self-organization and probabilistic thinking are included as descriptors of the process.[36] |
| Self-transcendence | Self-transcendence identifies **self-transcendence** as the major concept in the theory and refers to a basic human pattern of development linked to **well-being** and **vulnerability**.[34] |
| Women's anger | Women's anger includes the **appraisal** concepts of perceived stress, self-esteem, values, and perceived support; the **modifying factors** of trait anger, role responsibilities, demographics, health habits, and stress management; and the **outcome variables** of anger expression, depression, substance abuse, smoking, excessive eating, and health indicators.[8] |
| Caring | Caring is the process of **knowing**, **being with**, **doing for**, **enabling**, and **maintaining belief**. "Caring is a nurturing way of relating to a valued other toward whom one feels a personal sense of commitment and responsibility."[37(p165)] |
| Unpleasant symptoms | Unpleasant symptoms include the concepts of **symptoms**, **influencing factors**, and **performance outcomes**. Physiological, psychological, and situational factors influence the nature of the symptom experience. The symptom experience affects the performance outcomes of cognitive, physical, and social functioning.[28] |
| Transitions | Transitions proposes multidimensional and complex experiences that include **types and patterns**, **properties**, **conditions**, **process indicators**, **outcome indicators**, and **nursing therapeutics**. Types of transitions are developmental, situational, health/illness, and organizational. Patterns of transitions are single, multiple, sequential, simultaneous, related, and unrelated. Properties are awareness, engagement, change, time span, and critical points. Conditions of transitions are personal, community, and society. Process indicators are feeling connected, interacting, location and being situated, developing confidence, and coping. Outcome indicators are mastery and fluid integrative identities.[16] |
| Comfort | Comfort, based on holism and human needs, is described by 2 ideas, **type of comfort** (relief, ease, transcendence) and **context for comfort** (physical, psychospiritual, environmental, social). Patient comfort is defined as strengthening the immediate state of being through physical, psychospiritual, social, and environmental nursing interventions in the context of institutional outcomes.[38] |

(continues)

**Table 2.** Concepts From Middle Range Theories With Ongoing Use (*Continued*)

| Middle Range Theories | Theory Concepts |
|---|---|
| Inner strength | Inner strength describes **knowing and searching**, **nurturing through connection**, **dwelling in a different place** by creating the spirit within, **healing** through movement in the present, and **connecting with the future** by living a new normal.[39] |
| Nursing intellectual capital | Nursing intellectual capital describes **nursing knowledge**, influenced by the **work environment** that translates to **patient outcomes** and **organizational outcomes**. Nurse staffing, employer support, patient outcomes, and organization outcomes are noted in a model that incorporates nursing human capital and nursing structural capital.[39] |

**Theory name**

The first consideration when critiquing the theory name is consistency between the name and the central ideas that comprise the description of the theory. In the 9 theories noted in Table 2, there is correspondence between the theory name and its descriptors; however, identifying correspondence requires thoughtful review of theory content. Sometimes the descriptors are very broad as can be seen in examples such as the original theory of uncertainty in illness (antecedents; appraisal; coping), the theory of women's anger (appraisal; modifying factors; outcome variables), the theory of transitions (types and patterns; properties; conditions; process indicators; outcome indicators; nursing therapeutics), comfort theory (types of comfort; context for comfort), and nursing intellectual capital (nursing knowledge; work environment; patient outcomes; organizational outcomes). In these instances, the detail enabling evaluation between the name and the descriptors can be found in the author's elaboration of each of the descriptors (Table 2). In other cases, there is more specificity, such as the theories of caring and inner strength. Specificity limits the need for interpretation when assessing correspondence. Sometimes authors include the name of the theory as a central descriptor, such as self-transcendence and unpleasant symptoms. Therefore, the approach to

accomplishing this dimension of critique varies depending on the author's specificity when describing theory components. In Table 2, we have bolded what we believe are the central descriptors or concepts of each of the theories, but our interpretations may not always be in keeping with the ideas of the theory authors who seldom provide an explicit list of theory concepts.

The second consideration related to the theory name concerns the level of abstraction. In 1999, the names of 22 theories were grouped to distinguish the levels of discourse and the grouping included 9 at a lower level, as compared with 6 at a higher level and 7 at a middle range level of discourse. Considering the 9 middle range theories noted in the current critique, there was 1 at a higher level (self-transcendence)[34] and 2 at a lower level (women's anger[8] and intellectual capital[12]), but the majority were at the middle (uncertainty in illness,[35,36] caring,[37] unpleasant symptoms,[28] transitions,[16] comfort,[38] inner strength[39]).

One other consideration regarding naming that has surfaced in this critique is related to persistent identification of a theory as middle range. Even after designation as a middle range theory, it is common for scholars to eliminate the middle range specification in their future references. Sometimes, a conceptual structure at the middle range level of discourse is labelled as a model rather than as a middle range theory. Although the particular label may be irrelevant to usefulness for practice and research, the middle range theory label signals a level of discourse that makes research and practice guidance readily accessible. One wonders how the tilt in nursing values toward empirics[20] may be contributing to waffling around a theory label. We believe that this dimension of the "naming" criteria warrants watchfulness and reflection on relevance moving forward.

### Theory generation

All theories in the tables were built on a foundation of literature synthesis. Most authors note synthesis of nursing literature along with related threads from other disciplines, including psychology, ethics, and sociology. This multidisciplinary contribution to nursing middle range theory development, primarily from the human and social sciences, merits recognition. It seems that for a long time, nursing scholars have been "twisting and bending" theories from other disciplines[18(p85)] to serve the needs of the discipline.

In addition to literature synthesis, the theories in Table 1 indicate practice, concept analysis, and research as important contributors to theory formulation. One, self-transcendence, indicated a grand theory of nursing as a foundation.[34] Several scholars have woven together multiple theory-generating approaches in the process of developing middle range theory. Although not specifically noted in the tables, 3 of the theories, nursing intellectual capital,[12] comfort,[38] and inner strength,[39] began with dissertation research focused on the central idea of the theory.

### Disciplinary perspective

The disciplinary perspective emerges over time with nursing scholars proposing worldviews that stretch from the mechanistic to the transformational.[40] Newman and colleagues[41] synthesize the focus of the discipline in a way that encompasses worldviews in their description of nursing as caring in the human health experience. This disciplinary focus will be used to critique alignment of the 9 middle range theories using the theory names. The names of 8 of the theories directly describe specific dimensions of the human health experience: uncertainty in illness, self-transcendence, women's anger, caring, unpleasant symptoms, comfort, and inner strength. Although the theory name, intellectual capital, does not directly describe the human health experience, nursing intellectual capital does refer to delivering quality care leading to optimal patient outcomes. Patient outcomes, incorporating care maps and practice guidelines as described by the theory,[12] encompass patient health experiences even though the theory name does not reflect the focus of the discipline.

Caring in the human health experience can be viewed as how the nurse lives relationships with people regarding health. In the original article,[1] we identified 2 themes expressive of the disciplinary perspective suggested by the names of the 22 middle range theories that were reviewed: caring-healing processes and transforming struggle-growth. If one accepts the disciplinary perspective shared by Newman and colleagues as a meaningful synthesis, it is expected that all middle range nursing theories address caring in the human health experience, making the theme of caring-healing processes redundant. Most of the theory names in the current critique address the theme of transforming struggle-growth by highlighting either struggle (uncertainty in illness, unpleasant symptoms, women's anger, transitions) or growth (self-transcendence, inner strength). Although one dimension is highlighted, review of the theory details indicates juxtaposition with the other dimension of the transforming struggle-growth theme. For instance, while the theory of self-transcendence highlights growth in the theory name, vulnerability is a concept modelled in the theory.[42]

The middle range theories of caring and comfort are different because they are expressive of nursing intention to make a difference for another with a direct link to caring in the human health experience. Once again, the middle range theory name, intellectual capital stands alone, requiring extrapolation of theory ideas to arrive at a potentially relevant disciplinary perspective. The theory authors describe an appreciation for the relationship among environment-nurse-patient/organization outcomes, indicating a systems perspective that demands attention as a context for providing quality care.

In this critique of the disciplinary perspective of the 9 theories, caring in the human health experience surfaces as an overarching disciplinary perspective with 2 middle range theories (caring; comfort) directly linked as ones that are nurse-caring focused. Within the umbrella of this overarching perspective is the theme of transforming struggle-growth with 6 theories that can be described as human health focused (uncertainty in illness, unpleasant symptoms, women's anger, transitions, self-transcendence, inner strength). The middle range theory of intellectual capital is best described as system focused as it is currently described, leading to questions about how the disciplinary perspective is reflected in the theory.

### Use in practice

Description of middle range theory use in practice is scant. Five theories describe practice-relevant actions or outcomes including interventions such as nursing therapeutics (transitions) and processes for engaging (caring), or focus on patient outcomes expressed generally (intellectual capital) and specifically (unpleasant symptoms). Although authors often report general implications for use in practice in their theory-descriptive manuscripts, there is seldom an example of explicit use of middle range theory to guide practice with consideration of what can be learned from the example. In an article updating their original version of the theory, Lenz and colleagues[43] provide an exemplar of theory-guided practice use where the middle range theory of unpleasant symptoms shaped an intervention for breastfeeding women. Nursing circumstances readily allow for practice application, such as this. One wonders how this important use for middle range theory is generally missing from the literature.

Of the theory authors noted in the tables, Kolcaba[44] has most frequently described use in practice. Comfort theory has been used to guide practice at the unit level with hospitalized populations like pediatric patients, and the hospital-wide level with description of use in the Veterans Administration setting[45] and description of use by a hospital pursuing Magnet status.[46] The analysis of evidence supporting this criterion suggests that there is little documentation of middle range theory moving to the frontlines of nursing practice.

### Use in research

All but one theory in the tables documented ongoing use in research[28] and this is one of the theories that have described ongoing development and use in a middle range theory textbook.[31,32] Based on the CINAHL search, the middle range theory of uncertainty has been most often used in research with 14 studies reported since the introduction of the theory. This finding is not surprising given that the theory was introduced nearly 30 years ago, is accompanied by a reliable measure that has been used across a range of populations, and has acute and chronic illness versions expanding potential for application.[47] Several theories, including uncertainty, self-transcendence, comfort, and inner strength, have theory-derived instruments to quantify conceptual dimensions and one, women's anger, uses measures that are not theory-derived by closely matched to the central idea of the theory. Generally speaking, middle range theory continues to move to the front lines of nursing research.

## Limitations

We began with the intention of replicating a paper published in Advances in Nursing Science 18 years ago, formulating the 1999 recommendations as criteria to critique ongoing development and use of middle range theory, so that we could identify approaches for moving on. We replicated our previous approach by identifying publications and adding a layer of selection to capture ongoing use, recognizing that this was a flawed process, given the onset of publication of textbooks dedicated to the description of middle range theories. In spite of this limitation, there is something to be said for the importance of peer review as a gatekeeper for nursing knowledge development, including middle range theory, so we have opted to include only those theory publications that have been vetted with peer review processes.

Another limitation is the parameters set for ongoing use. We generously set 3 publications, including the original theory publication as the criteria that signaled ongoing use. We set no criteria regarding recent use such as publications occurring within the last 5 years. So, while some middle range theories in the tables have had no peer-reviewed published use that included the theory lead author in the past 5 years, they are still recognized as 1 of the 9.

Finally, the CINAHL search tapped only publications where the original theory lead author was included. It is possible that the theory had been used by other scholars with ensuing publications that did not include the theory author as one of the contributors.

In spite of these limitations, substantive information about the ongoing development and use of middle range theory has been culled from the literature and conclusions may provide direction for scholars wishing to contribute to the body of nursing knowledge through active engagement with middle range theory. Four conclusions are proposed.

### Stay with the theory

If middle range theory is to persist as a meaningful organizing structure in the body of nursing knowledge, it is imperative that authors continue to develop their theory through publishing in peer-reviewed journals. In addition, effort to include students and junior scholars through mentoring is warranted. Mentoring others to become engrossed in the understanding and application of middle range theory can ensure longevity and further use, thereby promising sustained knowledge development.

### Naming and development consistent with the disciplinary perspective

The disciplinary perspective shines through as the essential foundation for developing and naming. Being clear about the perspective that one holds enables a scholar to structure and name a theory that has relevance for making a difference in nursing's service to others. Even scholars who are systems-focused are challenged to consider the integral place of the nursing disciplinary perspective when developing and naming middle range theories.

### Move to the empirical level of discourse

While there is evidence that middle range nursing theory is being used to guide research, there is a pressing need for enhanced evidence of use in practice. Practice situations beg for a structure that enables reflective thinking about best approaches for promoting well-being. Scholars are encouraged to publish stories about practice viewed through the lens of a middle range theory and to critique the usefulness of the theory in the practice context.

### Bring middle range theory to the interdisciplinary table

When true collaboration exists among members of different disciplines, each member brings his or her unique knowledge perspective to the table for the good of the practice or research endeavor. When nursing is represented by a person who knows and understands a specific middle range theory, then caring in the human health experience comes alive at the table with the added possibility that middle range nursing theories become familiar to and used by other disciplines.

## CONCLUSION

In the spirit of celebrating the 40th anniversary of *Advances in Nursing Science,*

we have offered a snapshot of the knowledge tapestry currently created by middle range theory, critiquing a paper that welcomed the new millennium in 1999.[1] Like any snapshot, it is one view that generates interesting vistas but misses vistas outside the edge of the selected frame. We are inviting thoughtful engagement about the composition of this snapshot and once again, challenging nurse scholars to thoughtfully move to the future in a way that honors the discipline and makes a difference in the lives of the people we serve.

## REFERENCES

1. Liehr P, Smith MJ. Middle range theory: spinning research and practice to create knowledge for the new millennium. *Adv Nurs Sci*. 1999;21:81-91.
2. Merton RK. On sociological theories of the middle range. In: *Social Theory and Social Structure*. New York: Free Press; 1968:39-69.
3. Jacox A. Theory construction in nursing: an overview. *Nurs Res*. 1974;23:4-12.
4. Lenz ER. Role of middle range theory for nursing research and practice. Part 1: nursing research. *Nurs Leadersh Forum*. 1998;3:24-33.
5. Lenz ER. Role of middle range theory for nursing research and practice. Part 1: nursing practice. *Nurs Leadersh Forum*. 1998;3:62-66.
6. American Association of Colleges of Nursing. *The Doctor of Nursing Practice: Current Issues and Clarifying Recommendations*. Report from the Task Force on the Implementation of the DNP. Washington, DC: AACN; 2015, AACN, Washington DC.
7. American Nurses Credentialing Center. *2014 Magnet Application Manual: Revision 3.0*. Silver Spring, MD: American Nurses Credentialing Center; 2014.
8. Thomas SP. Toward a new conceptualization of women's anger. Issues Ment Health Nurs. 1991; 12:31-49.
9. Reigel B, Jaarsma T, Stromberg A. A middle range theory of self-care of chronic illness. *Adv Nurs Sci*. 2012;35:194-204.
10. Donaldson SK, Crowley DM. The discipline of nursing. *Nurs Outlook*. 1978;26:113-120.
11. Polit DF, Beck CT. *Essentials of Nursing Research: Appraising Evidence for Nursing Practice*. Philadelphia, PA: Wolters Kluwer/ Lippincott Williams & Wilkins; 2014.
12. Covell CL. The middle-range theory of nursing intellectual capital. *J Adv Nurs*. 2008;63:94-103.
13. Liehr P, Smith MJ. Concept building for research. In: *Middle Range Theory for Nursing*. New York: Springer; 2014:349-360.
14. Choi H. Theory of cultural marginality. In: *Middle Range Theory for Nursing*. New York: Springer; 2014, pp. 289-308.
15. Cody WK. Middle-range theories: do they foster the development of nursing science? *Nurs Sci Q*. 1999;12:9-14.
16. Meleis AI, Sawyer LM, Im E, Messias DKH, Schumacher K. Experiencing transitions. *Adv Nurs Sci*. 2000;23:12-28.
17. Im E. Theory of transitions. In: *Middle Range Theory for Nursing*. New York: Springer; 2014: 253-276.
18. Thorne S. Nursing as social justice: a case for emancipatory disciplinary theorizing. In: *Philosophies and Practices of Emancipatory Nursing: Social Justice as Praxis*. New York: Routledge Taylor & Francis; 2014, pp. 79-90.
19. Parse RR. Where have all the nursing theories gone? *Nurs Sci Q*. 2016;29:101-102.
20. Grace PJ, Willis DG, Roy C, Jones DA. Profession at the crossroads: a dialogue concerning the preparation of nursing scholars and leaders. *Nurs Outlook*. 2016;64:61-70.
21. Pink DH. *A Whole New Mind: Moving From the Information Age to the Conceptual Age*. New York: Riverhead; 2005.
22. Root-Bernstein RS. How scientists really think. *Perspect Biol Med*. 1989;32:472-488.

23. Liehr P, Smith MJ. Modeling the complexity of story theory for nursing practice. In: *Nursing, Caring and Complexity Science*. New York; Springer; 2011:241-248.

24. Nightingale F. *Notes on Nursing: What It Is and What It Is Not*. Philadelphia; JB Lippincott; 1992.

25. Newman MA, Smith MC, Pharris MD, Jones D. The focus of the discipline revisited. *Adv Nurs Sci*. 2008;31:E16-E27.

26. Varcoe C, Browne AJ, Cender LM. Promoting social justice and equity by practicing nursing to address structural inequities and structural violence. In: *Philosophies and Practices of Emancipatory Nursing: Social Justice as Praxis*. New York: Routledge Taylor & Francis; 2014:266-284.

27. Paley J. How not to clarify concepts in nursing. *J Adv Nurs*. 1996;24:572-578.

28. Lenz ER, Suppe F, Gift AG, Pugh LC, Milligan RA. Collaborative development of middle-range nursing theories: toward a theory of unpleasant symptoms. *Adv Nurs Sci*. 1995;17:1-13.

29. Meleis AI. *Transitions Theory*. New York: Springer; 2010.

30. Lenz ER, Pugh LC. The theory of unpleasant symptoms. In: *Middle Range Theory for Nursing*. New York: Springer; 2014.

31. Peterson S, Bredwo T. *Middle Range Theory: Application to Nursing Research*. Philadelphia, PA: Lippincott Williams & Wilkins; 2012.

32. Smith MJ, Liehr P. *Middle Range Theory for Nursing*. New York: Springer; 2014.

33. Smith M, Parker M. *Nursing Theories and Nursing Practice*. Philadelphia, PA: Lippincott Williams and Wilkins; 2015.

34. Reed PG. Toward a nursing theory of self-transcendence: deductive reformulation using developmental theories. *Adv Nurs Sci*. 1991;13:64-77.

35. Mishel MH. Uncertainty in illness. *Image*. 1988; 20:225-232.

36. Mishel MH. Reconceptualization in illness theory. *Image*. 1990;22:256-262.

37. Swanson KM. Empirical development of a middle range theory of caring. *Nurs Res*. 1991;40: 161-166.

38. Kolcaba K. Evolution of the midrange theory of comfort for outcomes research. *Nurs Outlook*. 2001;49:86-92.

39. Roux G, Dingley CE, Bush HB. Inner strength in women: metasynthesis of qualitative findings in theory development. *J Theory Constr Test*. 2002;6: 86-93.

40. Reed PG. A treatise on nursing knowledge development for the 21st century: beyond postmodernism. *Adv Nurs Sci*. 1995;17:70-84.

41. Newman M, Sime AM, Corcoran-Perry SA. The focus of the discipline of nursing. *Adv Nurs Sci*. 1991;14: 1-6.

42. Reed P. Theory of self-transcendence. In: *Middle Range Theory for Nursing*. New York: Springer; 2014:109-139.

43. Lenz ER, Pugh LC, Milligan R, Gift A, Suppe F. The middle range theory of unpleasant symptoms: an update. *Adv Nurs Sci*, 1997;19:14-27.

44. Kolcaba K, DiMarco MA. Comfort theory and its application to pediatric nursing. *Ped Nurs*. 2005;31:187-194.

45. Boudiab LD, Kolcaba K. Comfort theory: unraveling the complexities of veterans' health care needs. Adv Nurs Sci. 2015;38:270-278.

46. Kolcaba K, Tilton C, Drouin C. Comfort theory: a unifying framework to enhance the practice environment. *J Nurs Adm*. 2006;36:538-544.

47. Mishel M. Theories of uncertainty in illness. In: *Middle Range Theory for Nursing*. New York: Springer; 2014.

# APPENDIX

## Published Middle Range Theories: 1988–2017

The following academic databases were used in a search for middle range theories: Applied Social Sciences Index & Abstracts (ASSIA), CINAHL Plus with Full Text, Cochrane Library, Health and Psychosocial Instruments (HaPI), Health Reference Center-Academic, MEDLINE (ProQuest), MEDLINE (Web of Science), Nursing and Allied Health Collection, PsycArticles, and PubMed .gov. In articles added to the table, the author introduced the work as a middle range theory, mid-range theory, or middle range nursing theory in the abstract or title. The theory author(s)'s designation was given precedence for the purpose of table composition.

| Year | Full Citation (APA) | Name of Theory |
|------|---------------------|----------------|
| 1988 | Mishel, M. H. (1998). Uncertainty in illness. *Image: Journal of Nursing Scholarship, 20*(4), 225–232. | Uncertainty in illness |
| 1989 | Thompson, J. E., Oakley, D., Burke, M., Jay, S., & Conklin, M. (1989). Theory building in nurse-midwifery. The care process. *J Nurse Midwifery, 34*(3), 120–130. | Nurse-midwifery |
| 1990 | Kinney, C. K. (1990). Facilitating growth and development: A paradigm case for modeling and role-modeling. *Issues in Mental Health Nursing, 11,* 375–395. | Facilitating growth and development |
| 1991 | Burke, S. O., Kauffmann, E., Costello, E. A., & Dillon, M. C. (1991). Hazardous secrets and reluctantly taking charge: Parenting a child with repeated hospitalizations. *Image: Journal of Nursing Scholarship, 23*(1), 39–45. | Hazardous secrets and reluctantly taking charge |
| 1991 | Thomas, S. P. (1991). Toward a new conceptualization of women's anger. *Issues in Mental Health Nursing, 12,* 31–49. | Women's anger |

(*continued*)

| Year | Full Citation (APA) | Name of Theory |
|------|---------------------|----------------|
| 1991 | Reed, P. G. (1991). Toward a nursing theory of self-transcendence: Deductive reformulation using developmental theories. *Advances in Nursing Science, 13*(4), 64–77. | Self-transcendence |
| 1991 | Swanson, K. M. (1991). Empirical development of a middle range theory of caring. *Nursing Research, 40*(3), 161–166. | Caring |
| 1995 | Jezewski, M. A. (1995). Evolution of a grounded theory: Conflict resolution through culture brokering. *Advances in Nursing Science, 17*(3), 14–30. | Conflict resolution through culture brokering |
| 1995 | Lenz, E. R., Supple, F., Gift, A. G., Pugh, L. C., & Miligan, R. A. (1995). Collaborative development of middle-range nursing theories: Toward a theory of unpleasant symptoms. *Advances in Nursing Science, 17*(3), 1–13. | Unpleasant symptoms |
| 1995 | Tollett, J. H., &Thomas, S. P. (1995). A theory-based nursing intervention to instill hope in homeless veterans. *Advances in Nursing Science, 18*(2), 76–90. | Homelessness-hopelessness |
| 1996 | Good, M., & Moore, S. M. (1996). Clinical practice guidelines as a new source of middle-range theory: Focus on acute pain. *Nursing Outlook, 44*(2), 74–79. | Balance between analgesia and side effects |
| 1998 | Good, M. (1998). A middle range theory of acute pain management: Use in research. *Nursing Outlook, 46*(3), 120–124. | Acute pain management |
| 1997 | Acton, G. J. (1997). Affiliated-individuation as a mediator of stress and burden in caregivers of adults with dementia. *Journal of Holistic Nursing, 15*(4), 336–357. | Affiliated individuation as mediator of stress |
| 1997 | Auvil-Novak, S. E. (1997). A middle-range theory of chronotherapeutic intervention for postsurgical pain. *Nursing Research, 46*(2), 66–71. | Chronotherapeutic intervention for postsurgical pain |
| 1997 | Brooks, E. M., & Thomas, S. (1997). The perception and judgment of senior baccalaureate student nurses in clinical decision making. *Advances in Nursing Science, 19*(3), 50–69. | Perception and judgment of senior baccalaureate student nurses in clinical decision making |

(*continued*)

| Year | Full Citation (APA) | Name of Theory |
| --- | --- | --- |
| 1997 | Gerdner, L. (1997). An individualized music intervention for agitation. *Journal of the American Psychiatric Nurses Association*, 3(6), 177–184. | Individualized music intervention for agitation |
| 1997 | Olson, J., & Hanchett, E. (1997). Nurse-expressed empathy, patient outcomes, and development of a middle-range theory. *Image: Journal of Nursing Scholarship*, 29(1), 71–76. | Nurse-expressed empathy and patient distress |
| 1997 | Polk, L. V. (1997). Toward a middle-range theory of resilience. *Advances in Nursing Science*, 19(3), 1–13. | Resilience |
| 1998 | Burns, C. M. (1998). A retroductive theoretical model of the pathway to chemical dependency in nurses. *Archives of Psychiatric Nursing*, 21(1), 59–65. | Pathway to chemical dependency in nurses |
| 1998 | Eakes, G. G., Burke, M. L., & Hainsworth, M. A. (1998). Middle-range theory of chronic sorrow. *Image: Journal of Nursing Scholarship*, 30(2), 179–184. | Chronic sorrow |
| 1998 | Good, M. (1998). A middle-range theory of acute pain management: Use in research. *Nursing Outlook*, 46(3), 120–124. | Acute pain management |
| 1998 | Huth, M. M., & Moore, S. M. (1998). Prescriptive theory of acute pain management in infants and children. *Journal of the Society of Pediatric Nurses: JSPN*, 3(1), 23–32. | Theory of acute pain management in infants and children |
| 1998 | Kearney, M. H. (1998). Truthful self-nurturing: A grounded formal theory of women's addiction recovery. *Qualitative Health Research*, 8(4), 495–512. | Truthful self-nurturing |
| 1998 | Levesque, L., Ricard, N., Ducharme, F., Duquette, A., & Bonin, J. (1998). Empirical verification of a theoretical model derived from the Roy Adaptation Model: Findings from five studies. *Nursing Science Quarterly*, 11(1), 31–39. | Psychological adaptation |
| 1998 | Ruland, C. M., & Moore, S. M. (1998). Theory construction based on standards of care: A proposed theory of the peaceful end of life. *Nursing Outlook*, 46(4), 169–175. | Peaceful end of life |
| 1999 | Jirovec, M. M., Jenkins, J., & Isenberg, M. (1999). Urine control theory derived from Roy's conceptual framework. *Nursing Science Quarterly*, 12(3), 251–255. | Urine control theory |

*(continued)*

| Year | Full Citation (APA) | Name of Theory |
|------|---------------------|----------------|
| 1999 | Smith, A. A., & Friedemann, M. L. (1999). Perceived family dynamics of persons with chronic pain. *Journal of Advanced Nursing, 30*(3), 543–551. | Perceived family dynamics of persons with chronic pain |
| 1999 | Smith, M. J., & Liehr, P. (1999). Attentively embracing story: A middle-range theory with practice and research implications. *Scholarly Inquiry for Nursing Practice, 13*(3), 205–210. | Attentively embracing story |
| 2000 | August-Brady, M. (2000). Prevention as intervention. *Journal of Advanced Nursing, 31*(6), 1304–1308. | Prevention as intervention |
| 2000 | Doornbos, M. M. (2000). King's systems frameworks and family health: The derivation and testing of a theory. *The Journal of Theory Construction & Testing, 4*(1), 20–26. | Family health |
| 2000 | Leenerts, M. H., & Magilvy, J. (2000). Investing in self-care: A midrange theory of self-care grounded in the lived experience of low-income HIV-positive White women. *Advances in Nursing Science, 22*(3), 58–75. | Self-care |
| 2000 | Meleis, A. I., Sawyer, L. M., Im, E. O., Hilfinger Messias, D. K., & Schumacher, K. (2000). Experiencing transitions: An emerging middle-range theory. *Advances in Nursing Science, 23*(1), 12–28. | Experiencing transitions |
| 2000 | Sanford, R. C. (2000). Caring through relation and dialogue: A nursing perspective for patient education. *Advances in Nursing Science, 22*(3), 1–15. | Caring through relation and dialogue |
| 2001 | Engebretson, J., & Littleton, L. Y. (2001). Cultural negotiation: A constructivist-based model for nursing practice. *Nursing Outlook, 49*(5), 223–230. | Cultural negotiation |
| 2001 | Hills, R. G. S., & Hanchett, E. (2001). Human change and individuation in pivotal life situations: Development and testing the theory of enlightenments. *Visions, 9*(1), 6–19. | Enlightenments |
| 2001 | Kearney, M. H. (2001). A grounded formal theory of women's experience of domestic violence. *Research in Nursing & Health, 24*(4), 270–282 | Women's experience of domestic violence |

*(continued)*

| Year | Full Citation (APA) | Name of Theory |
|------|---------------------|----------------|
| 2001 | Kolcaba, K. (2001). Evolution of the mid range theory of comfort for outcomes research. *Nursing Outlook, 49*(2), 86–92. | Comfort |
| 2001 | Woods, S. J., & Isenberg, M. A. (2001). Adaptation as a mediator of intimate abuse and traumatic stress in battered women. *Nursing Science Quarterly, 14*(3), 215–221. | Adaptation as a mediator of intimate abuse and traumatic stress in battered women |
| 2001 | Wuest, J. (2001). Precarious ordering: Toward a formal theory of women's caring. *Health Care for Women International, 22,* 167–193 | Precarious ordering—women's caring |
| 2002 | Barnes, S., & Adair, B. (2002). The cognition-sensitive approach to dementia: Parallels with the science of unitary human beings. *Journal of Psychosocial Nursing and Mental Health Services, 40*(11), 30–37. | Cognition-sensitive approach to dementia |
| 2002 | Roux, G., Dingley, C. E., & Bush, H. A. (2002). Inner strength in women: Metasynthesis of qualitative findings in theory development. *Journal of Theory Construction and Testing, 6*(1), 86–93. | Inner strength in women |
| 2002 | Smith, C. E., Pace, K., Kochinda, C., Kleinbeck, S. V. M., Koehler, J., & Popkess-Vawter, S. (2002). Caregiving effectiveness model evolution to a midrange theory of home care: A process for critique and replication. *Advances in Nursing Science, 25*(1), 50–64. | Caregiving effectiveness |
| 2002 | Whittemore, R., & Roy, C. (2002). Adapting to diabetes mellitus: A theory synthesis. *Nursing Science Quarterly, 15*(4), 311–317. | Adapting to diabetes mellitus |
| 2003 | Dorsey, C. J., & Murdaugh, C. L. (2003). The theory of self-care management for vulnerable populations. *The Journal of Theory Construction & Testing, 7*(2), 43–49. | Self-care management for vulnerable populations |
| 2003 | Lawson, L. (2003). Becoming a success story: How boys who have molested children talk about treatment. *Journal of Psychiatric and Mental Health Nursing, 10,* 259–268. | Becoming a success story |
| 2003 | Tsai, P. F. (2003). A middle-range theory of caregiver stress. *Nursing Science Quarterly, 16*(2), 137–145. | Caregiver stress |

*(continued)*

| Year | Full Citation (APA) | Name of Theory |
|---|---|---|
| 2003 | Tsai, P., Tak, S., Moore, C., & Palencia (2003). Testing a theory of chronic pain. *Journal of Advanced Nursing, 43*(2), 158–169. | Chronic pain |
| 2004 | Dunn, K. S. (2004). Toward a middle-range theory of adaptation to chronic pain. *Nursing Science Quarterly, 17*(1), 78–84. | Adaptation to chronic pain |
| 2004 | Mefford, L. C. (2004). A theory of health promotion for preterm infants based on Levine's conservation model of nursing. *Nursing Science Quarterly, 17*(3), 260–266. | Health promotion for preterm infants |
| 2004 | Walton, J., & Sullivan, N. (2004). Men of prayer: Spirituality of men with prostate cancer. *Journal of Holistic Nursing, 22*(2), 133–151. | Spirituality |
| 2005 | Dunn, K. S. (2005). Testing a middle-range theoretical model of adaptation to chronic pain. *Nursing Science Quarterly, 18*(2), 146–156. | Adaptation to chronic pain |
| 2006 | Johansson, I., Hildingh, C., Wenneberg, S., Fridlund, B., & Ahlström, G. (2006). Theoretical model of coping among relatives of patients in intensive care units: A simultaneous concept analysis. *Journal of Advanced Nursing, 56*(5), 463–471. | Relatives' coping approaches |
| 2006 | Johnson, M. E., & Delaney, K. R. (2006). Keeping the unit safe: A grounded theory study. *Journal of the American Psychiatric Nurses Association, 12*(1), 13–21. | Violence prevention |
| 2006 | Peters, R. M. (2006). The relationship to racism, chronic stress emotions, and blood pressure. *Journal of Nursing Scholarship, 38*(3), 234–240. | Chronic stress emotions |
| 2006 | Register, M. E., & Herman, J. (2006). A middle range theory for generative quality of life for the elderly. *Advances in Nursing Science, 29*(4), 340–350. | Generative quality of life for the elderly |
| 2007 | Bu, X., & Jezewski, M. A. (2007). Developing a mid-range theory of patient advocacy through concept analysis. *Journal of Advanced Nursing, 57*(1), 101–110. | Patient advocacy |
| 2007 | Chen, H., & Boore, J. (2007). Establishing a super-link system: Spinal cord injury rehabilitation nursing. *Journal of Advanced Nursing, 57*(6), 639–648. | Super-link system for rehabilitation |

*(continued)*

| Year | Full Citation (APA) | Name of Theory |
|---|---|---|
| 2007 | Orticio, L. P. (2007). Sensing presence and sensing space: A middle range theory of nursing. *Insight (American Society of Ophthalmic Registered Nurses)*, *32*(4), 7–11. | Sensing presence and sensing space |
| 2007 | Penrod, J., Yu, F., Kolanowski, A., Fick, D. M., Loeb, S. J., & Hupcey, J. E. (2007). Reframing person-centered nursing care for persons with dementia. *Research and Theory for Nursing Practice: An International Journal*, *21*(1), 57–72. | Person-centered nursing care for persons with dementia |
| 2007 | Shanley, E., & Jubb-Shanley, M. (2007). The recovery alliance theory of mental health nursing. *Journal of Psychiatric & Mental Health Nursing*, *14*(8), 734–743. | Recovery alliance |
| 2008 | Janes, N., Sidani, S., Cott, C., & Rappolt, S. (2008). Figuring it out in the moment: A theory of unregulated care providers' knowledge utilization in dementia care settings. *Worldviews on Evidence-Based Nursing*, *5*(1), 13–24. | Unregulated care providers' knowledge utilization in dementia care settings |
| 2008 | Christie, J., Poulton, B. C., & Bunting, B. P. (2008). An integrated mid-range theory of postpartum family development: A guide for research and practice. *Journal of Advanced Nursing*, *61*(1), 38–50. | Post-partum parent development |
| 2008 | Covell, C. L. (2008). The middle-range theory of nursing intellectual capital. *Journal of Advanced Nursing*, *63*(1), 94–103. | Nursing intellectual capital |
| 2008 | Kelly, C. W. (2008). Commitment to health theory. *Research and Theory for Nursing Practice*, *22*(2), 148–160. | Commitment to health |
| 2009 | Murrock, C., & Higgins, P. A. (2009). The theory of music, mood and movement to improve health outcomes. *Journal of Advanced Nursing*, *65*(10), 2249–2257. | Music, mood and movement to improve health outcomes |
| 2009 | Ryan, P., & Sawin, K. J. (2009). The individual and family self-management theory: Background and perspectives on context, process and outcomes. *Nursing Outlook*, *57*, 217–225. | Individual and family self-management |
| 2010 | Davidson, J. E. (2010). Facilitated sensemaking: A strategy and new middle-range theory to support families of intensive care unit patients. *Critical Care Nurse*, *30*(6), 28–39. | Facilitated sensemaking |

*(continued)*

| Year | Full Citation (APA) | Name of Theory |
|---|---|---|
| 2010 | Hodges, H. F., Troyan, P. J., & Keeley, A. C. (2010). Career persistence in baccalaureate-prepared acute care nurses. *Journal of Nursing Scholarship*, *42*(1), 83–91. | Career persistence |
| 2010 | Reimer, A. P., & Moore, S. M. (2010). Flight nursing expertise: Towards a middle-range theory. *Journal of Advanced Nursing*, *66*(5), 1183–1192. | Flight nursing expertise |
| 2010 | Rasanen, P., Kanste, O., & Kyngas, H. (2010). Self-care of home-dwelling elderly: Testing the main structure of a middle-range theory. *Hoitotiede*, *22*(3), 218–230. | Self-care of home-dwelling elderly |
| 2010 | Trimm, D. R., & Sanford, J. T. (2010). The process of family waiting during surgery. *Journal of Family Nursing*, *16*(4), 435–461. | Maintaining balance during the wait |
| 2011 | Dobratz, M. C. (2011). Toward development of a middle-range theory of psychological adaptation in death and dying. *Nursing Science Quarterly*, *24*(4), 370–376. | Psychological adaptation in death and dying |
| 2012 | Dyess, S. M., & Chase, S. K. (2012). Sustaining health in faith community nursing practice: Emerging processes that support the development of a middle-range theory. *Holistic Nursing Practice*, *26*(4), 221–227. | Sustaining health in faith community nursing practice |
| 2012 | Riegel, B., Jaarsma, T., & Strömberg, A. (2012). A middle-range theory of self-care of chronic illness. *Advances in Nursing Science*, *35*(3), 194–204. | Self-care of chronic illness |
| 2013 | Elo, S., Kääriäinen, M., Isola, A., & Kyngäs, H. (2013). Developing and testing a middle-range theory of the well-being supportive physical environment of home-dwelling elderly. *Scientific World Journal*, *30*(4), 323–331. | Well-being supportive physical environment of home-dwelling elderly |
| 2013 | Phillippi, J. C., & Roman, M. W. (2013). The motivation-facilitation theory of prenatal care access. *Journal of Midfifery & Womens' Health*, *58*(5), 509–515. | Prenatal care access |
| 2014 | Carr, J. M. (2014). A middle range theory of family vigilance. *Medical Surgical Nurses*, *23*(4), 251–255. | Family vigilance |

(*continued*)

| Year | Full Citation (APA) | Name of Theory |
|------|---------------------|----------------|
| 2014 | García-Fernández, F. P., Agreda, J. J. S., Verdú, J., & Pancorbo-Hidalgo, P. L. (2014). A new theoretical model for the development of pressure ulcers and other dependence-related lesions. *Journal of Nursing Scholarship*, 46(1), 28–38. | Development of pressure ulcers and other dependence-related lesions |
| 2014 | Love, K. (2014). A midrange theory of empowered holistic nursing education: A pedagogy for a student-centered classroom. *Creative Nursing*, 20(1), 47–58. | Empowered holistic nursing education |
| 2014 | Morse, J. M., Pooler, C., Vann-Ward, T., Maddox, L. J., Olausson, J. M., Roche-Dean, M., . . . Martz K. (2014). Awaiting diagnosis of breast cancer: Strategies of enduring for preserving self. *Oncology nursing forum*, 41(4), 350–359. | Awaiting diagnosis: Enduring for preserving self |
| 2014 | Pickett, S., Peters, R. M., & Jarosz, P. A. (2014). Toward a middle-range theory of weight management. *Nursing Science Quarterly*, 27(3), 242–247. | Weight management |
| 2015 | Beck, C. T. (2015). Middle range theory of traumatic childbirth: The ever-widening ripple effect. *Global Qualitative Nursing Research*, 2, 1–13. | Traumatic childbirth |
| 2015 | Camargo-Sanchez, A., Nino, C., Sanchez, L., Echeverri, S., Gutierrez, D. P., Duque, A.F., . . . Vargas, R. (2015). Theory of inpatient circadian care (TICC): A proposal for a middle-range theory. *The Open Nursing Journal*, 9, 1–9. | Theory of inpatient circadian care (TICC) |
| 2015 | Fearon-Lynch, J., & Stover, C. M. (2015). A middle-range theory for diabetes self-management mastery. *Advances in Nursing Science*, 38(4), 330–346. | Diabetes self-management mastery |
| 2015 | Forsberg, A., Lennerling, A., Fridh, I., Karisson, V., & Nilsson, M. (2015). Understanding the perceived threat of the risk of graft rejections: A middle-range theory. *Global Qualitative Nursing Research*, 2, 1–9, doi:10.1177/2333393614563829 | Perceived threat of the risk of graft rejections |
| 2015 | Payne, L. K. (2015). Toward a theory of intuitive decision-making in nursing. *Nursing Science Quarterly*, 28(3), 223–228. | Intuitive decision-making in nursing |

*(continued)*

| Year | Full Citation (APA) | Name of Theory |
|------|---------------------|----------------|
| 2015 | Perry, D. J. (2015). Transcendent pluralism: a middle-range theory of nonviolent social transformation through human and ecological dignity. *Advances in Nursing Science, 38*(4), 317–329. | Transcendent pluralism |
| 2016 | DiMaria-Ghalili, R. A. (2016). Development of an integrated theory of surgical recovery in older adults. *Journal of Nutrition in Gerontology and Geriatrics, 35*(1), 1–14. | Integrated theory of surgical recovery in older adults |
| 2016 | Dobratz, M. C. (2016). Building a middle-range theory of adaptive spirituality. *Nursing Science Quarterly, 29*(2), 146–153. | Adaptive spirituality |
| 2016 | Walter, R. R. (2016). Emancipatory nursing praxis: A theory of social justice in nursing. *Advances in Nursing Science, 40*(3), 223–241. | Emancipatory nursing praxis |
| 2017 | Bloc, A. C. (2017). A middle-range explanatory theory of self-management behavior for collaborative research and practice. *Nursing Forum, 52*(2), 138–146. | Self-management behavior for collaborative research and practice |

# Index